# CUNNINGHAM'S MANUAL OF PRACTICAL ANATOMY

Volume 3

**Cunningham's Manual of Practical Anatomy**

Volume 1 General Anatomy, and Upper and Lower Limbs

Volume 2 Thorax and Abdomen

Volume 3 Head, Neck and Brain

# CUNNINGHAM'S MANUAL OF PRACTICAL ANATOMY

*Seventeenth edition*

**Volume 3** Head, Neck and Brain

**Dr Rachel Koshi** MBBS, MS, PhD

Professor, Department of Cellular Biology and Anatomy,
Medical College of Georgia-Savannah at Georgia Southern University,
Georgia, USA

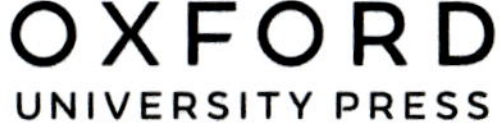

OXFORD
UNIVERSITY PRESS

Great Clarendon Street, Oxford, OX2 6DP,
United Kingdom

Oxford University Press is a department of the University of Oxford. It furthers the University's objective of excellence in research, scholarship, and education by publishing worldwide. Oxford is a registered trade mark of Oxford University Press in the UK and in certain other countries.



Thirteenth edition 1966
Fourteenth edition 1977
Fifteenth edition 1986
Sixteenth edition 2017



Published in the United States of America by Oxford University Press
198 Madison Avenue, New York, NY 10016, United States of America.

British Library Cataloguing in Publication Data
Data available

Library of Congress Control Number: 2026930057

ISBN 978–0–19–896035–5

DOI: 10.1093/med/9780198960355.001.0001

Printed in India by Manipal Technologies Limited

I fondly dedicate this book to the late Dr K. G. Koshi for his encouragement and support when I chose a career in anatomy, and to Dr Mary Jacob, under whose guidance I learnt the subject and developed a love for teaching.

Oxford University Press would like to dedicate this book to the memory of the late George John Romanes, Professor of Anatomy at Edinburgh University from 1954 to 1984, who brought his wisdom to previous editions of *Cunningham's*.

# Foreword to the sixteenth edition



It gives me great pleasure to pen down the Foreword to the 16th edition of *Cunningham's Manual of Practical Anatomy*. Just as the curriculum of anatomy is incomplete without dissection, so also is learning by dissection incomplete without a manual.

*Cunningham's Manual of Practical Anatomy* is one of the oldest dissectors, the first edition of which was published as early as 1893. Since then, the manual has been an inseparable companion to students during dissection.

I remember my days as a first MBBS student, the only dissector known in those days was *Cunningham's* manual. The manual helped me to dissect scientifically, step by step, explore the body, see all structures as mentioned, and admire God's highest creation—the human body—so perfectly. As a postgraduate student, I marvelled at the manual and learnt details of structures, in a way as if I had my teacher with me telling me what to do next. The clearly defined steps of dissection, and the comprehensive revision tables at the end, helped me personally to develop a liking for dissection and the subject of anatomy.

Today, as a Professor and Head of Anatomy, teaching anatomy for more than 30 years, I find *Cunningham's* manual extremely useful to all the students dissecting and learning anatomy.

With the explosion of knowledge and ongoing curricular changes, the manual has been revised at frequent intervals. The 16th edition is more student-friendly. The language is simplified, so that the book can be comprehended by one and all. The objectives are well defined. The clinical application notes at the end of each chapter are an academic feast to the learners. The lucidly enumerated steps of dissection make a student explore various structures, the layout, and relations and compare them with the simplified labelled illustrations in the manual. This helps in sequential dissection in a scientific way and for knowledge retention. The text also includes multiple-choice questions for self-assessment and holistic comprehension.

Keeping the concept of 'Adult Learning Principles' in mind, i.e. adults learn when they 'DO', and with a global movement towards 'competency-based curriculum', students learn anatomy when they dissect; *Cunningham's* manual will help students to dissect on their own, at their own speed and time, and become competent doctors, who can cater to the needs of the society in a much better way.

I recommend this invaluable manual to all the learners who want to master the subject of anatomy.

Dr Pritha S. Bhuiyan
Professor and Head, Department of Anatomy
Professor and Coordinator, Department of Medical Education
Seth GS Medical College and KEM Hospital, Parel, Mumbai

# Preface to seventeenth edition

*Cunningham's Manual of Practical Anatomy* has been the most widely used dissection manual in India for many decades. The 16th edition of this book was published in 2018. Later the same year the Medical Council of India published the comprehensive list of competencies (learning outcomes) to be achieved during graduate medical education, and in 2019 National Medical Commission of India (NMC) implemented this new competency-based curriculum all over the country.

The 17th edition of *Cunningham's Manual of Practical Anatomy Vol. 3* covers all the gross anatomy competencies required by the NMC and provides a list of where they are addressed in the text. One new chapter on the bones of the head and neck and another on surface marking have been added to address the related competencies.

Dissection forms an integral part of learning anatomy, and the practice of dissection enables students to retain and recall anatomical details learnt early in their training to their clinical practice. Each dissection section has a specific heading, learning objectives and easy-to-follow numbered stepwise instructions.

Each region also has numerous X-rays and magnetic resonance imaging to enable the student to visualize internal structures in the living. It retains the presentation of clinical application notes at the end of the chapter. Some of these notes focus on the anatomical basis of commonly used physical diagnostic tests such as corneal and gag reflex. Others deal with the underlying anatomy of clinical conditions such as stroke, otitis media and radiculopathy. Clinical anatomy of common procedures such as tracheostomy and laryngoscopy is described. The Q&A format of many of these challenge students to brainstorm the material covered in the chapter; and multiple-choice questions help them to assess their preparedness for the university examination.

It is hoped that this new edition respects the legacy of Cunningham in producing a text and manual that is accurate, student-friendly, comprehensive, and interesting, and that it will serve the community of students who are beginning their career in medicine to gain knowledge and appreciation of the anatomy of the human body.

Dr Rachel Koshi

# Contributors and reviewers

### Contributors to the 17th edition

**Dr J Suganthy**, Professor of Anatomy, Christian Medical College, Vellore, India.
*Dr Suganthy wrote the MCQs for the online material and Chapter 2 General Anatomy MCQs for Volume 1.*

**Dr Ritwik Baidya**, MD, Assistant Professor of Anatomy in Radiology, Weill Cornell Medicine, Radiology/Program of Gross Anatomy, New York, NY, USA.
*Dr Baidya wrote the online image-based questions.*

### Reviewers to the 17th edition

Oxford University Press would like to thank all those who read draft materials and provided valuable feedback during the writing process:

**C. S. Ramesh Babu**, *Associate Professor of Anatomy, Muzafffarnagar Medical College, Muzaffarnagar, India.*

**Dr Aby S. Charles**, *Senior Resident, Department of Anatomy, Christian Medical College, Vellore, India.*



**Professor Sunil Jonathan Holla**, *MBBS, MD (Anatomy), Professor of Anatomical Sciences, St Matthew's University School of Medicine, Grand Cayman, Cayman Islands (formerly of Christian Medical College, Vellore, India).*

### Contributors to the 16th edition

**Dr J Suganthy**, Professor of Anatomy, Christian Medical College, Vellore, India.
*Dr Suganthy wrote the MCQs, reviewed the manuscripts, and provided help and advice with the artwork.*

**Dr Aparna Irodi**, Professor of Radiology, Christian Medical College and Hospital, Vellore, India.
*Dr Irodi kindly researched, identified, and explained the radiology images.*

**Dr Ivan James Prithishkumar**, Professor of Anatomy, Christian Medical College, Vellore, India.
*Dr Prithishkumar wrote some of the clinical applications and reviewed the text as a critical reader.*

**Dr Tripti Meriel Jacob**, Associate Professor of Anatomy, Christian Medical College, Vellore, India.
*Dr Jacob wrote some of the clinical applications and reviewed the text as a critical reader.*

# Acknowledgements

Dr Koshi would like to thank the following:
Radiology Department, Christian Medical College, Vellore, India.
The Radiology Department kindly provided the radiology images.
Ms Geraldine Jeffers, Senior Commissioning Editor, Ms Fiona Sutherland, Senior Project Editor, Mr. Adam Brevik Project Editor, and the wonderful editorial and production teams of Oxford University Press and their partner company Newgen, for their assistance.

# Contents

## PART 3 Cross-sectional anatomy 405

# Additional MCQs available online

Enhance your understanding and be ready for anatomy examinations by visiting Oxford Academic, where you will find additional MCQs and image-based questions related to this resource.

Search for *Cunningham's Manual of Practical Anatomy Volume 3 Head, Neck, and Brain 17th edition* at https://academic.oup.com/ and go to the end matter to find the free online appendix at the end of the book. If you would like access to the whole book, or are interested in accessing other titles, you can recommend it to your librarian.

# Table of competencies required by the National Medical Commission of India gross anatomy curricula

See Tables 0.1 and 0.2 for competencies required by the National Medical Commission of India gross anatomy curricula.

**Table 0.1** Competencies in Head and Neck

| Competency No. | Competency | Chapter in 17th edition |
|---|---|---|
| AN26.1 | Demonstrate the anatomical position of the skull; identify and locate the individual skull bones in the skull | 2. Osteology of the head and neck |
| AN26.2 | Describe the features of the norma frontalis, verticalis, occipitalis, lateralis, and basalis | 2. Osteology of the head and neck |
| AN26.3 | Describe the cranial cavity, its subdivisions, the foramina, and the structures passing through them | 2. Osteology of the head and neck |
| AN26.4 | Describe the morphological features of the mandible | 2. Osteology of the head and neck |
| AN26.5 | Describe features of typical and atypical cervical vertebrae (atlas and axis) | 2. Osteology of the head and neck |
| AN26.6 | Explain the concept of bones that ossify in membrane | 2. Osteology of the head and neck |
| AN26.7 | Describe the features of the seventh cervical vertebra | 2. Osteology of the head and neck |
| AN27.1 | Describe the layers of the scalp, its blood supply, its nerve supply, and its surgical importance | 3. The scalp and face |
| AN27.2 | Describe the emissary veins with their role in spread of infection from the extracranial route to intracranial venous sinuses | 3. The scalp and face |
| AN28.1 | Describe and demonstrate the muscles of facial expression and their nerve supply | 3. The scalp and face |
| AN28.2 | Describe sensory innervation of the face | 3. The scalp and face |
| AN28.3 | Describe and demonstrate the origin/formation, course, and branches/tributaries of facial vessels | 3. The scalp and face |
| AN28.4 | Describe and demonstrate branches of the facial nerve with their distribution | 3. The scalp and face<br>13. The parotid region |
| AN28.5 | Describe cervical lymph nodes and lymphatic drainage of the head, face, and neck | 8. Deep dissection of the neck |
| AN28.6 | Identify superficial muscles of the face, and their nerve supply and actions | 3. The scalp and face |
| AN28.7 | Explain the anatomical basis of facial nerve palsy | 3. The scalp and face<br>12. Organs of hearing and equilibrium |
| AN28.8 | Explain the surgical importance of the deep facial vein | 3. The scalp and face<br>7. The cranial cavity |
| AN28.9 | Describe and demonstrate the parts, borders, surfaces, contents, relations, and nerve supply of the parotid gland with the course of its duct and its surgical importance | 13. The parotid region |
| AN28.10 | Explain the anatomical basis of Frey's syndrome | 13. The parotid region |

**Table 0.1** Continued

| Competency No. | Competency | Chapter in 17th edition |
|---|---|---|
| AN29.1 | Describe and demonstrate attachments, nerve supply, relations, and actions of the sternocleidomastoid | 5. The anterior triangle of the neck |
| AN29.2 | Explain the anatomical basis of Erb's and Klumpke's palsy | Vol. 1, Chapter 12 The nerves and nerve injuries of the lower limb |
| AN29.3 | Explain the anatomical basis of wry neck | 5. The anterior triangle of the neck |
| AN29.4 | Describe and demonstrate attachments of the: (1) inferior belly of the omohyoid; (2) scalenus anterior; (3) scalenus medius; and (4) levator scapulae | 5. The anterior triangle of the neck<br>6. The back<br>8. Deep dissection of the neck |
| AN30.1 | Describe the cranial fossae and identify related structures | 2. Osteology of head and neck<br>7. Cranial cavity |
| AN30.2 | Describe and identify major foramina with structures passing through them | 2. Osteology of the head and neck |
| AN30.3 | Describe and identify dural folds and dural venous sinuses | 7. The cranial cavity |
| AN30.4 | Describe the clinical importance of dural venous sinuses | 7. The cranial cavity |
| AN30.5 | Explain the effect of pituitary tumours on the visual pathway | 7. The cranial cavity<br>31. The cerebrum |
| AN31.1 | Describe and identify the extraocular muscles of the eyeball | 10. The orbit |
| AN31.2 | Describe and demonstrate nerves and vessels in the orbit | 10. The orbit |
| AN31.3 | Describe the anatomical basis of Horner's syndrome | 8. Deep dissection of the neck |
| AN31.4 | Enumerate the components of the lacrimal apparatus | 3. The scalp and face<br>10. The orbit |
| AN31.5 | Explain the anatomical basis of oculomotor, trochlear, and abducens nerve palsies, along with strabismus | 10. The orbit |
| AN32.1 | Describe the boundaries and subdivisions of the anterior triangle | 5. The anterior triangle of the neck |
| AN32.2 | Describe and demonstrate the boundaries and contents of the muscular, carotid, digastric, and submental triangles | 5. The anterior triangle of the neck |
| AN33.1 | Describe and demonstrate the extent, boundaries, and contents of the temporal and infratemporal fossae | 14. The temple and infratemporal regions |
| AN33.2 | Describe and demonstrate the attachments, direction of fibres, nerve supply, and actions of muscles of mastication | 14. The temple and infratemporal regions |
| AN33.3 | Describe and demonstrate the articulating surface, and type and movements of the temporomandibular joint | 14. The temple and infratemporal regions |
| AN33.4 | Explain the clinical significance of the pterygoid venous plexus | 14. The temple and infratemporal regions |
| AN33.5 | Describe the features of dislocation of the temporomandibular joint | 14. The temple and infratemporal regions |
| AN34.1 | Describe and demonstrate the morphology, relations, and nerve supply of the submandibular salivary gland and submandibular ganglion | 15. The submandibular region |
| AN34.2 | Describe the basis of formation of submandibular stones | 15. The submandibular region |
| AN35.1 | Describe the parts, extent, attachments, and modifications of the deep cervical fascia | 4. The posterior triangle of the neck<br>5. The anterior triangle of the neck<br>8. Deep dissection of the neck |
| AN35.2 | Describe and demonstrate the location, parts, borders, surfaces, relations, and blood supply of the thyroid gland | 8. Deep dissection of the neck |

*(continued)*

Table 0.1 Continued

| Competency No. | Competency | Chapter in 17th edition |
|---|---|---|
| AN35.3 | Demonstrate and describe the origin, parts, course, and branches of the subclavian artery | 4. The posterior triangle of the neck<br>8. Deep dissection of the neck |
| AN35.4 | Describe and demonstrate the origin, course, relations, tributaries, and termination of the internal jugular and brachiocephalic veins | 8. Deep dissection of the neck |
| AN35.5 | Describe and demonstrate the extent, drainage, and applied anatomy of cervical lymph nodes | 8. Deep dissection of the neck |
| AN35.6 | Describe and demonstrate the extent, formation, relations, and branches of the cervical sympathetic chain | 8. Deep dissection of the neck |
| AN35.7 | Describe the course and branches of cranial nerves IX, X, XI, and XII in the neck | 8. Deep dissection of the neck |
| AN35.8 | Describe the anatomically relevant clinical features of thyroid swellings | 8. Deep dissection of the neck |
| AN35.9 | Describe the clinical features of compression of the subclavian artery and lower trunk of the brachial plexus by the cervical rib | 4. The posterior triangle of the neck |
| AN35.10 | Describe the fascial spaces of the neck | 8. Deep dissection of the neck |
| AN36.1 | Describe the: (1) morphology, relations, blood supply, and applied anatomy of the palatine tonsil; and (2) composition of the soft palate | 16. The mouth and pharynx |
| AN36.2 | Describe the components and functions of Waldeyer's lymphatic ring | 16. The mouth and pharynx |
| AN36.3 | Describe the boundaries and clinical significance of the pyriform fossa | 16. The mouth and pharynx |
| AN36.4 | Describe the anatomical basis of tonsillitis, tonsillectomy, the adenoids, and peritonsillar abscess | 16. The mouth and pharynx |
| AN36.5 | Describe the clinical significance of Killian's dehiscence | 16. The mouth and pharynx |
| AN37.1 | Describe and demonstrate the features of the nasal septum, the lateral wall of the nose, and their blood supply and nerve supply | 18. The cavity of the nose |
| AN37.2 | Describe the location and functional anatomy of paranasal sinuses | 7. The cranial cavity<br>18. The cavity of the nose |
| AN37.3 | Describe the anatomical basis of sinusitis and maxillary sinus tumours | 18. The cavity of the nose |
| AN38.1 | Describe the morphology and identify the structure of the wall, nerve supply, blood supply, and actions of intrinsic and extrinsic muscles of the larynx | 19. The larynx |
| AN38.2 | Describe the anatomical aspects of laryngitis | 19. The larynx |
| AN38.3 | Describe the anatomical basis of recurrent laryngeal nerve injury | 19. The larynx |
| AN39.1 | Describe and demonstrate the morphology, nerve supply, embryological basis of nerve supply, blood supply, lymphatic drainage, and actions of extrinsic and intrinsic muscles of the tongue | 17. The tongue |
| AN39.2 | Explain the anatomical basis of hypoglossal nerve palsy | 17. The tongue |
| AN40.1 | Describe and identify the parts, blood supply, and nerve supply of the external ear | 12. Organs of hearing and equilibrium |
| AN40.2 | Describe and demonstrate the boundaries, contents, relations, and functional anatomy of the middle ear and auditory tube | 12. Organs of hearing and equilibrium |
| AN40.3 | Describe the features of the internal ear | 12. Organs of hearing and equilibrium |
| AN40.4 | Explain the anatomical basis of otitis externa and otitis media | 12. Organs of hearing and equilibrium |
| AN40.5 | Explain the anatomical basis of myringotomy | 12. Organs of hearing and equilibrium |
| AN41.1 | Describe and demonstrate the parts and layers of the eyeball | 11. The eyeball |

**Table 0.1** Continued

| Competency No. | Competency | Chapter in 17th edition |
|---|---|---|
| AN41.2 | Describe the anatomical aspects of cataract, glaucoma, and central retinal artery occlusion | 11. The eyeball |
| AN41.3 | Describe the position, nerve supply, and actions of intraocular muscles | 11. The eyeball |
| AN42.1 | Describe the contents of the vertebral canal | 20. The contents of the vertebral canal |
| AN42.2 | Describe and demonstrate the boundaries and contents of the suboccipital triangle | 6. The back |
| AN42.3 | Describe the position, direction of fibres, relations, nerve supply, and actions of the semispinalis capitis and splenius capitis | 6. The back |
| AN43.1 | Describe and demonstrate movements with muscles producing the movements of the atlanto-occipital and atlanto-axial joints | 21. The joints of the neck |
| AN43.6 | Demonstrate the surface projection of the thyroid gland, parotid gland and duct, pterion, common carotid artery, internal jugular vein, subclavian vein, external jugular vein, facial artery in the face, and accessory nerve | 22. Surface marking of the head and neck |
| AN43.7 | Identify the anatomical structures in: (1) plain X-ray of the skull—anteroposterior (AP) and lateral views; (2) plain X-ray of the cervical spine—AP and lateral views; and (3) plain X-ray of paranasal sinuses | 2. Osteology of the head and neck<br>18. The cavity of the nose |
| AN43.8 | Describe the anatomical route used for carotid angiography and vertebral angiography | 26. The blood vessels of the brain |
| AN43.9 | Identify the anatomical structures on a carotid angiogram and a vertebral angiogram | 26. The blood vessels of the brain |

**Table 0.2** Competencies in Brain and Spinal Cord

| Competency No. | Competency | Chapter in 17th edition |
|---|---|---|
| AN56.1 | Describe and identify the various layers of the meninges, with their extent and modifications | 25. The meninges of the brain |
| AN56.2 | Describe the circulation of cerebrospinal fluid, with its applied anatomy | 32. The ventricular system |
| AN57.1 | Identify the external features of the spinal cord | 20. The contents of the vertebral canal |
| AN57.2 | Describe the extent of the spinal cord in a child and an adult, with its clinical implication | 20. The contents of the vertebral canal |
| AN57.3 | Draw and label a transverse section of the spinal cord at the mid-cervical and mid-thoracic levels | 27. The spinal cord |
| AN57.4 | Enumerate the ascending and descending tracts at the mid-thoracic level of the spinal cord | 27. The spinal cord |
| AN57.5 | Describe the anatomical basis of syringomyelia | 27. The spinal cord |
| AN58.1 | Identify the external features of the medulla oblongata | 28. The brainstem |
| AN58.2 | Describe a transverse section of the medulla oblongata at the level of: (1) pyramidal decussation; (2) sensory decussation; and (3) ION | 28. The brainstem |
| AN58.3 | Enumerate the cranial nerve nuclei in the medulla oblongata, with their functional group | 28. The brainstem |
| AN58.4 | Describe the anatomical basis and effects of medial and lateral medullary syndrome | 28. The brainstem |
| AN59.1 | Identify the external features of the pons | 28. The brainstem |
| AN59.2 | Draw and label a transverse section of the pons at the upper and lower levels | 28. The brainstem |

*(continued)*

**Table 0.2** Continued

| Competency No. | Competency | Chapter in 17th edition |
|---|---|---|
| AN59.3 | Enumerate the cranial nerve nuclei in the pons, with their functional group | 28. The brainstem |
| AN60.1 | Describe and demonstrate the external and internal features of the cerebellum | 29. The cerebellum |
| AN60.2 | Describe the connections of the cerebellar cortex and intracerebellar nuclei | 29. The cerebellum |
| AN60.3 | Describe the anatomical basis of cerebellar dysfunction | 29. The cerebellum |
| AN61.1 | Identify the external and internal features of the midbrain | 28. The brainstem |
| AN61.2 | Describe the internal features of the midbrain at the level of the superior and inferior colliculi | 28. The brainstem |
| AN61.3 | Describe the anatomical basis and effects of Benedikt's syndrome and Weber's syndrome | 28. The brainstem |
| AN62.1 | Enumerate the cranial nerve nuclei, with their functional component | 28. The brainstem |
| AN62.2 | Describe and demonstrate the surfaces, sulci, gyri, poles, and functional areas of the cerebral hemisphere | 31. The cerebrum |
| AN62.3 | Describe the white matter of the cerebrum | 31. The cerebrum |
| AN62.4 | Enumerate the parts and major connections of the basal ganglia and limbic lobe | 31. The cerebrum |
| AN62.5 | Describe the boundaries, parts, gross relations, major nuclei, and connections of the dorsal thalamus, hypothalamus, epithalamus, metathalamus, and subthalamus | 30. The diencephalon |
| AN62.6 | Describe and identify the formation, branches, and major areas of distribution of the circle of Willis | 26. The blood vessels of the brain |
| AN63.1 | Describe and demonstrate the parts, boundaries, and features of the third, fourth, and lateral ventricles | 32. The ventricular system |
| AN63.2 | Describe the anatomical basis of congenital hydrocephalus | 32. The ventricular system |

# PART 1

# Head and neck

## CHAPTER 1

# Introduction to the head and neck

The section on head and neck deals with the bones, cavities, organs, muscles, vessels, and nerves of the head and neck. It does not include the study of the brain, which is dealt with in a separate section devoted to the brain and spinal cord.

The head and neck section begins with a description of the bones of the region—the cervical vertebrae and skull. The dissectors should study these bones and the bony prominences in the living, as a preliminary to the dissection of the head and neck.

The next few chapters (the scalp and face, anterior triangle, posterior triangle, and back of the neck) complete the superficial dissection of the head and neck. The cranial cavity and deeper structures of the head and neck (the orbit, ear, oral cavity, nasal cavity, pharynx, and larynx) are then dissected and described. The joints of the neck and contents of the vertebral canal are discussed last.

# CHAPTER 2
# Osteology of the head and neck

## Skull

The skeleton of the head is the skull. It is formed by a number of separate bones, almost all of which meet each other at linear fibrous joints—the sutures. Sutures are narrow gaps between adjacent bones, filled with dense fibrous tissue in early life. Bony fusion across the fibrous tissue begins after 30 years of age. The mandible (bone of the lower jaw) articulates with the skull at a synovial joint—the temporomandibular joint—the only movable joint in the skull. The skull without the mandible is the **cranium**. For descriptive purposes, the cranium is divided into the neurocranium and viscerocranium. The neurocranium surrounds the brain and its coverings. It is divided into the cranial vault, which provides a roof for the brain, and the skull base, which increases in depth from anterior to posterior. The viscerocranium is the facial skeleton and lies inferior to the shallow, anterior part of the neurocranium.

A number of bony foramina are present in the skull, especially at the base. These give passage to nerves and vessels entering and leaving the skull. You should note the positions of these foramina and relate them to the structures which pass through them as you proceed with the study of the head, neck, and brain.

The different views of the skull are described as: the **norma frontalis**, the skull as seen from in front; the **norma verticalis**, the skull as seen from the top; the **norma lateralis**, the skull as seen from the side; the **norma occipitalis**, the skull as seen from the back; and the **norma basalis**, the skull as seen from below.

### General features of norma frontalis

Examine the frontal or anterior aspect of the skull, and identify the orbit, nasal aperture, and bones seen in this view. The bones seen in the anterior view are the frontal, ethmoid, lacrimal, maxilla, zygomatic, nasal bone, and mandible [Fig. 2.1A]. The **frontal bone** is the bone of the forehead. It consists of the right and left halves, which usually fuse together early in life. At the lower margin of the forehead, the frontal bone forms part of the roof of the orbits (the sockets for the eyeballs) and the roof of the nasal cavities.

The main elements of the facial skeleton are the right and left **maxillae**. The body of each maxilla lies below the orbit, lateral to the nasal cavity. It is shaped like a three-sided pyramid with an anterolateral or anterior surface, a posterolateral surface, and a superior surface. The base is directed medially and forms the lateral wall of the nasal cavity. The apex points laterally and is overlapped by the **zygomatic bone** (cheek bone). The anterior surface of the body of the maxilla projects on the face; the posterolateral surface forms the anterior wall of the infratemporal fossa, and the superior surface forms the floor of the orbit.

The curved alveolar processes of the maxillae project down from the body and bear the sockets for the upper teeth. Medial to the orbit, the maxilla articulates with the frontal bone through the **frontal process of the maxilla**. This process forms part of the medial margin of the orbit.

The zygomatic bone forms the prominence of the cheek and articulates with the apex of the maxilla. The **frontal process** of the zygomatic bone extends upwards along the lateral margin of the

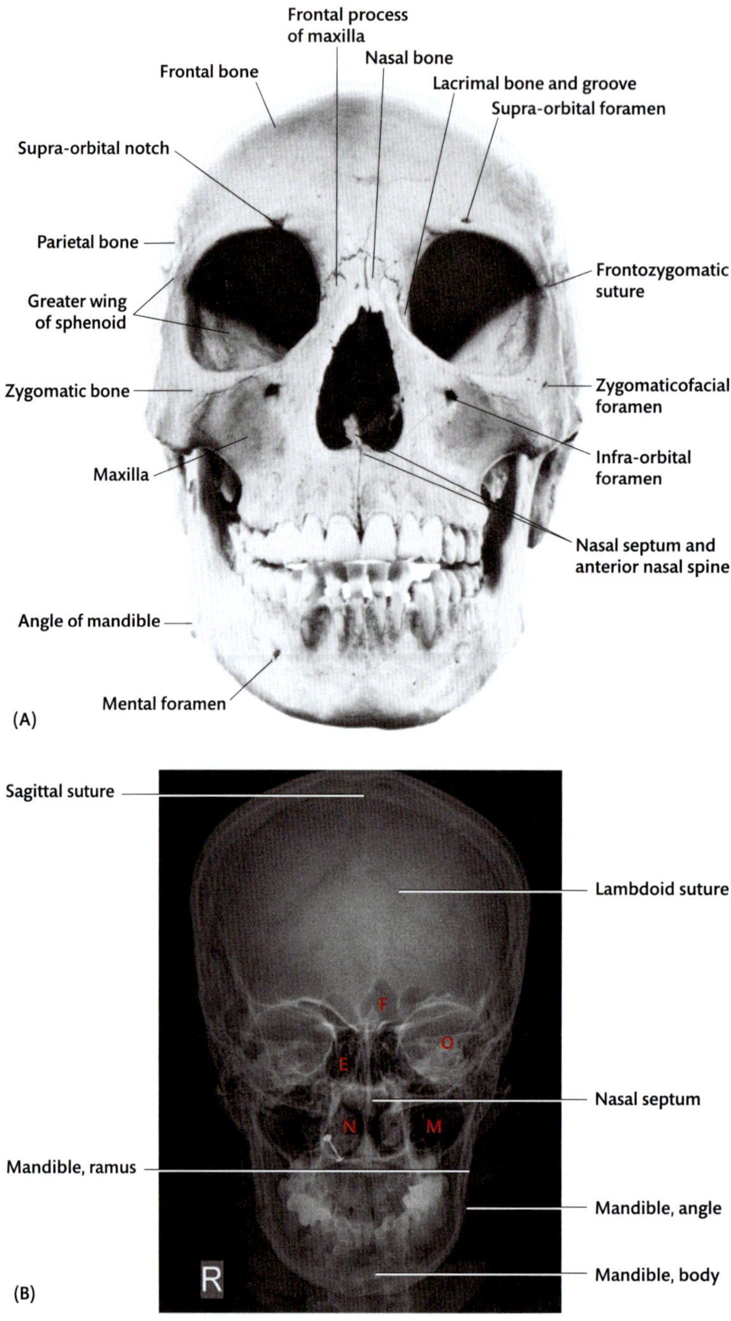


**Fig. 2.1** (A) Anterior view of the skull. The alveolar bone has been worn away from the roots of the anterior teeth in the mandible. (B) Plain X-ray of the skull—anteroposterior view. E = ethmoid air sinus. F = frontal air sinus. M = maxillary air sinus. N = nasal cavity. O = orbit. (A nose pin is seen on the right side.)

orbit to meet the zygomatic process of the frontal bone. The anterior nasal aperture lies in the midline and is pear-shaped. The inferior and lateral margins of the aperture are formed by the maxilla. The superior margin is formed by the two **nasal** bones, which articulate with each other in the midline. The bony nasal septum is seen between the two nasal cavities and is formed partly by the perpendicular plate of **ethmoid bone**. The ethmoid bone also forms parts of the lateral wall of the nasal cavities. Inferior to the nasal aperture, the two maxillae are firmly united in the midline by the intermaxillary suture.

The bone of the lower jaw is the **mandible**. Identify the horizontal **body** of the mandible which bears the alveolar sockets for the lower teeth. The lower border of the body extends laterally to the **angle** of the mandible. The two halves of the mandible are fused together in the adult at the **symphysis menti**. Fig. 2.1B is a plain radiograph of the skull in the anteroposterior view.

## Bony landmarks and muscle attachments on norma frontalis

The right and left **frontal eminences** are the most prominent and convex parts of the frontal bone. The supraorbital margin is formed by the frontal bone and is notched in the medial part by the **supraorbital notch**. The supraorbital notch transmits the supraorbital vessels and nerve. It may be converted to a foramen by a spicule of bone at its inferior aspect. Between the two orbits, the inferior margin of the frontal bone articulates with the two nasal bones, which form the superior margin of the nasal aperture. The point where the frontonasal and internasal sutures meet is the **nasion**.

The frontal process of the maxilla forms part of the medial margin of the orbit. It articulates anteriorly with the **nasal bone** and posteriorly with the **lacrimal bone**. The body of the maxilla forms part of the inferior margin of the orbit. The **infraorbital foramen** lies on the anterior surface of the maxilla and transmits the infraorbital nerve. The body of the maxilla contains the **maxillary air sinus**. The zygomatic bone forms part of the inferior margin and the lateral margin of the orbit. A small foramen on the zygomatic bone transmits the zygomaticofacial nerve.

The **mental foramen** lies about 4 cm lateral to the midline between the alveolar border and the lower border of the body of the mandible. In the living, it is felt as a slight depression.

The **bony orbit** is pyramidal in shape. The base is directed anteriorly and lies at the orbital margin; the apex is directed posteriorly. The **roof** of the orbit is formed mainly by: (1) the orbital plate of the frontal bone and (2) the lesser wing of the sphenoid [Fig. 2.2]. The **medial wall** is formed mainly by: (1) the orbital plate of the ethmoid; and (2) the lacrimal and (3) frontal processes of the maxilla [Fig. 2.3A]. At the lacrimo-maxillary suture is a shallow depression—the fossa for the lacrimal sac. The **floor** of the orbit is formed by: (1) the maxilla and (2) the zygomatic bone [Fig. 2.3B]. The **lateral wall** is formed mainly by: (1) the greater wing of the sphenoid and (2) the frontal process of the zygomatic bone [Fig. 2.2].

The muscles of facial expression are attached to the anterior surface of the skull [Fig. 2.4]. The three parts of the orbicularis are attached to the frontal, ethmoid, and maxilla. The procerus is attached to the nasal bone. The zygomaticus major, zygomaticus minor, and part of the levator

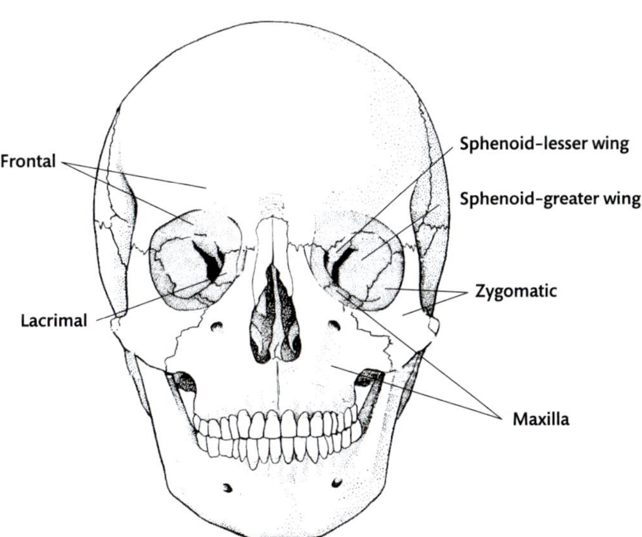


**Fig. 2.2** Anterior view of the skull showing bones forming the orbit.

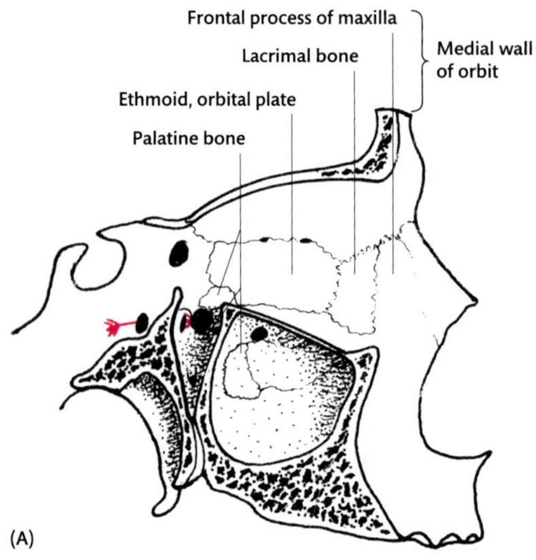


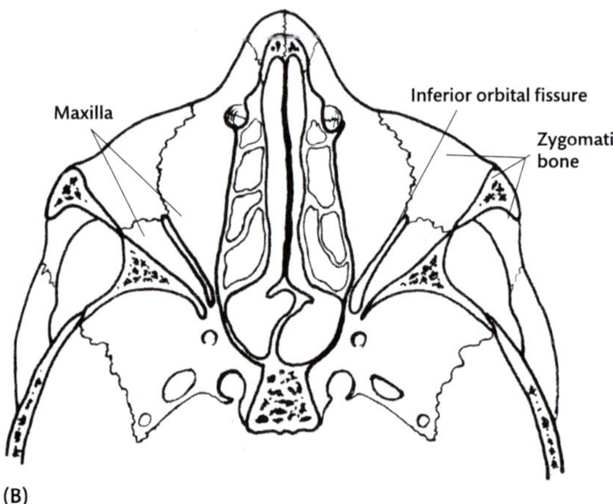


**Fig. 2.3** (A) Medial wall of the orbit. (B) Horizontal section of the anterior part of the skull showing the floor of the orbits.

labii superioris are attached to the zygomatic bone. The zygomatic bone also gives origin to the masseter, a muscle of mastication. The muscles of the upper lip and nose that are attached to the maxilla are the levator anguli oris, levator labii superioris, and nasalis. The maxilla also gives attachment to the buccinator. The mandible gives attachment to the masseter, buccinator, depressor labii inferioris, depressor anguli oris, and mentalis.

## General features of norma verticalis

The vault, or roof of the skull, is formed by the frontal bone in front, the two parietal bones laterally, and the occipital bone at the back [Fig. 2.5]. The frontal bones have been described in the anterior view. The two **parietal bones** articulate anteriorly with the frontal bone at the **coronal suture**, and with each other in the midline at the **sagittal suture**. From the sagittal suture, the parietal bones arch downwards and laterally and form the greatest and widest part of the dome of the skull. Posteriorly, the parietal bones articulate with the **squamous part of the occipital bone** at the **lambdoid suture**.

## Bony landmarks on norma verticalis

Paired parietal foramina are seen on either side of the sagittal suture. The paired **parietal eminence** is the most convex and prominent part of the parietal bone [Fig. 2.5]. The meeting point of the coronal and sagittal sutures is the **bregma**. It represents the position of the **anterior fontanelle** in the infant. The meeting point of the sagittal and lambdoid sutures is the **lambda**. It represents the position of the **posterior fontanelle** in the infant [Fig. 2.5].

➲ The fontanelles are fibrous, membranous gaps between the bones of the vault of the cranium. They are present in the infant and are found at the four angles of the parietal bone where ossification is not yet complete.

➲ The anterior fontanelle is the largest of the four. It is diamond-shaped and situated at the junction of the sagittal and coronal sutures. It usually closes by 18 months of age. Palpation of the anterior fontanelle is an important clinical examination in the infant. A tense, bulging fontanelle may indicate raised intracranial pressure due to meningitis or obstruction to flow of cerebrospinal fluid (CSF). A sunken fontanelle is a sign of dehydration. Delayed closure of the anterior fontanelle commonly occurs in achondroplasia, rickets, and hypothyroidism.

## General features of norma occipitalis

Most of the posterior aspect of the skull is made up of the parietal and occipital bones, with a small contribution from the temporal bone [Fig. 2.6]. The parietal bones make up the superior and lateral aspects. The upper part of the squamous part of the occipital bone lies in the interval between the diverging posterior margins of the parietal bones. The **mastoid process of the temporal bone** is seen at the inferolateral corner.

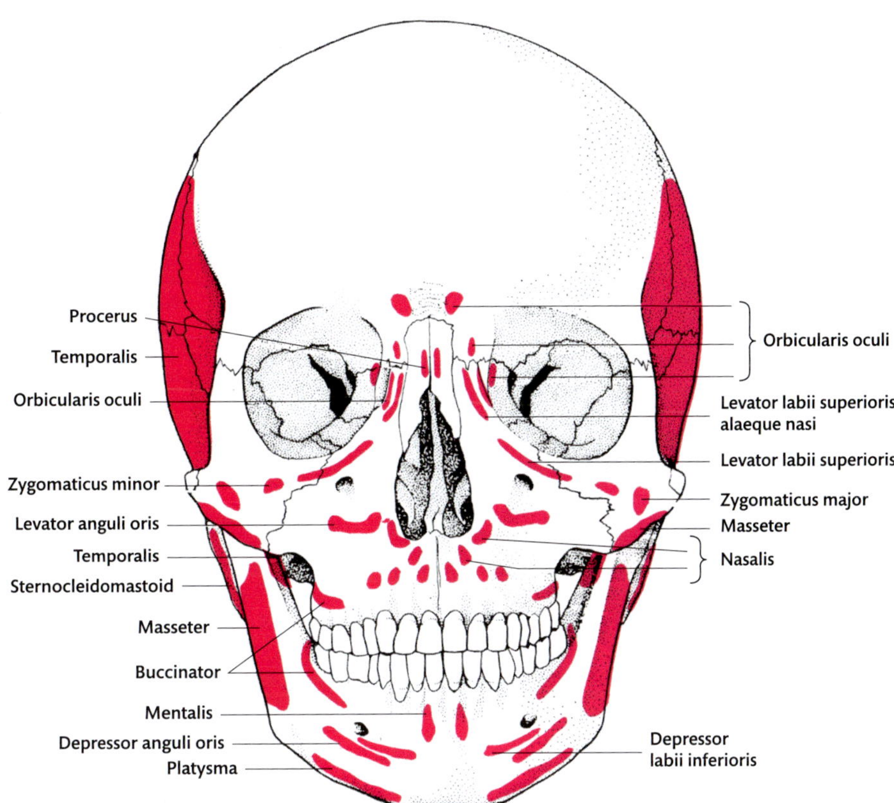


**Fig. 2.4** Anterior view of the skull showing muscle attachments.



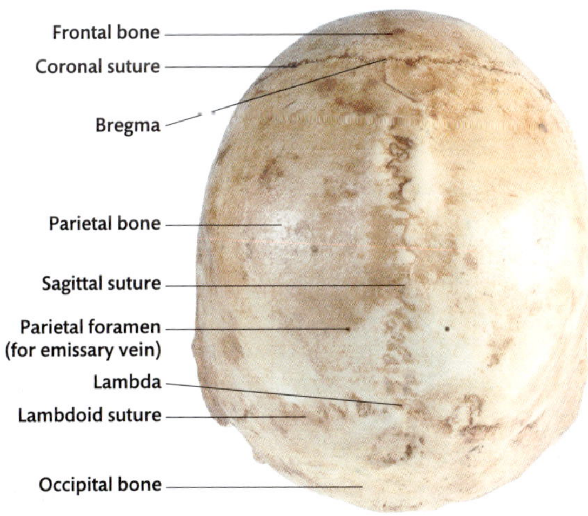


**Fig. 2.5** Superior view of the skull.



## Bony landmarks and muscle attachments on norma occipitalis

In the lambdoid suture, small bones called **sutural bones**, or Wormian bones, are often present. The **external occipital protuberance** is a midline projection seen at the lower part of the posterior view. On either side of the external occipital protuberance, bony linear elevations—the **superior nuchal lines**—extend laterally. Parallel and approximately 1 cm superior to the superior nuchal lines are faint bony ridges—the **highest nuchal lines**. The **external occipital crest** extends inferiorly in the midline from the external occipital protuberance. It is better seen on the inferior aspect of the skull.

At the lower end, the lambdoid suture is continuous with the parietomastoid suture between the parietal bone and the mastoid process, and with the occipitomastoid suture between the occipital bone and the mastoid process [Fig. 2.6].

The trapezius and occipital belly of the occipitofrontalis are attached to the superior nuchal line.

## General features of norma lateralis

The bones seen on the lateral view of the skull are the frontal, zygomatic, maxilla, mandible, greater

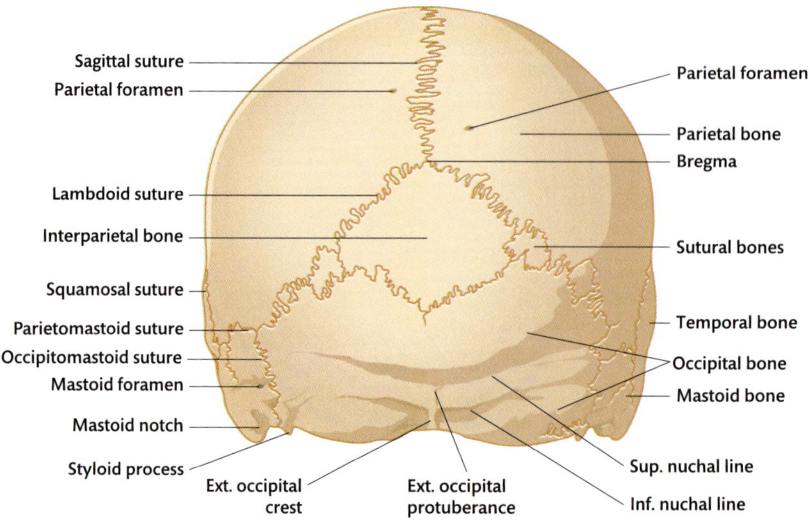


**Fig. 2.6** Posterior view of the skull. Note the presence of the sutural bone and the large interparietal bone.

wing of the sphenoid, temporal, and occipital. Start your study of the norma lateralis by identifying the parts of the frontal, parietal, occipital, maxilla, and zygomatic bones described in the anterior and superior views [Fig. 2.7A]. Review the zygomaticofrontal suture on the lateral wall of the orbit, and the coronal, lambdoid, parietomastoid, and occipitomastoid sutures.

The **temporal process** of the zygomatic bone joins the **zygomatic process** of the temporal bone to form the **zygomatic arch**, inferolateral to the orbit. The **greater wing of the sphenoid** forms the lateral wall of the skull behind the orbit. The **squamous part of the temporal bone** lies inferior to the parietal bone. Anteriorly, it articulates with the greater wing of the sphenoid. Superiorly and posteriorly, it articulates with the parietal bone, at the **squamosal suture**. Posteriorly, the squamous part of the temporal bone is fused with the mastoid part.

Below the root of the zygomatic process, the inferior surface of the squamous part of the temporal bone has a large notch—the **mandibular fossa**—for articulation with the head of the mandible (the mandibular fossa is better seen on the basal view of the skull). Behind the mandibular fossa is a bony canal—the **external acoustic meatus**—and more posteriorly the **mastoid process of the temporal bone**. A ridge of bone—the **supramastoid crest**—extends posteriorly from the zygomatic arch and separates the squamous part of temporal bone from the mastoid process. The **squamous part of the occipital bone** is seen behind the lambdoid and the occipitomastoid sutures.

Below the zygomatic arch is the ramus of the mandible—a wide, flat plate of bone, which extends superiorly from the posterior part of the body. It ends superiorly in the **condylar** and **coronoid processes** of the mandible. The condylar process projects upwards from the posterior margin of the ramus and continues with the **neck** and **head of the mandible** [Fig. 2.7A]. Fig. 2.7B is a lateral radiograph of the skull.

## Bony landmarks and muscle attachments on norma lateralis

The temporal line arises from the zygomatic process of the frontal bone and extends upwards and backwards to cross the coronal suture. On the parietal bone, it splits into the **superior** and **inferior temporal lines**. The superior temporal line becomes indistinct posteriorly, but the inferior temporal line curves downwards and forwards to continue with the supramastoid crest of the temporal bone. The shallow area bounded by the temporal lines above and the zygomatic arch below is the temporal fossa.

The greater wing of the sphenoid articulates anteriorly with the frontal and zygomatic bones, superiorly with the frontal and parietal bones, and posteriorly with the squamous part of the temporal bone. The 'H'-shaped area where the frontal, parietal, temporal, and sphenoid bones meet is called the **pterion**. It represents the position of the

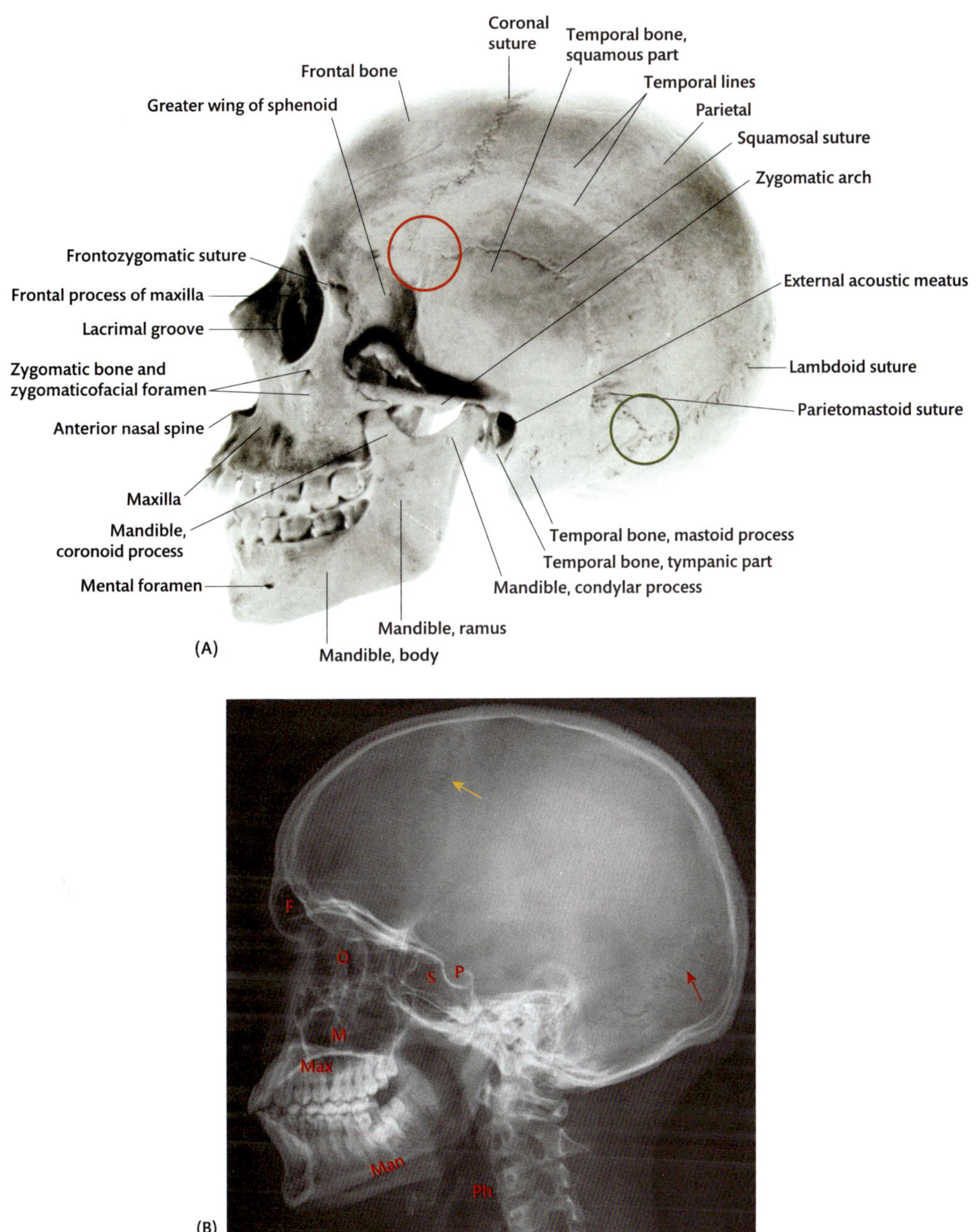


**Fig. 2.7** (A) Lateral view of the skull. Red circle: pterion. Green circle: asterion. (B) Lateral radiograph of the skull. F = frontal sinus. M = maxillary sinus. Man = mandible. Max = maxilla. O = orbit. P = pituitary fossa. Ph = pharynx. S = sphenoid sinus. Yellow arrow = coronal suture. Red arrow = lambdoid suture.

**sphenoidal fontanelle** in the fetus. At the root of the zygomatic process of the temporal bone is the **articular tubercle**.

The **tympanic part** of the temporal bone forms the anterior, inferior, and lower part of the posterior wall of the **external acoustic meatus**. Anteriorly, the **tympanic bone** meets the squamous part in the posterior wall of the mandibular fossa at the **squamotympanic fissure**. Posteriorly, it fuses with the mastoid process. Also seen in this view is the **styloid process of the temporal bone**, projecting downwards and forwards from the base of the skull [Fig. 2.8]. The squamosal suture continuous posteriorly with the **parietomastoid suture**. Trace the parietomastoid suture back to its junction with the lambdoid and occipitomastoid sutures.

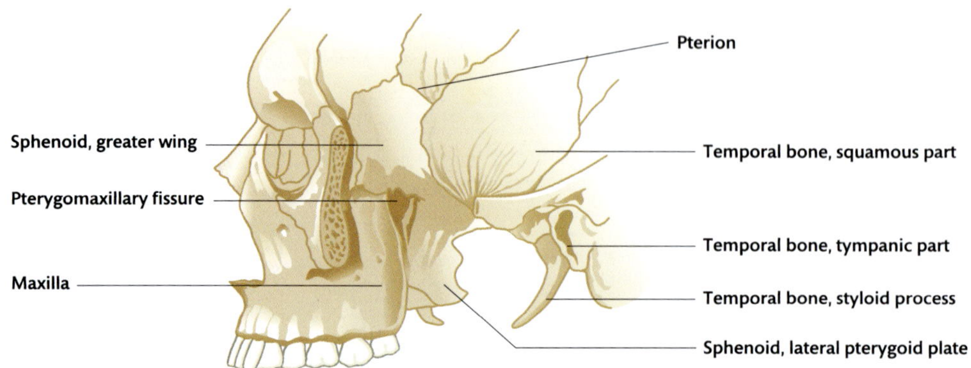


**Fig. 2.8** Lateral view of the cranium. (The mandible and zygomatic arch have been removed.)

This region at the posterior–inferior corner of the parietal bone is the **asterion** and marks the place where the temporal, parietal, and occipital bones come together. It represents the position of the **mastoid fontanelle** in the fetus.

The **supramastoid crest** is a blunt ridge which begins immediately above the external acoustic meatus and curves posterosuperiorly. It is continuous superiorly with the **inferior temporal line**, which curve forwards, marking the upper limit of the temporal region. (The temporal fossa is limited above by the inferior temporal line and below by the zygomatic arch [Fig. 2.7A].)

Remove the mandible to study the part of the normal lateralis which lies medial to it. The **maxillary tuberosity** is a small blunt elevation directed backwards from the area just above the socket for the last molar. Behind the maxilla, two plates of bone—the **medial** and **lateral pterygoid plates** or **laminae**—extend downwards and forwards from the junction of the body and greater wings of the sphenoid. Together they form the **pterygoid process** of the sphenoid bone. The medial pterygoid plate is not seen in the lateral view. The lower part of the anterior border of the lateral pterygoid plate articulates with the palatine bone in front. The upper part of this border forms the posterior boundary for the **pterygomaxillary fissure**. The region lateral to the lateral pterygoid lamina is the **infratemporal fossa** [Fig. 2.8].

The temporalis takes origin from the parts of the sphenoid, frontal, parietal, and temporal bones bounded by the inferior temporal line. The temporal fascia is attached to the superior temporal line. The attachments of the levator labii superioris, zygomaticus major, and zygomaticus minor to the zygomatic bone, the attachments of the levator anguli oris, nasalis, levator labii superioris, and buccinator to the maxilla, and the attachments of the buccinator, depressor labii inferioris, depressor anguli oris, and mentalis to the mandible were seen in the norma frontalis and should be reviewed here. The temporalis is inserted into the coronoid process of the mandible, and the masseter to a wide area on the lateral surface of the ramus of the mandible. The platysma is attached to the lower border of the body of the mandible. The lateral pterygoid takes origin from the lateral pterygoid plate and greater wing of the sphenoid, and is inserted on the neck of the mandible. The stylohyoid, stylopharyngeus, and styloglossus muscles are attached to the styloid process of the temporal bone. The sternocleidomastoid, longissimus capitis, and splenius capitis are attached to the mastoid process, and the trapezius and occipitalis are attached to the occipital bone [Fig. 2.9].

## General features of norma basalis

The inferior surface of the skull is described without the mandible. It extends from the upper central incisors anteriorly to the external occipital protuberance posteriorly, and is arbitrarily divided into anterior, middle, and posterior parts [Fig. 2.10]. The bones seen in this view are the maxilla, palatine, parts of the sphenoid—pterygoid process and greater wing of the sphenoid, parts of the occipital—basilar and squamous parts, and parts of the temporal bone—petrous, mastoid, tympanic plate, and styloid process.

The anterior part of the norma basalis is formed by the **hard palate** and the **alveolar arch** in the

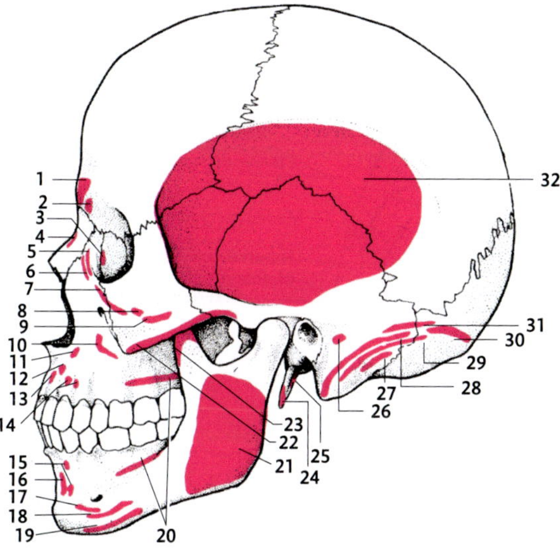


**Fig. 2.9** Lateral view of the skull showing muscle attachments. 1, 2, and 3 = orbicularis oculi. 4 = procerus. 5 = orbicularis oculi. 6 = levator labii superioris alaeque nasi. 7 = levator labii superioris. 8 = zygomaticus minor. 9 = zygomaticus major. 10 = levator anguli oris. 11 and 12 = nasalis. 13 = depressor septi. 14 and 15 = incisive Mm. 16 = mentalis. 17 = depressor labii inferioris. 18 = depressor anguli oris. 19 = platysma. 20 = buccinator. 21 and 22 = masseter. 23 = temporalis. 24 = styloglossus. 25 = stylohyoid. 26 = auricularis posterior. 27 = longissimus capitis. 28 = sternocleidomastoid. 29 = splenius capitis. 30 = trapezius. 31 = occipitalis. 32 = temporalis.

midline. Lateral to the alveolar arch lie the maxillary and zygomatic bones.

The middle part of the norma basalis is the **pharyngeal part** of the base of the skull in the midline. It is formed by the **body of the sphenoid** (which is overlapped by the **vomer**) and the **basilar part of the occipital bone**. Lateral to the basilar part, two **pterygoid processes** descend from the body of the sphenoid. Each pterygoid process is formed by a **medial** and a **lateral pterygoid plate**, which are fused together anteriorly, but separated from each other by the **pterygoid fossa** posteriorly [Fig. 2.11]. Lateral to the lateral pterygoid plate is the **greater wing of the sphenoid**. Lateral and posterior to the greater wing are the **squamous** and **petrous parts of the temporal bone**. The petrous part of the temporal bone lies immediately lateral to the basilar part of the occipital bone.

Posterior to the pharyngeal area on the base of the skull is the large **foramen magnum**. The anterolateral margin of the foramen magnum has an oval, curved articular facet—the **occipital condyle**—for articulation with the superior articular facets of the first cervical vertebra. Posterior to the foramen




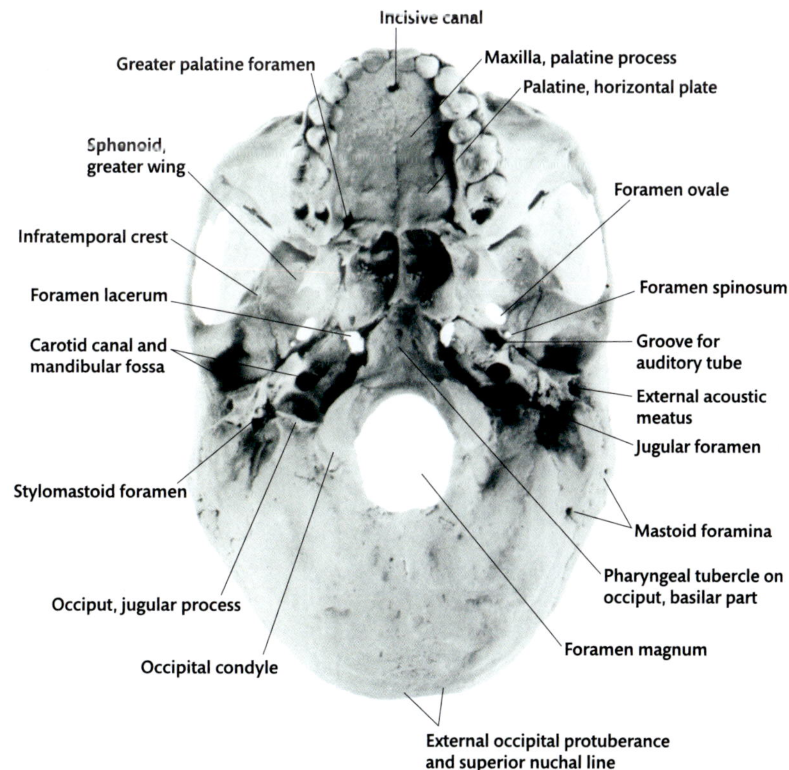


**Fig. 2.10** The external surface of the base of the skull. Two molar teeth are missing on the left of the picture, and one-and-a-half on the right.

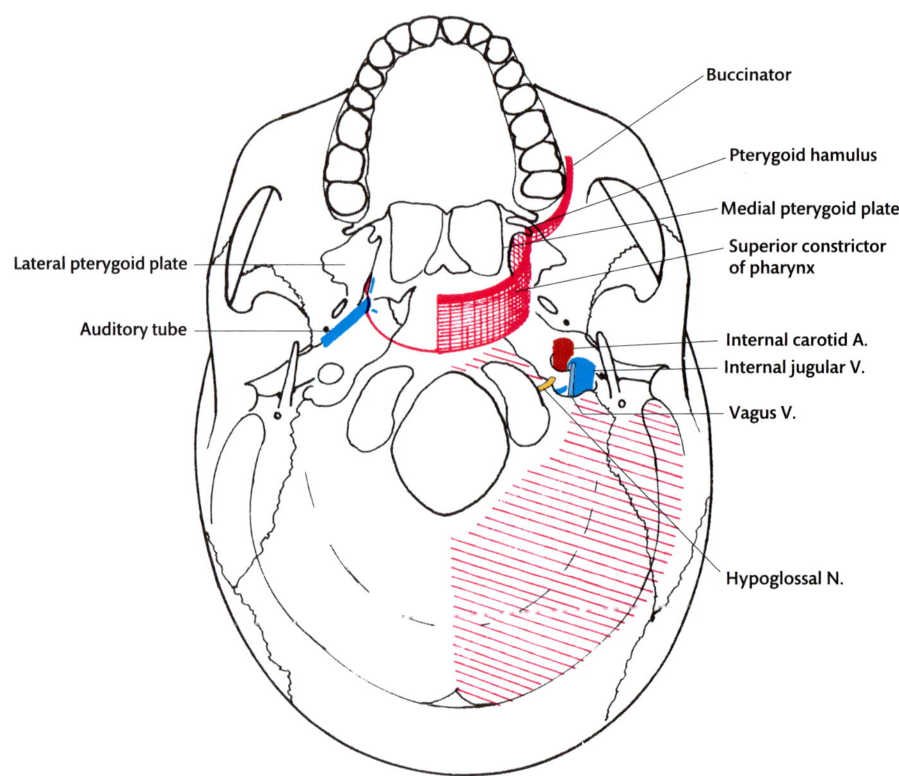


**Fig. 2.11** External surface of the base of the skull showing the position of the superior constrictor, buccinator, and auditory tube.

magnum, the greater part of the inferior surface of the cranium is formed by the occipital bone. This surface is roughened by the attachment of the muscles of the back of the neck.

## Bony landmarks and muscle attachments on norma basalis

The hard palate is formed by two bones on either side, which meet each other in the midline. In the anterior part, the **palatine processes of the maxillae** extend horizontally inwards from the upper margins of the alveolar processes and meet in the midline. Posteriorly, the palatine processes of the maxilla articulate with the **horizontal plates of the palatine bone** to complete the hard palate. Each half of the alveolar arch has eight tooth sockets for the two incisors, one canine, two premolars, and three molars. The opening of the incisive canal lies in the midline, posterior to the incisors. It marks the embryological junction of the premaxilla and the definitive hard palate, and transmits the terminal branches of the nasopalatine nerves, sphenopalatine arteries, and the terminal part of the greater palatine nerves. The greater palatine foramina lie in the horizontal plate of the palatine bone, close to the molars. They transmit the greater palatine nerves and arteries. The lesser palatine foramina lie behind the greater palatine foramina.

The **pharyngeal tubercle** is a small midline prominence on the basilar part of the occipital bone, 1 cm anterior to the foramen magnum. The **pterygoid hamulus** is the hook-shaped projection from the lower end of the posterior margin of the medial pterygoid plate [Fig. 2.11]. Lateral to the lateral pterygoid plate is the **greater wing of the sphenoid**. Traced laterally, this plate of bone turns sharply at the **infratemporal crest** to continue on the lateral surface of the skull. Between the infratemporal crest on the greater wing of the sphenoid and the lateral pterygoid lamina is the **infratemporal fossa**. The **spine of the sphenoid** is a small, sharp bony projection at the posterolateral angle of the greater wing. The **auditory tube** lies in the groove at the junction of the greater wing of the sphenoid and petrous temporal bone [Fig. 2.11].

A number of important foramina are seen in this part. On the greater wing of the sphenoid are the

**foramen ovale** and **foramen spinosum**. The **foramen lacerum** lies at the apex of the petrous part of the temporal bone and is bounded by that bone, the basilar part of the occiput, and the body of the sphenoid. On the inferior aspect of the petrous part of the temporal bone is the **carotid canal**. The **stylomastoid foramen** lies between the styloid and the mastoid processes of the temporal bone [Fig. 2.10]. The bony part of the auditory tube lies in the groove between the greater wing of the sphenoid and the petrous temporal bone [Fig. 2.11].

The foramen magnum is oval, longer than it is wide, and overlapped at the anterolateral margin by the occipital condyle. Lateral to the condyle is the jugular process of the occipital bone, which articulates with the temporal bone to form the **jugular foramen**. The jugular foramen lies immediately posterior to the carotid canal. The **hypoglossal canal** for the twelfth cranial nerve lies immediately above the occipital condyles.

Posterior to the foramen magnum, the **squamous part of the occipital bone** is limited posteriorly by the **external occipital protuberance** in the midline and the **superior nuchal line** which extends laterally from it [Fig. 2.10]. The **external occipital crest** runs between the posterior margin of the foramen magnum and the external occipital protuberance. The **inferior nuchal line** extends laterally from the middle of the external occipital crest.

The buccinator is attached on the surface of the maxilla, immediately lateral to the molars. The buccopharyngeal fascia and superior constrictor of the pharynx are attached to the pharyngeal tubercle and basilar part of the occipital bone [Fig. 2.11]. The medial and lateral surfaces of the lateral pterygoid plates give attachment to the medial and lateral pterygoid muscles. Some fibres of the medial pterygoid have an additional attachment to the maxillary tuberosity. The small muscles of the soft palate—the tensor veli palatini, levator veli palatini, and musculus uvulae—and one muscle of the ear—the tensor tympani—take attachment from the hard palate, the pterygoid fossa, and the margins on the groove for the auditory tube.

The prevertebral muscles—the rectus capitis superior and longus capitis—are attached to the basilar part of the occipital bone immediately in front of the foramen magnum [Fig. 2.12].

The part of the occipital bone anterior to the inferior nuchal line gives attachment to the rectus capitis posterior minor medially and the rectus capitis posterior major laterally. The area between the two nuchal lines gives attachment to the semispinalis capitis medially and the obliquus capitis superior laterally. The lateral part of the superior nuchal line gives attachment to the sternocleidomastoid and splenius capitis. The rectus capitis lateralis is attached to the occipital bone immediately behind and lateral to the jugular foramen [Fig. 2.12].





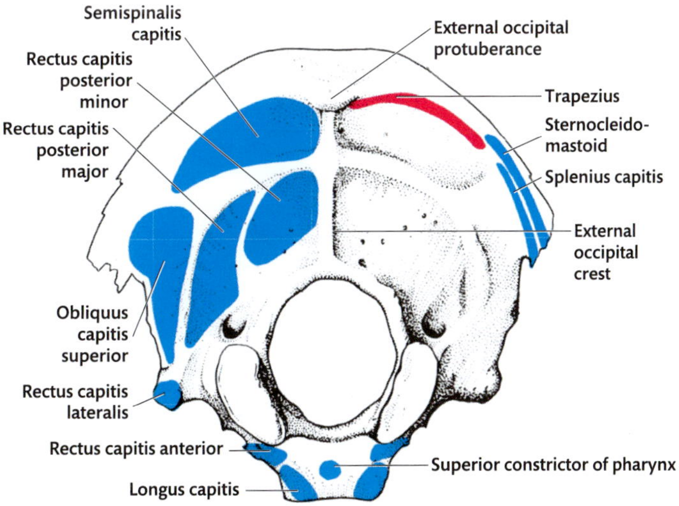


**Fig. 2.12** Muscle attachments to the occipital bone. Red = origins; blue = insertions.

**Table 2.1** Structures passing through foramina seen on the norma basalis

| Name of foramen | Structures passing through |
|---|---|
| Incisive foramen | • Nasopalatine nerve<br>• Sphenopalatine artery |
| Greater palatine foramen | • Greater palatine nerves and vessels |
| Foramen ovale | • Mandibular nerve<br>• Lesser petrosal nerve<br>• Accessory meningeal artery |
| Foramen spinosum | • Middle meningeal artery |
| Foramen lacerum | • Emissary veins |
| Jugular foramen | • Sigmoid sinus<br>• Inferior petrosal sinus<br>• Glossopharyngeal nerve<br>• Vagus nerve<br>• Accessory nerve |
| Stylomastoid foramen | • Facial nerve |
| Carotid canal | • Internal carotid artery |
| Foramen magnum | • Medulla-spinal cord junction<br>• Vertebral arteries<br>• Spinal root of accessory nerve<br>• Spinal meninges |

The 12 pairs of cranial nerves, internal carotid and vertebral arteries, and internal jugular vein and other structures pass through foramina in the skull. Table 2.1 lists the structures passing through each foramen seen in this view. (The extra- and intracranial courses of these structures are described in subsequent chapters.)

## Anatomical position of the skull

### Exercise 2.1: To hold the skull in the anatomical position

Hold the skull such that:

1. The orbits and nasal aperture are directed anteriorly
2. The upper margin of the external auditory meatus and the inferior margin of the orbit lie in the same horizontal plane.

## Internal features of the skull

The internal features of the skull are best studied on a skull bone that has been cut horizontally to separate the vault from the base. The following section describes the bony features of the vault and the cranial fossae [Figs. 2.13, 2.14]; markings for the attachment of the dural folds and soft tissue impressions are seen on the bones.

### Internal features of the vault

The cranial vault, or calvaria, is oval in shape. The internal surface is deeply concave and is made up of the squamous part of the frontal bone in front, the two parietal bones behind it, and the squamous part of the occipital bone behind. Note the coronal

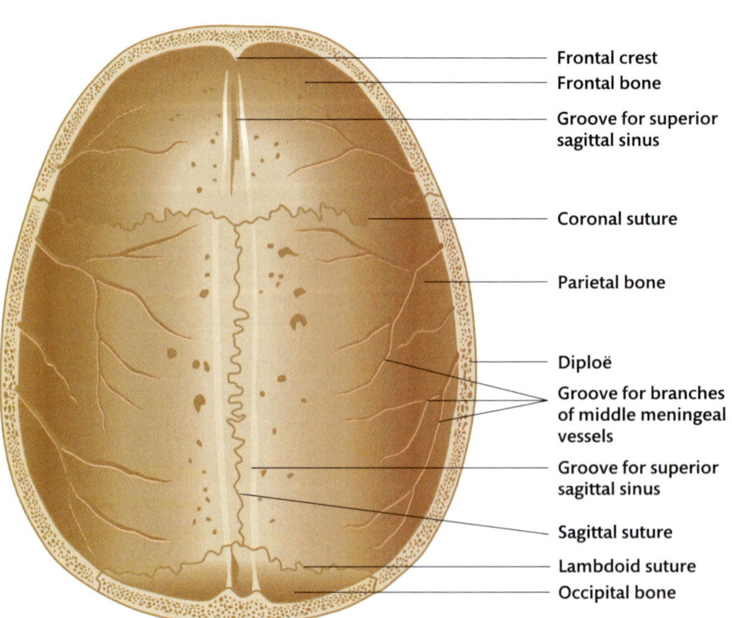


**Fig. 2.13** Internal surface of the calvaria.

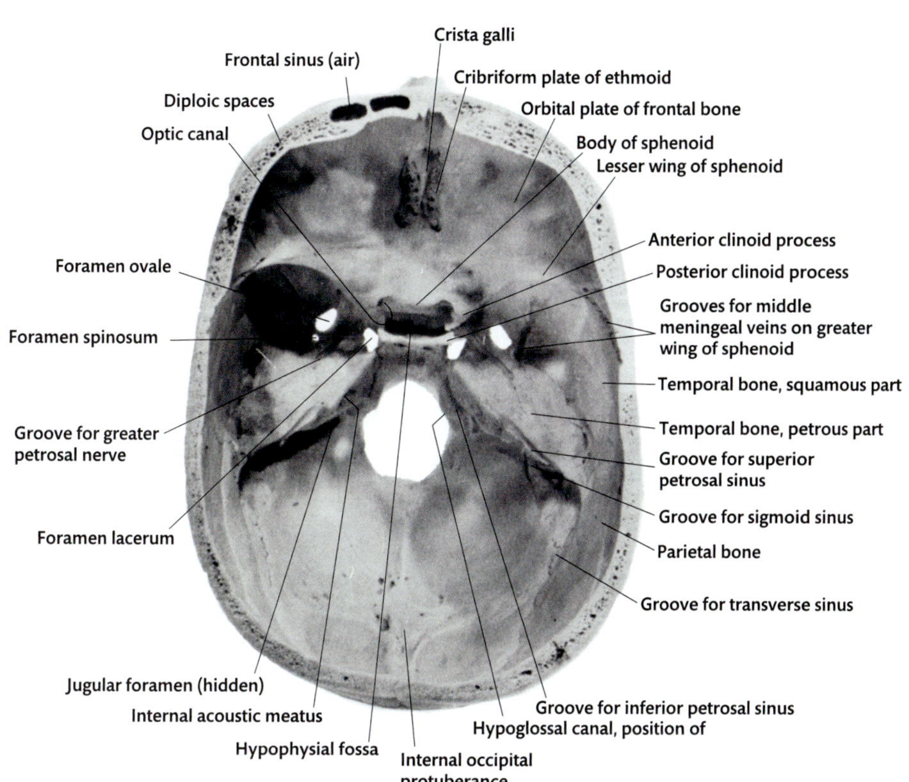


**Fig. 2.14** Internal surface of the base of the skull.

suture between the frontal and parietal bones, the sagittal suture between the two parietal bones, and the lambdoid suture between the occipital and parietal bones. Anteriorly in the midline is the frontal crest. The shallow groove for the superior sagittal sinus extends posteriorly in the midline from the frontal crest [Fig. 2.13].

## Internal features of the base of the cranial cavity

The inferior aspect of the cranial cavity supports the brain. It is divided into three distinct fossae—the **anterior**, **middle**, and **posterior** cranial fossae [Fig. 2.14].

### Anterior cranial fossa

The floor of the anterior cranial fossa is formed by the **orbital plates of the frontal bone**, parts of the **ethmoid**, and the **body and lesser wings of the sphenoid**. The orbital plates of the frontal bone project posteriorly above the orbit. They are separated from each other by the **cribriform plate** of the ethmoid which lies in the roof of the nasal cavities. In the midline, a bony ridge—the **crista galli**—projects upwards from the cribriform plate. A small foramen—the **foramen caecum**—lies anterior to the crista galli and transmits an emissary vein. Posteriorly, the ethmoid and orbital plates of the frontal bone articulate with the body and lesser wings of the sphenoid to complete the floor of the anterior cranial fossa. The floor of the anterior cranial fossa has the impressions of the sulci and gyri on the orbital surface of the frontal lobe of the brain.

Each lesser wing has a free curved posterior margin which forms the posterior limit of the anterior cranial fossa and ends medially in the **anterior clinoid process**. The anterior clinoid process lies immediately lateral to a rounded opening—the **optic canal**. Laterally, the tip of each lesser wing fuses with the corresponding greater wing of the sphenoid bone. Between the greater and lesser wings of the sphenoid is the **superior orbital fissure**.

### Middle cranial fossa

The floor of the middle cranial fossa is formed by parts of the sphenoid—the body and greater wing—and the **petrous part of the temporal bone**. In the midline, the floor of the **middle cranial fossa** is narrow and formed by the **body of the sphenoid**. The central part of the body is hollowed out to form the **hypophysial fossa**, which lodges the pituitary gland [Fig. 2.7B]. The hypophysial fossa is limited posteriorly by a rectangular plate of bone—the **dorsum sellae**. The superolateral corners of the dorsum sellae project upwards as the **posterior clinoid processes**. Anteriorly, the fossa is limited by the **tuberculum sellae**, with the horizontal **sulcus chiasmatis** in front of it. On each side, the sulcus leads into the **optic canal**, which transmits the corresponding optic nerve and ophthalmic artery.

The lateral part of the middle cranial fossa is formed mainly of the greater wing of the sphenoid. Each greater wing is roughly rectangular in shape and projects laterally from the body. The anterior part of the greater wing is upturned and articulates with the lesser wing of the sphenoid and the inferior margins of the frontal and parietal bones. The **foramen rotundum** is an opening on the greater wing of the sphenoid, close to the body near the medial end of the superior orbital fissure. More posteriorly are two other foramina—the **foramen ovale** and **foramen spinosum**. The anterior surface of the **petrous part of the temporal bone** articulates with the greater wing of the sphenoid and forms the posterior boundary of the middle cranial fossa. The apex of the petrous temporal bone is directed towards the body of the sphenoid. The **foramen lacerum** lies between the apex of the petrous temporal bone and the body of the sphenoid [Fig. 2.14]. The floor of the middle cranial fossa is marked by impressions created by the branches of the middle meningeal vessels and the greater petrosal nerve.

## Posterior cranial fossa

The posterior cranial fossa is large and deep. The floor is made up by the basilar and squamous parts of the occipital bone, the petrous part of the temporal bone, and a small part of the parietal bone [Fig. 2.14]. In the midline, it is made up of the posterior surface of the dorsum sellae, the body of the sphenoid, the basilar part of the occipital bone, and the squamous part of the occipital bone (the **foramen magnum** lies between the basilar and the squamous parts of the occipital bone). The sloping surface of the sphenoid and occipital bones in front of the foramen magnum are together known as the **clivus**.

Laterally, the posterior surface of the **petrous part of the temporal bone** forms the anterior limit of the posterior cranial fossa. The lateral margin of the basilar part of the occipital bone articulates with the petrous temporal bone at the **petro-occipital fissure**. The **jugular foramen** is a large opening situated at the posterior end of this petro-occipital fissure. The **internal acoustic meatus** opens on the posterior surface of the petrous temporal bone. The **hypoglossal canal** lies medial to the jugular foramen, immediately above the anteromedial margin of the foramen magnum.

The medial surface of the **mastoid part of the temporal bone** and the posteroinferior corner of the parietal bone form the lateral wall of the posterior cranial fossa.

Behind the foramen magnum and the petrous temporal bone, the **squamous part of the occipital bone** forms the floor of the posterior cranial fossa. The **internal occipital protuberance** is a bony midline prominence on the internal aspect of the posterior cranial fossa, at the same level as the external occipital protuberance on the external aspect of the occiput. Extending laterally from the internal occipital prominence to the mastoid angle of the parietal bone is a groove for the transverse sinus. At the lateral end, the groove for the transverse sinus continues with the groove for the sigmoid sinus on the petrous temporal bone. A linear elevation—the **internal occipital crest**—extends inferiorly from the internal occipital protuberance. Four shallow fossae are present—two below the groove for the transverse sinus, and two above it. The occipital lobes of the cerebrum lie in the fossae above the groove for the transverse sinus, and the lobes of the cerebellum lie in the fossae below [Fig. 2.14].

The twelve pairs of cranial nerves, the internal carotid and vertebral arteries, and the internal jugular vein and other structures pass through foramina in the skull. Table 2.2 lists the structures passing through each foramen seen in the cranial cavity. (The extra- and intracranial courses of these structures are described in subsequent chapters.)

**Table 2.2** Structures passing through foramina in the cranial fossae

| Name of foramen | Structures passing through it |
|---|---|
| Cribriform plate of ethmoid | • Olfactory nerve (cranial nerve I) |
| Foramen caecum | • Emissary veins |
| Superior orbital fissure | • Oculomotor nerve<br>• Trochlear nerve<br>• Frontal nerve<br>• Lacrimal nerve<br>• Nasociliary nerve<br>• Abducens nerve<br>• Superior and inferior ophthalmic veins |
| Inferior orbital fissure | • Zygomatic nerve |
| Optic canal | • Optic nerve enclosed in the meninges<br>• Ophthalmic artery |
| Foramen rotundum | • Maxillary nerve |
| Foramen ovale | • Mandibular nerve<br>• Accessory meningeal artery |
| Foramen spinosum | • Middle meningeal artery |
| Foramen lacerum | • Emissary veins |
| Jugular foramen | • Sigmoid sinus<br>• Inferior petrosal sinus<br>• Glossopharyngeal nerve<br>• Vagus nerve<br>• Accessory nerve |
| Internal acoustic meatus | • Facial nerve<br>• Vestibulocochlear nerve |
| Hypoglossal canal | • Hypoglossal nerve |
| Foramen magnum | • Medulla oblongata*<br>• Vertebral arteries<br>• Spinal root of accessory nerve<br>• Spinal meninges |

* The spinal cord begins just below the foramen magnum.

## Ossification of skull bones

The skull is formed by bones that develop in membrane (intramembranous ossification) and in cartilage (endochondral ossification).

### Skull bones that ossify fully in membrane

The bones forming the cranial vault and viscerocranium develop in membrane. These include the frontal, parietal, upper part of the occipital, squamous portion of the temporal, maxilla, zygomatic, and mandible.

### Skull bones that ossify in cartilage

The bones of the base of the skull develop in cartilage. These include the lower portion of the occipital, petrous part of the temporal, and sphenoid bone.

## Mandible

### General features of the mandible

The mandible forms the lower jaw. Review the features of the mandible seen in the frontal and side views of the skull [Figs. 2.1, 2.7]. The **body** of the mandible lies horizontally. The **ramus** of the mandible is a wide, flat plate of bone, which extends superiorly from the posterior part of the body. The part where the lower border of the mandible turns upwards to continue as the posterior border of the ramus is the **angle** of the mandible. The ramus ends superiorly in the **condylar** and **coronoid processes** of the mandible. The condylar process projects upwards from the posterior margin of the ramus and forms the **neck** and **head** of the mandible. The coronoid process is thin and pointed, and continuous with the anterior border of the ramus [Fig. 2.15A]. The coronoid and condylar processes are separated by the deep mandibular notch. The head of the mandible articulates with the temporal bone in the temporomandibular joint. The neck of the mandible has a shallow depression—the **pterygoid fovea**—on the anterior aspect.

### Bony landmarks and muscle attachments on the mandible

The upper border of the body of the mandible bears the sockets for the lower teeth. On each half of the jaw, there are sockets for two incisors, one canine, two premolars, and three molars. The two halves of the mandible are united in the midline by the **symphysis menti**. The prominence seen in the midline at the junction of the two halves is the **mental protruberance**. The **mental foramen** is felt as a slight depression on the anterior surface of the body, 4 cm from the midline, halfway between the edge of the socket and the lower border of the mandible [Fig.

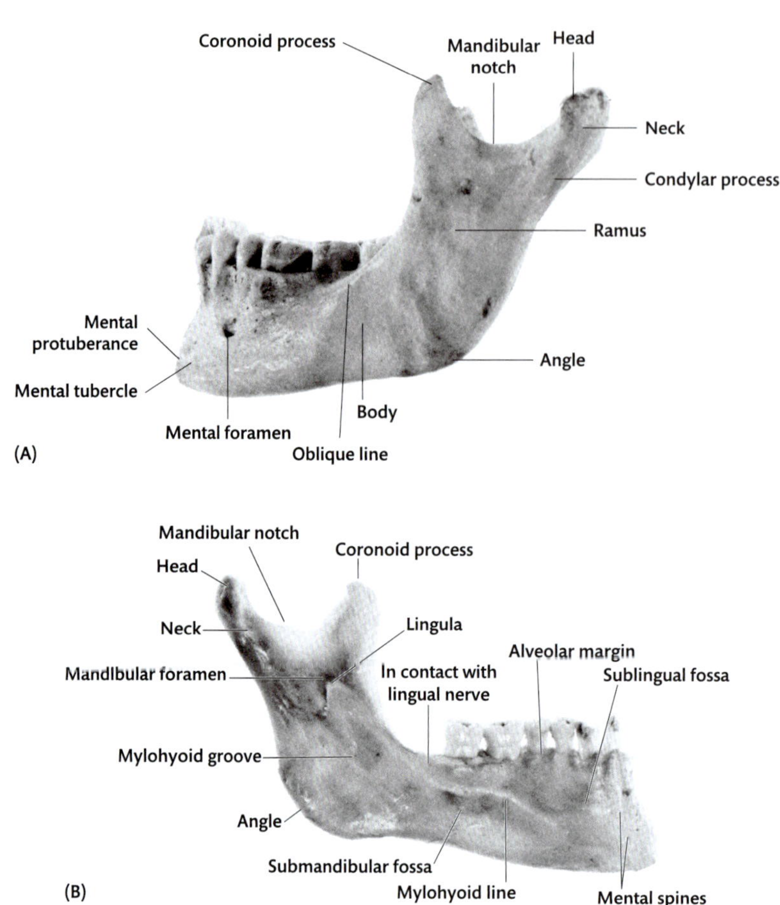


Fig. 2.15 (A) Mandible viewed from the left side. (B) The medial surface of the mandible. The third molar is missing.

2.15A]. The oblique line extends downwards and forwards across the body of the mandible from the upper margin immediately behind the third molar.

The lateral surface of the ramus of the mandible is roughened by muscle attachments. The neck lies immediately anterior to the lobule of the auricle, and the head lies anterior to the tragus. Place your fingertip in front of your own tragus, and open your mouth. The fingertip slips into a shallow depression created when the head of the mandible glides downwards and forwards. Note that the mouth cannot be closed while the finger remains in this fossa.

The medial surface of the ramus of the mandible is roughened by muscle attachments. The **mandibular foramen** is seen approximately 1 cm below the mandibular notch. A sharp spicule of bone—the **lingula**—is directed upwards and backwards, medial to the mandibular foramen. The mandibular foramen leads into the mandibular canal, which transmits the inferior alveolar vessels and nerves. On the medial surface of the body is the **mylohyoid line**, a sharp bony elevation which runs downwards and forwards. The **submandibular fossa** lies below and behind the mylohoid line, and the **sublingual fossa** lies above and in front of this line. The **superior** and **inferior mental spines** lie in the midline on the internal aspect of the symphysis menti [Fig. 2.15B].

Review the attachment of the buccinator, mentalis, depressor labii inferioris, depressor anguli oris, and platysma on the body of the mandible. The masseter is attached to the greater part of the lateral surface of the ramus. The lateral pterygoid muscle is attached to the pterygoid fovea on the neck of the mandible. The coronoid process and upper part of the anterior margin of the ramus give attachment to the temporalis [Fig. 2.16A]. On the medial surface, the mylohyoid muscle is attached to the

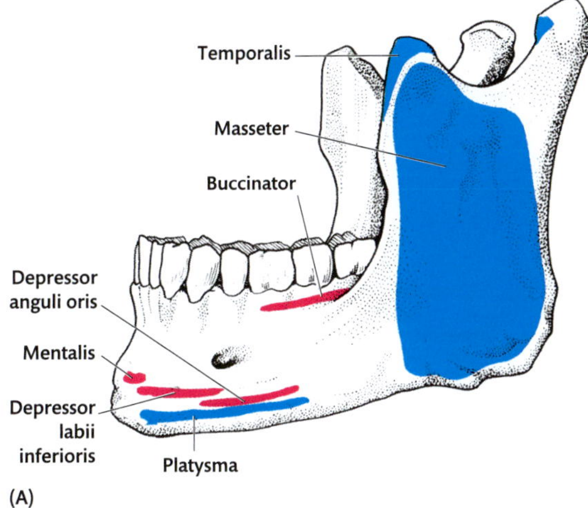


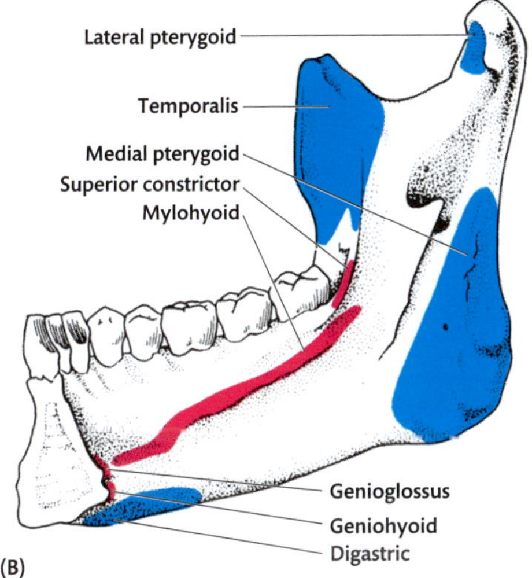


**Fig. 2.16** (A) Muscle attachments to the superficial surface of the mandible. Red = origins; blue = insertions. (B) Muscle attachments to the medial surface of the mandible. Red = origins; blue = insertions.

mylohyoid line. The genioglossus and geniohyoid are attached to the upper and lower mental spines, and the anterior belly of the digastric is attached on the inferior border of the body. The superior pharyngeal constrictor is attached on the internal surface of the ramus of the mandible immediately behind the third molar [Fig. 2.16B].

### Exercise 2.2: To hold the mandible in the anatomical position

Hold the mandible such that:

1. The alveolar margin is directed up
2. The ramus of the mandible is directed posteriorly.

## Hyoid

The hyoid bone is U-shaped and opens posteriorly. It has a body and paired lesser and greater horns [Fig. 2.17A]. It lies between the root of the tongue and the thyroid cartilage, and forms a movable base for the tongue. It does not articulate with any other bone in the body but is held in position by the muscles and ligaments attached to it.

The outer surface of the U-shaped hyoid gives attachment to a number of muscles [Fig. 2.17B]. The mylohyoid, geniohyoid, and anterior belly of the digastric attach the hyoid to the mandible. The stylohyoid muscle, stylohyoid ligament, and posterior belly of the digastric attach it to the skull. The thyrohyoid, sternohyoid, and omohyoid attach the hyoid to the thyroid cartilage, sternum, and scapula.

### Exercise 2.3: To hold the hyoid in the anatomical position

Hold the hyoid such that:

1. The body of the hyoid is directed anteriorly
2. The lesser horns are directed upwards.

## The cervical vertebrae

Review the features of a typical vertebra described in *Cunningham's Manual of Practical Anatomy*, Vol. 2, Chapter 1. The bodies of the cervical vertebrae are smaller and more delicate than those in the thoracic and lumbar regions, as they carry less weight. They have a larger vertebral foramen to accommodate the cervical swelling of the spinal cord [Fig. 2.18].

There are seven cervical vertebrae. The third to the sixth are typical cervical vertebrae. The first and second are modified to permit movements of the head on the neck. The seventh shows some features of a thoracic vertebra. All seven cervical vertebrae have a foramen—the **transverse foramen**—in the transverse process.

### General features of the typical cervical vertebrae

The **body** of the cervical vertebra is oval in shape, with a long transverse axis [Fig. 2.18]. The superior surface is concave from side to side, and the lateral

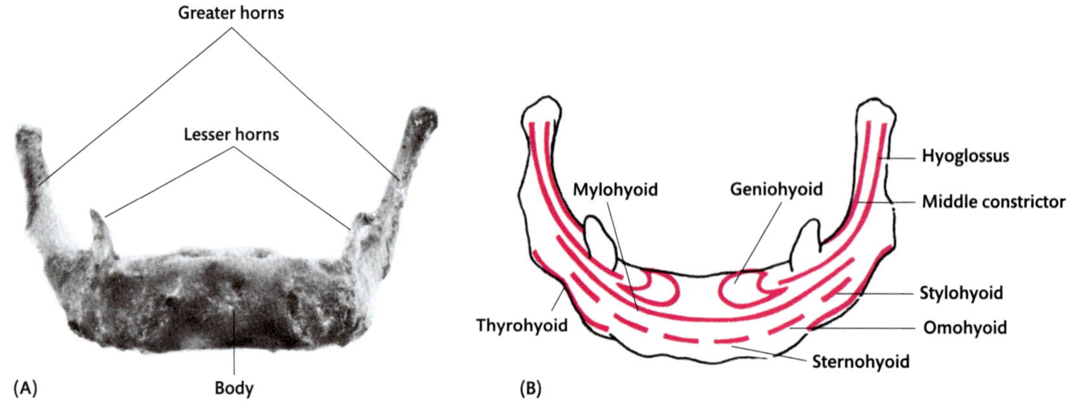


**Fig. 2.17** (A) Anterior view of the hyoid bone. (B) Anterior view of the hyoid bone to show muscle attachments.

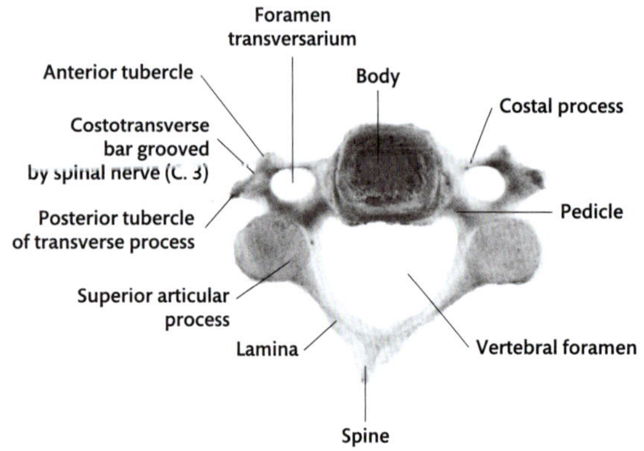


**Fig. 2.18** The third cervical vertebra, superior surface.

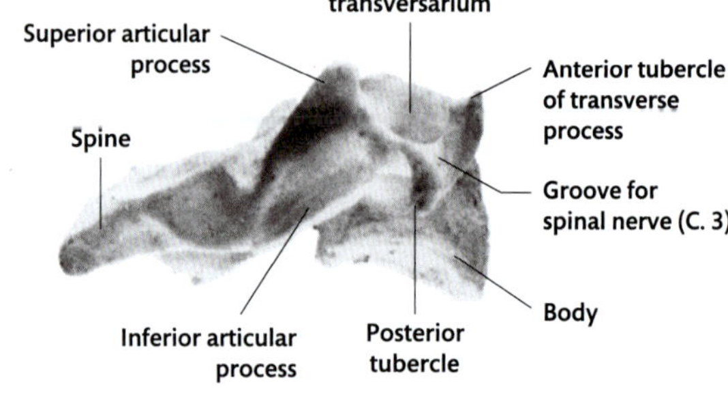


**Fig. 2.19** The third cervical vertebra, right surface.

margins project upwards to articulate with the cut-away inferolateral margins of the body above. The **pedicles** are short and directed laterally and backwards from the middle of the posterolateral part of the body. Each **transverse process** is short and perforated by the transverse foramen. The pedicles form the posteromedial wall of the transverse foramen. Anterior to the transverse foramen, a bar of bone—the **costal process**—projects laterally from the body and ends as the **anterior tubercle**. Behind the foramen, the true transverse process projects laterally from the junction of the pedicle and lamina and ends as the **posterior tubercle**. The anterior and posterior tubercles are united by the **costotransverse bar**.

The laminae are long and rectangular, and almost overlap the adjacent vertebrae in extension. The spines are short and bifid. The superior and inferior articular processes are short bars of bone at the junction of the pedicle and lamina on each side [Fig. 2.19]. The vertebral foramen is large and triangular in shape [Fig. 2.18].

## Bony landmarks and muscle attachments on the typical cervical vertebrae

The superior and inferior aspects of the two paired articular processes are cut obliquely to form the articular facets. The **superior articular facets** face upwards and backwards, and the **inferior articular facets** face downwards and forwards.

The costal process corresponds to the ribs in the thoracic region. They give origin to the anterior scalene and longus capitis. The posterior tubercle gives attachment to the middle and posterior scalene. The costotransverse bar is concave superiorly and has the ventral ramus of the corresponding spinal nerve lying on it. The transverse foramen transmits the vertebral artery (C. 1–C. 6 only), vertebral veins, and sympathetic plexus. The cervical spines give attachment to the ligamentum nuchae. The cervical spines, lamina, and transverse process give attachment to the cervical parts of the erector spinae muscles.

### Exercise 2.4: To hold a typical cervical vertebra in the anatomical position

Hold the typical cervical vertebra such that:

1. The body of the vertebra is directed anteriorly
2. The concave surface of the body is directed upwards.

## General features of the atlas (C. 1)

The first cervical vertebra has no body. It consists of two **lateral masses** united by the **anterior** and posterior **arches** [Fig. 2.20]. (The body of C. 1 is represented by a tooth-like projection—the **dens** from the superior surface of the body of C. 2.) Each lateral mass has **superior** and **inferior articular facets** on it. The **transverse process** of the atlas is long and thick, and lacks an anterior tubercle. Its **transverse foramen** is lateral to those of the vertebrae below. The **posterior tubercle** on the posterior arch represents the spine.

## Bony landmarks on the atlas

The posterior arch is grooved on its superior surface by the vertebral artery and the first cervical ventral ramus. The superior articular facet is concave and kidney-shaped for articulation with the occipital condyles. The inferior facet is almost circular and slightly concave, and faces downwards and medially to articulate with the axis. An inward projection from each lateral mass gives attachment to the **transverse ligament of the atlas**, which divides the vertebral foramen into a small anterior compartment for the dens, and a larger posterior compartment for the spinal cord and its coverings. The **transverse process of the atlas** is palpable through the anterior border of the sternocleidomastoid immediately below the tip of the mastoid process.

Fig. 2.20 The upper surface of the atlas. The course of the vertebral artery is indicated by a broken line.

## Second cervical vertebra or axis (C. 2)

The most prominent feature on the second cervical vertebra is the upward projection of the **dens** or the **odontoid process** from the body [Fig. 2.21].

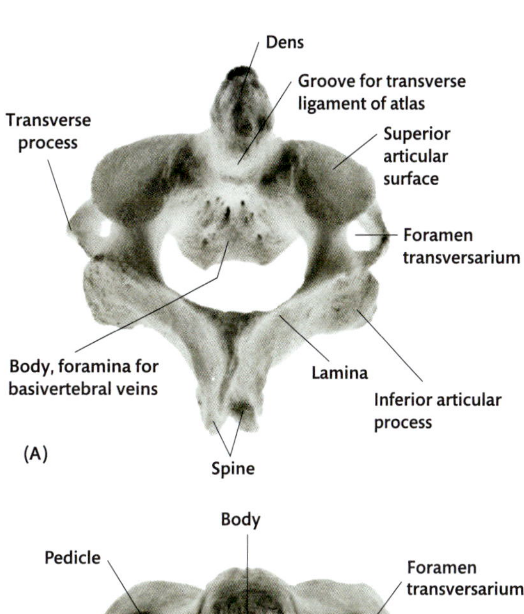


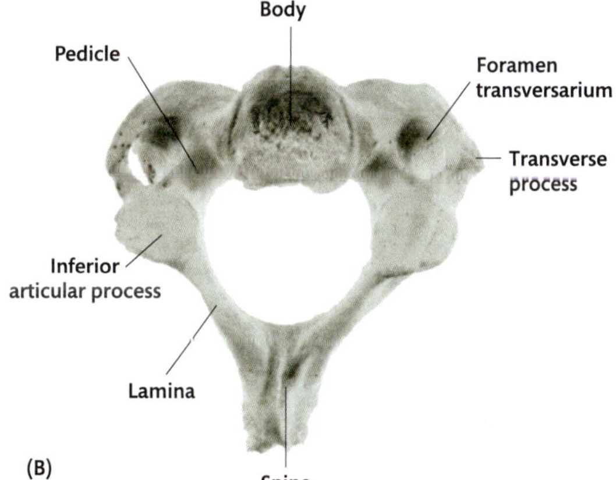


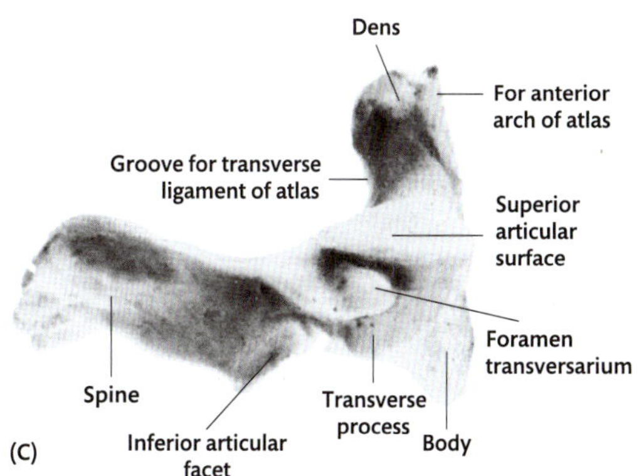


Fig. 2.21 The axis vertebra seen (A) from behind and above, (B) from below, and (C) from the right side.

The dens articulates with the anterior arch of the atlas and is held against it by the transverse ligament of the atlas, which grooves the posterior surface of the dens. The thick **pedicle** projects posterolaterally from the side of the body. The **superior articular facet** overhangs the pedicle, part of the body, and part of the transverse foramen. The **inferior articular facet** is typical and articulates with the third cervical vertebra. The **laminae** of the axis are thickened for muscle attachments and unite to form a massive **spine**. The **transverse foramen** turns laterally through 90 degrees under the superior articular facet and is better seen from the lateral aspect. The **spine of the axis** is palpable at the nape of the neck about 5 cm below the external occipital protuberance.

## Seventh cervical vertebra or axis (C. 2)

The **spine** of the seventh cervical vertebra is long and non-bifid, and is felt as a prominence at the root of the neck—the vertebra prominence. The **transverse process** does not have an anterior tubercle, and the **transverse foramen** transmits only veins (not the vertebral artery).

Fig. 2.22A and B are radiographs of the cervical vertebrae.

See Clinical Applications 2.1 and 2.2 for the practical implications of the anatomy discussed in this chapter.

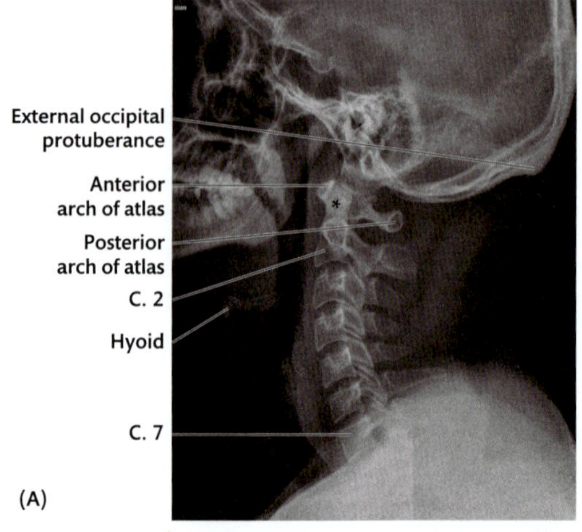


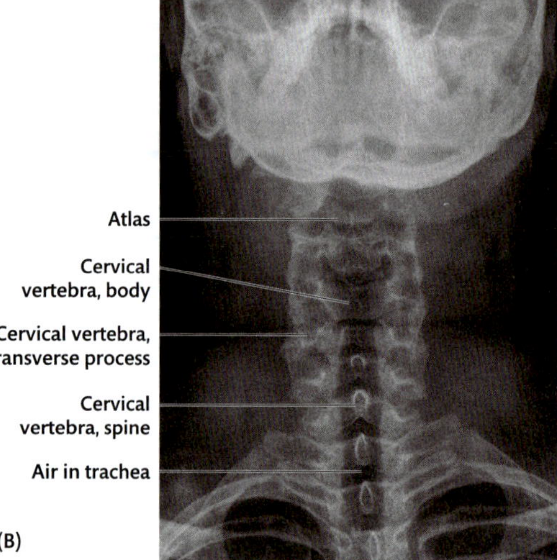


**Fig. 2.22** (A) Lateral radiograph and (B) anteroposterior (AP) view of the neck. C. 2, C. 7 = second and seventh cervical vertebrae, respectively. * = dens.

**CLINICAL APPLICATION 2.1 Fracture of mandible**

A 24-year-old male presented with multiple facial lacerations, following a road traffic accident. Examination revealed severe pain and swelling of the lower jaw, intra-oral bleeding, and an inability to open the mouth. Examination revealed a deformity of the lower jaw and loss of sensation over the lower lip.

Study question 1: what is the likely diagnosis? (Answer: fracture of the mandible.)

Study question 2: which are the common sites of fracture of the mandible? (Answer: the mandible is the most common facial bone to be fractured in facial trauma. The second is the maxilla. Common sites of fracture of the mandible include the coronoid process, and the body and angle of the mandible. Fractures involving the coronoid process cause swelling over the temporomandibular joint, severe limitation of mouth opening, and deviation of the jaw to the affected side on opening the mouth.)

Study question 3: why is there loss of sensation of the lower lip? (Answer: injury to the mental branch of the inferior alveolar nerve causes paraesthesiae or loss of sensation over the lower lip [Chapter 3].)

Study question 4: how are fractures of the mandible treated? (Answer: the aim of fracture reduction is functional alignment of bone fragments and restoration of normal occlusion. This can be achieved by reduction, followed by immobilization. Reduction and alignment of fractured segments can be done by using surgical incisions of the oral mucosa (open reduction) or by simple manipulation without any incision (closed reduction). Immobilization can be achieved with the help of plates and screws or wires.)

**CLINICAL APPLICATION 2.2 Fracture of cervical vertebrae**

A 23-year-old biker sustained severe injuries on the face and multiple injuries to the body in a road traffic accident. He was semi-conscious, but completely unable to move both upper and lower limbs. On examination, he had pain and tenderness of the neck, with radiation of pain from the neck to the shoulder. He was carefully moved from the accident site by trained paramedics.

Study question 1: what diagnosis should you consider? (Answer: fracture of the cervical vertebrae with compression of the spinal cord. Cervical vertebral injury usually occurs in high-velocity impact in road traffic accidents, sports, and bullet injury to the cervical vertebrae.)

Study question 2: what measures should be undertaken while shifting the patient from the accident site? (Answer: fracture of the cervical vertebrae can cause compression of the cervical spinal cord. Hence, the neck should be immobilized during transfer. X-rays or computerized tomography (CT) may need to be done to assess fracture of the cervical vertebrae.)

Study question 3: what are the complications of cervical fracture? (Answer: fracture of the cervical vertebrae can cause damage to the spinal cord, leading to spinal shock, quadriplegia, or even death.) Spinal shock is caused by a concussion injury to the spinal cord. It manifests as transient, flaccid quadriplegia, with complete loss of reflexes that slowly begin to recover after 24 hours. Recovery is usually complete in spinal shock. Quadriplegia is irreversible partial or complete loss of motor and sensory function involving all four limbs.

Study question 4: what is the cause for the radiating pain? (Answer: pain radiating from the neck to the shoulder indicates compression of nerve roots by fractured segments.)

Study question 5: how is cervical fracture treated? (Answer: mild compression fractures may be treated with just a cervical brace. More severe fractures may require surgery and traction.)

# CHAPTER 3
# The scalp and face

## Introduction

We begin the study of the head with dissection of the scalp, including the temple, and the face. The chapter also includes the study of the lacrimal apparatus.

## Surface anatomy

Begin by identifying the bony and soft tissue landmarks of the head in the living.

### Face

#### External nose

The term 'nose' includes the paired nasal cavities which extend posteriorly from the nostrils to the pharynx. The mobile anterior part of the external nose consists of skin and cartilage [Fig. 3.1]. The rigid upper part—the bridge of the nose—is formed by the two **nasal bones** and the two **frontal processes of the maxillae**. The skin is adherent to the cartilages but is mobile over the bones. The part of the nasal cavity immediately above each nostril is the **vestibule of the nose**. The vestibule is lined by hairy skin, and its lateral wall is expanded to form the **ala** of the nose.

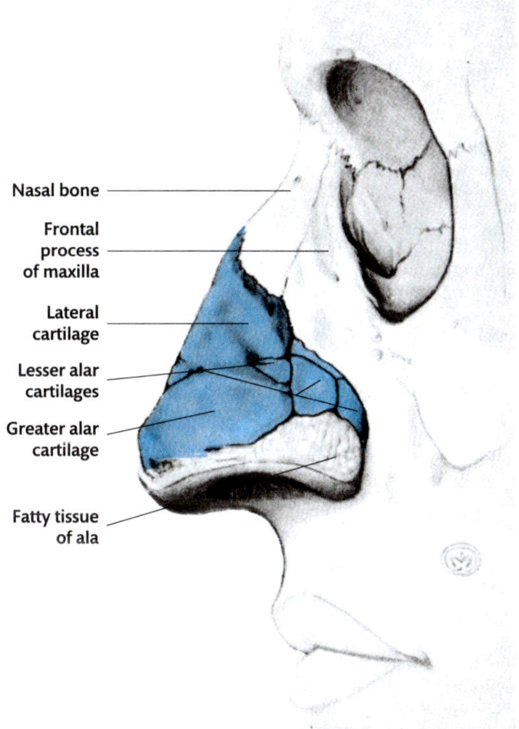


**Fig. 3.1** Cartilages of the external nose.

#### Lips, cheeks, and teeth

The lips and cheeks are composed primarily of muscle and fat. They are covered on the external surface with skin and are lined on the internal surface with mucous membrane. The space that separates the lips and cheeks from the teeth and gums is the **vestibule of the mouth**. A full set of adult **teeth** consists of 32 teeth, 8 in each half of the jaw. From before backwards, these are: two incisors, one canine, two premolars, and three molars. There are 20 teeth in the primary dentition—that is, five in each half of the jaw: two incisors, one canine, and two molars, also called 'milk' molars. The **oral fissure**, the gap or space between the lips, is opposite the biting edge of the upper teeth. The corner, or angle, of the mouth is opposite the first premolar tooth. The median groove on the external surface of the upper lip is the **philtrum**. In the midline, the internal surface of each lip is attached to the gum by a fold of mucous membrane—the **frenulum of the lip**.

## Mandible

Palpate the horizontal **body** of the mandible below the lower lip and cheeks, the **angle** of the mandible, and the **ramus** of the mandible. The ramus of the mandible is covered laterally by the masseter muscle. The condylar process projects upwards from the posterior margin of the ramus and forms the **neck** and **head** of the mandible. The neck lies immediately anterior to the lobule of the auricle; the head lies anterior to the tragus.

## Zygomatic arch

Palpate the zygomatic arch which extends over the interval between the ear and the eye. The narrow posterior part is formed by the zygomatic process of the temporal bone, and the anterior part by the zygomatic bone.

## Orbit

The bony structure of the orbit has been described in part in Chapter 2. Palpate the orbital margins on yourself, and find: (1) the **supraorbital notch** on the highest point of the superior margin, about 2.5 cm from the midline; and (2) the **frontozygomatic suture** at the superolateral angle.

## Eyebrow

The hairy skin above the supraorbital margin is the eyebrow. Over its medial end is a curved ridge of bone—the superciliary arch. This is well formed only in males and is separated from its fellow on the other side by a smooth median area—the **glabella**.

## Eye

The white of the eye is the **sclera**. The transparent part of the front of the eye is the **cornea**. The coloured **iris** (usually black or dark brown) is seen through the cornea and has a dark, circular central aperture—the **pupil**. The visible part of the sclera is covered with a moist, transparent membrane—the **conjunctiva**. The conjunctiva passes from the sclera on to the deep surface of the eyelids. The reflection of the conjunctiva onto the eyelids is the **fornix of the conjunctiva**, and the entire conjunctiva encloses the **conjunctival sac**. The sac opens anteriorly between the eyelids through the palpebral fissure [Fig. 3.2].

## Eyelids

The eyelids, or palpebrae, are folds which protect the front of the eye. Each time we blink, the eyelids moisten the exposed surface of the eyeball by spreading lacrimal fluid over it. The upper lid is larger and more mobile than the lower one, and the upper conjunctival fornix is much deeper. When the eyes are closed, the **palpebral fissure** is nearly horizontal and lies opposite the lower margin of the cornea. When the eyes are open, the margins of the eyelids overlap the cornea slightly, with the upper eyelid more than the lower.

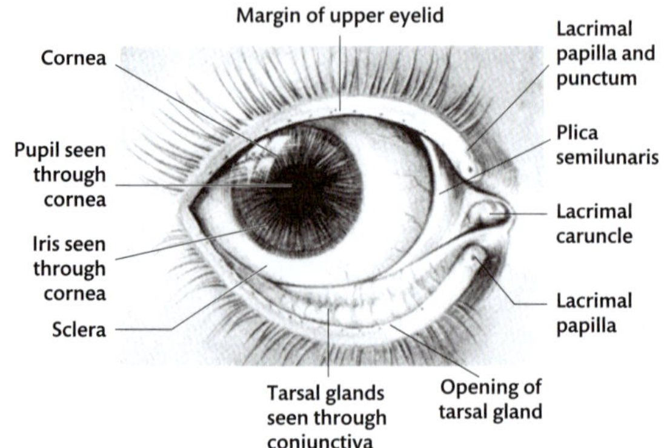


**Fig. 3.2** Eyeball and eyelids. The eyelids are slightly everted to show part of the conjunctival sac.

At the medial angle of the eye is a small, triangular area known as the **lacus lacrimalis**, with a reddish elevation—the **lacrimal caruncle**—near its centre. The lacus carries a few fine hairs which filter the lacrimal fluid passing to the lacrimal canaliculi. Just lateral to the lacus is a small, vertical fold of conjunctiva—the **plica semilunaris** [Fig. 3.2].

The lower eyelid is easily everted by pulling down the skin below it, and the lower fornix is exposed by turning the eyeball upwards. The upper lid is difficult to evert because of the rigid **tarsal plate** buried in it. Once everted, the upper eyelid tends to remain so. Even with the upper eyelid everted, the deep superior fornix is not exposed.

Eyelashes (**cilia**) project from the anterior edge of the free margin of the eyelid. On the deep surface of the eyelids are a number of yellowish, parallel streaks produced by the tarsal glands [Fig. 3.2]. The ducts of these glands open near the posterior edge of the free margin of the eyelids. The free margin of the lids is rounded medially and has a small elevation—the **lacrimal papilla**. Each papilla is surmounted by a tiny aperture—the **lacrimal punctum**. The puncta lead into the lacrimal canaliculus, which drains the lacrimal fluid from the conjunctival sac. Note that the puncta face posteriorly into the conjunctival sac, and that the eyelids move medially when the eye is forcibly closed. This action moves the lacrimal fluid towards the puncta at the medial angle of the eye.

Press a fingertip on the skin between the nose and the medial angle of the eye and feel the rounded, horizontal cord—the **medial palpebral ligament**. This ligament connects the upper and lower eyelids (and their muscle—the orbicularis oculi) to the medial margin of the orbit. If the eyelids are gently pulled laterally, the medial palpebral ligament is more easily felt and may be seen as a small skin ridge.

## Side of the head

At the lateral end of the eyebrow, feel for the anterior end of the **temporal line**. The **parietal** and **frontal eminences** are the most convex parts of the parietal and frontal bones. The **vertex** is the topmost part of the head.

### Auricle

The auricle is that part of the ear which is seen on either side of the head [Fig. 3.3]. It consists of a thin plate of elastic cartilage covered with skin. (The lobule is devoid of cartilage.) The external ear lies nearer the back of the head than the front and is at the level of the eye and nose. The main parts of the auricle, or external ear—the **lobule**, **helix**, **antihelix**, **tragus**, **antitragus**, and **intertragic notch**—are shown in Fig. 3.3. The cartilage of the auricle is continuous with the cartilage of the external acoustic meatus.

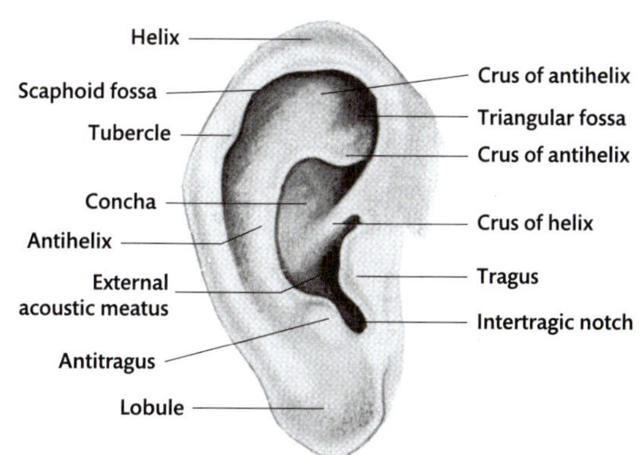


**Fig. 3.3** The auricle.

## Back of the head

The **external occipital** protuberance is the midline bony elevation felt where the back of the head joins the neck. From this protuberance, an indistinct, curved ridge—the **superior nuchal line**—extends laterally on each side between the scalp and the neck. The superior nuchal line passes towards the corresponding **mastoid process**—a rounded bony elevation behind the lower part of the auricle. Press your finger into the surface depression below and in front of the mastoid process. The resistance felt is the transverse process of the atlas. It is covered by the lower part of the parotid salivary gland, the anterior border of the sternocleidomastoid muscle, and the accessory nerve.

# The scalp

The scalp extends from the eyebrows in front to the superior nuchal lines behind. Side to side, it extends between the right and left superior temporal lines. The scalp covers the vault of the skull.

## Layers of the scalp

The scalp consists of five layers: (1) skin; (2) superficial fascia; (3) epicranial aponeurosis; (4) loose connective tissue; and (5) the pericranium [Fig. 3.4]. The **epicranial aponeurosis** is a flat aponeurotic sheet uniting the frontal and occipital bellies of the occipitofrontalis muscle. The superficial fascia is adherent to the epicranial aponeurosis. The skin is also adherent to the epicranial aponeurosis by dense strands of fibrous tissue which run through the superficial fascia and divide it into a number of separate pockets filled with fat. The blood vessels and nerves of the scalp lie in this superficial layer. Deep to the aponeurosis is a relatively avascular layer of **loose areolar tissue** which allows the scalp to slide freely on the **pericranium**. The pericranium is the periosteum on the external surface of the skull [Fig. 3.4].

The **temple** is the area bounded by the superior temporal line above and the zygomatic arch below. The skull is thin in this region and covered by the temporalis muscle, the temporal fascia, and a thin extension of the epicranial aponeurosis.

Using the instructions given in Dissection 3.1 (and Figs. 3.5, 3.6, 3.7, 3.8), dissect the scalp.

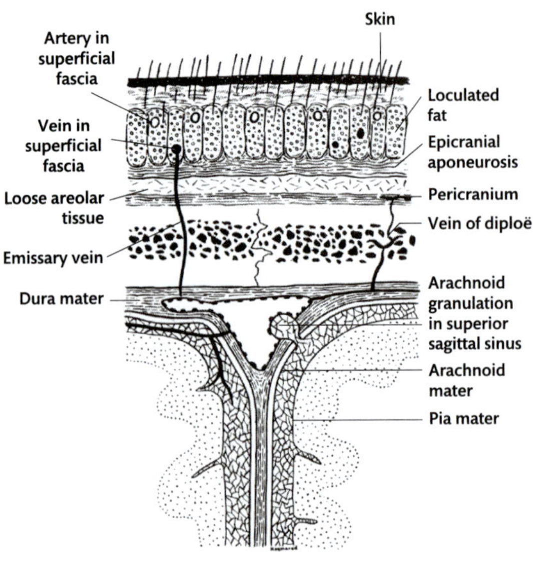


**Fig. 3.4** Schematic section through the scalp, skull, meninges, and brain. Note the venous connections through the skull.

## Occipitofrontalis muscle

The occipitofrontalis has the occipital belly on the back of the skull, and the frontal belly anteriorly [Figs. 3.5, 3.8]. **Origin of occipital belly**: the occipital belly arises from the lateral part of the superior nuchal line [see Fig. 2.9]. The occipital bellies are shorter and narrower than the frontal bellies, and are widely separated by the aponeurosis.

Each frontal belly lies in the forehead and adjoining part of the scalp. **Origin of frontal belly**: the frontal belly has no attachment to bone but runs between the skin of the forehead and the epicranial aponeurosis. The medial parts of the frontal bellies lie close together and are attached to the skin of the nose. **Action**: when the frontal belly contracts, it raises the eyebrows and wrinkles the forehead and the skin of the nose. **Nerve supply**: the facial nerve.





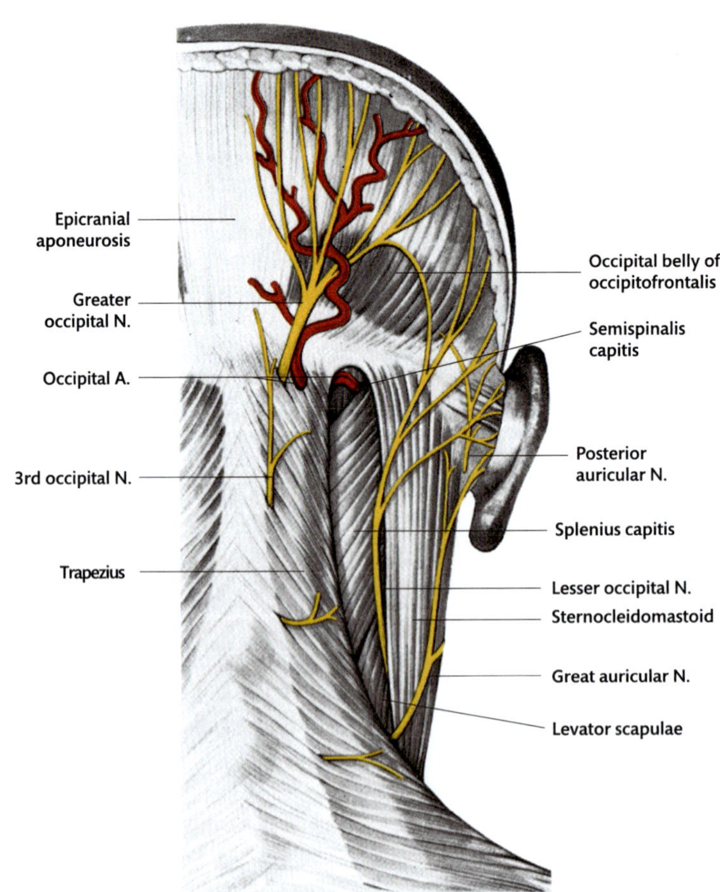


**Fig. 3.5** Cutaneous nerves and vessels of the posterior part of the scalp.

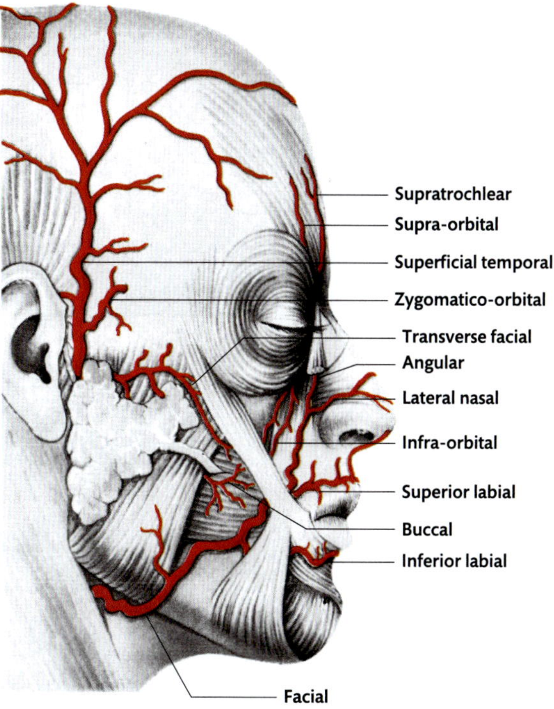


**Fig. 3.6** The arteries of the face.





## Epicranial aponeurosis

The **epicranial aponeurosis** is the aponeurosis of the occipitofrontalis. It is attached loosely to the superior temporal lines and firmly to the superior nuchal lines. Between these attachments, it slides freely on the pericranium because of the loose connective tissue deep to it.

## Nerves of the scalp and temple

The muscles of the scalp receive motor innervation from the **facial nerve** [Fig. 3.7]. Sensory innervation to the scalp comes from the **trigeminal nerve** and the **second** and **third cervical spinal nerves** [Figs. 3.7, 3.9]. Sympathetic innervation to

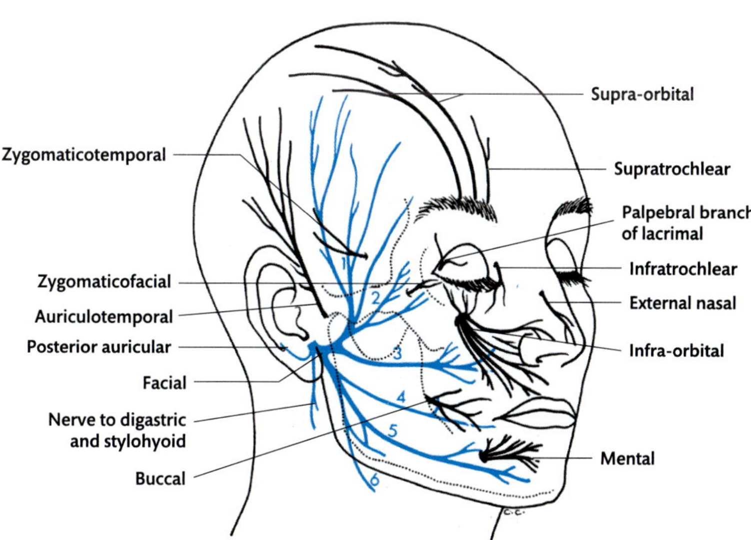


**Fig. 3.7** The nerves of the face. The facial nerve (motor) is shown in blue, and the branches of the trigeminal nerve (sensory) in black.
1 = temporal branches of facial nerve. 2 and 3 = zygomatic branches. 4 = buccal branch. 5 = marginal mandibular branch. 6 = cervical branch.

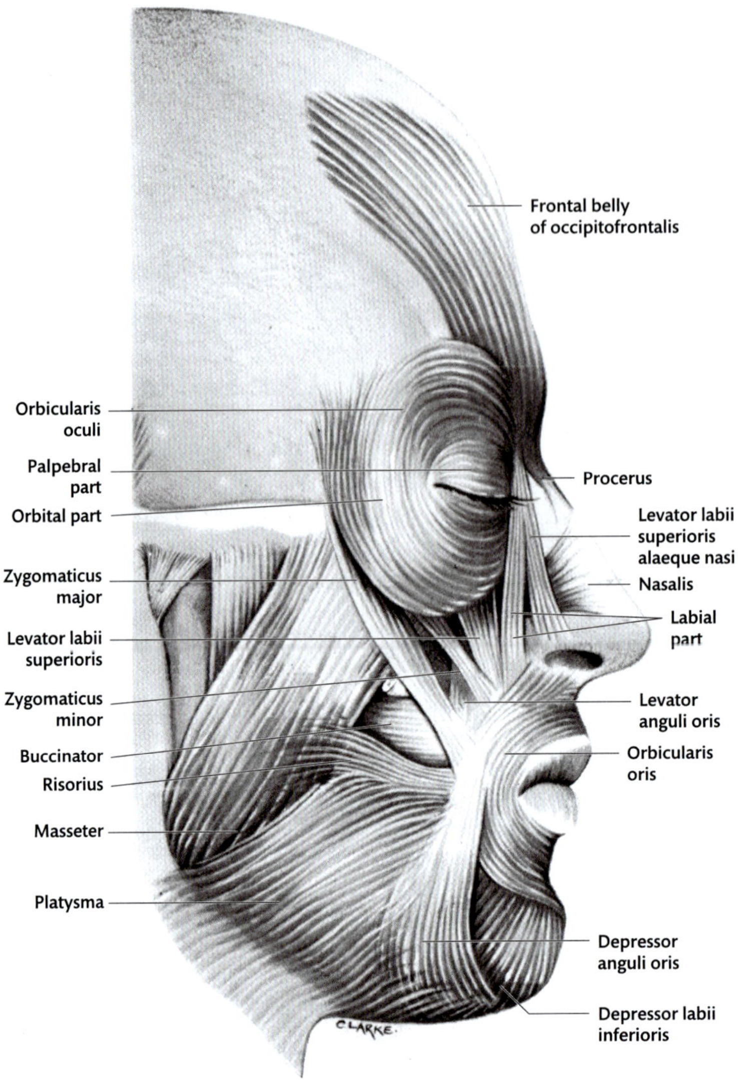


**Fig. 3.8** The facial muscles and masseter.

## DISSECTION 3.1 The scalp

### Objectives

**I.** To reflect the skin of the scalp and trace the vessels and nerves supplying it. **II.** To expose the upper part of the orbicularis oculi and the frontal and occipital bellies of the occipitofrontalis.

### Instructions

1. Place a block under the back of the head to raise it to a convenient angle. Make a median incision in the skin of the scalp, from the root of the nose to the external occipital protuberance. Make a coronal incision from the middle of the first incision to the root of each auricle.
2. Continue the coronal incision behind the auricle to the mastoid process, and in front of the auricle to the root of the zygomatic arch. Avoid cutting deeper than the skin to preserve the vessels, nerves, and muscles in the subcutaneous tissue. Reflect the skin flaps superficial to these structures.
3. Make use of Figs. 3.5, 3.6, and 3.7 to identify the positions of the main structures in the scalp—the greater occipital nerve, lesser occipital nerve, third occipital nerve, great auricular nerve, superficial temporal artery, supraorbital and supratrochlear arteries and nerves, and temporal branches of the facial nerve—so that they are not damaged.
4. Expose the upper part of the orbicularis oculi [Fig. 3.8].

5. Follow the frontal belly of the occipitofrontalis from below upwards [Fig. 3.8].
6. Find the branches of the supratrochlear and supraorbital vessels and nerves. The supratrochlear vessels and nerve lie about a finger-breadth from the midline, and the supraorbital vessels and nerve another finger-breadth further laterally. The supraorbital vessels and nerve ascend from the supraorbital notch.
7. Expose the anterior part of the epicranial aponeurosis, and note its extension downwards into the temple.
8. Find two or more **temporal branches of the facial nerve** which cross the zygomatic arch 2 cm or more in front of the auricle [Fig. 3.7]. Trace them upwards to the deep surface of the orbicularis oculi.
9. Find the **superficial temporal artery** [Fig. 3.6] and **veins** and the **auriculotemporal nerve**. These structures cross the root of the zygomatic arch, immediately anterior to the auricle, along with the small branch of the facial nerve to the superior auricular muscles. Trace these structures into the scalp, uncovering this part of the temporal fascia. (The auriculotemporal nerve may be very slender and difficult to find.)
10. Inferior and posterior to the auricle, find the great auricular and lesser occipital nerves [Fig. 3.5], and the posterior auricular vessels and nerve which lie immediately behind the root of the auricle. Trace the branches of these nerves.
11. Look for small terminal branches of the **third occipital nerve** in the fascia over the external occipital protuberance [Fig. 3.5].
12. Cut through the dense superficial fascia over the superior nuchal line, 2.5 cm lateral to the external occipital protuberance, and find the occipital vessels and greater occipital nerve which pierce the deep fascia here. Trace them superiorly towards the vertex [Fig. 3.5].
13. Lateral to the greater occipital nerve, find the occipital belly of the occipitofrontalis, and expose the posterior part of the epicranial aponeurosis.
14. Make a small incision through the aponeurosis near the vertex. Introduce a blunt probe through it into the loose areolar tissue beneath the aponeurosis, and expose the extent of this tissue by moving the probe in all directions. Note that the aponeurosis is adherent to the periosteum near the temporal and nuchal lines.





blood vessels and the skin run in the plexuses on the arteries.

## Sensory nerves of the scalp

The area behind the imaginary line from the auricle to the vertex is supplied by C. 2 and C. 3, through the large **greater occipital nerve** (C. 2), the **third occipital nerve** (C. 3), and branches of the **great auricular** and **lesser occipital nerves** (C. 2, C. 3) [Fig. 3.9]. The greater occipital nerve enters the scalp with the occipital artery by piercing the trapezius and deep fascia, 2.5 cm lateral to the external occipital protuberance. The third occipital nerve pierces the trapezius, 2–3 cm inferior to this [Fig. 3.5].

Anterior to an imaginary line from the ear to the vertex, the sensory supply is mainly from the trigeminal nerve. The trigeminal nerve is the fifth cranial nerve, named so because it divides into three large nerves—ophthalmic, maxillary, and mandibular. Each of the three divisions supplies sensory branches to the skin of the anterior half of the scalp [Fig. 3.9].

The **ophthalmic nerve** gives two cutaneous branches—the supratrochlear and supraorbital nerves. The **supratrochlear nerve** emerges at the supraorbital margin, a finger-breadth from the midline. It supplies the paramedian part of the forehead and the medial part of the upper eyelid. The **supraorbital nerve** emerges more laterally through the supraorbital notch, supplies the upper eyelid, and then divides into lateral and medial branches. Each branch sends a twig through the bone to the mucous lining of the **frontal sinus** (the cavity in the frontal bone above the nose and orbit). The supratrochlear and supraorbital nerves together supply the skin of the forehead of the anterior part of the scalp as far as the vertex [Fig. 3.7].

The **maxillary nerve** gives rise to the slender **zygomaticotemporal nerve**, which arises from the zygomatic branch of the maxillary nerve in the orbit. It pierces the zygomatic bone and temporal fascia to supply the skin of the anterior part of the temple [Fig. 3.7].

The **auriculotemporal** branch of the **mandibular nerve** emerges from the upper end of the parotid gland, close to the auricle, at the root at the zygomatic arch. It supplies the upper part of the auricle, the external acoustic meatus, and the skin of the side of the head [Fig. 3.7].

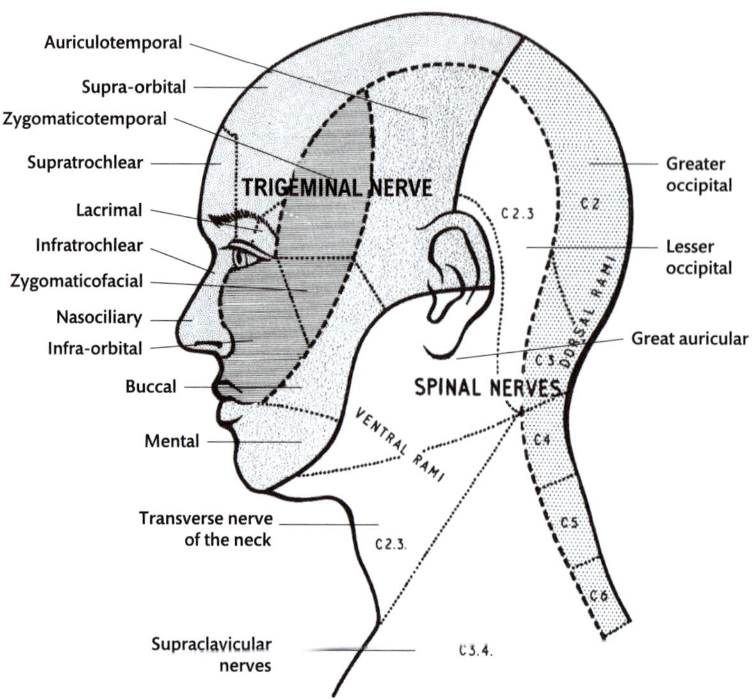


**Fig. 3.9** Distribution of cutaneous nerves to the head and neck. The ophthalmic, maxillary, and mandibular divisions of the trigeminal nerve here are indicated by different shading.





### Motor nerves of the scalp

The **facial nerve** is the seventh cranial nerve. It supplies the muscles of the scalp and auricle.

The **temporal branches** of the facial nerve emerge from the upper part of the parotid gland, cross the zygomatic arch obliquely, and supply the frontal belly of the occipitofrontalis, the upper part of the orbicularis oculi, and the anterior and superior auricular muscles [Fig. 3.7].

The **posterior auricular nerve** arises from the facial nerve, as it emerges from the stylomastoid foramen. It curves posterosuperiorly below the root of the auricle and runs above the superior nuchal line to supply the occipital belly of the occipitofrontalis and the posterior and superior auricular muscles [Figs. 3.5, 3.7].

## Arteries of the scalp and temple

The scalp and temple are mostly supplied by branches of the **external carotid artery**, except for the forehead which is supplied by the supraorbital and supratrochlear branches of the internal carotid artery. These arteries run with the supraorbital and supratrochlear nerves.

### Branches from the external carotid artery

The **superficial temporal artery** is a large terminal branch of the external carotid artery. It begins behind the neck of the mandible in, or deep to, the parotid gland. It runs upwards with the auriculotemporal nerve and divides into anterior and posterior branches which run towards the frontal and parietal eminences. The anterior branch is frequently seen through the skin in elderly individuals and is often very tortuous.

➲ The pulse of the superficial temporal artery can be felt above the zygomatic arch, above and in front of the tragus of the ear. It is often assessed during a full physical examination.

Small branches of the superficial temporal artery supply the temple and anterior part of the scalp. The **transverse facial branch** [Fig. 3.6] runs forwards on the masseter muscle, below the zygomatic arch. The **middle temporal branch** crosses the root of the zygomatic arch, pierces the temporal fascia, and runs vertically upwards. The **zygomatico-orbital branch** runs anteriorly above the zygomatic arch between the two layers of the temporal fascia. It anastomoses with branches of the ophthalmic artery.

The small **posterior auricular branch** of the external carotid artery curves posterosuperiorly below and behind the root of the auricle, with the posterior auricular nerve.

The **occipital artery** is a large branch of the external carotid artery. It arises deep to the angle of the mandible and runs posterosuperiorly. It pierces the trapezius with the greater occipital nerve [Fig. 3.5] and supplies the muscles of the neck and the back of the head.

The arteries of the scalp anastomose freely with each other and with those of the opposite side.

## Veins of the scalp and temple

Like the arteries, the veins of the scalp anastomose freely. The main tributaries accompany the arteries of the scalp, but their proximal parts drain by different routes.

The **supratrochlear** and **supraorbital veins** unite at the medial angle of the eye to form the **facial vein**. They communicate with veins within the orbit. The **superficial temporal vein** joins the **maxillary vein** at the root of the zygomatic arch to form the **retromandibular vein**. The **occipital veins** join the suboccipital plexus, deep to the semispinalis capitis muscle at the back of the neck.

**Emissary veins** pierce the skull and connect the extracranial veins with the venous sinuses within the cranium. Usually, one emissary vein passes through each parietal foramen to the superior sagittal sinus, and another through each mastoid foramen to the corresponding sigmoid sinus [see Fig. 2.10].

## Lymph vessels of the scalp and temple

Lymph vessels cannot be demonstrated by dissection. Lymph from the area in front of the ear drains into small **parotid lymph nodes** buried in the surface of the parotid gland. Those from the region behind the ear drain into lymph nodes on the upper end of the trapezius **(occipital nodes)** and the sternocleidomastoid (**retroauricular nodes**).

## Applied anatomy of the scalp

➲ Common skin conditions like dandruff, dermatitis, and psoriasis involve the skin of the scalp. The abundant hair follicles make this a common site for sebaceous cysts and also for infestations like pediculosis (lice).

➲ The dense connective tissue in the superficial fascia (second layer) of the scalp contains numerous blood vessels and nerves. The dense fibres in this layer attach to the walls of the blood vessels and prevent vasoconstriction following lacerations of the scalp. As a result, wounds of the scalp bleed profusely but heal rapidly. Also, if a large piece of scalp is torn downwards from the skull, it will survive and heal satisfactorily, provided the peripheral attachment containing an artery is intact.

➲ Traction injuries of the scalp separate the epicranial aponeurosis from the pericranium. This leads to bleeding from the emissary veins, which pass through the loose areolar tissue, and collection of blood in this tissue.

➲ The loose connective tissue of the scalp is continuous with the space between the skeletal muscle and the tarsal plate of the eyelid, and bleeding into the loose connective tissue tracks into the eyelid and presents as a **black eye**.

➲ Infections from the loose areolar tissue can potentially spread into the cranial cavity through the numerous valveless emissary veins that connect the veins of the scalp to intracranial venous sinuses. The spread of infection into the cranial cavity may lead to meningitis or dural venous thrombosis.

➲ **Cephalhaematoma** is a subperiosteal bleed beneath the periosteum of the parietal (rarely occipital) bone during childbirth. This is the result of rupture of minute periosteal arteries, leading to a localized swelling over the parietal bone which does not extend beyond its bony margins.

➲ **Caput succedaneum**, on the other hand, is more diffuse oedema of the subcutaneous tissue of the entire scalp, due to prolonged compression of the fetal head against the bony pelvis of the mother during labour.

# Superficial dissection of the face

The face extends from the hairline on the scalp to the chin, and from one auricle to the other. (The forehead is common to the face and the scalp.)

Anterior to an imaginary line from the ear to the vertex, the sensory supply to the face is from the trigeminal nerve, except for the skin over the posteroinferior part of the jaw and the lower part of the auricle. The area over the posteroinferior part of the jaw and the lower part of the auricle is supplied by the **great auricular** and **lesser occipital nerves** (ventral rami of C. 2 and C. 3 [Fig. 3.9]).

Dissection 3.2 provides instructions on dissection of the face.

**DISSECTION 3.2 Face**

**Objectives**

**I.** To identify the muscles of facial expression. **II.** To identify and trace the vessels and nerves of the face.

**Instructions**

Before you begin, stretch the skin of the eyelids and cheeks by packing the conjunctival sacs and the vestibule of the mouth with cloth or cotton wool soaked in preservative. When the skin of the face is reflected, the attachments of the facial muscles to it are inevitably damaged. This can be minimized by keeping the knife as close to the skin as possible.

1. Make a median incision from the root of the nose to the point of the chin. Make a horizontal incision from the angle of the mouth to the posterior border of the mandible. Reflect the lower flap downwards to the lower border of the mandible, and the upper flap backwards to the auricle.
2. Expose the major facial muscles [Fig. 3.8], taking care not to cut through them and damage major branches of the nerves and vessels. Refer to Fig. 2.9 to see the bony attachments of the muscles.
3. Pull the eyelids laterally and identify the medial palpebral ligament; then expose the orbital part of the orbicularis oculi, subsequently following the palpebral part to the margins of the eyelids.
4. Attempt to find the small palpebral branch of the lacrimal nerve entering the lateral part of the upper eyelid through the orbicularis oculi.
5. The orbicularis oris is more difficult to expose because of the large number of facial muscles which fuse with, and help to form, it [Fig. 3.8]. At the side of the nose, find the **levator labii superioris alaeque nasi**, with the facial vein lying on its surface.
6. Trace the facial vein downwards till it passes deep to the zygomaticus major. Expose that muscle, and then the levator labii superioris, following it upwards to its origin deep to the orbicularis oculi [Fig. 3.8].
7. At the lower border of the mandible, expose the broad, thin sheet of muscle—the **platysma**—which ascends over the mandible from the neck. Note that its posterior fibres curve forwards towards the angle of the mouth to form part of the **risorius muscle** [Fig. 3.8].
8. Find the depressor anguli oris and the depressor labii inferioris [Fig. 3.8].

(The buccinator muscle lies in a deeper plane, immediately external to the mucous membrane of the cheek. It is continuous with the lateral part of the orbicularis oris and will be dissected later.)

## Facial muscles

The facial muscles are known collectively as the '**muscles of facial expression**'. They are the orbicularis oculi, corrugator supercilii, frontal belly of the occipitofrontalis, procerus, levator labii superioris, levator labii superioris alaeque nasi, zygomaticus major, zygomaticus minor, nasalis, levator anguli oris, orbicularis oris, buccinator, depressor anguli oris, depressor labii inferioris, mentalis, platysma, and risorius. Many of the muscles are named according to their actions, and the actions of others may be inferred from their positions. The muscles of facial expression take origin from the underlying bones [see Figs. 2.4, 2.9] and are inserted into the skin of the face. These muscles are supplied by the facial nerve [Fig. 3.7].

The larger muscles—the orbicularis oculi, buccinator, and orbicularis oris—are described in detail. The attachments and action of the smaller muscles are tabulated in Table 3.1.

### Orbicularis oculi

The **orbicularis oculi** has three parts: the orbital part, palpebral part, and lacrimal part.

#### Orbital part

**Origin** and **insertion**: the fibres of the orbital part arise from the medial palpebral ligament and the adjacent part of the orbital margin [see Figs. 2.4, 2.9]. They form complete loops on and around the orbital margin. Muscle fibres sweep superiorly into the forehead (mingling with fibres of the frontalis), laterally into the temple, and inferiorly into the cheek, before returning to their point of origin. A few fibres which arise from the bone superior to the medial palpebral ligament end in the skin of the eyebrow, but the remainder are only loosely attached to the skin [Fig. 3.8].

#### Palpebral part

**Origin** and **insertion**: the palpebral part of the orbicularis oculi consists of thin fibres which arise from the medial palpebral ligament and form similar

**Table 3.1** The attachments and actions of the smaller muscles of facial expression [the origin of these muscles is shown in Fig. 2.4]

| Name | Attachments | | Action/actions |
|---|---|---|---|
| | Origin | Insertion | |
| Corrugator supercilii | Frontal bone | Skin on supraorbital margin | Draws eyebrows medially |
| Procerus | Nasal bone | Skin between eyebrows | Draws medial angle of eyebrows down |
| Levator labii superioris | Maxilla and zygomatic bone | Skin of upper lip | Elevate and/or evert upper lip |
| Levator labii superioris alaeque nasi | Maxilla, frontal process | Skin over alar of nose and upper lip | Elevate and/or evert upper lip |
| Zygomaticus major | Zygomatic bone | Skin of angle of mouth | Elevate angle of lip |
| Zygomaticus minor | Zygomatic bone | Skin of upper lip | Elevate and/or evert upper lip |
| Nasalis | Maxilla, below the nasal aperture | Skin on bridge of nose and of nasolabial folds | - Upper fibres compress nasal aperture<br>- Lower fibres dilate nasal aperture |
| Levator anguli oris | Maxilla, body | Skin at and below angle of mouth | Elevate angle of lip |
| Depressor anguli oris | Mandible, body | Skin of angle of mouth | Depress angle of lip |
| Depressor labii inferioris | Mandible, body | Skin of lower lip | Depress and/or evert lower lip |
| Mentalis | Mandible, body | Skin of chin | Tense skin of chin |
| Platysma | Skin of neck | Lateral half of lower lip | Depress and/or evert lower lip |
| Risorius | Zygomatic arch, parotidomasseteric fascia | Skin of angle of mouth | Pulls angle of mouth laterally |





loops within the eyelids. They form a continuous layer with the orbital part. A small, partially isolated bundle of muscle fibres—the ciliary bundle—lies in the margin of the eyelid and runs posterior to the roots of the eyelashes.

### Lacrimal part

**Origin** and **insertion**: the lacrimal part of the orbicularis oculi is a small sheet of muscle fibres which arises from the posterior margin of the fossa for the lacrimal sac and from the sac itself. It forms slips which pass laterally into the eyelids.

**Actions**: a number of different actions are attributed to the orbicularis oculi. (1) The palpebral part, acting alone, closes the eye lightly, as in sleep or blinking. (2) The orbital part screws up the eye to give partial protection from bright light, sun, or wind. (3) The fibres passing to the eyebrows draw them together, as in frowning. (4) The orbital and palpebral parts contract together to close the eye forcibly, protecting it from a blow, and in strong expiratory efforts such as coughing, sneezing, or crying in a child. Tight closure of the eyes during strong expiratory movements prevents overdistension of the orbital veins by compressing the orbital contents. (5) The muscle draws the skin and eyelids medially towards the bony attachments and promotes the flow of lacrimal fluid towards the lacrimal canaliculi. (6) The lacrimal part probably also dilates the lacrimal sac and promotes the flow of fluid through it. **Nerve supply**: facial nerve—temporal and zygomatic branches.

➲ Paralysis of the orbicularis oculi prevents the eye from being closed. This results in a number of clinical conditions: (1) the exposed cornea becomes dry, sore, and opaque; (2) the lower eyelid falls away from the eyeball, creating a space where tears collect and spill over onto the face; and (3) dirt entering the conjunctival sac is not moved to the caruncular filter and the sac rapidly becomes infected.

## Buccinator

The **buccinator** will be dissected later, but it is described here as it contributes significantly to the orbicularis oris. **Origin**: the buccinator muscle is made up of horizontal fibres which take origin from the outer surfaces of the maxilla and mandible,

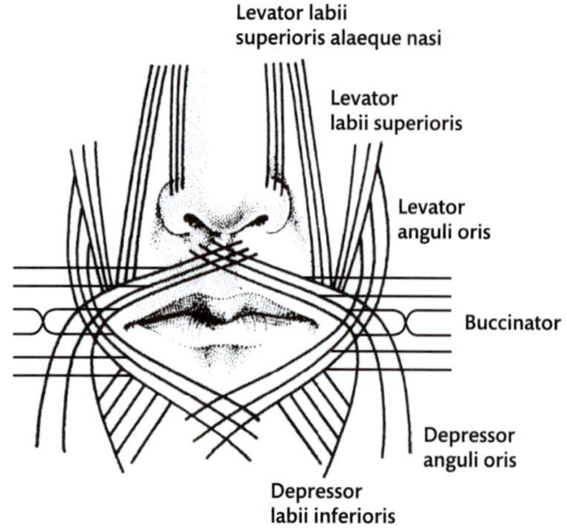


Fig. 3.10 Schematic diagram of the orbicularis oris muscle.

opposite the sockets of the molar teeth, and the **pterygomandibular raphe** [see Fig. 2.9]. The pterygomandibular raphe is formed by the interlacing tendinous fibres of the buccinator and the superior constrictor muscle of the pharynx where these muscles meet edge to edge [Fig. 3.8; see also Fig. 5.6]. (The superior constrictor will be seen later when the pharynx is dissected.)

**Insertion**: anteriorly, fibres of the buccinator converge on the corner of the mouth and blend with the orbicularis oris to form a large part of it [Fig. 3.10]. Its middle fibres interlace near the corner of the mouth to form a marginal bundle and enter the lips. The upper and lower fibres enter the corresponding lip and interdigitate with fibres of the opposite muscle in the midline. Some of the posterior fibres pass almost vertically downwards from the maxilla to the mandible.

**Nerve supply**: the buccal branch of the facial nerve. **Actions**: the buccinator is used during mastication to press the cheek against the teeth and prevent food from collecting in the vestibule of the mouth. It also compresses the blown-out cheek (as when blowing a balloon) and raises the intra-oral pressure [Fig. 3.8; see also Figs. 5.6, 16.6].

### Orbicularis oris

The orbicularis oris is the sphincter muscle of the mouth. It is a complex muscle which forms the greater part of the lips. It is composed mainly of interlacing fibres of muscles which converge on the mouth. These muscles include the buccinator, levator labii superioris, levator labii superioris alaeque nasi, levator anguli oris, zygomaticus major, zygomaticus minor, risorius, depressor labii inferioris, and depressor anguli oris [Fig. 3.10]. The fibres of the various muscles converging on the mouth mingle and sweep in curves through the lips.

**Actions**: the muscles of the orbicularis oris confer a wide variety of movements on the lips. They elevate the upper lip, depress the lower lip, and evert or retract both lips. They act as sphincters at the oral fissure. **Nerve supply**: facial nerve, upper and lower buccal branches.

➲ Paralysis of one-half of the orbicularis oris prevents proper closure of the mouth and affects movements of the lips on that side. Speech is slurred. Food and fluids collect in the vestibule or fall out of the mouth. The lips are pulled towards the normal side by the unopposed action of those muscles. When the patient attempts to blow against resistance, the cheek and lips are blown out and air escapes on the paralysed side.

➲ Damage to the facial nerve at, or distal to, the stylomastoid foramen causes weakness or paralysis on one or both sides of the face. The patient will have loss of control over muscles of facial expression, difficulty in blinking and eating, and drooping of the eyelids, eyebrows, and mouth.

➲ (When the facial nerve is affected in the brain, in the internal acoustic meatus, or at the level of the genicular ganglion, in addition to paralysis of facial muscles, the patient will also have loss of taste on the anterior two-thirds of the tongue, hyperacusis, and decreased secretion of the submandibular, sublingual, lacrimal, nasal, palatine, and oral glands. The anatomical basis of these symptoms is described in Chapter 12.)

Dissection 3.3 provides instructions on deep dissection of the vessels and nerves of the face.

## Arteries of the face

The face has a rich arterial supply. The facial and transverse facial arteries anastomose freely with the smaller arteries which accompany the branches of the trigeminal nerve into the face, and with the arteries of the opposite side, especially in the lips. ➲ As such, wounds of the face bleed a lot but also heal rapidly.

**DISSECTION 3.3 Vessels and nerves of the face**

**Objectives**

**I.** To find and trace the facial artery and vein. **II.** To find and trace the parotid duct. **III.** To find and trace the branches of the facial nerve. **IV.** To find and trace the infraorbital and auriculotemporal nerves.

**Instructions**

1. Detach the risorius, and reflect it with the remains of the platysma towards the corner of the mouth. Avoid injury to the underlying vessels and nerves.
2. Find the cut end of the great auricular nerve, and trace it upwards over the lower part of the parotid gland.
3. Expose the facial artery and vein at the anteroinferior angle of the masseter, but do not trace them further at the moment [Fig. 3.6].
4. Cut through the fascial covering of the **parotid gland** immediately in front of the auricle from the zygomatic arch to the angle of the mandible. Dissect the fascia carefully forwards to the margins of the gland, looking for the nerves, the vessels, and the duct of the gland which emerge at the anterior border.
5. The **parotid duct** appears at the anterior border of the parotid, about a finger-breadth below the zygomatic arch. It is large [Fig. 3.6] and readily palpated in the living by rolling it against the anterior border of the tightened masseter.
6. Above the duct, find: (1) a small detached part of the parotid gland—the **accessory parotid**; (2) the transverse facial artery and vein [Fig. 3.6]; and (3) the zygomatic branches of the facial nerve [Fig. 3.7].
7. Find the **branches of the facial nerve** emerging from the anterior border of the parotid gland, and trace them forwards. This is difficult because they communicate with each other and with the branches of the trigeminal nerve in the face. (The facial nerve is motor to the muscles of the face; the trigeminal nerve is sensory.)
8. Identify the muscles of facial expression: the zygomaticus major, zygomaticus minor, levator labii superioris, and depressor anguli oris.
9. Follow the upper zygomatic branches of the facial nerve. They pass deep to the lateral part of the orbicularis oculi. At this point, the zygomaticofacial nerve (sensory) may be found emerging from the zygomatic bone.
10. Trace the lower zygomatic branches of the facial nerve forwards, inferior to the orbit and deep to the zygomatic muscles. Find their communications with the **infraorbital nerve** (sensory).
11. Trace the branches of the infraorbital nerve.
12. Cut through the zygomaticus major and minor, and levator labii superioris at their origins, and turn them downwards to expose the facial artery and vein. Trace these vessels and their branches.
13. Find the **buccal branch of the facial nerve** at the anterior border of the parotid gland. Trace it forwards through the fat of the cheek to the buccinator muscle.
14. Attempt to find the communications between the buccal branch of the facial nerve and the buccal (sensory) branch of the trigeminal nerve. Follow the buccal branch of the trigeminal nerve posteriorly, till it disappears deep to the ramus of the mandible.
15. Trace the marginal mandibular branch of the facial nerve forwards from the lower border of the parotid gland to the depressor anguli oris. Cut through the depressor anguli oris, and trace the communication of the nerve with the **mental nerve** (sensory) which emerges through the mental foramen. Follow the branches of the mental nerve to the chin and lower lip.
16. At the upper border of the parotid gland, identify: (1) the superficial temporal artery and veins; (2) the **auriculotemporal nerve** close to the auricle; and (3) the temporal branches of the facial nerve anterior to the vessels.
17. At the lower border of the gland, identify again: (1) the anterior and posterior branches of the retromandibular vein; and (2) the cervical branch of the facial nerve.
18. Trace the facial vein downwards, till it joins the anterior branch of the retromandibular vein [see Fig. 4.4].

## Transverse facial artery

The transverse facial artery arises from the superficial temporal artery under cover of the parotid gland. It emerges near the upper end of the gland and runs forwards over the masseter below the zygomatic arch [Fig. 3.6].

## Facial artery

The facial artery is a branch of the external carotid artery. It is the main artery of the face. It enters the face by turning around the lower border of the mandible and piercing the deep fascia at the anteroinferior angle of masseter. (It can be palpated against the mandible at this point.) It runs anterosuperiorly to a point 1.5 cm lateral to the angle of the mouth, and then ascends more vertically to end near the medial angle of the eye [Fig. 3.6]. It has a sinuous course on the face.

The facial artery gives large branches to the chin, lips (**inferior labial** and **superior labial**), and nose (**lateral nasal**), and smaller branches to the adjacent muscles. An important anastomosis is present at the medial angle of the eye between the facial vessels and those of the orbit. Through this arterial anastomosis, blood from the external carotid artery can reach the internal carotid artery in the skull. Similarly, venous blood from the face can drain into the orbit and skull.

## Veins of the face

The face is drained by veins that accompany the arteries that supply it. The veins of the face anastomose freely with each other.

### Facial vein

The facial vein is formed by the union of the supraorbital and supratrochlear veins at the medial angle of the eye. The initial segment of the vein (near the angle of the eye) is also known as the **angular vein**. It runs posteroinferiorly, behind and in the same plane as the artery, but takes a straighter course, close to the anterior border of the masseter. It lies close to the artery again on the surface of the mandible. The vein then descends into the neck, pierces the deep fascia, and receives the anterior branch of the retromandibular vein. It crosses the carotid arteries and drains into the internal jugular vein.

The facial vein receives tributaries which correspond to the branches of the facial artery. On the surface of the buccinator, it gives off the **deep facial vein**, which passes medial to the masseter to join the **pterygoid plexus of veins**.

➲ The wide communication channel between the deep facial vein and the pterygoid plexus makes it possible for infections from the face to spread to the pterygoid plexus, and from there to the cavernous sinus. Facial infections can easily become intracranial when they occur in the '**danger triangle of the face**', or '**triangle of death**', and can lead to serious complications like cavernous sinus thrombosis, meningitis, or brain abscess. The dangerous area of the face is a triangular area from the bridge of the nose to the corners of the mouth.

## Nerves of the face

### Sensory nerves of the face

The great auricular nerve and trigeminal nerve supply sensory innervation to the face [Fig. 3.9]. The trigeminal nerve is the main sensory nerve of the face. It gives rise to three nerves—ophthalmic, maxillary, and mandibular—each of which supplies cutaneous branches to one of three roughly concentric areas of the face [Figs. 3.7, 3.9]. The trigeminal cutaneous area abuts on that supplied by the ventral and dorsal rami of the second cervical nerve. (The first cervical nerve does not supply skin).

#### Great auricular nerve

The skin over the parotid gland and the angle of the mandible are supplied by the **great auricular nerve** (ventral rami of C. 2, C. 3) [Fig. 3.9].

#### Ophthalmic nerve

The **ophthalmic division of the trigeminal nerve** supplies the area of skin between the angle of the eye and the vertex of the head [Figs. 3.7, 3.9] through the lacrimal, frontal, and nasociliary branches. These branches pass through the orbit and give rise to five nerves on the face:

1. The **palpebral branch of the lacrimal nerve** supplies the lateral part of the upper eyelid.

2, 3. The **supraorbital** and **supratrochlear** branches of the frontal nerve supply the forehead and anterior scalp.

4. The **infratrochlear branch** of the nasociliary nerve supplies the medial parts of the eyelids and the root of the nose.

5. The **external nasal nerve** emerges between the nasal bone and the lateral nasal cartilage [Fig. 3.1] and supplies the skin of the lower half of the dorsum of the nose. It is a branch of the **anterior ethmoidal nerve** which arises from the nasociliary nerve in the orbit, and enters the nasal cavity through the cribriform plate of the ethmoid.

### Maxillary nerve

The **maxillary division of the trigeminal nerve** supplies an area of skin inferior and lateral to the eye by three branches [Figs. 3.7, 3.9].

1. The **infraorbital nerve** emerges from the infraorbital foramen under cover of the orbicularis oculi and levator labii superioris. It gives the **labial**, **palpebral**, and **nasal branches** which supply the skin and mucous membrane of the upper lip, the lower eyelid, the skin between them, and the skin on the side of the nose. These nerves form a **plexus** with the zygomatic branches of the facial nerve. Such plexuses are not the site of union of nerve fibres, but merely places where the nerve fibres run together, so that sensory nerves from the muscles of the face can enter the trigeminal nerve.
2. The **zygomaticofacial nerve** supplies the skin over the bony part of the cheek. It passes from the orbit through the zygomatic bone on to its facial surface [Fig. 3.7].
3. The **zygomaticotemporal nerve** also pierces the zygomatic bone and emerges from its temporal surface. It passes through the temporal fascia and supplies the skin over the anterior part of the temple.

### Mandibular nerve

The **mandibular division of the trigeminal nerve** supplies an area of skin posterior and inferior to the previous areas, by three branches [Figs. 3.7, 3.9].

1. The **auriculotemporal nerve** emerges from the upper border of the parotid gland beside the auricle. It supplies the upper part of the auricle, the external acoustic meatus, and the skin of the side of the head [Fig. 3.7].
2. The **buccal nerve** passes anteroinferiorly, deep to the masseter and the ramus of the mandible. It supplies the skin over the buccinator and sends branches through it to the mucosa of the mouth [Fig. 3.7].
3. The **mental nerve** is a branch of the inferior alveolar nerve. It appears on the face through the mental foramen of the mandible. It divides into branches deep to the depressor anguli oris. These branches supply the skin and mucous membrane of the lower lip, and the skin over the mandible from the symphysis to the anterior border of the masseter [Fig. 3.7].

## Motor nerves of the face

The facial nerve is the motor nerve to the muscles of facial expression. It has five terminal branches, or groups of branches—temporal, zygomatic, buccal (upper and lower buccal), marginal mandibular, and cervical—which emerge from the parotid gland [Fig. 3.7].

1. The **temporal branches** have been described in the scalp.
2. Small **zygomatic branches** run across the zygomatic arch to supply the orbicularis oculi. Larger branches run forwards below the arch to supply the muscles of the nose—the nasalis and levator labii superioris alaeque nasi—and those between the eye and the mouth—the zygomaticus major, zygomaticus minor, and levator labii superioris.
3. The **buccal branches** run towards the angle of the mouth and supply the muscles of the cheek—the buccinator.
4. The **marginal mandibular branches** run forwards along the mandible and usually curve down into the neck, before running with the inferior labial branch of the facial artery to supply the muscles of the lower lip—the depressor labii inferioris, depressor anguli oris, and mentalis.
5. The **cervical branch** leaves the lower border of the parotid gland and runs forwards and downwards into the neck, to supply the platysma and communicate with the transverse nerve of the neck [Fig. 3.7].

Dissection 3.4 provides instructions on dissection of the buccinator.

## Structures in the cheek and lips

The bulk of the cheek and lips is formed by muscles. The muscles are covered externally by skin, and internally by the mucous membrane of the mouth. In addition, the cheek and lips contain buccal and labial salivary glands, few lymph nodes, fascia enclosing the buccinator, and the buccal pad of fat.

## Buccopharyngeal fascia

The buccopharyngeal fascia covers the external surface of the buccinator and continues backwards over the constrictor muscles of the pharynx. The

**DISSECTION 3.4 Buccinator**

**Objective**

**I.** To expose and study the buccinator.

**Instructions**

1. Expose the levator anguli oris and buccinator.
2. Remove the buccal fat from the buccinator, avoiding injury to the buccal nerve. Note the small buccal glands that lie in the fat.
3. Remove the fascia covering the buccinator. Define its attachments to the maxilla and mandible, and trace its fibres towards the angle of the mouth.

parotid duct pierces the buccopharyngeal fascia and the buccinator, and opens into the vestibule of the mouth, opposite the upper second molar tooth. The fascia and muscle are also pierced by the nerves and vessels of the mucous membrane.

## Molar glands and buccal lymph nodes

Four to five small molar mucous salivary glands lie on the buccopharyngeal fascia around the parotid duct. Their ducts follow the parotid duct to the vestibule of the mouth. The buccal lymph nodes are found on the buccopharyngeal fascia.

## Buccal pad of fat

An encapsulated mass of fat—the buccal pad of fat—lies on the buccopharyngeal fascia. It is traversed by the buccal nerve and parotid duct. It adds bulk to the cheek to help to resist the external pressure during sucking. This pad is relatively large in infants when the cheeks are not supported by teeth, and accounts for the fullness of the cheeks in them.

## Labial and buccal glands

These are small, closely set mucous salivary glands that lie in the submucosa of the lips and cheek. They are palpable as small nodules when the tongue is pressed against them. Their ducts open into the vestibule of the mouth.

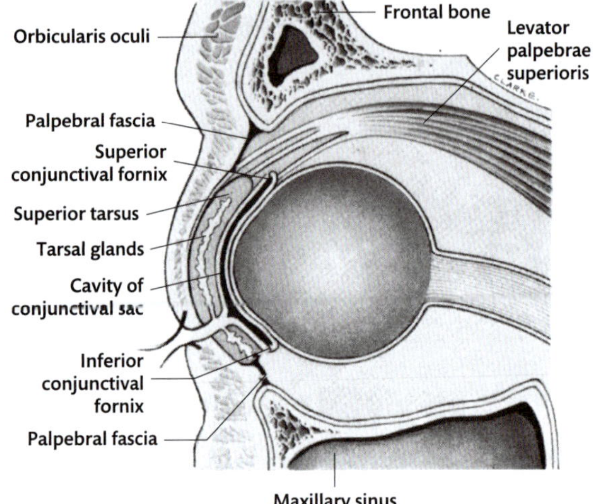


**Fig. 3.11** Structure of the eyelids seen in section.

# Eyelids

The eyelids, or palpebrae, consist of the: (1) skin and superficial fascia; (2) orbicularis oculi; (3) tarsi and palpebral fascia; and (4) conjunctiva [Fig. 3.11]. The skin of the eyelids is very thin. The superficial fascia is thin, loose, and devoid of fat. It allows the skin to move freely over the lid and can become greatly swollen with fluid or blood after an injury.

Using the instructions given in Dissection 3.5, identify the palpebral fascia and tarsi.

**DISSECTION 3.5 Palpebral fascia and tarsi**

**Objective**

**I.** To identify the medial palpebral ligament, palpebral fascia, and tarsal plates.

**Instructions**

1. Separate the palpebral part of the orbicularis oculi from the remainder of the muscle by a circular incision.
2. Turn the palpebral part towards the palpebral fissure. Avoid injury to the palpebral fascia, vessels, and nerves.
3. Deep to the muscles, identify the medial palpebral ligament at the medial angle of the eye, and the palpebral fascia and tarsi elsewhere.

## Tarsal plates

The tarsal plates and the palpebral fascia together form a continuous layer of the eyelid known as the **orbital septum** [Figs. 3.11, 3.12]. The tarsi are two thin plates of condensed fibrous tissue in the eyelids. They stiffen the eyelids and extend up to the free margin. The **inferior tarsus** is narrow and attached to the inferior orbital margin by the palpebral fascia. The **superior tarsus** is much larger and can be felt if the upper lid is pinched sideways between the finger and the thumb. The deep surface is adherent to the palpebral conjunctiva. The palpebral fascia is attached to its anterior surface some distance below its upper border. The tendon of the **levator palpebrae superioris** (a muscle of the upper eyelid) is attached to the deep surface of the palpebral fascia and the superior tarsus [Figs. 3.11, 3.12]. The lower edge of the superior tarsus is adherent to the skin of the margin of the upper eyelid. (The levator palpebrae superioris is described in Chapter 10.)

The **tarsal glands** lie in furrows on the deep surfaces of the tarsi. They appear as closely placed, parallel yellow streaks running at right angles to the margin of the lid. Their ducts open on the margin of the eyelid behind the eyelashes. The **ciliary glands** are arranged in several rows immediately behind the roots of the eyelashes. Their ducts open on the margin close to the lashes. (They are too small to be seen by dissection.) ➲ When infected, they produce a red swelling of the margin of the eyelid known as a **stye** or **hordeolum**.

The **palpebral fascia** is a thin fibrous membrane which connects the tarsi to the orbital margins. Medially, it passes posterior to the lacrimal sac to be attached to the bone. In the lower eyelid, it is attached to the inferior margin of the inferior tarsus. In the upper eyelid, it is attached to the anterior surface of the superior tarsus, close to the superior margin. The palpebral fascia is pierced by nerves and vessels which pass from the orbit to the exterior [Figs. 3.11, 3.12].

## Palpebral ligaments

The **medial** palpebral ligament is a strong fibrous band that connects the superior and inferior tarsi with the medial margin of the orbit. It lies under the skin, anterior to the lacrimal sac, and gives origin to fibres of the orbicularis oculi [Fig. 3.12].

The **lateral** palpebral ligament is a slender fibrous band which lies posterior to the palpebral fascia and connects the lateral ends of the two tarsi to a small tubercle on the lateral orbital margin [Fig. 3.12].

## Vessels and nerves of eyelids

The **arteries** of the eyelids are derived from the ophthalmic artery. They pierce the palpebral fascia to enter the eyelids and anastomose with each other to form arches near the margins of the lids. These arterial arches lie between the tarsus and the orbicularis oculi.

The **veins** of the eyelids run medially and end in the supratrochlear and facial veins.

The **motor supply** to the orbicularis oculi come from the temporal and upper zygomatic branches of the facial nerve. The **sensory supply** to the upper

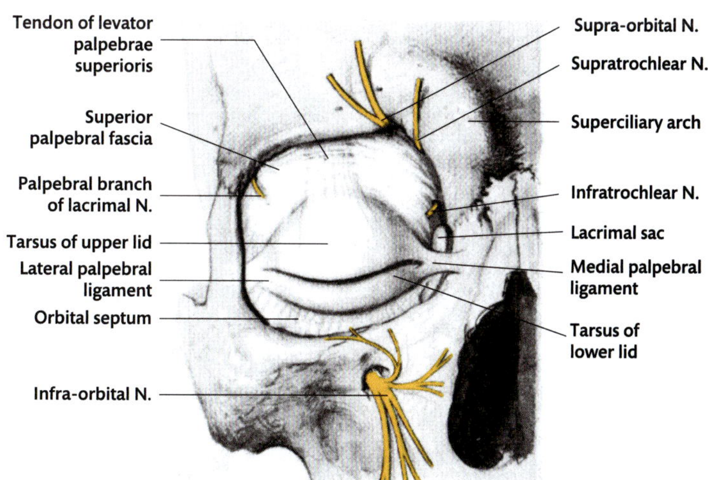


**Fig. 3.12** Dissection of the right eyelid. The orbicularis oculi has been removed.

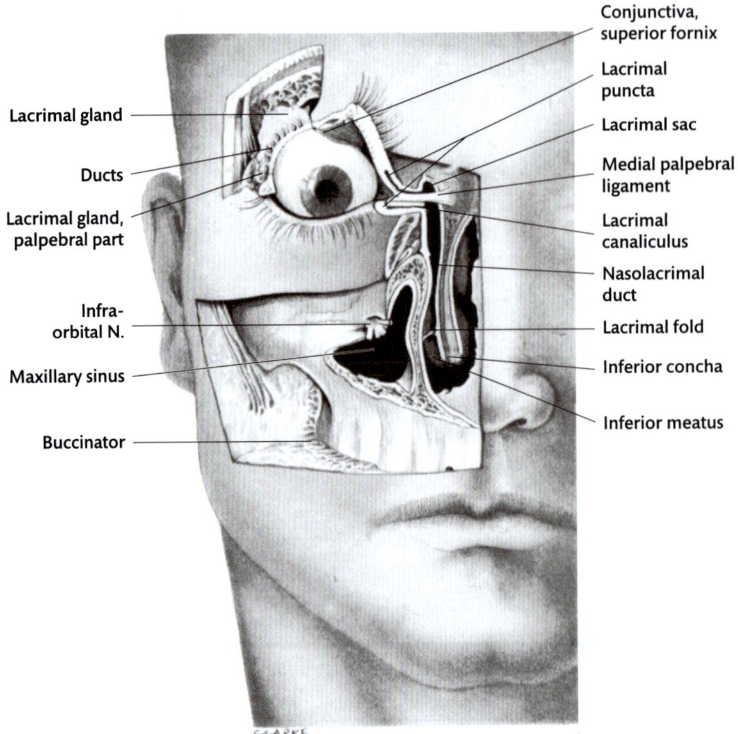


**Fig. 3.13** Dissection of the lacrimal apparatus.

lid is from the palpebral branch of the lacrimal nerve and branches of the supraorbital, supratrochlear, and infratrochlear nerves. The lower lid is supplied by the infraorbital and infratrochlear nerves.

## The lacrimal apparatus

The lacrimal apparatus consists of the lacrimal gland, lacrimal canaliculi, lacrimal sac, and nasolacrimal duct [Fig. 3.13]. The lacrimal gland produces lacrimal fluid which enters the superolateral part of the conjunctival sac. In the conjunctival sac, it flows over the conjunctiva towards the medial angle of the eye, aided by the contraction of the orbicularis oculi [Fig. 3.2]. At the medial angle, the lacrimal fluid enters the lacrimal canaliculi and passes through the lacrimal sac and nasolacrimal duct to drain into the nose [Figs. 3.2, 3.13].

Using the instructions given in Dissection 3.6, explore the lacrimal apparatus.

### DISSECTION 3.6 Lacrimal apparatus

#### Objectives

**I.** To expose the lacrimal gland. **II.** To explore the lacrimal puncta, lacrimal canaliculi, lacrimal sac, and nasolacrimal duct.

#### Instructions

1. Cut through the superolateral part of the palpebral fascia, and expose the lacrimal gland.
2. Raise the gland, and find its ducts by moving the points of a pair of fine forceps up and down in the loose tissue below the gland.
3. Find the lacrimal papillae at the medial ends of the eyelids, and attempt to pass a fine bristle into the lacrimal canaliculi through the puncta.
4. Identify the medial palpebral ligament and the lacrimal sac which lies posterior to it.
5. Note the lacrimal part of the orbicularis oculi passing around the lateral side of the sac.
6. Make an opening into the sac. Pass a probe into it and explore its extent.
7. Then pass the probe downwards into the nose through the nasolacrimal duct. Confirm its orifice in the nasal cavity.

## Lacrimal gland

The lacrimal gland [Fig. 3.13; see Fig. 10.2] lies mainly in the superolateral corner of the anterior part of the orbit. A small part of it—the **palpebral process**—extends into the upper eyelid lateral to the tarsus, between the conjunctiva and the palpebral fascia. When the eyelid is everted, it may be seen as a bulge in the conjunctiva. The **ducts** of the lacrimal gland (10 or fewer) are short and thin. They open into the conjunctival sac near the superior fornix. Small **accessory lacrimal glands** lie near the conjunctival fornices. They can be effective in moistening the conjunctiva if the lacrimal gland is removed.

## Conjunctival sac

The conjunctiva lines the deep surfaces of the eyelids—the **palpebral conjunctiva**—and covers the exposed surface of the eyeball—the **bulbar conjunctiva**. At the corneoscleral junction, the bulbar conjunctiva becomes continuous with the anterior epithelium of the cornea. The **conjunctival fornices** are produced where the thick, vascular palpebral part of the conjunctiva is reflected from the eyelids onto the eyeball. On the eyeball, the conjunctiva is thin and transparent, and is loosely attached to the sclera. The space bounded by the bulbar and palpebral conjunctivae is known as the **conjunctival sac**. The conjunctival sac is no more than a capillary interval moistened by lacrimal fluid. It opens to the exterior through the **palpebral fissure** and drains into the lacrimal sac through the canaliculi [Fig. 3.13].

## Lacrimal canaliculi

The lacrimal canaliculi are two thin tubes about 1 cm in length. Each begins at a tiny hole (the **lacrimal punctum**) on the summit of a lacrimal papilla. It runs medially in the margin of the eyelid and opens into the lacrimal sac, posterior to the medial palpebral ligament [Fig. 3.13].

## Lacrimal sac

The **lacrimal sac** lies posterior to the medial palpebral ligament in the lacrimal groove. It is approximately 1 cm long and 0.5 cm wide. The upper end of the sac is closed. Its lower end is continuous with the nasolacrimal duct [Fig. 3.13]. It receives the lacrimal fluid through the lacrimal canaliculi.

## Nasolacrimal duct

The **nasolacrimal duct** is 1.5 cm long and 0.5 cm wide. It begins at the anteromedial part of the floor of the orbit as a continuation of the lacrimal sac, and descends in a bony canal to the inferior meatus of the nasal cavity. The mucous membrane at the medial side of its opening is raised to form the **lacrimal fold**. This fold acts as a flap valve which prevents air and secretions from being blown up the nasolacrimal duct when the intranasal pressure is raised (e.g. when blowing the nose or sneezing) [Fig. 3.13; see Fig. 18.5].

See Clinical Applications 3.1 and 3.2 for the practical implications of the anatomy discussed in this chapter.





**CLINICAL APPLICATION 3.1 Sensory nerve blocks in the face**

Individual branches of the trigeminal nerve can be blocked by using anaesthetic agents for doing surgical procedures in the face. The connective tissue around a sensory nerve is injected with an anaesthetic agent, which then temporarily stops transmission of pain. Knowledge of the course and area supplied by the nerve is essential for achieving proper anaesthesia.

1. Supraorbital and supratrochlear nerve blocks to anaesthetize the forehead and anterior scalp are done by infiltrating the nerve at the supraorbital margin.
2. Infraorbital nerve block to anaesthetize the mid-face region is done by infiltrating the nerve at the infraorbital foramen, either intra-orally or through the skin of the face.
3. Posterior superior alveolar nerve blocks to anaesthetize the maxillary molar teeth are done by infiltrating the nerve at the maxillary tuberosity.
4. Anterior superior alveolar nerve block to anaesthetize the upper canine and incisors is done by infiltrating the nerve where the mucobuccal fold meets the apex of the canine tooth.
5. Inferior alveolar nerve block to anaesthetize all the mandibular teeth is done by infiltrating the nerve at the lingula of the mandible.
6. Mental nerve block to anaesthetize the lower lip and skin of the chin is done by infiltrating the nerve as it emerges from the mental foramen.
7. Lingual nerve block to anaesthetize the anterior two-thirds of the tongue is done by infiltrating the nerve next to the second mandibular molar tooth.

#### CLINICAL APPLICATION 3.2 Lacrimal fluid

Under ordinary conditions, the lacrimal fluid flows downwards over the eyeball and most of it evaporates. The remaining is carried medially by the frequent involuntary contractions of the orbicularis oculi which move the eyelids and the lacrimal fluid medially, due to the attachment of the muscle to the medial palpebral ligament. Excessive secretion by the lacrimal gland, due to irritation of the conjunctiva or in response to strong emotions, floods the conjunctiva and the lacrimal fluid overflows as tears. When the orbicularis oculi is paralysed, the eyes remain open; the lacrimal fluid is not spread, and the cornea becomes dry. Tears pool in the sagging, paralysed lower lid and spill over onto the face.

CHAPTER 4

# The posterior triangle of the neck

## Introduction to the neck

The **side of the neck** is limited inferiorly by the clavicle, and superiorly by the lower border of the mandible, the mastoid process of the temporal bone, and the superior nuchal line of the occipital bone. It extends from the midline in front to the anterior border of the trapezius at the back. The sternocleidomastoid muscle runs obliquely across the side of the neck and divides it into **anterior** and **posterior triangles** [Fig. 4.1].

(Chapter 6 on the back of the neck deals with the structures under cover of the trapezius and includes the erector spinae, muscles of the suboccipital region, other back muscles, and their blood vessels and nerves.)

In this dissection manual, the neck is described in four chapters. The superficial structures of the neck are described in Chapters 4 and 5—the posterior and anterior triangles. The deep structures of the neck are described in Chapter 8. Finally, the muscles of the prevertebral region, which lie most posteriorly, are described in Chapter 9. When necessary, cross-references are provided to help the reader navigate between these chapters.

## Surface anatomy of the posterior triangle of the neck

The upper 3–4 cervical vertebrae are overlapped anteriorly by the facial skeleton, as the cervical vertebrae extend to a much higher level than the chin. The first cervical vertebra lies at the level of the tip of the mastoid process—the same level as the hard palate. The second lies at the level of the oral cavity, and the third lies at the level of the symphysis menti.

The **sternocleidomastoid muscle** extends from the manubrium sternum and the medial third of the clavicle to the mastoid process of the temporal bone behind the ear. It raises a low ridge diagonally across the side of the neck. This ridge is made prominent when the face is turned towards the opposite side. The **external jugular vein** is seen crossing the surface of the sternocleidomastoid, almost vertically from a point behind the angle of the mandible to the clavicle [Fig. 4.1].

The **lesser supraclavicular fossa** is a shallow depression between the sternal and clavicular parts of the sternocleidomastoid. It is above the medial end of the clavicle and overlies the internal jugular vein. The **greater supraclavicular fossa** is a larger depression above the intermediate third of the clavicle, between the lower parts of the trapezius and sternocleidomastoid. It overlies the cervical part of the brachial plexus and the third part of the subclavian artery. It is made obvious when the shoulders are shrugged.

## Cervical fascia and arrangement of neck structures

The major structures of the neck are surrounded by the **investing layer of the deep fascia**. This fascia encloses the trapezius and sternocleidomastoid muscles and forms the superficial covering of

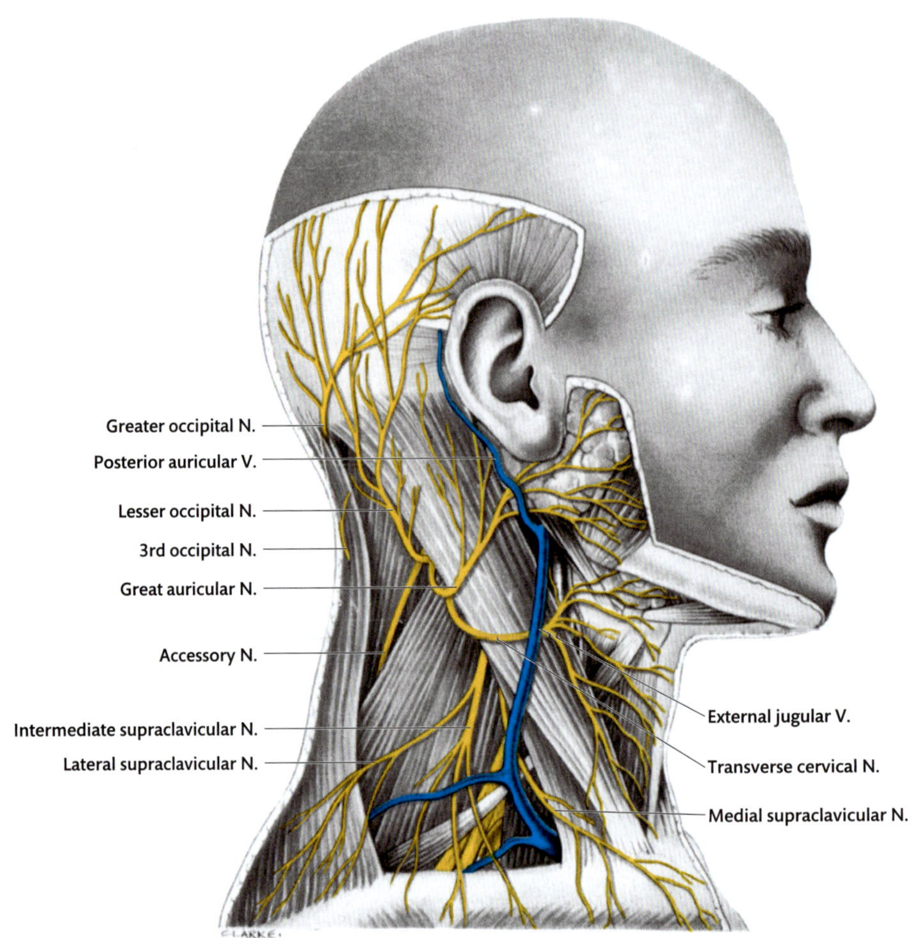


**Fig. 4.1** Cutaneous branches of the cervical plexus.

the posterior triangle. Deep to this layer of fascia are two compartments. (1) The larger posterior compartment consists of the vertebral column and the muscles which immediately surround it. This compartment is enclosed in a sleeve of fascia, which passes anterior to the vertebral bodies and is known as the **prevertebral fascia**. Laterally, this fascia covers the muscles which form the floor of the posterior triangle, and the erector spinae muscles. (2) The smaller anterior compartment contains the pharynx, larynx, oesophagus, and trachea, and their associated muscles. These structures are covered anteriorly by the **pretracheal fascia**. This compartment also contains the vertical neurovascular bundle of the neck. The ventral rami of the **cervical nerves** emerge from the vertebral canal between the muscles attached to the anterior and posterior tubercles of the transverse processes [Fig. 4.2]. Since these nerves arise within the prevertebral fascia, they may either carry a sheath of this fascia outwards with them—the fascia of the cervico-axillary canal [see Fig. 4.8]—or continue to remain within the fascia (the phrenic nerve).

## The posterior triangle—boundaries and contents

The boundaries of the posterior triangle are the posterior margin of the sternocleidomastoid, the anterior margin of the trapezius, and the intermediate third of the clavicle [Fig. 4.3].

The investing layer of the deep fascia forms the roof of the triangle and is pierced by the external jugular vein, the cutaneous branches of the cervical

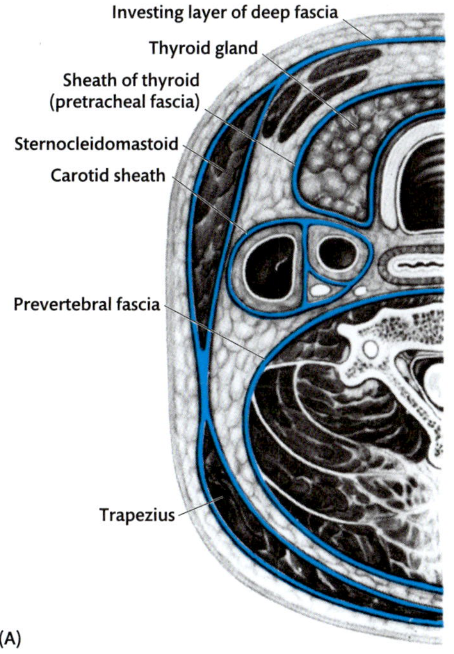


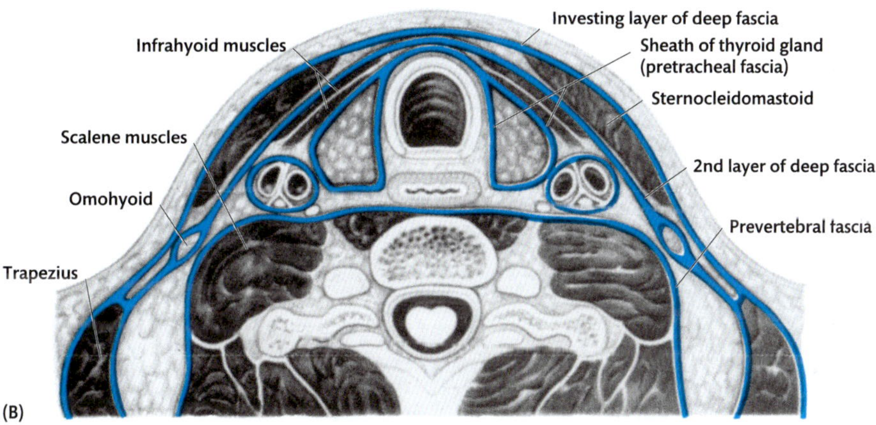


**Fig. 4.2** (A) Cervical fascia (blue) in transverse section at the level of the thyroid isthmus. (B) Cervical fascia (blue) in transverse section of the lower part of the neck.

plexus, and lymph vessels passing from the superficial structures to the nodes in the triangle.

The floor of the triangle is formed from above downwards by the splenius capitis, levator scapulae, and middle scalene, covered by the prevertebral fascia [Fig. 4.4].

Using the instructions given in Dissection 4.1, reflect the skin of the posterior triangle and begin tracing the cutaneous nerves and veins.

## Platysma

This thin sheet of muscle lies in the superficial fascia, superficial to the cutaneous branches of the cervical plexus and the external jugular vein. It extends down from the face to the upper part of the chest over the superior part of the anterior triangle and the antero-inferior part of the posterior triangle [Fig. 4.5].

The platysma takes origin from the skin and fascia over the upper parts of the pectoralis major and deltoid. The muscle fibres run superomedially over the sternocleidomastoid and anterior triangle. The anterior fibres either are attached to the lower border of the anterior part of the mandible or meet with the fibres of the opposite side below the chin. The posterior fibres curve upwards over the mandible to the skin of the lower face and mingle with

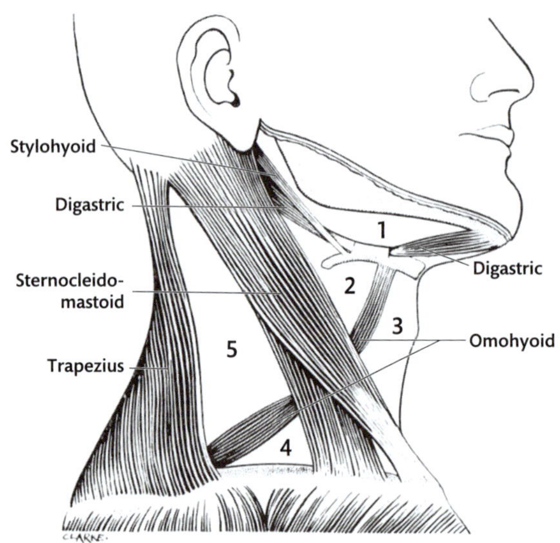


**Fig. 4.3** The triangles of the neck. Anterior triangle: 1 = digastric triangle; 2 = carotid triangle; 3 = muscular triangle. Posterior triangle: 4 = subclavian triangle, 5 = occipital triangle.



the muscles of the lips, helping to form the risorius [see Fig. 3.8].

**Nerve supply**: the cervical branch of the facial nerve. **Action**: it pulls down the corner of the mouth, elevates the skin over the upper part of the chest, and tenses the skin of the neck. It contracts most obviously in strenuous inspiratory effort and may prevent compression of the airway by the skin.

## Deep fascia of the posterior triangle

The **roof** of the posterior triangle is formed by the investing layer of the deep cervical fascia. It extends from the intermediate third of the clavicle to the superior nuchal line. It is a thin sheet which splits inferiorly into superficial and deep layers. The superficial layer fuses with the clavicle. The deep layer splits to enclose the posterior belly of the omohyoid muscle [Figs. 4.2B, 4.4], passes deep to the clavicle, and is attached to its lower surface. It holds the inferior belly of the omohyoid in place. The space between the two layers of fascia extends medially deep to the sternocleidomastoid behind the clavicle, and contains the terminal parts of the external jugular and transverse cervical veins and the suprascapular vessels. The **accessory nerve** enters the triangle at the posterior border of the sternocleidomastoid and runs posteroinferiorly across the triangle embedded in the investing fascia [Fig. 4.4]. The fascia is pierced by: (1) cutaneous branches of the cervical plexus;

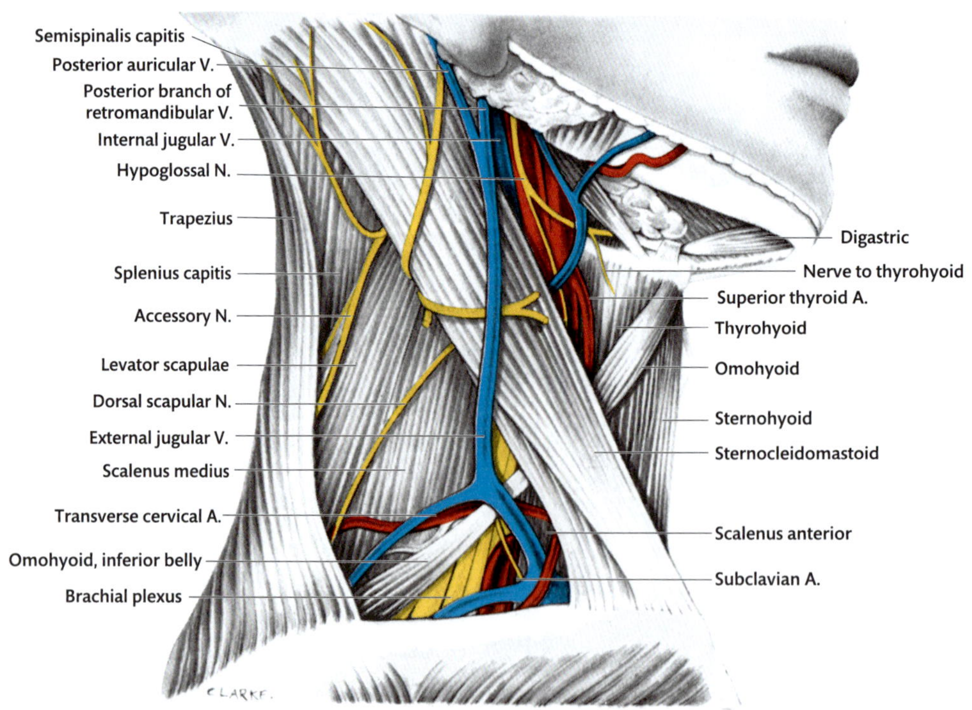


**Fig. 4.4** Lateral view of the superficial structures in the neck.

**DISSECTION 4.1 Skin reflection and cutaneous nerves and veins of the posterior triangle-1**

**Objectives**

**I.** To reflect the skin of the posterior triangle. **II.** To identify and trace the great auricular nerve, lesser occipital nerve, transverse cutaneous nerve of the neck, and supraclavicular nerves. **III.** To identify and trace the external jugular vein [Fig. 4.1].

**Instructions**

1. Reflect the skin of the posterior triangle. Avoid damage to the supraclavicular nerves, which lie deep to the platysma in the lower part of the triangle, and to the accessory nerve, which is in the investing layer of the deep fascia in the upper part of the triangle.
2. Make an incision through the skin along the middle of the sternocleidomastoid muscle from the mastoid process to the sternal end of the clavicle. Do not cut into the superficial fascia, or the great auricular nerve, transverse nerve of the neck, and external jugular vein will be damaged.
3. Extend the incision along the clavicle to its acromial end, and reflect the flap of skin back to the anterior border of the trapezius.
4. Turn the platysma upwards and forwards from the clavicle, superficial to the supraclavicular nerves and the **external jugular vein**. Find this vein, and trace it upwards till it is joined by the posterior auricular vein, and downwards till it pierces the deep fascia.
5. Find the three cutaneous nerves which pierce the deep fascia at the middle of the posterior border of the sternocleidomastoid. (1) The **lesser occipital nerve** runs upwards along the posterior border of the sternocleidomastoid. (2) The **great auricular nerve** crosses the sternocleidomastoid obliquely towards the auricle. (3) The **transverse nerve of the neck** passes horizontally forwards across the sternocleidomastoid.
6. Find the medial, intermediate, and lateral **supraclavicular nerves**, either individually or by finding one branch and tracing it back to the trunk.





(2) the external jugular vein; and (3) small cutaneous arteries.

The **floor** of the posterior triangle is formed by the **prevertebral fascia**, which passes in front of the cervical vertebrae and prevertebral muscles [Fig. 4.2]. It covers the muscles on the floor of the posterior triangle—the levator scapulae, anterior scalene, medius, and posterior.

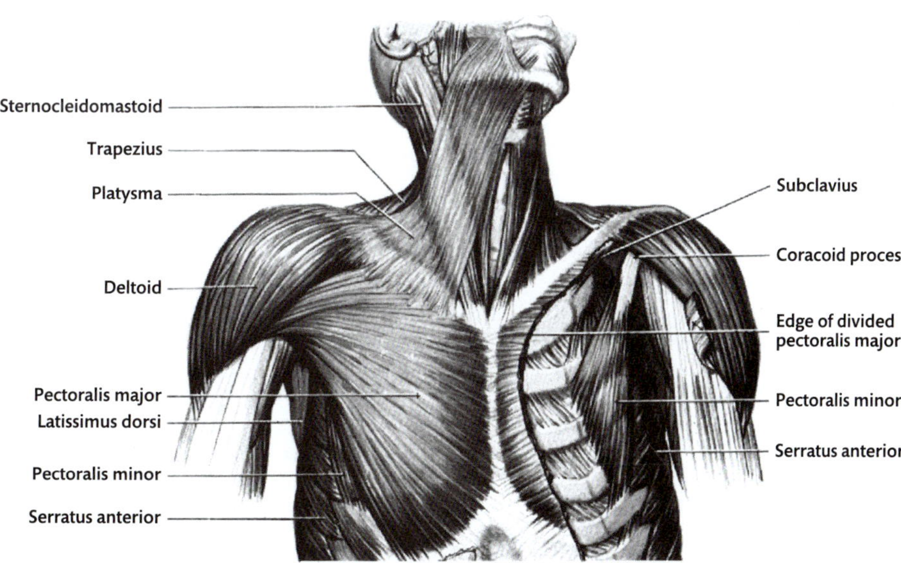


**Fig. 4.5** The platysma is seen on the right side of the neck.

## DISSECTION 4.2 Cutaneous nerves and veins of the posterior triangle-2

### Objectives

**I.** To identify and trace the nerve to the subclavius, and the accessory nerve. **II.** To identify and trace the transverse cervical and suprascapular veins.

### Instructions

1. Follow the supraclavicular nerves to their common trunk.
2. Cut through the investing fascia above the clavicle and along the posterior border of the sternocleidomastoid to expose its deeper layer.
3. Find the external jugular, transverse cervical, and suprascapular veins in the space between the two layers, and trace the veins to their termination.
4. Find the **nerve to the subclavius** on the lateral side of the external jugular vein, and trace it in both directions. It may give an accessory branch to the phrenic nerve.
5. Find the entry of the anterior jugular vein into the external jugular vein, and the **suprascapular artery** deep to the clavicle. Trace the artery and its vein deep to the trapezius by pushing the fat out of the way. They run towards the scapular notch beside the attachment of the inferior belly of the omohyoid.
6. Follow the cutaneous nerves emerging at the middle of the posterior border of the sternocleidomastoid. Take care not to damage the accessory nerve where the lesser occipital nerve hooks round it.

Dissection 4.2 continues the study of the cutaneous nerves and veins of the posterior triangle.

## Cutaneous branches of the cervical plexus

The cervical plexus is formed by the ventral rami of the upper four cervical nerves. It lies in the upper part of the neck, deep to the internal jugular vein and the sternocleidomastoid muscle. Its cutaneous branches emerge at the middle of the posterior border of the sternocleidomastoid [see Fig. 4.9; Figs. 4.4, 4.6].

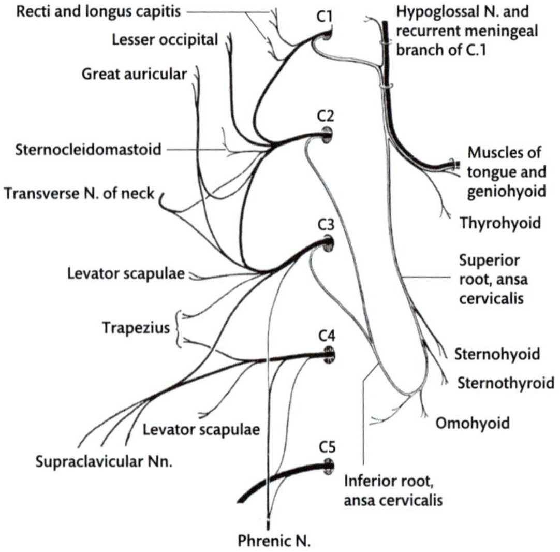

**Fig. 4.6** Cervical plexus and ansa cervicalis. C. 1–C. 5, ventral rami of the upper five cervical nerves. Note that the nerves to the geniohyoid and thyrohyoid muscles and the superior root of the ansa are derived from the first cervical ventral ramus (although they appear to arise from the hypoglossal nerve).

### Lesser occipital nerve (C. 2)

The lesser occipital nerve ascends on the posterior border of the sternocleidomastoid, giving small branches to the skin of the neck. It pierces the deep fascia and supplies the upper part of the cranial surface of the auricle and the skin over the mastoid process. It may communicate with the greater occipital nerve [Fig. 4.1].

### Great auricular nerve (C. 2, 3)

The great auricular nerve turns around the posterior border of the sternocleidomastoid, pierces the deep fascia, and runs towards the parotid gland behind and parallel to the external jugular vein. The **posterior branch** supplies the skin on both surfaces of the auricle and on the mastoid process. The **anterior branch** supplies the skin over the angle of the mandible and the parotid gland, and communicates with the facial and auriculotemporal nerves in that gland [Fig. 4.1].

### Transverse nerve of the neck (C. 2, 3)

The transverse nerve of the neck passes forwards towards the anterior triangle of the neck on the superficial surface of the sternocleidomastoid. Its upper and lower branches supply most of the skin on the side and front of the neck. The upper branch communicates with the cervical branch of the facial nerve [Fig. 5.1].

## Supraclavicular nerves (C. 3, 4)

The medial, intermediate, and lateral supraclavicular nerves arise as a single trunk. Diverging as they descend, they send small branches to the skin of the neck and pierce the deep fascia a little above the clavicle. The nerves pass over the corresponding thirds of the clavicle and supply the skin on the front of the chest, down to the level of the sternal angle, and over the upper half of the deltoid muscle [Fig. 4.1].

## External jugular vein

The external jugular vein varies greatly in size and is often conspicuous in the neck. It begins by the union of the posterior branch of the retromandibular vein and the posterior auricular vein on the surface of the sternocleidomastoid, behind the angle of the mandible. It passes vertically downwards in the superficial fascia, deep to the platysma [Fig. 4.4]. It pierces the investing layer of the deep fascia at the posterior border of the sternocleidomastoid, 2–3 cm above the clavicle. In the posterior triangle, it descends beside the sternocleidomastoid, crosses the lower roots of the brachial plexus and the third part of the subclavian artery, and drains into the subclavian vein behind the clavicle. It receives the transverse cervical, suprascapular, and anterior jugular veins.

Dissection 4.3 provides instructions on dissection of the posterior triangle.

## Accessory nerve (eleventh cranial)

The accessory nerve consists of nerve fibres which arise in the cervical part of the spinal cord. These fibres, the **spinal part of the spinal accessory**, enter the cranium through the foramen magnum. In the cranial cavity, they join with the nerve fibres arising from the medulla oblongata (**cranial part of the spinal accessory**), and together they exit from the skull through the jugular foramen.

The spinal part immediately separates from the cranial part of the nerve [see Fig. 8.12]. It passes posteroinferiorly across the transverse process of the atlas, supplies the sternocleidomastoid muscle, and pierces its deeper part. It emerges from the posterior border of the sternocleidomastoid a little above its middle, runs in the investing layer of the deep fascia covering the posterior triangle, and passes deep to the trapezius about 5 cm above the clavicle. It is

### DISSECTION 4.3 Posterior triangle

**Objectives**

**I.** To identify and clean the inferior belly of the omohyoid. **II.** To trace the accessory nerve and branches of the third and fourth cervical nerves to the trapezius. **III.** To clean the brachial plexus, and identify and trace the branches in the posterior triangle. **IV.** To expose the subclavian vessels.

**Instructions**

1. Remove the fat and fascia from the posterior triangle, starting at the apex where the occipital artery crosses it.
2. Find the accessory nerve [Fig. 4.4] at the posterior border of the sternocleidomastoid, and follow it and the branches from the third and fourth cervical nerves near it, to the trapezius. Branches of the same nerves may be found entering the levator scapulae.
3. Remove the fascia from the inferior belly of the omohyoid, and turn the muscle forwards to expose the nerve entering its deep surface near the sternocleidomastoid.
4. Expose the upper part of the brachial plexus, and trace it backwards to its roots. Avoid damage to the nerves arising from the roots. (1) The **suprascapular nerve** runs posteroinferiorly immediately above the plexus, under cover of the omohyoid. (2) Slightly above the supraclavicular nerve, the thin **dorsal scapular nerve** (C. 5) runs posteroinferiorly deep to the trapezius. (3) The three roots of the **long thoracic nerve** arise from the back of the roots of the plexus (C. 5, 6, 7) and descend behind it. The upper two pierce the middle scalene muscle. Find the long thoracic nerve in the axilla, and trace it up to the three roots of origin.
5. Find the superficial cervical artery at the upper border of the omohyoid. Follow it across the posterior triangle to its origin from the thyrocervical trunk by removing the deeper layer of the investing fascia.
6. Follow the nerve to the subclavius to its termination.
7. Expose the subclavian vessels and the brachial plexus posterior to them.

**DISSECTION 4.4 Deep dissection of the posterior triangle**

**Objective**

**I.** To expose the anterior scalene and the vessels and nerves in relation to it.

**Instructions**

1. Cut through the clavicular attachment of the sternocleidomastoid, and reflect this part of the muscle forwards.
2. Remove the underlying fatty tissue to expose the anterior scalene in front of the brachial plexus.
3. Define the borders of the anterior scalene, and expose the omohyoid muscle, superficial cervical artery, anterior and internal jugular veins, and phrenic nerve anterior to it.
4. Depress the clavicle, and expose the subclavian vein.

the only motor supply to the sternocleidomastoid and trapezius. The branches from the cervical plexus (C. 2, 3, 4) are sensory [Fig. 4.4].

Dissection 4.4 provides instructions on deep dissection of the posterior triangle.

## Anterior scalene

The anterior scalene arises from the anterior tubercles of the third to sixth cervical transverse processes and is inserted into the scalene tubercle on the medial margin of the first rib, posterior to the subclavian vein. It lies anterior to the ventral rami of the fourth to eighth cervical nerves, the cervical pleura, and the subclavian artery. Anteriorly, the phrenic nerve and internal jugular vein descend obliquely in front of the muscle from its lateral to medial borders. The muscle is also crossed more horizontally by the superficial cervical and suprascapular vessels and the anterior jugular vein [see Figs. 8.9, 8.17, 9.1; Fig. 4.7].

**Nerve supply**: the ventral rami of adjacent nerves C. 4–C. 6. **Action**: it raises the first rib (inspiration) and produces lateral flexion of the neck.

## Omohyoid, inferior belly

The inferior belly of the omohyoid is a slender muscle which arises from the transverse scapular ligament and the adjacent part of the scapula [see Fig. 4.6 in Vol. 1]. It runs anterosuperiorly across the posterior triangle, a short distance superior to the clavicle. It joins the tendon which links it to the superior belly of the omohyoid, deep to the sternocleidomastoid.

**Nerve supply**: a branch of the ansa cervicalis [p. 68]. **Action**: it helps to steady or depress the hyoid bone in speaking and swallowing.

## Subclavian artery, third part

The right subclavian artery arises from the brachiocephalic trunk, posterior to the right sternoclavicular joint. The left arises from the arch of the aorta and enters the neck behind the left sternoclavicular joint. In the root of the neck, both arteries arch laterally in front of the cervical pleura and continue

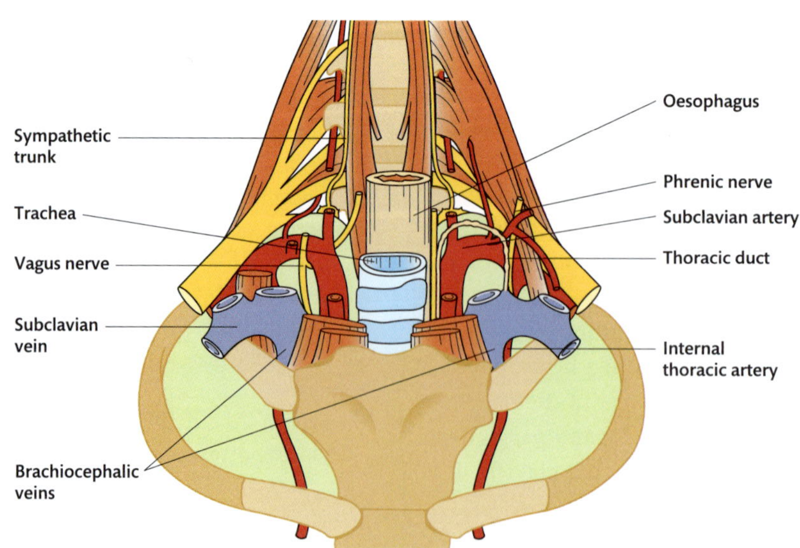


**Fig. 4.7** Dissection of the root of the neck to show the structures adjacent to the cervical pleura (green shading).

as the axillary artery at the outer border of the first rib. The anterior scalene lies in front of the artery at its highest part and divides it into three parts—a first part medial to the anterior scalene, a second part behind it, and a third part lateral to it. The first and second parts of the artery are described in Chapter 8.

The third part of the subclavian artery begins about a finger-breadth above the clavicle. It descends across the cervical pleura and lies in the subclavian groove of the first rib, anterior to the lower trunk of the brachial plexus and middle scalene. It ends at the outer border of the first rib, behind the middle of the clavicle. The suprascapular artery and the external jugular vein and its tributaries lie in front of the artery, between it and the clavicle [Fig. 4.7].

## Subclavian vein

The subclavian vein is the continuation of the axillary vein from the outer border of the first rib. It passes medially, anteroinferior to the third part of the subclavian artery and the anterior scalene. It unites with the internal jugular vein behind the sternoclavicular joint to form the brachiocephalic vein. The external jugular vein is the only tributary of the subclavian vein. It joins the subclavian vein at the lateral border of the anterior scalene. The subclavian vein has a valve near its junction with the brachiocephalic vein [Fig. 4.7].

## Suprascapular and superficial cervical vessels

The suprascapular and superficial cervical arteries arise from the **thyrocervical trunk**—a short branch of the first part of the subclavian artery. (The inferior thyroid artery is the other branch of the thyrocervical trunk.)

The **superficial cervical artery** runs laterally, anterior to the anterior scalene, phrenic nerve, upper and middle trunks of the brachial plexus, and suprascapular nerve, to the anterior border of the levator scapulae [Fig. 4.4].

The **suprascapular artery** passes inferolaterally behind the clavicle, in front of the anterior scalene and the subclavian artery. It accompanies the suprascapular nerve at the posteroinferior angle of the posterior triangle and descends with it to the scapular notch [see Fig. 4.4 in Vol. 1].

The corresponding veins end in the external jugular vein.

## The brachial plexus

The **supraclavicular part** of the brachial plexus lies in the lower part of the posterior triangle. It continues behind the clavicle into the axilla as the **infraclavicular part**.

The brachial plexus is formed by the union of the ventral rami of C. 5–T. 1, at the lateral border of the anterior scalene, deep to the lower third of the sternocleidomastoid. It ends in the axilla by dividing into the nerves of the upper limb. The supraclavicular (cervical) part of the brachial plexus consists of the roots, trunks, and divisions [Fig. 4.8].

Using the instructions given in Dissection 4.5, dissect the supraclavicular part of the brachial plexus.

### Roots of the brachial plexus

The roots of the brachial plexus are the ventral rami of the lower four cervical and first thoracic nerves (C. 5–T. 1). In addition to these, the plexus receives a variable contribution from the fourth cervical and second thoracic nerves as well.

### Trunks of the brachial plexus

The fifth and sixth cervical ventral rami (with a small contribution from the fourth) unite to form the upper trunk. The seventh cervical ventral ramus continues as the middle trunk. The eighth cervical and first thoracic ventral rami (with a small contribution from the second thoracic ventral ramus) unite to form the lower trunk [Fig. 4.8].

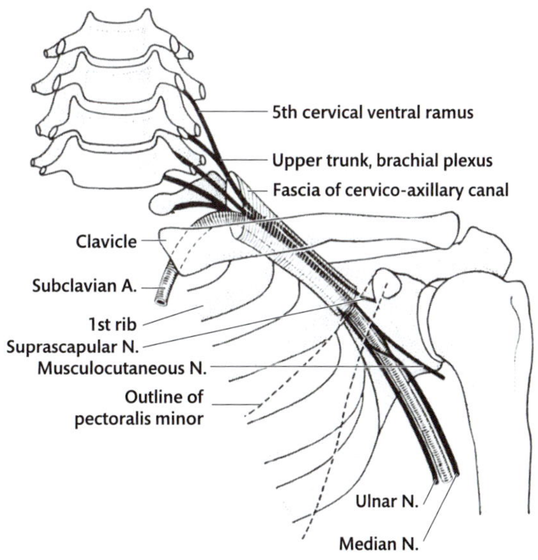

Fig. 4.8 The brachial plexus and axillary artery in the cervico-axillary canal.

**DISSECTION 4.5 Supraclavicular part of the brachial plexus**

**Objective**

**I.** To expose the roots and trunks of the brachial plexus.

**Instructions**

The brachial plexus should be dissected in conjunction with the dissection of the axilla. To expose the brachial plexus in its full extent, the clavicle should be divided between drill holes placed in its intermediate third. This allows the shoulder to fall back and opens the cervico-axillary canal. Subsequently, the clavicle should be wired together through the drill holes to replace the parts in their normal relationships.

1. Clean the fascia overlying the anterior and middle scalene, and find the ventral rami of C. 5, C. 6, C. 7, C. 8, and T. 1. These are the roots of the brachial plexus.
2. Trace C. 5 and C. 6 laterally to the formation of the upper trunk.
3. Note that C. 7 continues as the middle trunk.
4. Trace C. 8 and T. 1 laterally to the formation of the lower trunk.
5. Find the long thoracic nerve on the medial wall of the axilla, and trace it back to its origin from the roots.
6. Find and trace the nerve to the subclavius and the suprascapular nerve to the upper trunk.
7. Trace the phrenic nerve from where it has been identified on the anterior scalene to the roots.

## Divisions of the brachial plexus

Each trunk splits into an anterior and a posterior division. The three posterior divisions unite to form the **posterior cord**. The anterior divisions of the upper and middle trunks unite to form the **lateral cord**. The anterior division of the lower trunk forms the **medial cord**.

## Relations of the brachial plexus

The **supraclavicular part** of the brachial plexus lies on the middle scalene. The lower trunk lies on the superior surface of the first rib, posterior to the subclavian artery [Fig. 4.7]. The roots of the long thoracic nerve are posterior to the plexus. The external jugular vein, the inferior belly of the omohyoid, and the suprascapular and superficial cervical vessels are anterior to it.

## Brachial plexus branches in the neck

All five roots of the brachial plexus receive **grey rami communicantes** from the sympathetic trunk. The upper two roots receive from the middle cervical ganglion, and the others from the cervicothoracic ganglion.

Most of the branches in the neck are muscular and pass to the upper limb. Small nerves also pass to the scalene muscles, the longus colli [see Fig. 5.18 in Vol. 1; see Fig. 9.1], and the phrenic nerve.

The **dorsal scapular nerve** passes backwards from the fifth cervical ventral ramus through the middle scalene. It runs inferolaterally, anterior to the levator scapulae and the rhomboids major and minor, supplying all three.

The thin **nerve to the subclavius** arises where the fifth and sixth cervical ventral rami unite. It descends across the brachial plexus and subclavian vessels, and enters the posterior surface of the subclavius. It often sends a branch to the **phrenic nerve**, which may replace the C. 5 contribution to phrenic nerve.

The **suprascapular nerve** arises from the junction of the fifth and sixth cervical ventral rami. It runs posteroinferiorly on the middle scalene, lateral to the plexus. It descends with the suprascapular vessels over the scapula and supplies the supraspinatus, infraspinatus, and shoulder joint.

The **long thoracic nerve** arises by a series of branches from the upper three roots of the plexus. It descends on the surface of the middle scalene and enters the axilla over the serratus anterior on the first rib. It supplies the serratus anterior.

➲ Review the anatomical basis of Erb's and Klumpke's palsy described in *Cunningham's Manual of Practical Anatomy* 17th edition, Vol. 1, Chapter 12.

➲ Rarely, a supernumerary rib may project laterally from the transverse process of the seventh cervical vertebra. The presence of such a cervical rib may cause compression of the lower trunk of the brachial plexus and the subclavian artery. It may cause pain and tingling on the medial aspect of the forearm and hand due to pressure on the lower trunk, and ischaemia of the hand due to pressure on the subclavian artery. [See Clinical Application 4.2.]

See Clinical Applications 4.1 and 4.2 for the practical implications of the anatomy discussed in this chapter.

**CLINICAL APPLICATION 4.1 External jugular vein laceration**

A young man sustained a cut on the right side of his neck in a street fight and was found bleeding heavily on the road. He was rushed to a hospital. On arrival in the Emergency Unit, he was bleeding heavily from the site of injury, and was cyanotic and dyspnoeic. On examination, it was found that his external jugular vein had been lacerated.

Study question 1: how and where is the external jugular vein formed? And how and where does it terminate? (Answer: the external jugular vein begins by the union of the posterior branch of the retromandibular and posterior auricular veins on the surface of the sternocleidomastoid. It ends by draining into the subclavian vein in the posterior triangle.)

Study question 2: name the layer of the deep cervical fascia pierced by the vein before its termination. (Answer: investing layer of the deep fascia.)

The tight attachment of the fascia to the wall of the vein causes the wound to be pulled open. The negative intrathoracic pressure causes air to enter into the vein, leading to an air embolus.

Study question 3: from your knowledge of anatomy, in which chamber of the heart would the air embolus in the external jugular vein enter? (Answer: the embolus will go through the external jugular vein, subclavian vein, right brachiocephalic vein, and superior vena cava into the right atrium. The air embolus in the right atrium accounts for the cyanosis and dyspnoea.)

Study question 4: speculate on what steps could be taken to prevent a fatal air embolism in this case. (Answer: pressure on the vein will help control the bleeding and prevent air from entering into it.)

**CLINICAL APPLICATION 4.2 Anterior scalene syndrome**

A 43-year-old painter presented with a history of pain and tingling sensation in the medial aspect of his forearm and hand, especially while lifting his arm above his shoulder to paint a wall.

Study question 1: what is the likely diagnosis? (Answer: compression of the lower part of the brachial plexus. The scalene triangle is formed by the anterior scalene anteriorly, the middle scalene posteriorly, and the first rib inferiorly, and contains the brachial plexus and subclavian artery. Compression of the brachial plexus in the scalene triangle is a probable diagnosis.)

Study question 2: what factors often lead to compression of the contents? (Answer: any clinical conditions which decrease the space within the scalene triangle can cause compression. Common conditions include hypertrophied anterior scalene muscle, cervical rib, and fibromuscular bands between the two scalene muscles.)

Study question 3: what are the symptoms that arise due to compression? (Answer: compression of the lower trunk of the brachial plexus causes pain, numbness, or tingling sensation of the medial aspect of the forearm and arm. Compression of the subclavian artery can cause ischaemia, leading to pain and blanching of the hand.)

Study question 4: how is the diagnosis of the anterior scalene syndrome confirmed? (Answer: several manoeuvres can be done to precipitate symptoms and confirm the diagnosis of the anterior scalene syndrome. The Wright's test stimulates change in the radial pulse with hyperabduction of the arm. A fall in the radial pulse on hyperabduction of the arm indicates compression of the subclavian artery above the shoulder joint. More conclusive results are obtained by X-ray, magnetic resonance imaging, and subclavian Doppler sonography.)

# CHAPTER 5
# The anterior triangle of the neck

## Introduction

The anterior triangle of the neck is the area bound by the midline, the mandible, and the sternocleidomastoid muscle [Figs. 5.1, 5.2].

## Surface anatomy

Draw a finger in the midline from the chin to the sternum. Identify in sequence: (1) the body of the hyoid bone approximately 1 cm below, and 6 cm behind, the chin; (2) the **laryngeal prominence**, the sharp protuberance formed at the fusion of the thyroid laminae; (3) the rounded arch of the **cricoid cartilage**; and (4) the rings of the trachea, which are partly masked by the isthmus of the thyroid gland.

Grasp the U-shaped **hyoid bone** between the finger and the thumb. Trace it backwards to the greater horns. The tips of the greater horn may be overlapped by the sternocleidomastoid muscles. Trace the superior border of the **thyroid cartilage** posteriorly from its midline notch. Note that it ends in a projection—the superior horn—immediately anterior to the sternocleidomastoid. The superior border of the thyroid cartilage lies at the level of the fourth cervical vertebra C. 4. The arch of the cricoid cartilage lies at the level of sixth cervical vertebra and can be felt below the thyroid cartilage. The **isthmus of the thyroid gland** [Fig. 5.1] forms a soft mass on the second, third, and fourth tracheal rings.

Press the tip of your fingers into the side of the neck from the mastoid process downwards. The deep bony resistances felt are the **transverse processes of the cervical vertebrae**. Only the transverse process of the first cervical vertebra can be felt clearly, immediately anteroinferior to the tip of the mastoid process. The fourth is at the level of the upper border of the thyroid cartilage. The sixth is at the level of the cricoid cartilage.



Using the instructions given in Dissection 5.1, open the anterior triangle and study its superficial content.

## Superficial fascia

The superficial fascia in this region contains a variable amount of fat. It is only loosely connected to the skin and deep fascia, so the skin is freely movable. The superficial fascia contains the anterior jugular veins, the decussating fibres of the platysma, and a few small **submental lymph nodes**. These nodes lie on the deep fascia and drain lymph from the anterior part of the floor of the mouth.

### Platysma

The platysma lies in the superficial fascia. It extends down from the face to the upper part of the chest over the superior part of the anterior triangle and the anteroinferior part of the posterior triangle [refer to Chapter 4].

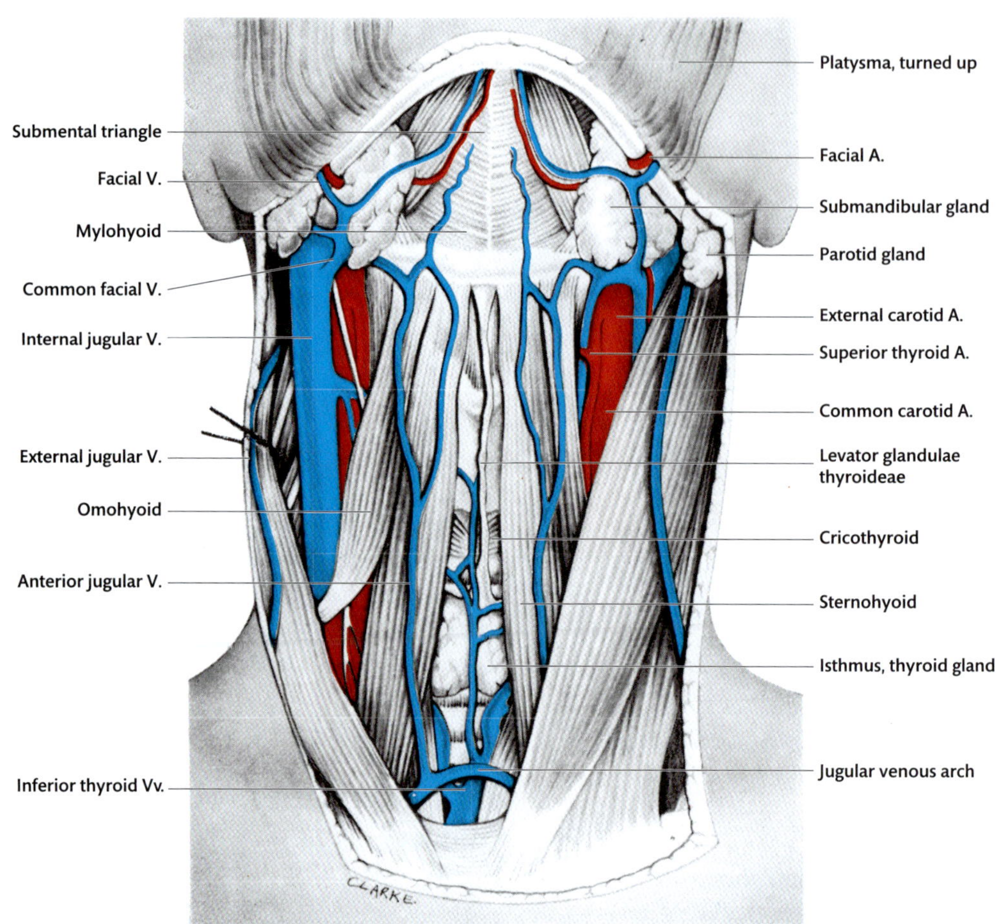


**Fig. 5.1** Dissection of the front of the neck. The right sternocleidomastoid has been retracted.

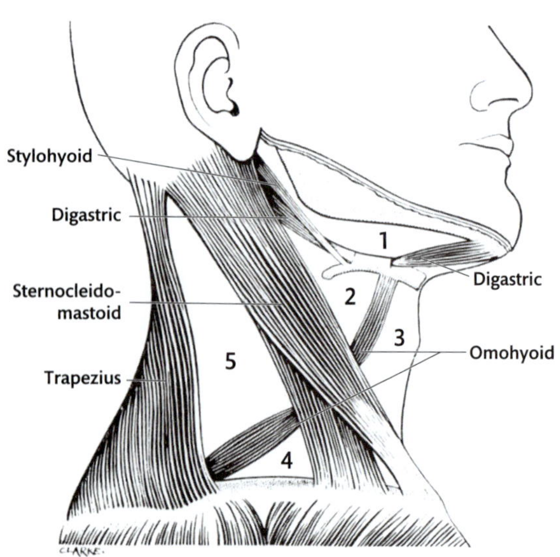


**Fig. 5.2** The triangles of the neck. Anterior triangle: 1 = digastric triangle; 2 = carotid triangle; 3 = muscular triangle. Posterior triangle: 4 = subclavian triangle; 5 = occipital triangle.

## Cervical branch of the facial nerve

The **cervical branch of the facial nerve** emerges from the lower border of the parotid gland and pierces the deep fascia. Branches arising from it spread on the deep surface of the platysma to supply it. Some fibres go over the border of the mandible to supply the muscles of the lower lip.

## Anterior jugular vein

The anterior jugular vein is usually the smallest of the three jugular veins—the internal, external, and anterior jugular veins. It varies inversely in width with the external jugular vein. It begins below the chin and descends in the superficial fascia, about 1 cm from the midline [Fig. 5.1]. Approximately 2 cm above the sternum, it pierces the first layer of the deep fascia, runs laterally in the suprasternal space, passes deep to the sternocleidomastoid, and joins the external jugular vein. It is united to

**DISSECTION 5.1 Skin reflection of the anterior triangle**

**Objectives**

**I.** To reflect the skin over the anterior triangle. **II.** To expose the platysma. **III.** To identify and trace the vessels and nerves in the superficial tissue. **IV.** To explore the suprasternal space.

**Instructions**

1. Make a midline skin incision from the chin to the sternum, and reflect the flap of skin inferolaterally. Do not cut deep, but remain superficial to the fibres of the platysma in the posterosuperior part.
2. Reflect the platysma upwards, keeping close to its deep surface and dividing any nerves which enter it.
3. Find the branches of the transverse cervical nerve [see Fig. 4.1] as they cross the sternocleidomastoid, and follow them anteriorly to their termination.
4. Identify the cervical branch of the facial nerve as it leaves the lower border of the parotid gland, and trace it anteroinferiorly.
5. Find the **anterior jugular vein** near the midline. Trace it inferiorly till it pierces the deep fascia about 2 cm above the sternum.
6. Expose the deep fascia of the anterior triangle.
7. Make a transverse incision through the first layer of the deep fascia immediately above the sternum, and extend the incision 4 cm upwards along the anterior border of the sternocleidomastoid. Reflect this fascia to open the **suprasternal space** between the first (superficial) and second (deep) layers of the fascia.
8. Trace the anterior jugular vein and the deeper layer of the fascia laterally deep to the sternocleidomastoid. Follow the fascia upwards till it fuses with the first layer (midway between the sternum and the thyroid cartilage). Follow it downwards to its fusion with the back of the sternum.

its fellow in the suprasternal space through the **jugular arch**, which may be large, and forms an important anterior relation to the trachea and thyroid gland.

The two anterior jugular veins may be replaced by a single median vein, or the anterior and external jugular veins may be partly or completely replaced by a single vein, which descends along the anterior border of the sternocleidomastoid to the jugular arch [Fig. 5.1].

Dissection 5.2 provides instructions on cleaning the sternocleidomastoid and identifying the accessory nerve.

## Sternocleidomastoid

This important landmark muscle of the neck is easily seen in the living. When contracted, it stands out as a well-defined ridge between the anterior and posterior triangles [Fig. 5.2].

The sternocleidomastoid originates by two heads: a rounded, tendinous **sternal head** from the upper part of the anterior surface of the manubrium sternum, and a thin, fleshy **clavicular head** from the upper surface of the medial third

**DISSECTION 5.2 Sternocleidomastoid and accessory nerve**

**Objectives**

**I.** To remove the fat and fascia off the sternocleidomastoid. **II.** To identify the accessory nerve and blood vessels in relation to it.

**Instructions**

1. Remove the fat and fascia from the superficial surface and margins of the sternocleidomastoid, but retain the nerves and vessels in contact with it.
2. In the anterosuperior part of the anterior triangle, push the parotid gland forwards and find the accessory nerve at the anterior border of the sternocleidomastoid.
3. Now lift the sternocleidomastoid, and note the vessels which enter it anteriorly and the structures which lie deep to it.

of the clavicle. The sternal head ascends across the medial part of the sternoclavicular joint. It widens rapidly and overlaps the clavicular head a short distance above the clavicle. The two heads fuse with each other about halfway up the neck. The thick anterior border of the sternocleidomastoid is inserted into the anterior surface of the mastoid process. The posterior part is thin and aponeurotic, and is attached to the lateral surface of the mastoid process and the lateral half of the superior nuchal line. The deep part of the sternocleidomastoid is pierced by the accessory nerve. It receives its main blood supply from the occipital and superior thyroid arteries.

**Nerve supply**: the accessory nerve is the motor nerve to the muscle. The ventral ramus of the second cervical nerve is sensory. **Actions**: acting alone, the sternocleidomastoid tilts the head to its own side and rotates the head, so that the face is turned towards the opposite side. Acting together, the two muscles flex the neck. In forced inspiration, the two muscles act together and raise the sternum when neck flexion is prevented by the extensors.

➲ Damage of the spinal part of the accessory nerve paralyses the sternocleidomastoid, causing the neck to be flexed to the opposite side and the face turned to the paralysed side by the unopposed action of the normal sternocleidomastoid. This condition is known as **wry neck**.

## Deep fascia of the neck

Review the details of the three layers of the deep fascia described in Chapter 4. In the midline, the **investing layer** of the cervical deep fascia is attached to the mandible, hyoid bone, and sternum. Superiorly, it encloses the anterior bellies of the digastric muscles. Inferiorly, it encloses the **suprasternal space**, which contains the jugular arch, the sternal head of the sternocleidomastoid, the lowest parts of the anterior jugular veins, and an occasional lymph node [Fig. 5.3]. The deeper **pretracheal fascia** descends from the thyroid and cricoid cartilages to invest the **thyroid gland** and cover the front and side of the trachea. It fuses with the back of the pericardium in the thorax [Fig. 5.3].

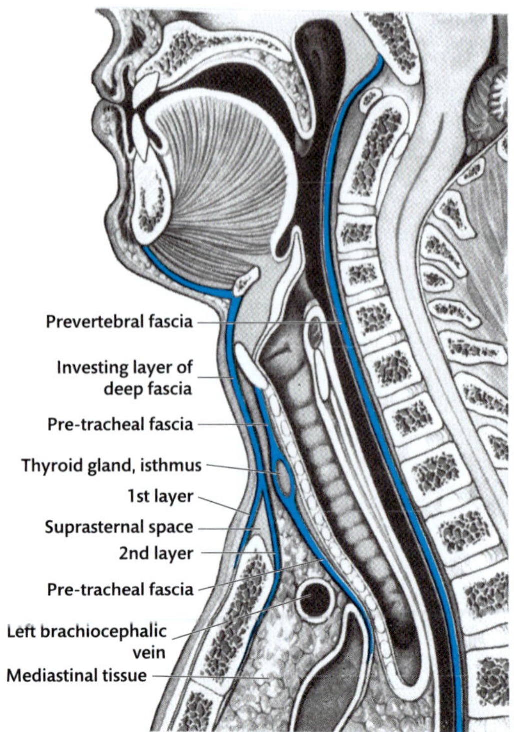


**Fig. 5.3** Diagram of the cervical fascia (blue) in sagittal section.

Dissection 5.3 describes the dissection of the midline structures of the neck.

## Midline structures in the neck

A number of midline structures lie between the infrahyoid muscles of the two sides [Fig. 5.1]. The bones and cartilages are easily palpable as described in the preceding surface marking section. From above downwards, these are:

1. The **thyrohyoid ligament**, which unites the upper border of the thyroid cartilage and the upper border of the hyoid bone. It passes deep to the hyoid bone and is separated from it by a bursa. The bursa permits the upper edge of the thyroid cartilage to ascend inside the concavity of the hyoid bone during swallowing.
2. The **laryngeal prominence** is formed by the thyroid cartilage. The cartilage is notched on its superior margin.
3. The **cricothyroid ligament** attaches the thyroid cartilage to the arch of the cricoid cartilage. On the side of the ligament, the **cricothyroid**

**DISSECTION 5.3 Midline structures of the neck**

**Objective**

**I.** To clean and identify the midline structures in the front of the neck.

**Instructions**

1. Remove the deep fascia from the anterior bellies of the digastric muscles and from the area between them. This exposes parts of the two mylohyoid muscles, which are inserted into a median raphe.
2. Continue the removal of this fascia below the hyoid. This exposes the infrahyoid muscles between the hyoid and the sternum on each side of the midline.
3. Separate these muscles in the midline to expose the pretracheal fascia.
4. Below the isthmus of the thyroid gland [Fig. 5.1], remove this fascia to expose the trachea and the inferior thyroid veins. The small thyroidea ima artery may be seen ascending to the thyroid in this region.
5. At the upper border of the isthmus, look for the slender fibromuscular band–the **levator glandulae thyroideae**–which, when present, extends between the isthmus and the hyoid bone.
6. Remove the pretracheal fascia from the isthmus.
7. Find the **cricothyroid ligament** between the median parts of the cricoid and thyroid cartilages. The small cricothyroid muscle covers it on each side.
8. Find the **median thyrohyoid ligament** between the thyroid cartilage and the hyoid bone, and the anastomosis of the infrahyoid arteries on it. Follow the ligament upwards behind the body of the hyoid bone.





**muscle** radiates posterosuperiorly from the cricoid to the thyroid cartilage. The cricothyroids are important muscles of speech and the only intrinsic laryngeal muscles to be located on the external surface of the larynx.

4. The **isthmus of the thyroid gland** usually lies on the second to fourth tracheal rings and has a rich vascular anastomosis on its surface. Occasionally, a small lobe—the **pyramidal lobe**—projects upwards from it and may give rise to a slender slip of fibromuscular tissue—the **levator glandulae thyroideae**—which attaches it to the hyoid bone. The levator glandulae thyroideae is the embryological remnant of the tubular downgrowth from the tongue—the **thyroglossal duct**.
5. Below the isthmus of the thyroid gland is the trachea with the **jugular arch** and the **inferior thyroid veins** anterior to it. Occasionally, the left brachiocephalic vein and the brachiocephalic artery extend high enough to appear in front of the trachea at the root of the neck.

## Suprahyoid muscles

The suprahyoid muscles are the anterior and posterior bellies of the digastric, mylohyoid, stylohyoid, and hyoglossus. They are described in Chapter 15.

## Subdivisions of the anterior triangle

The anterior triangle may be divided into four subsidiary triangles: the submental, carotid, muscular, and digastric triangles [Fig. 5.2].

### Submental triangle–boundaries and contents

The **submental triangle** lies in the midline and is bound by the hyoid bone and the anterior bellies of the digastric muscles. The floor of the triangle is formed by the muscular floor of the mouth (i.e. the mylohyoid muscles). The **submental lymph nodes** lie in the superficial fascia of the triangle [Fig. 5.1].

Dissection 5.4 (and Figs. 5.4, 5.5) provides instructions to dissect the digastric triangle.

### Digastric triangle–boundaries and contents

The digastric triangle is part of the submandibular region [Chapter 15]. It is bound by the anterior belly of the digastric in front, the posterior belly of the digastric and stylohyoid behind, and the lower border of the mandible above. Its floor is formed by the mylohyoid and hyoglossus muscles [Figs. 5.1, 5.2, 5.4, 5.6].

## DISSECTION 5.4 Digastric triangle

### Objective

**I.** To identify the boundaries and contents of the digastric triangle [Fig. 5.4].

### Instructions

1. Identify the facial artery and vein at the lower border of the mandible.
2. Cut the deep fascia from the mandible and turn it downwards, exposing part of the submandibular gland.
3. Identify the anterior and posterior bellies of the digastric muscle at the lower border of the gland.
4. Follow the facial vein posteroinferiorly, superficial to the gland and the posterior belly of the digastric.
5. At the lower border of the mandible, find the **submental branch of the facial artery**. Trace it forwards by pushing the submandibular gland aside and removing the fat and lymph nodes beside it. (The artery runs with the mylohyoid nerve, which supplies the mylohyoid and the anterior belly of the digastric.)
6. Pull the submandibular gland laterally to expose the intermediate tendon of the digastric, the fascial sling which attaches it to the hyoid, and the stylohyoid muscle. The stylohyoid muscle splits to enfold the intermediate tendon of the digastric and lies on the upper surface of the posterior belly of the digastric.
7. Follow the stylohyoid and the posterior belly of the digastric as far as the angle of the mandible.
8. Pull the submandibular gland back to expose the posterior border of the mylohyoid.
9. Find the hypoglossal nerve and one of the veins of the tongue passing above the free border of the mylohyoid.
10. Identify the hyoglossus, a thin sheet of muscle deep to the hypoglossal nerve [Fig. 5.5].
11. Remove the fascia from the rest of the mylohyoid and from the hyoglossus.

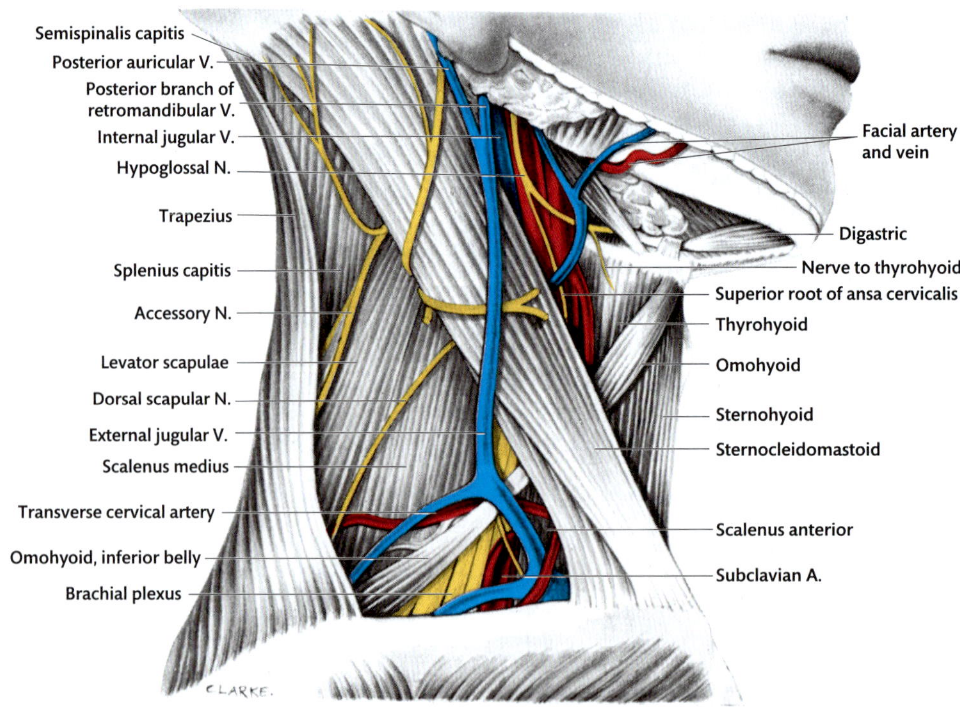


**Fig. 5.4** Lateral view of the triangles of the neck.

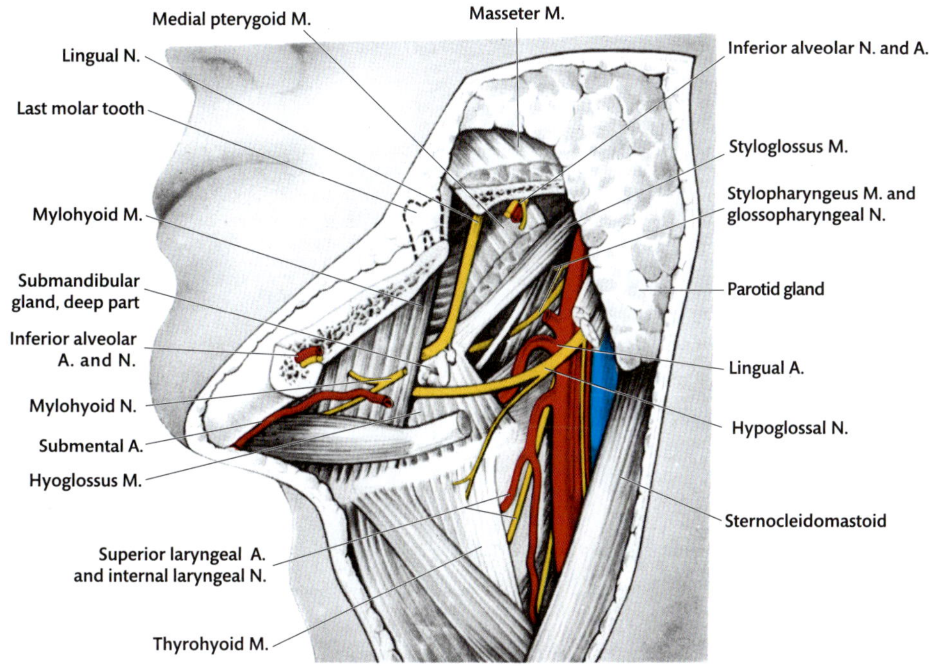


**Fig. 5.5** Deep dissection of the submandibular region.





A number of important structures lie in the digastric triangle. The lower (superficial) part of the **submandibular gland** almost fills the triangle. The **submandibular lymph nodes** lie on the surface of the gland, especially along the lower border of the mandible. These nodes drain lymph from the side of the tongue, teeth, lips, and cheek to the deep cervical lymph nodes beneath the sternocleidomastoid.

The **facial vein** pierces the deep fascia covering the triangle at the lower border of the mandible. It crosses the submandibular gland, unites with the anterior branch of the retromandibular vein, and drains into the internal jugular vein. The **facial artery** curves round the lower border of the mandible, gives off the submental artery, and pierces the deep fascia. The **submental artery** passes forwards with the corresponding vein and the mylohyoid nerve [Fig. 5.1].

The **mylohyoid nerve** lies on the inferior surface of the mylohyoid near the mandible. It supplies the mylohyoid and the anterior belly of the digastric. The **hypoglossal nerve** lies in a deeper plane, passes above the mylohyoid, and lies on the hyoglossus. The **intermediate tendon of the digastric** lies on the hyoglossus, immediately above the hyoid bone, and is held to the bone by a loop of fascia which forms a pulley for it. This arrangement permits anteroposterior movements of the hyoid when it is elevated by the digastric muscles [Fig. 5.1].

## Carotid triangle—boundaries and contents

The carotid triangle is bound by the sternocleidomastoid behind, the posterior belly of the digastric superiorly, and the superior belly of the omohyoid inferiorly [Fig. 5.2]. It contains the vertical neurovascular bundle of the neck—the common carotid and external and internal carotid arteries, internal jugular vein, and vagus nerve—covered by the sternocleidomastoid. The floor of the triangle is formed by the hyoglossus and thyrohyoid muscles anteriorly and by the middle and inferior constrictor muscles of the pharynx posteriorly [Figs. 5.4, 5.6].

Dissection 5.5 (and Fig. 5.7) provides instructions to dissect the carotid triangle.

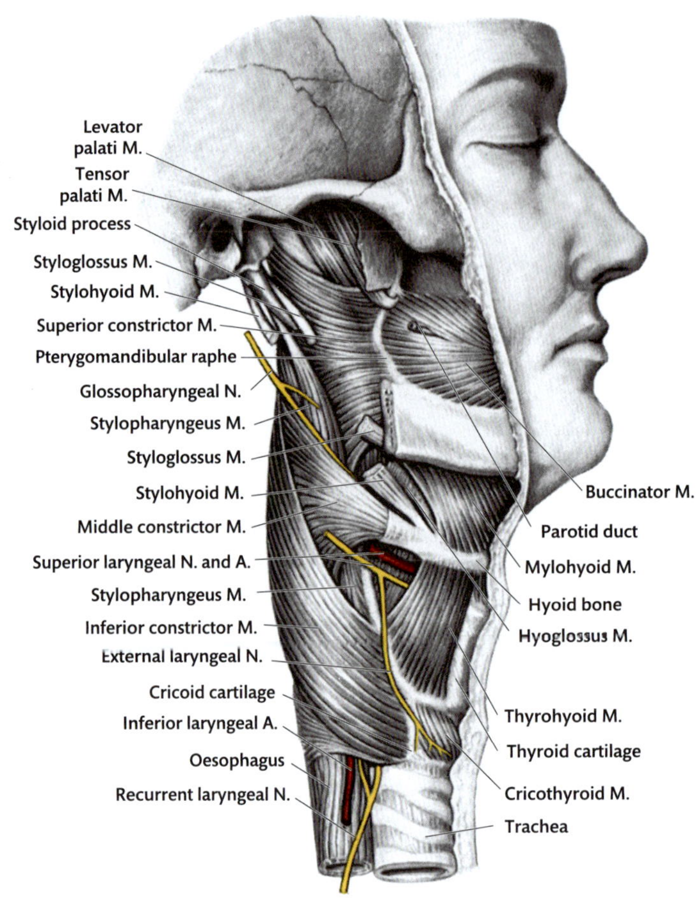


**Fig. 5.6** Lateral view of the constrictors of the pharynx and associated muscles.

## DISSECTION 5.5 Carotid triangle

### Objective

**I.** To study the boundaries and contents of the carotid triangle [Fig. 5.4].

### Instructions

1. Remove the fat and fascia from the area between the posterior belly of the digastric and the superior belly of the omohyoid [Fig. 5.2].
2. Expose the internal jugular vein laterally, the common and internal carotid arteries medial to it, and the external carotid artery anteromedial to the internal carotid artery.
3. Find the facial and lingual veins entering the internal jugular vein in the upper part of the triangle, and the superior thyroid vein entering it in the lower part.
4. Between the vein and the internal carotid artery, find the **hypoglossal nerve**. Follow it forwards across the external carotid artery, and find the following branches in the carotid triangle: (1) the superior root of the ansa cervicalis, given off where the nerve hooks round the occipital artery to enter the triangle; and (2) the branch to the thyrohyoid muscle, given off as the hypoglossal leaves the carotid triangle [Fig. 5.4].
5. Remove the superficial part of the carotid sheath which surrounds the internal jugular vein, carotid arteries, and vagus nerve. Avoid injury to the superior root of the **ansa cervicalis** anterior to the vein and to its inferior root lateral to the vein. (The inferior root of the ansa cervicalis arises from the second and third cervical ventral rami. The two roots unite to form a loop—the ansa cervicalis—at a lower level.)
6. Expose the **external carotid artery** and its branches [Figs. 5.5, 5.7]. The superior thyroid is the lowest branch in the carotid triangle [Fig. 5.7]. The lingual, facial, and occipital arteries arise in the upper part

of the triangle; the occipital artery arises opposite the facial artery [Fig. 5.7].

7. Find the internal laryngeal nerve in the interval between the hyoid bone and the thyroid cartilage [Fig. 5.5]. Trace it posterosuperiorly, deep to the carotid arteries, to the parent stem, the superior laryngeal branch of the vagus. From the superior laryngeal nerve, follow the slender external laryngeal nerve downwards, deep to the superior thyroid artery [Fig. 5.6].
8. Expose the part of the hyoglossus which lies in the carotid triangle immediately above the hyoid bone. Note the hypoglossal nerve on its surface, and the **lingual artery** lying deep to it. The lingual artery lies on the middle constrictor of the pharynx [Fig. 5.6], which separates it from the mucous membrane of the pharynx.
9. Raise the posterior belly of the digastric to expose the middle constrictor at the hyoid bone [Fig. 5.6].
10. Find the thyrohyoid muscle in the floor of the carotid triangle.
11. Push the superior thyroid and carotid arteries posteriorly, and remove the fat surrounding the external laryngeal nerve. This exposes a part of the inferior constrictor muscle which passes backwards from the side of the thyroid cartilage.
12. Separate the internal and common carotid arteries from the internal jugular vein, and expose the vagus nerve in the posterior part of the carotid sheath between them. Pull the arteries anteromedially, and find the sympathetic trunk posteromedial to the sheath.

## Carotid sheath

The **carotid sheath** is a fascial sheath enclosing the internal jugular vein, the common and internal carotid arteries, the vagus nerve, and the superior and inferior roots of the ansa cervicalis [see Fig. 4.2A]. The sympathetic trunk is on the posteromedial wall of the sheath, and many **lymph nodes** lie on its superficial surface.

The common carotid artery divides at the level of the upper border of the thyroid cartilage into the internal and external carotid arteries. The internal jugular vein descends vertically, first with the internal and then with the common carotid artery medial to it.

## External carotid artery

The external carotid artery begins at the upper border of the thyroid cartilage as a branch of the common carotid artery. It ascends along the side of the pharynx, anteromedial to the internal carotid artery. It gives off the following branches in the carotid triangle [Fig. 5.7]. (The full extent of the external carotid artery and details of its branches are described with the deeper dissection of the neck in Chapter 8.)

1. The **superior thyroid artery** curves anteroinferiorly and disappears deep to the omohyoid.
2. The **ascending pharyngeal artery** arises from the lowest part of the external carotid artery. It ascends deep to the internal carotid artery on the lateral side of the pharynx.
3. The **lingual artery** arises behind the tip of the greater horn of the hyoid bone. It runs forwards on the middle constrictor of the pharynx, hooks above the tip of the greater horn, and passes medial to the hyoglossus.
4. The **facial artery** arises above the lingual artery and leaves the triangle by looping upwards deep to the posterior belly of the digastric.
5. The **occipital artery** runs posterosuperiorly along the lower border of the posterior belly of the digastric.

## Veins in the carotid triangle

The **facial vein** enters the carotid triangle superficial to the posterior belly of the digastric. It unites with the anterior branch of the retromandibular vein, as it crosses the carotid arteries, and drains into the internal jugular vein [Fig. 5.4]. It may receive the lingual and superior thyroid veins.

The **lingual vein** is formed at the posterior border of the hyoglossus by the union of veins which run with the lingual artery and the hypoglossal nerve. It crosses the carotid arteries and drains into either the internal jugular vein or the facial vein.

The **superior thyroid vein** drains into either the internal jugular vein or the facial vein.

## Nerves in the carotid triangle

The **accessory nerve** runs posteroinferiorly across the upper angle of the triangle, either superficial or deep to the internal jugular vein.

The **hypoglossal nerve** (which supplies the muscles of the tongue) appears at the lower border of the posterior belly of the digastric, curves forwards on the carotid arteries at the root of the occipital artery and the curve of the lingual artery,

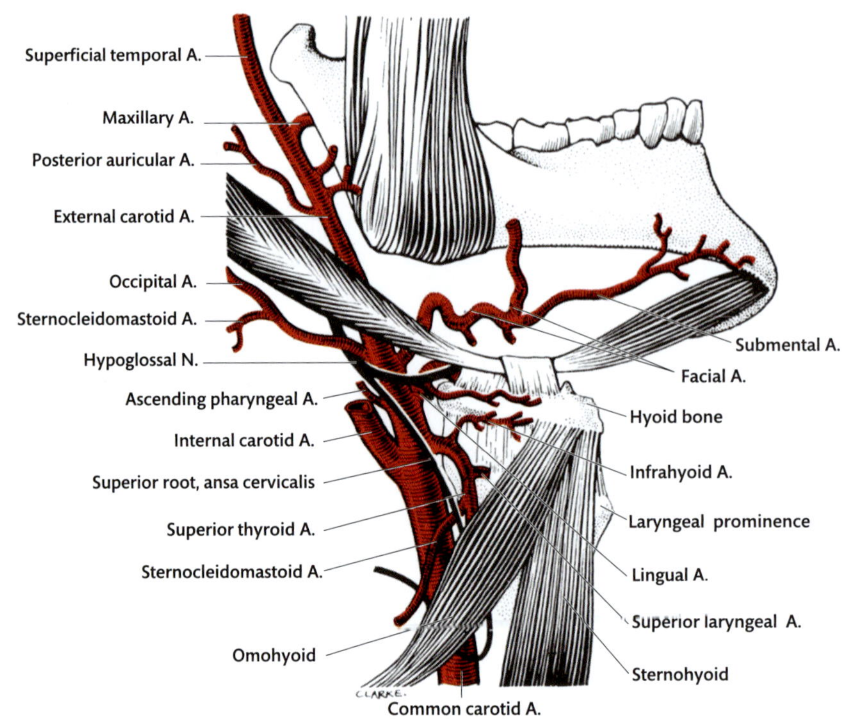


**Fig. 5.7** External carotid artery and its branches. The mandible has been tilted upwards.

and leaves the triangle by passing deep to the posterior belly of the digastric. In the carotid triangle, the hypoglossal nerve gives off the **superior root of the ansa cervicalis** (which descends on the internal and common carotid arteries) and the thyrohyoid branch which passes forwards to that muscle. Both branches are composed of fibres of the ventral ramus of the first cervical nerve, which join the hypoglossal nerve close to the skull [Figs. 5.4, 5.5, 5.7]. Further details of the hypoglossal nerve are given in Chapters 8 and 15.

### Ansa cervicalis

The ansa cervicalis is formed by two roots which unite with each other to form a loop. The slender **inferior root of the ansa cervicalis** arises from the ventral rami of the second and third cervical nerves behind the internal jugular vein. It curves forwards, usually on the lateral surface of the vein, and passes down on the common carotid artery. Here it joins the superior root from the hypoglossal nerve. The loop lies at the level of the lower part of the larynx.

The ansa cervicalis consists of nerve fibres from the cervical ventral rami of C. 1, C. 2, and C. 3. It supplies the **infrahyoid muscles**—sternohyoid, sternothyroid, and omohyoid. The thyrohyoid and geniohyoid are supplied by C. 1 fibres which run along with the hypoglossal nerve [see Fig. 15.3]. (In this way, the hypoglossal and first three cervical ventral rami form a secondary plexus which supply a ventral strip of muscles from the tongue to the sternum.)

## Muscular triangle—boundaries and contents

This triangle is bound by the sternocleidomastoid inferolaterally, the superior belly of the omohyoid superolaterally, and the midline anteriorly. It contains the infrahyoid muscles and the midline structures of the neck [Figs. 5.1, 5.2].

Dissection 5.6 provides instructions to dissect the muscular triangle.

### Infrahyoid muscles

The infrahyoid muscles—sternohyoid, sternothyroid, thyrohyoid, and omohyoid—form two layers of ribbon-like muscles extending from the sternum to the hyoid bone [Fig. 5.1]. The deeper muscle layer (sternothyroid and thyrohyoid) is interrupted at the thyroid cartilage. The muscles lie on the

**DISSECTION 5.6 Muscular triangle**

**Objective**

**I.** To study the boundaries and contents of the muscular triangle.

**Instructions**

1. Pull back the sternal head of the sternocleidomastoid to expose the anterior jugular vein deep to it.
2. Find the intermediate tendon of the omohyoid, and raise the superior belly to expose its nerve. Trace this nerve to the ansa cervicalis, and expose the entire ansa and its branches.
3. Remove the fascia from the infrahyoid muscles, but retain their nerves.
4. Define the attachments of the sternohyoid. To define the sternal attachment, pass the handle of a knife down between it and the sternum. Then divide the muscle low down, and reflect it upwards to the hyoid. This exposes the sternothyroid, the thyrohyoid, and their attachments.

trachea, thyroid gland, larynx, and thyrohyoid membrane. The thin fascia which encloses them is thickened around the intermediate tendon of the omohyoid and holds it down to the sternum and clavicle.

The **sternohyoid** lies superficial to the sternothyroid and thyrohyoid. It extends from the posterior surface of the manubrium and the medial end of the clavicle to the lower border of the hyoid bone adjacent to the midline [Fig. 5.1].

The superior belly of the **omohyoid** is attached to the inferior surface of the body and the greater horn of the hyoid, immediately lateral to the sternohyoid [Fig. 5.1]. Inferiorly, it continues with the inferior belly of the omohyoid at the intermediate tendon. The intermediate tendon lies on the internal jugular vein under the sternocleidomastoid, at the level of the cricoid cartilage. The inferior belly of the omohyoid extends from the intermediate tendon to the scapular notch [see Fig. 4.4 in Vol. 1].

The **sternothyroid** is shorter and wider, and is situated deep to the sternohyoid. It arises from the sternum and first costal cartilage below the attachment of the sternohyoid. It ascends to the oblique line on the lateral surface of the thyroid cartilage [see Fig. 19.2], superficial to the attachment of the pre-tracheal fascia and the cricothyroid muscle. It is anterior to the large vessels of the thorax at the root of the neck, and to the thyroid gland.

The **thyrohyoid** seems like the upward continuation of the sternothyroid. It extends from the oblique line on the thyroid cartilage to the lower border of the greater horn of the hyoid bone [Fig. 5.6]. It is deep to the omohyoid and sternohyoid, and covers the entry of the internal laryngeal nerve to the larynx.

**Nerve supply**: the ventral rami of the first three cervical nerves supply the omohyoid, sternohyoid, and sternothyroid muscles through the ansa cervicalis. The thyrohyoid nerve, C. 1 fibres which run with the hypoglossal, supplies the thyrohyoid. **Actions**: the infrahyoid muscles move the larynx and hyoid bone in speech and swallowing. They can: (1) depress the hyoid bone or, when acting with the suprahyoid muscles, fix the hyoid to form a stable base for the tongue; (2) draw the larynx towards the hyoid (thyrohyoid), as in the early phase of swallowing; and (3) depress the larynx, leaving the hyoid in position (sternothyroid), as in the last phase of swallowing.

See Clinical Application 5.1 for the practical implications of the anatomy discussed in this chapter.

### CLINICAL APPLICATION 5.1 Carotid artery stenosis

A 75-year-old woman was brought to the hospital by relatives, with a history of disorientation and memory loss. On examination, the woman was well oriented in time and space, and could recall events that occurred in the distant past, as well as events that occurred earlier that day. She, however, recounted that she had no clear recollection of events that happened two days ago—the day the relatives reported disorientation. The physician made a tentative diagnosis of transient ischaemic attack and ordered a colour Doppler study.

Study question 1: what is a transient ischaemic attack? (Answer: a sudden, focal loss of neurological function which disappears within 24 hours is a transient ischaemic attack.)

Study question 2: from your knowledge of anatomy, involvement of which vessel could have caused this ischaemia? (Answer: the internal carotid artery or vertebral artery. However, disorientation and memory loss are more likely to occur with involvement of the internal carotid artery.)

Colour Doppler of the neck vessels showed stenosis (narrowing) of the internal carotid artery in the neck by an atherosclerotic plaque. A carotid endarterectomy was performed to remove the plaque, and the patient had an uneventful recovery.

Study question 3: what important structures lie close to the internal carotid artery in the neck? (Answer: cranial nerves IX, X, XI, and XII, and the laryngeal and pharyngeal branches of X and XI lie close to the internal carotid artery in the neck. They are bound to the artery by the carotid sheath.)

CHAPTER 6

# The back

## Introduction to the back

This chapter describes the muscles, vessels, and nerves of the posterior aspect of the trunk, with special attention to the back of the neck. The contents of the vertebral column are discussed separately in Chapter 20.

## Back of the neck

Begin the study of this region by reviewing the surface anatomy of the back [Vol. 1, p. 73]. The investing layer of the deep cervical fascia encloses the trapezius and is attached in the midline to the external occipital protuberance, ligamentum nuchae, and spine of the seventh cervical vertebra.

Dissection 6.1 (and Fig. 6.1) gives instructions on skin reflection and identification of cutaneous nerves of the back.

## General arrangement of muscles of the back

The muscles of the back are classified into two groups: the **extrinsic** and **intrinsic** muscles. The extrinsic muscles are posterior (superficial) to the intrinsic muscles and act on the upper limb and rib cage. They include the trapezius, latissimus dorsi, levator scapulae, rhomboids major and minor, and serratus posterior superior and serratus posterior inferior.

The intrinsic muscles of the back are confined to the back and are supplied by the dorsal rami of the spinal nerves. They include the splenius, erector spinae, semispinalis, and muscles of the suboccipital triangle. They are arranged in layers [Table 6.1]. The interspinales are short muscles which extend between adjacent spinous processes, and the intertransversarii extend between adjacent transverse processes. Detailed dissection and description of all the muscles of the back is beyond the scope of this book.



### Extrinsic muscles

The upper limb muscles on the back are described in Vol. 1, Chapter 6. The cervical parts of the trapezius, levator scapulae, and serratus posterior superior and inferior are described here.

#### Trapezius

The trapezius arises from the medial third of the superior nuchal line, external occipital protuberance, ligamentum nuchae, spines of the seventh cervical, and all the thoracic vertebrae. At the cervicothoracic junction, it arises from an aponeurosis which spreads laterally into the muscle [see Fig. 6.2 in Vol. 1].

The upper fibres run downwards and laterally, and are inserted into the lateral third of the clavicle. They form the slope of the shoulder. The middle fibres run horizontally to the medial edge of the acromion and the lateral part of the superior margin of the crest of the spine of the scapula. The lower fibres run upwards and laterally to the superior margin of the crest of the spine of the scapula [Figs. 6.1, 6.2].

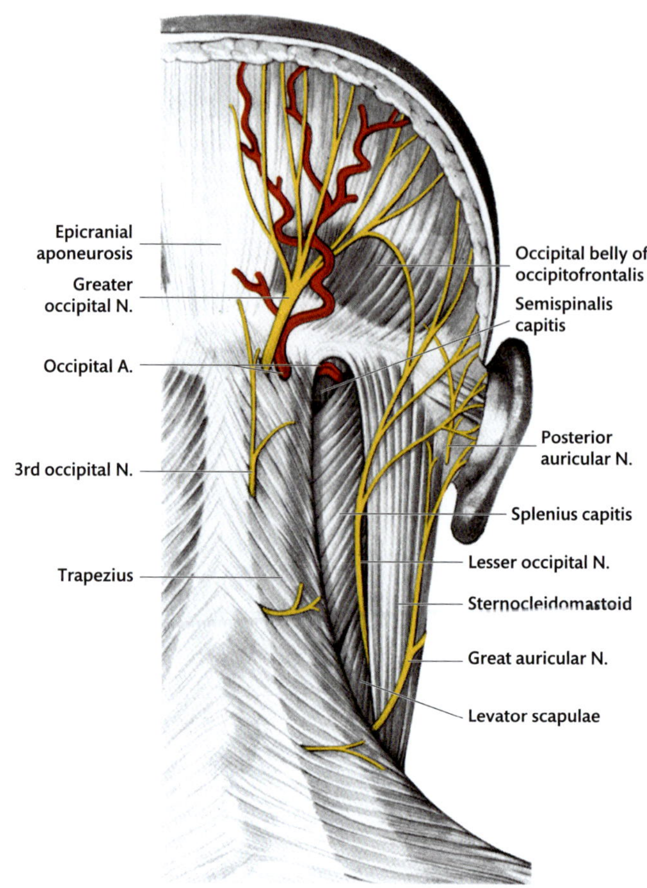


**Fig. 6.1** Superficial structures of the back of the neck.

## DISSECTION 6.1 Skin reflection and cutaneous nerves of the back

### Objectives

**I.** To reflect the skin on the back of the neck. **II.** To identify and trace the posterior auricular, greater occipital, and third occipital nerves.

### Instructions

1. Make a vertical midline incision through the skin from the external occipital protuberance to the seventh cervical spine. Make a horizontal incision laterally from the lower end of the first incision. Reflect the skin flap, and examine the posterior triangle from behind.
2. Expose the occipital belly of the occipitofrontalis, with the occipital branch of the **posterior auricular nerve** (branch of the facial nerve) running across it near its attachment [Fig. 6.1].
3. Find a branch of the occipital artery on the back of the scalp, and a branch of the greater occipital nerve beside it. Trace both downwards to the main stem of the nerve and artery. The **greater occipital nerve** pierces the deep fascia 2–3 cm lateral to the external occipital protuberance with the occipital artery [Fig. 6.1].
4. The **third occipital nerve** lies in the superficial fascia, medial to the greater occipital nerve. Find and follow it in both directions. Like the cutaneous branches of the other cervical dorsal rami, it pierces the trapezius and the deep fascia close to the midline.
5. Remove the superficial and deep fascia from the surface of the trapezius.

**Table 6.1** Intrinsic muscles of the back

| Layer | Muscles |
|---|---|
| Superficial layer | Splenius |
| Intermediate layer (erector spinae) | 1. Spinalis |
| | 2. Longissimus |
| | 3. Iliocostalis |
| Deep layer (spinotransverse group) | 1. Rotators |
| | 2. Multifidus |
| | 3. Semispinalis |

**Nerve supply**: motor fibres are from the spinal accessory nerve, the eleventh cranial nerve. Sensory fibres are from the third and fourth cervical nerves. **Actions**: the middle fibres pull the scapula medially, bracing the shoulder backwards. The upper fibres elevate the scapula. The lower fibres depress the medial part of the scapula. Acting together, the upper and lower parts rotate the scapula laterally, turning the glenoid cavity upwards, as in raising the arm above the head. The trapezius also extends the head on the neck.

Using the instructions given in Dissection 6.2, complete the superficial dissection of the neck.

### DISSECTION 6.2 Superficial dissection of the back of the neck

#### Objectives

**I.** To reflect the trapezius and trace the vessels and nerves deep to it. **II.** To reflect the levator scapulae and trace the vessels and nerves deep to it.

#### Instructions

1. Reflect the trapezius laterally by separating it from the superior nuchal line and dividing it vertically 1 cm from the vertebral spines.
2. Find the accessory nerve on its deep surface with the branches from the third and fourth cervical nerves. Find the superficial transverse cervical artery which runs with the accessory nerve.
3. Define the attachments of the levator scapulae, and follow the deep cervical artery and the dorsal scapular nerve on its deep surface.

## Levator scapulae

The levator scapulae arise from the transverse processes of the upper four cervical vertebrae. It descends as two or more slips and is inserted into the medial border of the scapula from the upper angle to the spine of the scapula [see Fig. 6.2 in Vol. 1].

**Nerve supply**: ventral rami of the third and fourth cervical nerves and the dorsal scapular nerve. **Actions**: elevation and medial rotation of the scapula. It also helps to hold the scapula steady in movements of the upper limb.

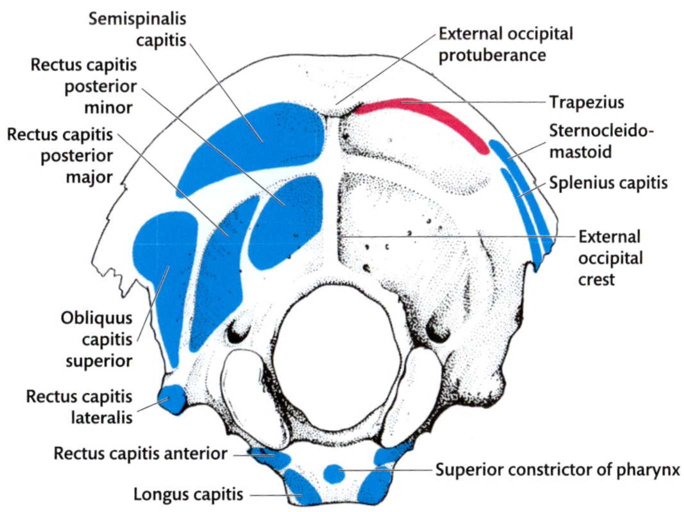


**Fig. 6.2** Muscle attachments to the occipital bone. Red = origins; blue = insertions.

### Serratus posterior

The serratus posterior muscles are exposed when the trapezius, latissimus dorsi, and rhomboid muscles are removed and the scapula is pulled laterally. They are thin musculo-aponeurotic sheets on the back of the thorax.

The serratus posterior superior runs inferolaterally from the seventh cervical and upper two or three thoracic spines to the second to fifth ribs.

The serratus posterior inferior passes superolaterally from the lumbar fascia and the lower two thoracic spines to the last four ribs.

**Nerve supply**: the serratus posterior superior receives branches from the second to fourth intercostal nerves. The serratus posterior inferior receives branches from the lower intercostal and subcostal nerves. **Actions**: both muscles are inspiratory muscles; the superior elevates the upper ribs, and the inferior holds down the lower ribs against the pull of the diaphragm.

## Intrinsic muscles

Using the instructions given in Dissection 6.3 (and Fig. 6.3), identify some of the intrinsic muscles.

## Superficial layer–splenius

The splenius is most superficially placed among the intrinsic muscles of the back. It covers the deeper muscles of the neck like a blanket. **Origin**: it arises from the lower part of the ligamentum nuchae, and the spines of the seventh cervical and upper six thoracic vertebrae. **Insertion**: the muscle fibres run superolaterally, and the lower fibres—the **splenius cervicis**—are inserted into the transverse processes of the upper two or three cervical vertebrae, deep to the levator scapulae. The upper fibres—the **splenius capitis**—are inserted into the lower part of the mastoid process and the lateral part of the superior nuchal line, deep to the sternocleidomastoid [Figs. 6.1, 6.2, 6.3, 6.4].

**Nerve supply**: the dorsal rami of the cervical nerves. **Actions**: acting together, the muscles of both sides extend the neck and the head on it. Acting on one side only, the splenius turns the face to the same side.

## Intermediate layer–erector spinae and thoracolumbar fascia

### Thoracolumbar fascia

The thoracolumbar fascia is a strong aponeurotic layer which extends from the ilium and dorsal surface of the sacrum to the upper thoracic region. It binds down the erector spinae group of muscles and is particularly thick in the lumbar and sacral regions [Vol. 2, Chapter 12].

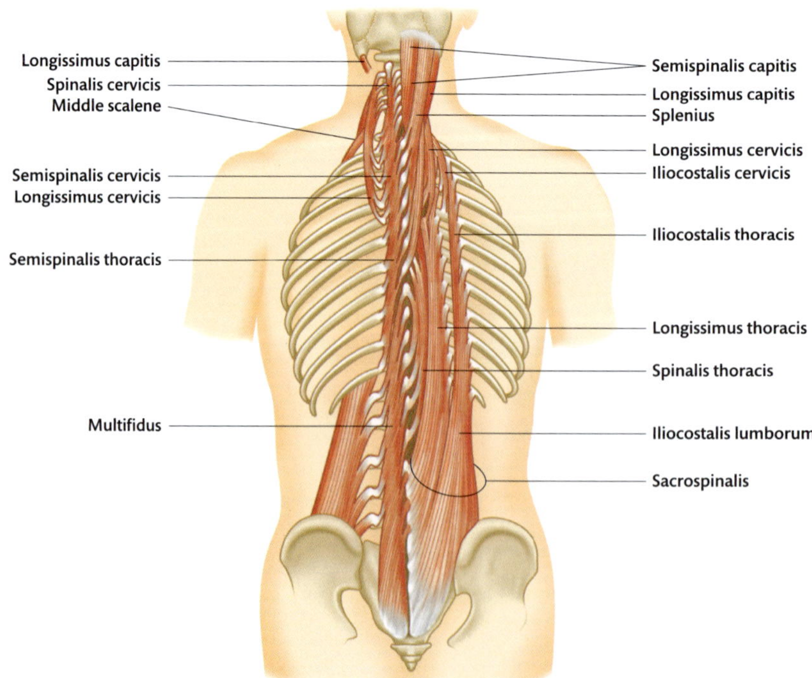


**Fig. 6.3** Intrinsic muscles of the back.

**DISSECTION 6.3 Intrinsic muscles of the back-1**

**Objective**

**I.** To identify the splenius, erector spinae, semispinalis, and longissimus [Fig. 6.3].

**Instructions**

1. Reflect the serratus posterior superior, and find the nerves entering its deep surface.
2. Remove the thoracic part of the thoracolumbar fascia to expose the longitudinal erector spinae muscles, with the splenius curving superolaterally across it above the mid-thoracic region.
3. Define the attachments of the splenius, and find the nerves piercing it. Then separate the splenius from the vertebral spines, and turn it superolaterally.
4. Remove the thoracic part of the thoracolumbar fascia to expose the erector spinae muscles.
5. Examine the semispinalis (part of the spinotransverse group of muscles) and longissimus muscles (part of the erector spinae).
6. Identify the part of the obliquus capitis superior which is exposed.
7. Detach the sternocleidomastoid from the superior nuchal line, and expose the insertion of the splenius capitis.

The thoracic part of this fascia is relatively thin and transparent. It extends from the tip of the spine of the vertebrae and supraspinous ligaments to the angles of the ribs. Superiorly, the fascia passes deep to the serratus posterior superior and fades out into the neck. Inferiorly, it is continuous with the posterior layer of the lumbar part, deep to the serratus posterior inferior [Fig. 6.5].

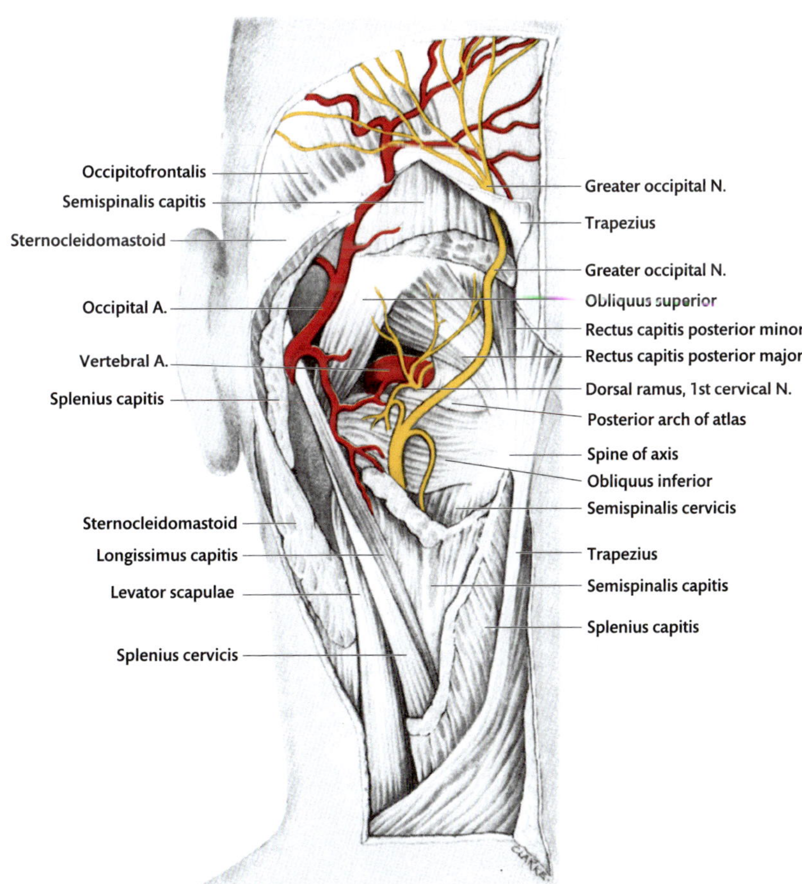


**Fig. 6.4** The suboccipital region. Deep structures of the back of the neck.

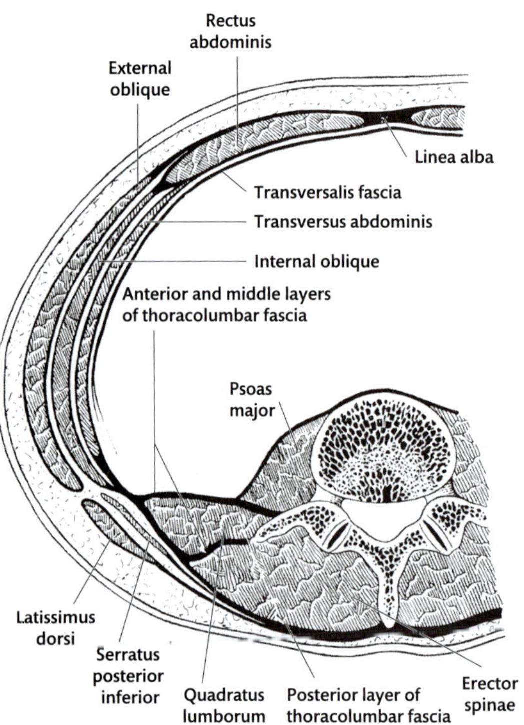


**Fig. 6.5** Diagram of a section through the abdominal wall at the level of the second lumbar vertebra to show the arrangement of the thoracolumbar fascia.

## Erector spinae

The major part of the erector spinae muscle takes origin from the sacrum and ascends into the lumbar, thoracic, and cervical regions [Fig. 6.3]. It fills the space between the spines and transverse processes of the vertebrae and splits into three vertical columns of muscles. From lateral to medial, the three columns are: the **iliocostalis**, **longissimus**, and **spinalis**. The iliocostalis is inserted into the lower ribs and cervical transverse processes. The longissimus is inserted into the cervical transverse processes and the mastoid process. The spinalis is inserted into the spinous process. At the insertion into the spine and transverse process, fresh slips arise from the same situations and continue upwards. The longissimus cervicis and capitis are described in further detail below.

## Deep layer

Deep to the erector spinae are the muscles which connect the sacrum with the transverse processes, laminae, and spines. They are known as the **spinotransverse muscles** and include the **semispinalis**, **multifidus**, and **rotatores** [Fig. 6.3]. The semispinalis cervicis and capitis are described in further detail below.

**Nerve supply**: dorsal rami of the spinal nerves. **Actions**: these muscles act on the vertebral column to bring about: (1) extension; (2) rotation; and (3) lateral flexion. In addition, they help to balance the vertebral column on the pelvis and maintain an erect posture during all movements.

Using the instructions given in Dissection 6.4, dissect the semispinalis, longissimus, and suboccipital muscles.

## Longissimus

This slender muscle is part of the erector spinae. In the neck, it lies under cover of the splenius, immediately posterior to the transverse processes [Fig. 6.3]. It has two parts—the **longissimus cervicis** and **longissimus capitis**. The longissimus takes origin from the upper thoracic transverse processes. The longissimus capitis is inserted to the back of the mastoid process under cover of the splenius

### DISSECTION 6.4 Intrinsic muscles of the back-2

#### Objectives

**I.** To expose the semispinalis and longissimus and study their attachments. **II.** To identify and trace the occipital and deep cervical arteries. **III.** To identify the suboccipital muscles.

#### Instructions

1. Remove the fascia from the semispinalis capitis and from the longissimus. (Do not disturb the nerves which pierce the semispinalis close to the midline.)
2. Determine the attachments of these muscles.
3. Reflect the longissimus capitis from the skull, and follow the occipital artery deep to the mastoid process over the obliquus capitis superior.
4. Trace the obliquus capitis superior to the transverse process of the atlas and to the skull [Fig. 6.4].
5. Detach the semispinalis capitis from the occipital bone, and turn it laterally, preserving the nerves which pierce it.
6. Identify the suboccipital muscles and semispinalis cervicis, with the dorsal rami running over them.
7. Identify the **deep cervical artery** ascending on the semispinalis capitis to anastomose with the occipital artery. (If a branch from the first cervical dorsal ramus enters the semispinalis capitis, it should be retained by cutting out a piece of the muscle with the nerve, as this makes the dissection of that ramus much easier.)
8. Define the attachments of the semispinalis cervicis.

and sternocleidomastoid. The longissimus cervicis lies anterior to the longissimus capitis. It is inserted into the posterior surfaces of the cervical transverse processes of C. 2–C. 7 vertebrae.

## Occipital artery

The occipital artery arises from the external carotid artery in the front of the neck. It runs posterosuperiorly deep to the posterior belly of the digastric. It grooves the skull deep to the mastoid notch and the insertion of the posterior belly of the digastric. It then passes posteriorly immediately deep to the muscles attached to the superior nuchal line, crosses the apex of the posterior triangle, and pierces the trapezius 2–3 cm from the midline with the greater occipital nerve. It ramifies on the back of the head, supplying the posterior half of the scalp [Fig. 6.1].

**Branches**: in the back, the artery gives off mainly (1) muscular branches. In addition, it gives: (2) a mastoid branch which enters the mastoid foramen to supply the bone and dura mater; and (3) a descending branch which passes deep to the semispinalis capitis and anastomoses with the deep cervical branch of the subclavian artery.

### Semispinalis capitis

This long muscle is part of the deep layer. It produces the rounded ridge on either side of the median furrow in the back of the neck, even though it is deep to the trapezius and splenius. It has the same origin as the longissimus capitis—the upper thoracic transverse processes—and is inserted into the medial half of the area between the superior and inferior nuchal lines [Figs. 6.2, 6.3, 6.4].

**Nerve supply**: dorsal rami of the upper cervical nerves. **Action**: it extends the neck and the head on the neck.

### Semispinalis cervicis

This bulky muscle lies deep to the semispinalis capitis and has the same origin—the upper thoracic transverse processes. It passes superomedially to the spines of the second to fifth cervical vertebrae, principally the second—a feature which partly accounts for the size of the spine of the axis.

## Ligamentum nuchae

The ligamentum nuchae is a median fibrous septum between the muscles of the back of the neck. It is a continuation of the supraspinous and interspinous ligaments uniting the cervical vertebrae. It extends from the spine of the seventh cervical vertebra to the external occipital protuberance and crest. Anteriorly, it is attached to the posterior tubercle of the atlas and the spines of the other cervical vertebrae [Fig. 6.6].



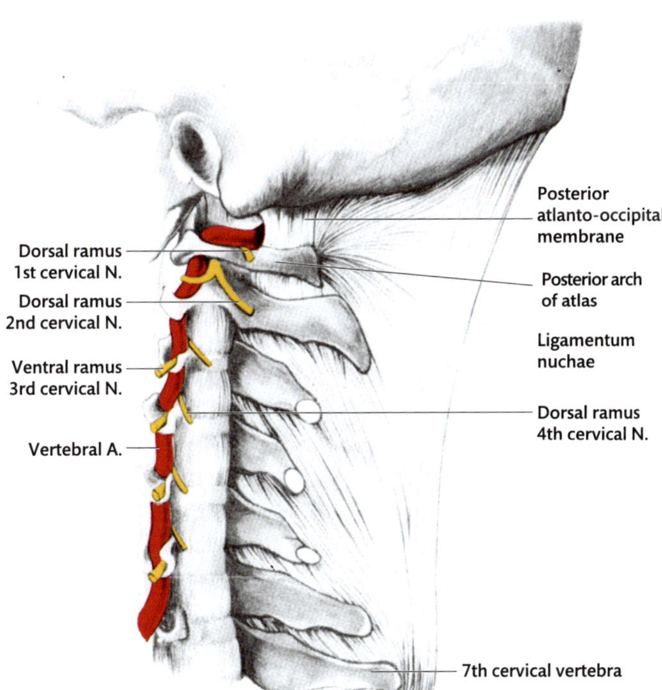


**Fig. 6.6** Dissection of the ligamentum nuchae and of the vertebral artery in the neck. The neck is slightly flexed.

## Deep cervical artery

The deep cervical artery arises from the costocervical trunk of the subclavian artery. It passes into the back of the neck between the seventh cervical transverse process and the neck of the first rib. It ascends deep to the semispinalis capitis and anastomoses with the descending branch of the occipital artery [see Fig. 8.8].

## Suboccipital triangle—boundaries and content

This small intermuscular triangle is formed by the **rectus capitis posterior major** superomedially, the **obliquus capitis inferior** inferiorly, and the **obliquus capitis superior** superolaterally. The **rectus capitis posterior minor** lies medial to the major. These muscles hold the skull to the axis and atlas. The triangle is roofed over by the semispinalis capitis and crossed by the greater occipital nerve, which hooks around the lower border of the obliquus capitis inferior. The floor of the triangle is formed by the posterior atlanto-occipital membrane and the posterior arch of the atlas, with the first cervical nerve and the vertebral artery lying on it. The triangle contains the suboccipital plexus of veins which drain to the vertebral and deep cervical veins and the dorsal ramus of the first cervical nerve [Fig. 6.4].

Using the instructions given in Dissection 6.5, dissect the suboccipital triangle.

### DISSECTION 6.5 Suboccipital triangle

#### Objectives

**I.** To identify the dorsal ramus of the first cervical nerve. **II.** To expose the muscles of the suboccipital triangle.

#### Instructions

1. Identify the dorsal ramus of the first cervical nerve, as it emerges between the vertebral artery and the posterior arch of the atlas. (The suboccipital triangle is difficult to dissect because of the dense fibrous tissue in it. If the branch of the dorsal ramus of the first cervical nerve to the semispinalis capitis has been retained, it can be followed to the ramus and the other branches traced from there. Alternatively, a communicating branch to the greater occipital nerve or the branch to one of the muscles of the triangle may be found and followed.)
2. Remove the fascia from the triangle and surrounding muscles.

### Dorsal ramus of the first cervical (suboccipital) nerve

The dorsal ramus of the first cervical nerve emerges from the vertebral canal between the posterior arch of the atlas and the vertebral artery. It gives branches to the muscles of the suboccipital triangle—rectus capitis posterior major, rectus capitis posterior minor, obliquus capitis superior, obliquus capitis inferior, and semispinalis capitis—and a communicating branch to the greater occipital nerve [Fig. 6.4].

### Vertebral artery

The third part of the vertebral artery leaves the transverse foramen of the atlas and hooks posteromedially on the posterior surface of the lateral mass of the atlas. It grooves the lateral mass and the lateral part of the posterior arch of the atlas. It passes anterior to the thickened lateral edge of the **posterior atlanto-occipital membrane** and enters the vertebral canal [Figs. 6.4, 6.6; see Figs. 7.15, 8.8].

### Suboccipital plexus of veins

The suboccipital plexus of veins lies in and around the suboccipital triangle. It forms a route of communication between the occipital veins, the internal vertebral venous plexuses [see Fig. 15.2 in Vol. 2], an emissary vein from the sigmoid sinus, muscular veins, the deep cervical vein, and the plexus of veins around the vertebral artery. As it unites many different veins, it provides a number of alternative routes for venous drainage when any of the venous channels are blocked.

### Suboccipital muscles

The following four muscles attach the atlas and axis to the occiput and stabilize the head on the cervical vertebra. The first three form the boundaries of the suboccipital triangle.

The **rectus capitis posterior major** passes superolaterally from its origin on the spine of the axis to the lateral half of the area below the inferior nuchal line on the occiput [Figs. 6.2, 6.4].

The **obliquus capitis inferior** takes origin from the spine of the axis and is inserted into the transverse process of the atlas [Figs. 6.2, 6.4].

The **obliquus capitis superior** runs posterosuperiorly from its origin on the transverse process of the atlas and to the lateral half of the area between the superior and inferior nuchal lines [Figs. 6.2, 6.4].

The **rectus capitis posterior minor** passes from its origin on the tubercle of the posterior arch of the atlas to the insertion on the medial part of the area below the inferior nuchal line, under cover of the rectus capitis posterior major [Figs. 6.2, 6.4].

**Nerve supply**: the dorsal ramus of C. 1. **Action**: the main function of these muscles is to stabilize the head on the atlas and axis, by acting as ligaments of variable length and tension.

## Dorsal rami of spinal nerves

The dorsal rami of the spinal nerves are the nerves of the back. They supply the intervertebral joints, ligaments and muscles of the back (but not the muscles of the upper limb which extend over the back), and the overlying skin.

The general arrangement and distribution of the dorsal rami follow the pattern shown in Fig. 6.7, with the following exceptions.

1. The first cervical, fourth and fifth sacral, and coccygeal nerves do not divide into medial and lateral branches.
2. Above the mid-thoracic region, the cutaneous branches arise from the medial branches of the dorsal rami and emerge close to the midline (2–3 cm). Below the mid-thoracic region, the cutaneous branches arise from the lateral branches and emerge 8–9 cm from the midline (in line with the angles of the ribs) [see Fig. 6.2 in Vol. 1]. The cutaneous branches of the small dorsal rami of the sacral nerves emerge on an imaginary line between the posterior superior iliac spine and the tip of the coccyx.
3. The cutaneous branches of some dorsal rami are large and supply an extended area of skin. The dorsal rami of C. 2 (greater occipital nerve) supply a large part of the scalp. Those of T. 1 and 2 extend laterally over the scapula. Those of L. 1, 2, and 3 extend over the buttock to the level of the greater trochanter.

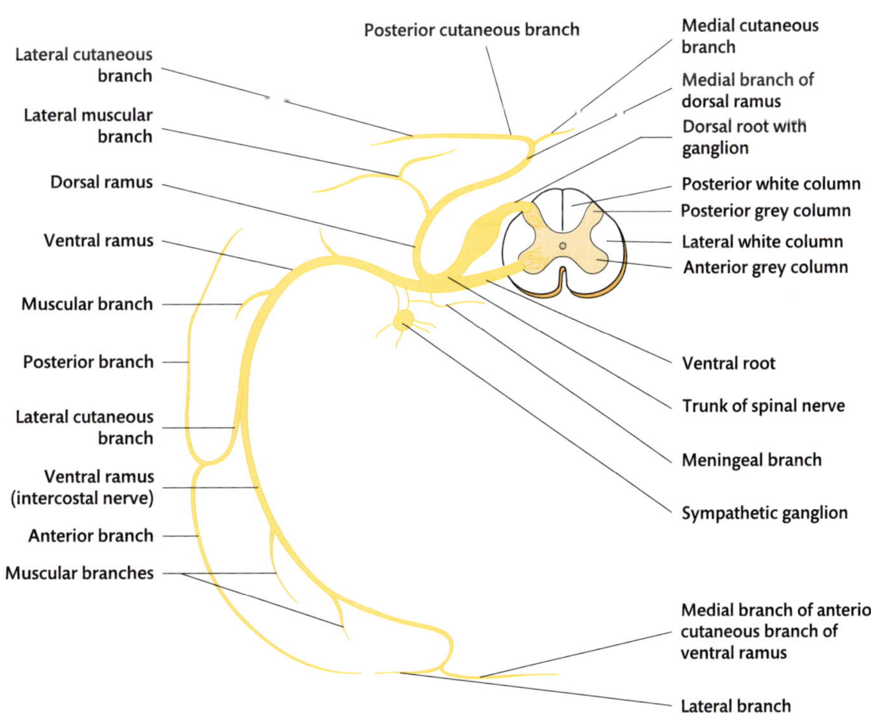


Fig. 6.7 Diagram of a typical spinal nerve.

4. The upper cervical dorsal rami and the sacral dorsal rami form simple looped plexuses. The cervical plexus is deep to the semispinalis capitis, and the sacral plexus is deep to the gluteus maximus.

## Greater occipital nerve

The **greater occipital nerve** is the cutaneous branch of the dorsal ramus of C. 2. It is the thickest cutaneous nerve in the body. It emerges below the middle of the obliquus capitis inferior, curves superomedially across the suboccipital triangle, and pierces the semispinalis capitis. It ascends on the semispinalis capitis, pierces the trapezius 2–3 cm lateral to the external occipital protuberance, and spreads out on the back of the scalp, reaching as far as the vertex. Though it is mainly cutaneous, it also supplies the semispinalis capitis [see Fig. 3.9; Figs. 6.1, 6.4].

## Third occipital nerve

The third occipital nerve is the small cutaneous branch of the dorsal ramus of C. 3. It pierces the semispinalis capitis and trapezius, and supplies the skin at the back of the neck up to the external occipital protuberance [Fig. 6.1].

# Arteries of the back

## Arteries of the cervical region

The main arterial supply to the cervical region comes from the **deep cervical** branch of the costocervical trunk of the subclavian artery. It anastomoses with the descending branch of the **occipital artery** deep to the semispinalis capitis, and with the **superficial cervical artery**. In addition, small branches of the vertebral artery supply the muscles of the back of the neck.

In the thorax, the posterior branches of the **intercostal arteries** supply the muscles and skin of the back, together with branches from the deep cervical artery.

Posterior branches of the lumbar arteries supply the back in the lumbar region.

# Veins of the back

The veins follow the corresponding arteries. They drain into the vertebral and deep cervical veins in the neck, and to the intercostal and lumbar veins in the thoracic and lumbar regions. These veins are also linked to the posterior vertebral and internal vertebral venous plexuses.

The extensive **posterior vertebral venous plexus** lies posterior to the vertebral arches. It drains the veins of the back into the vessels indicated above.

See Clinical Application 6.1 for the practical implications of the anatomy discussed in this chapter.

### CLINICAL APPLICATION 6.1 Occipital neuralgia

Occipital neuralgia is a form of headache characterized by severe pain that begins in the upper neck and back of the head. This pain is typically one-sided and can be throbbing, aching, or sharp and stabbing. It is in the distribution of the occipital nerves.

Study question 1: name the sensory nerves which supply the upper part of the neck and back of the head, and give their root values. (Answer: greater occipital nerve, dorsal ramus of C. 2; third occipital nerve, dorsal ramus of C. 3. A portion of the back of the head near the auricle is supplied by the lesser occipital nerve, ventral ramus of C. 2.) The cause of occipital neuralgia is poorly understood. It is thought to result from irritation or inflammation of the C. 2 fibres by arthritis of the atlanto-axial joint, or from entrapment of the nerve in muscles or surrounding fascia.

CHAPTER 7
# The cranial cavity

## Introduction

In this chapter, the soft tissue structures seen on the interior of the cranium after removing the brain are described. The sutural ligaments and endosteum of the skull are also described.

Start the study of this region by removing the skull cap, as described in Dissection 7.1.

## Skull cap or calvaria

### Sutural ligaments

The periosteum on the external surface of the skull is continuous with the endosteal layer of the dura mater on the internal surface, through sutural ligaments at the sutures. These ligaments hold the bones together and allow growth between them. Starting in the third to fourth decades of life, the adjacent skull bones unite by ossification of the sutural ligaments—a process known as **synostosis**. This process begins at the internal surface [see Figs. 2.5, 2.6].

## The meninges

The brain and spinal cord are enclosed in three membranes or meninges—the dura mater, the arachnoid, and the pia mater. The membranes are separated from each other by two spaces—the subdural and subarachnoid spaces [Fig. 7.1].

### Dura mater

This outermost layer of meninges is a thick, fibrous layer. In the cranium, the dura mater has two layers—an inner or **meningeal layer**, and an outer or **endosteal layer**. The meningeal layer covers the brain, and the endosteal layer is adherent to the surrounding bone.

When the skull cap is detached, the outer surface of the endosteal layer is exposed. It is rough because of the fine fibrous and vascular processes which pass between this layer and the bones. Blood vessels are most numerous, close to the midline where one of the largest intracranial venous channels—the superior sagittal sinus—lies deep to the endocranium. If a blunt instrument is pressed on the sinus, blood oozes from the numerous small veins which have been ruptured when the skull cap was removed. The endosteal layer is more firmly attached to the base of the cranial cavity than to the vault, with the degree of adhesion varying with age and from individual to individual.

A number of branching vessels ascend on the outer surface of the dura mater towards the vertex. These are the branches of the **middle meningeal artery**. The corresponding veins lie on the external surface of the artery. They groove the inner table of the skull and stand out on the surface of the dura. These vessels supply the skull (particularly the red bone marrow in its diploë) and the dura mater which is fused to its internal surface. The meningeal vessels do not supply the pia-arachnoid or the brain itself.

The two layers of the dura are firmly adherent to each other, except: (1) where the meningeal layer

**DISSECTION 7.1 Removal of the skull cap**

**Objective**

**I.** To remove the skull cap in preparation to expose the brain.

**Instructions**

1. Support the head on a block, and make a sagittal cut through the epicranial aponeurosis from the root of the nose to the external occipital protuberance. Pull each half of the scalp laterally, and detach it from the temporal lines.
2. Strip the periosteum (**pericranium**) from the external surface of the vault of the skull down to a level of the upper attachment of the temporalis muscle [see Fig. 2.9]. (At the **sutures**, it will be necessary to cut through the periosteum which is continuous through the sutures with the dura lining the interior of the skull.)
3. Turn the scalp, periosteum, and upper parts of the temporalis muscles down over the auricles.
4. To remove the skull cap, or **calvaria**, first make a horizontal mark on the skull by encircling it with a piece of string. The line should pass no more than 1 cm above the orbital margins and external occipital protuberance.
5. Using a saw, cut along this line, but avoid cutting deeper than the marrow cavity. (You will know when you reach the marrow cavity as the sawdust will turn red.) The outer table of the skull has now been divided. In the temporal region, the skull is very thin and there may be no **marrow cavity** (**diploë**), so proceed with caution.
6. Introduce a blunt chisel into the saw cut, and split the inner table by a series of short, sharp taps with a hammer. Even when the inner table is broken, the calvaria will not lift free because it is firmly adherent to the underlying dura mater.
7. Introduce the thick part of the chisel into the cut, and force the skull cap upwards. The dura will tear away from the skull, taking the vessels of the skull with them.
8. Examine the calvaria.

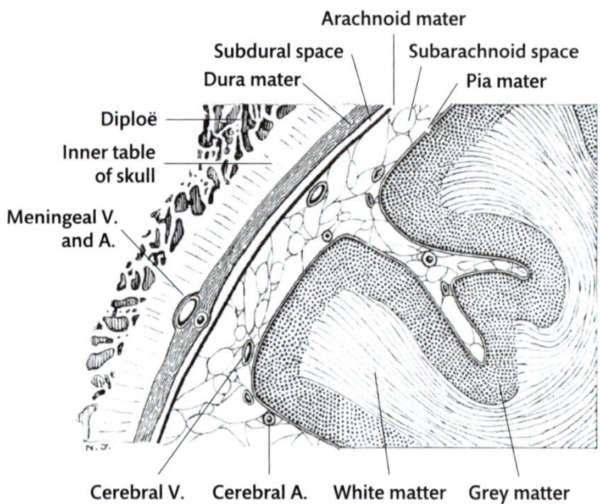


Fig. 7.1 Diagrammatic section to show the relation of the meninges to the skull and brain. Note that the meningeal vessels lie on the external surface of the dura mater and are in the endocranium, whereas the cerebral vessels lie in the subarachnoid space.

forms rigid folds or partitions between the major parts of the brain (these folds incompletely subdivide the cranial cavity and support the brain); and (2) where the venous sinuses of the dura mater lie between the endosteal and meningeal layers [Fig. 7.2]. At the foramen magnum, the spinal dura fuses with the meningeal layer of the cranial dura.

The internal surface of the dura mater is smooth and glistening. It is separated from the equally smooth external surface of the arachnoid by a capillary interval—the **subdural space**. This space encloses the brain and spinal cord, except at a few points. It is absent where structures pierce the meninges to enter or leave the brain and spinal cord, and where arachnoid villi [p. 84] are present. The space allows movement between the dura and the structures it encloses.

## The arachnoid and subarachnoid space

The arachnoid and pia mater lie inside the dura mater and develop from a single mass of loose connective tissue immediately surrounding the central nervous system. The two layers are separated by the subarachnoid space. The arachnoid mater is applied to the inner surface of the dura mater, and the pia mater is applied to the outer surface of the central nervous system [Fig. 7.1]. Cerebrospinal fluid (CSF) from the cavities of the brain circulates in the subarachnoid space. Strands of tissue—the **trabeculae**—extend between the arachnoid and the pia. In places where the arachnoid and pia are close together, the trabeculae are numerous so that the subarachnoid space is like

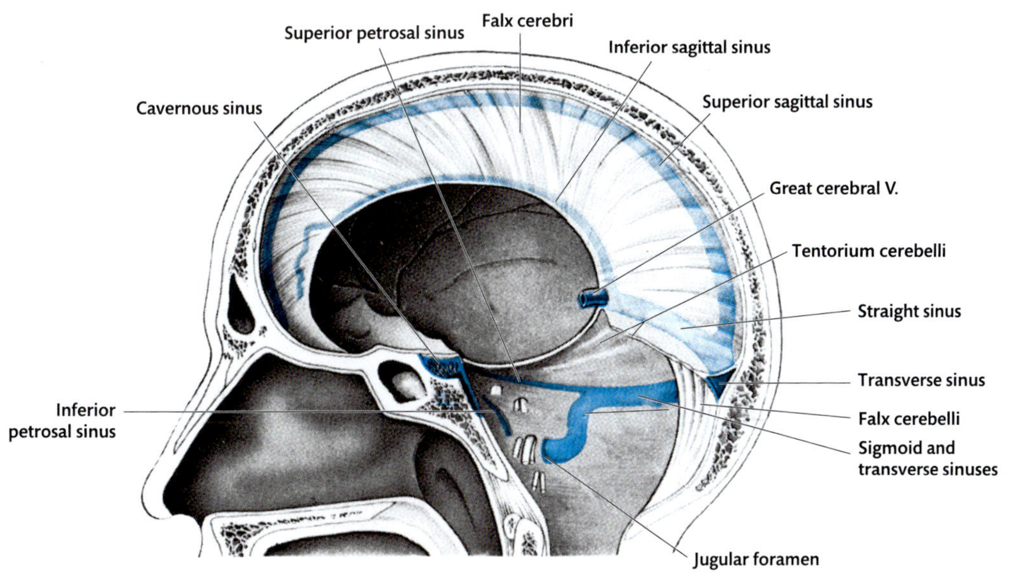


**Fig. 7.2** Sagittal section through the skull to the left of the falx cerebri. The brain has been removed to show the folds of the dura mater which incompletely partition the cranial cavity.





a fluid-filled sponge protecting the brain. Where the arachnoid and pia are more widely separated, the trabeculae are fewer and a simple fluid-filled space exists. Such larger subarachnoid spaces are known as **cisterns**.

The **arachnoid** is a thin, transparent, avascular membrane, with trabeculae passing to the pia mater from its deep surface. In a few places, notably at the superior sagittal sinus, the arachnoid pierces the dura in a number of finger-like or cauliflower-shaped projections. These finger-like projections are **arachnoid villi**; the more bulbous ones are **arachnoid granulations** [Figs. 7.3, 7.4]. The tip of the arachnoid villi is perforated and CSF from the subarachnoid space drains into the venous sinus [p. 77]. Like the dura, the arachnoid extends along the nerves which arise from the central nervous system for a short distance, before becoming continuous with the **epineurium**.

## Pia mater

The pia mater is a vascular membrane which covers the surface of the central nervous system and follows most of the irregularities of the surface [Fig. 7.1]. The pia mater is thicker than the arachnoid, especially on the spinal cord and the

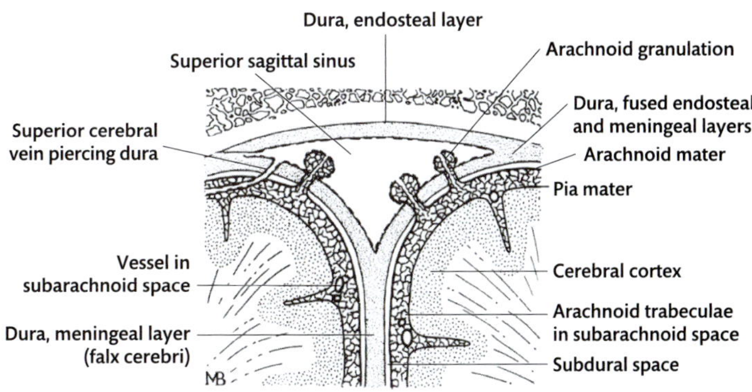


**Fig. 7.3** Diagrammatic transverse section through the superior sagittal sinus and surrounding brain.

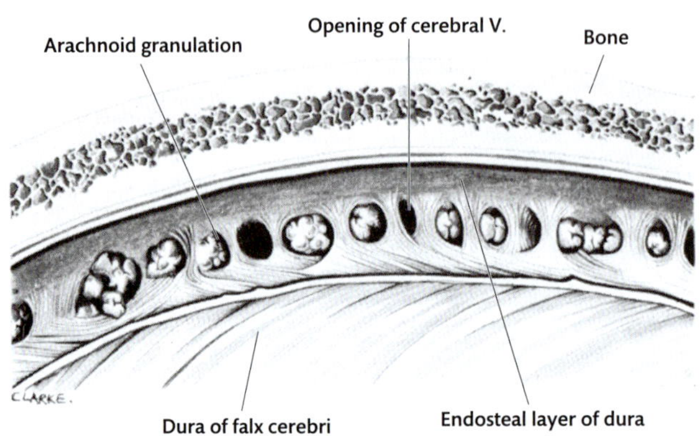


**Fig. 7.4** Median section through the skull and superior sagittal sinus. Note the arachnoid granulations protruding into the sinus.





medulla oblongata of the brain. The blood vessels of the central nervous system lie on the external surface of the pia mater. Their branches carry a sleeve of the pia mater and an extension of the subarachnoid space with them for a short distance into the central nervous system. This extension of the subarachnoid space is the **perivascular space**. Also, each rootlet of nerves entering or leaving the brain carries an extension of the pia mater as it crosses the subarachnoid space. These extensions become continuous with the perineurium of the nerves. Another modification of the pia mater—the **denticulate ligament** of the spinal cord—is described in Chapter 20.

## Cerebrospinal fluid

CSF is produced by the **choroid plexuses** in the cavities of the brain (the ventricles). It leaves the ventricular system from the fourth ventricle and enters the subarachnoid space.

Using the instructions given in Dissection 7.2, open the superior sagittal sinus.

### DISSECTION 7.2 Exploration of the superior sagittal sinus

**Objective**

**I.** To open the superior sagittal sinus.

**Instructions**

1. Make a median sagittal incision through the endocranium, and open the superior sagittal sinus as far as possible.

## Structure of dural venous sinuses

Dural venous sinuses are venous channels lined with endothelium. Use Figs. 7.2 and 7.5 to identify the superior and inferior sagittal sinuses, straight sinus, transverse sinuses, sigmoid sinuses, and cavernous sinuses. Most of the sinuses lie between the endosteal layer of the dura externally and the meningeal layer internally. Two sinuses—the straight and inferior sagittal sinuses—are entirely enclosed in the meningeal layers of the dura. The dural venous sinuses drain venous blood from the brain and surrounding bone, and communicate with the external veins through many foramina. The superior sagittal sinus also drains CSF. There are no valves in this system, so blood can flow in either direction, depending on the pressure gradient. The venous blood eventually drains into the internal jugular veins. Most of the sinuses form shallow grooves on the internal surface of the cranial cavity [see Figs. 2.13, 2.14].

## Arachnoid villi and granulations

These small, granular bodies lie along the sides of the superior sagittal sinus. They are protrusions of the arachnoid mater through the dura into the superior sagittal sinus and its lateral lacunae [Figs. 7.3, 7.4]. The granulations are normal enlargements of the arachnoid villi which are smaller and finger-shaped. In the elderly, the arachnoid granulations may reach considerable proportions and even erode the inner table of the skull. Small perforations on the surface of the arachnoid villi and granulations allow for the passage of CSF from the

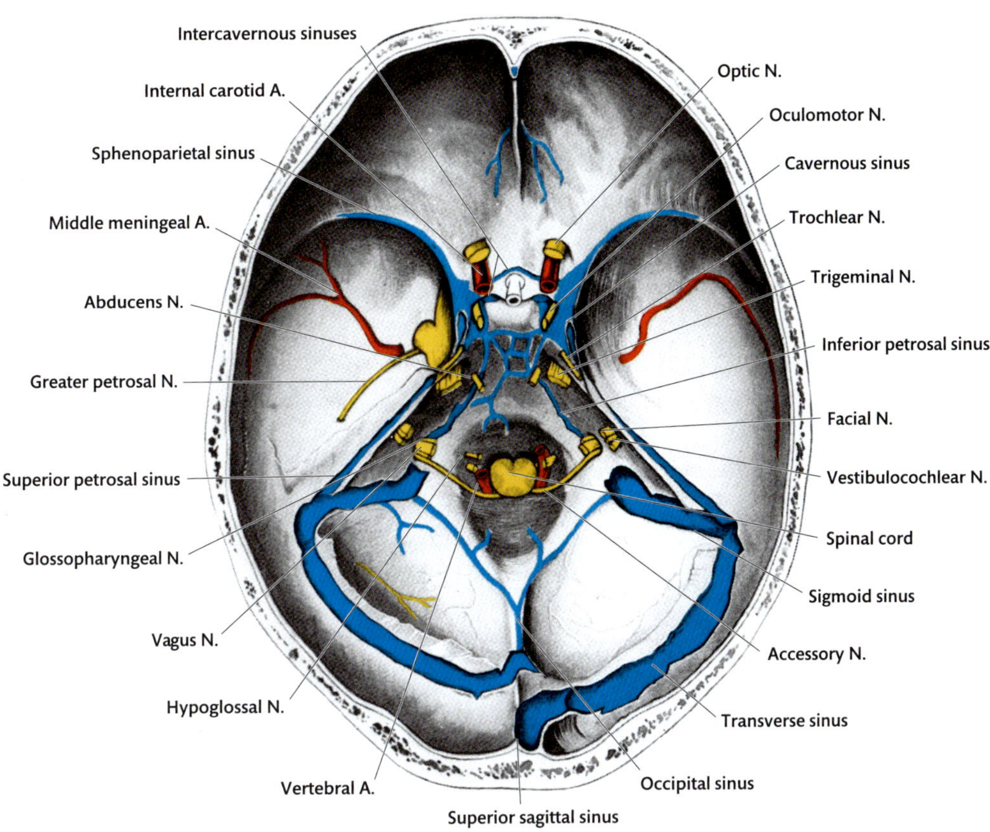


**Fig. 7.5** Dissection of the floor of the cranial cavity after removal of the brain.

subarachnoid space into the superior sagittal sinus. (At the same time, they prevent the reflux of blood into the subarachnoid space.) ➲ Clotting of blood in the superior sagittal sinus blocks the drainage of CSF and causes a rapid rise in intracranial pressure due to the build-up of CSF.

Using the instructions given in Dissection 7.3, cut through the dura and open into the subdural space.

## Superior cerebral veins

These thin-walled veins lie in the subarachnoid space immediately superficial to the pia mater. (The meningeal veins lie superficial to the dura.) They run upwards towards the midline and converge on the superior sagittal sinus [see Fig. 26.1]. They have a short course in the subdural space before piercing the dura to enter the sinus.

### DISSECTION 7.3 Reflection of the dura

**Objective**

**I.** To cut and reflect the dura covering the brain.

**Instructions**

1. Make two longitudinal incisions through the dura mater along each side of the superior sagittal sinus. From the midpoint of each incision, make another incision down to the cut edge of the skull above the auricle. As these cuts are made, raise the dura to avoid incising the underlying arachnoid, pia, and brain.
2. Turn the four flaps of dura down over the cut edges of the skull, to avoid its sharp edges injuring the brain or your fingers during subsequent dissection.
3. The subdural space is now opened and should be examined.
4. Examine the pia-arachnoid and blood vessels on the upper parts of the cerebral hemispheres now exposed.

## Superior sagittal sinus

The superior sagittal sinus is a dural venous sinus. It begins anteriorly at the crista galli. At the origin, it communicates with the veins of the frontal sinus and nose, through the foramen caecum. The sinus runs posteriorly, forming a median groove on the cranial vault. It becomes continuous with the right transverse sinus at the internal occipital protuberance [Fig. 7.2].

### Lateral lacunae

**Lateral lacunae** are cleft-like lateral extensions of the superior sagittal sinus, between the endosteal and meningeal layers of the dura mater. The largest lacuna is 2–3 cm in diameter and overlies the upper part of the motor area of the brain. Lacunae and arachnoid granulations both increase in size with age and may produce shallow depressions in the skull vault on both sides of the groove for the superior sagittal sinus.

Expose the falx cerebri following the instructions provided in Dissection 7.4.

**DISSECTION 7.4 Exposure of the falx cerebri**

**Objective**

**I.** To expose the falx cerebri.

**Instructions**

1. Expose the falx cerebri by dividing the superior cerebral veins on one side, and displacing the upper part of that cerebral hemisphere laterally.

## Falx cerebri

The falx cerebri is a median, sickle-shaped fold of the dura mater, which lies between the two cerebral hemispheres [Fig. 7.2]. The superior margin of the falx is attached to the lips of the groove for the superior sagittal sinus on the calvaria. Anteriorly, the falx is narrow and attached to the crista galli. Posteriorly, it increases in depth and becomes continuous with the upper surface of the tentorium cerebelli—an approximately horizontal fold of the dura mater [Fig. 7.2]. (The tentorium cerebelli lies between the posterior parts of the cerebral hemispheres and the cerebellum.) From this attachment, the falx descends between the two cerebral hemispheres. The lower border of the falx is free and concave, and overhangs the corpus callosum of the brain. The **superior sagittal sinus** lies in the fixed upper margin of the falx, and the **inferior sagittal sinus** lies in its free margin. The **straight sinus** lies at the attachment to the falx cerebri to the tentorium cerebelli [Fig. 7.2].

## Removal of the brain

Dissection 7.5 (and Figs. 7.6, 7.7, 7.8, 7.9) provides information on how to detach the brain from the base of the skull and remove it.

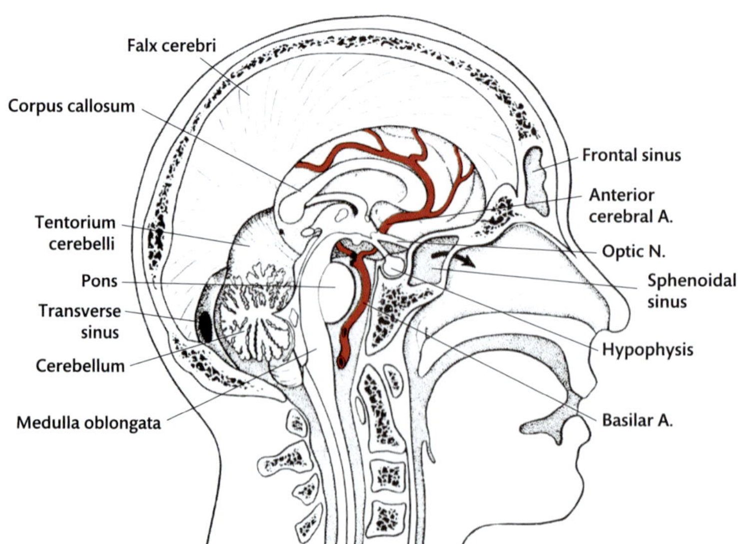


**Fig. 7.6** Sagittal section through the head and neck, slightly to the right of the median plane.

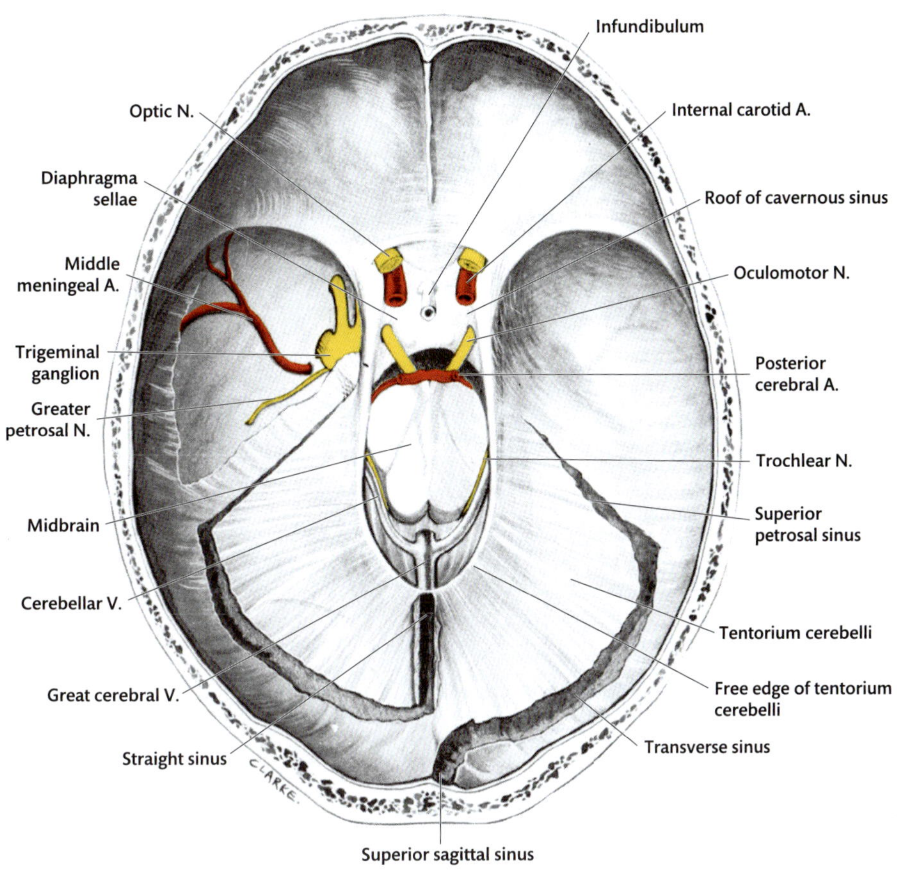


**Fig. 7.7** Interior of the cranium after removal of the cerebrum. The transverse, straight, and superior petrosal sinuses have been opened, and the dura mater has been removed from the floor of the left middle cranial fossa.

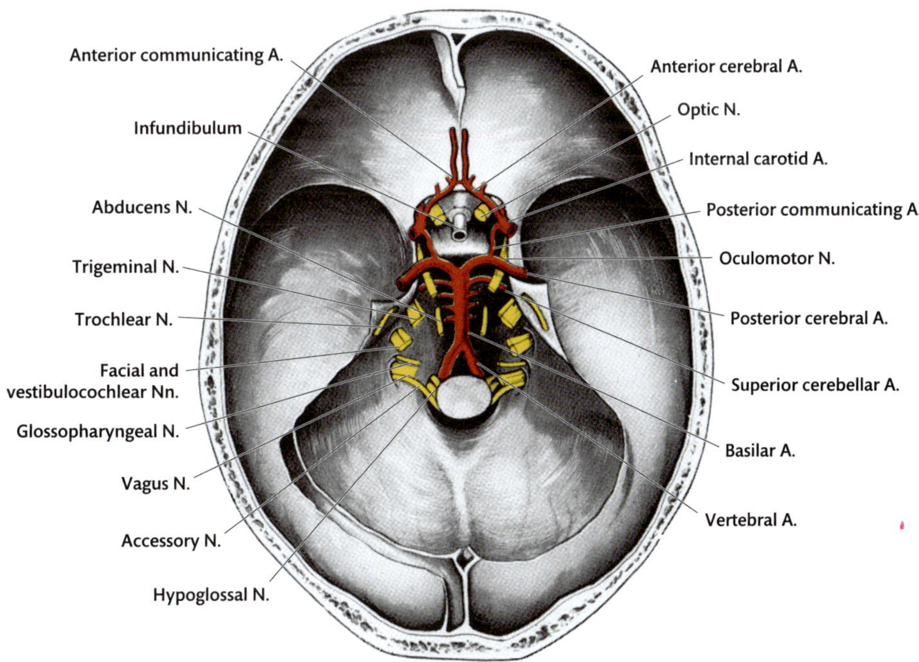


**Fig. 7.8** The floor of the cranial cavity after removal of the brain, but with the arteries at the base of the brain ***in situ***.

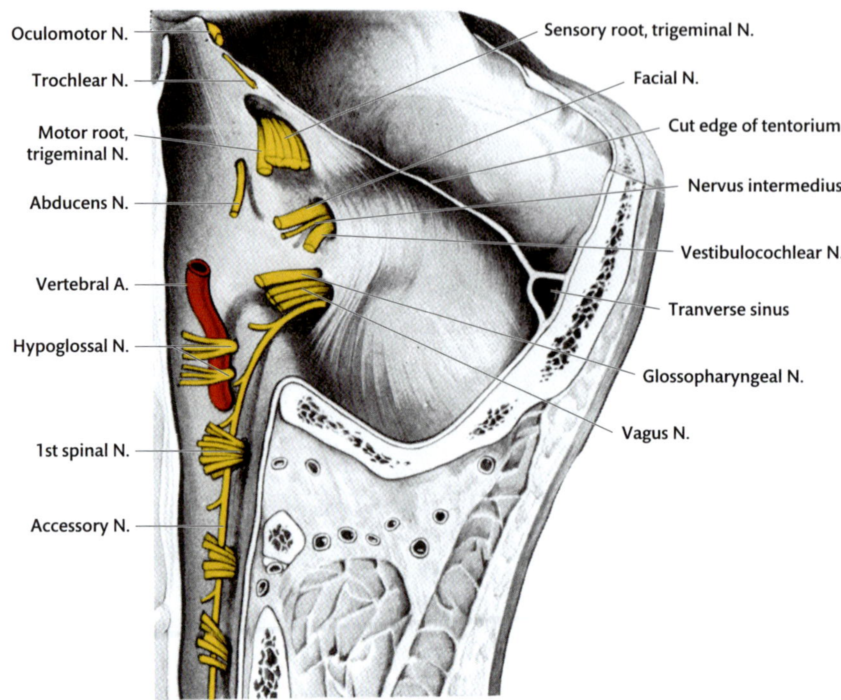


**Fig. 7.9** Oblique section through the posterior cranial fossa. The brain and spinal cord have been removed.

## DISSECTION 7.5 Removal of the brain

### Objective

**I.** To remove the brain in one piece.

### Instructions

Fig. 7.6 is a sagittal section of the head which shows the relationship of the main parts of the brain to the dural folds and the base of the brain. Identify the cerebrum (largely hidden by the falx cerebri), cerebellum, pons, and medulla on this section prior to starting the dissection.

1. Detach the falx cerebri from the crista galli, and pull the falx up posteriorly from between the hemispheres.
2. Place a block under the shoulders to allow the head to fall back. This makes the frontal lobes fall away from the anterior cranial fossae and exposes the **olfactory bulbs**. Elevate the olfactory bulbs gently from the cribriform plate of the ethmoid, tearing the olfactory nerves which pierce them.
3. The large **optic nerves** then come into view and should be divided close to the optic canal [Fig. 7.7].
4. The internal carotid arteries, with the infundibulum passing vertically to the hypophysis between them, are now seen. Divide all three structures [Fig. 7.7].
5. Allow the brain to fall backwards as each structure is divided, but support it posteriorly so as to avoid damaging it on the skull.
6. Posterior to the infundibulum, identify the dorsum sellae with a posterior clinoid process at each lateral extremity [Fig. 7.7] and the **oculomotor nerves** passing forwards, one on each side of it [Fig. 7.7].
7. Lateral to each oculomotor nerve is the **free edge of the tentorium cerebelli**. Turn the margin of the tentorium laterally, and divide the slender **trochlear nerve** which lies just under its free margin [Fig. 7.5].
8. Turn the head forcibly to one side, and raise the posterior part of the cerebral hemisphere from the tentorium with your fingers. Divide the **tentorium** along its attachment to the petrous temporal bone [Figs. 7.7, 7.8], taking care not to injure the cerebellum beneath.
9. Then turn the head to the opposite side, and repeat the procedure on the other side.
10. Let the brain fall backwards, so as to draw the brainstem away from the anterior wall of the posterior cranial fossa, and bring the lower cranial nerves into view.

11. Divide the oculomotor nerves and, allowing the brain to fall first to one side and then to the other, identify and divide the trigeminal, abducens, facial, and vestibulocochlear nerves. The last two enter the internal acoustic meatus [Figs. 7.5, 7.8].
12. Identify and cut the nerves passing to the jugular foramen [Figs. 7.5, 7.9], but leave the accessory nerve on one side by detaching it from the brain.
13. Look for the hypoglossal nerves which are deeper and more medial, and cut them [Fig. 7.9].
14. Press the pons [Fig. 7.6] further posteriorly, and identify the two vertebral arteries ascending to form the basilar artery on its surface.
15. Pass a knife into the vertebral canal in front of the medulla oblongata, and cut the spinal cord and vertebral arteries.
16. Remove the brain from the cranial cavity, dividing any roots of the accessory nerve still attached to the spinal cord.
17. Removal of the brain in this way, without complete separation of the tentorium from the skull, ruptures the great cerebral vein. Find the cut end of the great cerebral vein where it enters the straight sinus at the junction of the free margins of the falx and tentorium.

## Structures seen after removal of the cerebrum

With the help of a skull, identify the boundaries of the anterior and middle cranial fossae and the taut, but resilient, tentorium cerebelli [Fig. 7.7].

In the **anterior cranial fossa**, note:

1. The **crista galli** with the falx cerebri attached to it.
2. The **cribriform plate of the ethmoid** which lodges the olfactory bulb. The olfactory nerves pass from the nasal mucosa through the cribriform plate into the olfactory bulb.
3. The **orbital part of the frontal bone** which forms most of the floor of the anterior cranial fossa. It is closely fitted to the irregularities of the orbital surface of the frontal lobe which it separates from the orbit.
4. The **lesser wing of the sphenoid bone**, with the sphenoparietal venous sinus running along its posterior margin towards the **anterior clinoid process**. The free margin of the tentorium is attached to the anterior clinoid process [Figs. 7.5, 7.7].

In the middle cranial fossa, note:

1. The deep depression for the tip of the temporal lobe of the brain, posterolateral to the orbit.
2. The **middle meningeal vessels** seen through the dural floor of the lateral part of the fossa. Note that there are no branches piercing the dura mater.
3. The **diaphragma sella**, a raised central area formed by the dura stretched between the four clinoid processes of the sphenoid bone. The diaphragma sella is perforated by:
   (i) The **infundibulum** as it passes to the hypophysis.
   (ii) The **oculomotor nerves** as they pierce the dura, medial to the free border of the tentorium.
   (iii) The **optic nerves** and **internal carotid arteries** as they pierce the dura, medial to the anterior clinoid processes [Fig. 7.7].

### Tentorium cerebelli

The **tentorium cerebelli** is a wide, sloping fold of the dura matter. It has a free, curved margin surrounding the midbrain, and a fixed margin attached to the skull at the edge of the posterior cranial fossa. The free margin of the tentorium extends almost horizontally backwards from each anterior clinoid process, forming the **tentorial notch**. At the notch, the posterior cranial fossa continues with the supratentorial compartments of the cranial cavity [Fig. 7.7].

At the attached margin, the two layers of the dural fold diverge to enclose: (1) the wide **transverse sinus** between the internal occipital protuberance and the base of the petrous temporal bone; and (2) the superior petrosal sinus on the superior margin of the petrous temporal bone [Figs. 7.5, 7.8].

At the apex of the petrous temporal bone, the free and attached margins of the tentorium cross each other. The free margin passes forwards to the **anterior clinoid process** above the attached margin. The attached margin passes medially to the **posterior clinoid process**. The dura mater which unites these two margins, anteromedial to the crossing, forms the roof of the hypophysial fossa and the lateral wall of the cavernous sinus [Fig. 7.7].

The **great cerebral vein** pierces the dura mater of the tentorium cerebelli and joins the inferior sagittal sinus to form the **straight sinus** [Figs. 7.2, 7.7].

### Functions of the falx cerebri and tentorium cerebelli

The falx cerebri and tentorium cerebelli are tough folds of the dura mater which play an important part in stabilizing the brain within the cranial cavity. They prevent the brain from moving freely when the head is moved suddenly.

Dissection 7.6 provides instructions on dissection of the straight, transverse, and sigmoid sinuses.

## Dural venous sinuses

### Inferior sagittal sinus

The narrow inferior sagittal sinus lies in the posterior two-thirds of the free margin of the falx cerebri.

#### DISSECTION 7.6 Straight, transverse, and sigmoid sinuses

**Objective**

**I.** To open and explore the extent of the straight, transverse, sigmoid, and superior petrosal sinuses.

**Instructions**

1. Open the straight sinus by incising the falx cerebri along the left side of its union with the tentorium. Carry this incision forwards along the free edge of the falx to open the small inferior sagittal sinus.
2. Open the transverse sinus by continuing the first incision laterally from the internal occipital protuberance along the fixed margin of the tentorium cerebelli [Figs. 7.5, 7.7].
3. Carry the incision down from the lateral end of the transverse sinus along the edge of the sigmoid sinus [Fig. 7.5].
4. Open the superior petrosal sinus by cutting along the fixed margin of the tentorium cerebelli [Figs. 7.5, 7.7].
5. On the right side, follow the superior sagittal sinus into the transverse sinus, and check for continuity of all the sinuses at the internal occipital protuberance.

It drains the falx and part of the medial surface of the hemisphere into the straight sinus [Fig. 7.2].

### Straight sinus

The straight sinus is formed by the union of the great cerebral vein and the inferior sagittal sinus at the point where the free margins of the falx cerebri and tentorium cerebelli meet. It runs posteroinferiorly in the line of union of these two folds. At the internal occipital protuberance, it becomes continuous with one of the transverse sinuses, usually the left [Figs. 7.2, 7.10]. It drains the posterior and central parts of the cerebrum, part of the cerebellum, the falx, and the tentorium.

### Transverse sinus

On each side, a transverse sinus runs horizontally in the fixed margin of the tentorium, from the internal occipital protuberance to the base of the petrous temporal bone. It grooves the occipital, parietal, and temporal bones. Usually, the right transverse sinus is a continuation of the superior sagittal sinus, and the left a continuation of the straight sinus. The transverse sinus which receives the superior sagittal sinus is larger than the other, but if the sinuses communicate, they may be of equal size. The transverse sinus receives veins from the cerebrum (occipital lobe) and cerebellum, the occipital diploic vein, and the superior petrosal sinus. Anteriorly, it drains into the sigmoid sinus [Figs. 7.2, 7.5, 7.10].

The four sinuses (superior sagittal, straight, and right and left transverse sinuses) may meet in the **confluence of the sinuses** at the internal occipital protuberance.

### Superior petrosal sinus

The narrow superior petrosal sinus drains the posterior end of the cavernous sinus [p. 93] to the junction of the transverse and sigmoid sinuses. It lies in that margin of the tentorium cerebelli which is fixed to the petrous temporal bone [Fig. 7.5].

## Paranasal air sinuses

The paranasal air sinuses are air-filled spaces within bones surrounding the nasal cavities. They replace the marrow cavities of the maxilla, ethmoid, frontal, and sphenoid bones, either partly or completely. Each sinus is lined by mucosa which is

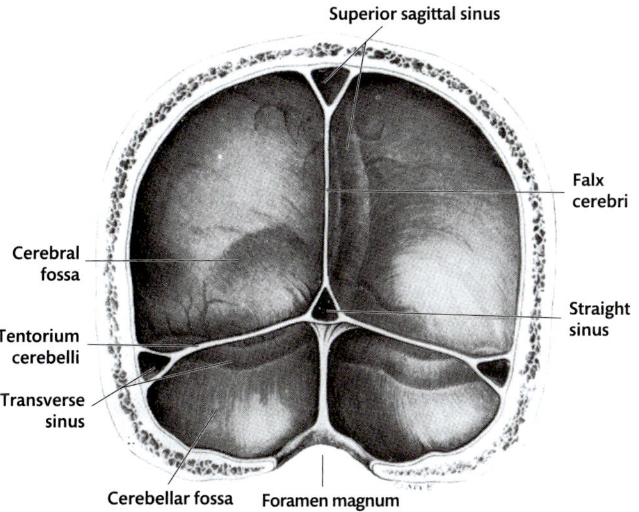


**Fig. 7.10** Coronal section through the skull at the level of the foramen magnum. The brain has been removed to show the fossae which lodge the occipital lobes of the hemispheres and the cerebellum.





adherent to the endosteum lining the bone—a **muco-endosteum**. Cilia on the mucous membrane move the surface mucus towards the opening of the sinus into the nasal cavity and keep the sinus empty of secretions. ➲ The openings of the sinuses are relatively narrow and easily obstructed, even by swelling of the vascular endosteum. When blocked, the sinus tends to fill with secretions which readily become infected.

The frontal air sinus is described and dissected in this chapter. The ethmoid air sinuses with the orbit [Chapter 10], and the maxillary and sphenoid air sinuses with the nasal cavity [Chapter 18].

## Frontal air sinuses

Dissection 7.7 provides instructions on exploring the frontal air sinus.

### DISSECTION 7.7 Frontal air sinus

**Objective**

**I.** To explore the frontal air sinus.

**Instructions**

1. One or other of frontal sinuses was probably opened when the calvaria was removed. If not, chisel off part of the frontal bone close to the median plane till one of the sinuses is opened.
2. Explore the cavity with a probe, and attempt to find its opening into the nasal cavity.

The frontal sinuses are paired, asymmetrical cavities in the frontal bone, immediately above the root of the nose and the upper margins of the orbits. They lie between the inner and outer tables of the frontal bone and are separated from each other by a bony septum [see Figs. 2.1B, 2.14; Fig. 7.6]. The sinuses are normally about 2–3 cm in height and width. In addition to expanding into the forehead, they may pass posteriorly between the two tables of the roof of the orbit. The sinuses drain into the nasal cavity through a funnel-shaped passage called the **infundibulum**.

## Anterior cranial fossa

Expose the cribriform plate of the ethmoid and the anterior ethmoidal nerve, using the instructions given in Dissection 7.8.

## Anterior ethmoidal nerve

The **anterior ethmoidal nerve** is a terminal branch of the nasociliary branch of the ophthalmic nerve. It arises in the orbit and enters the cranial cavity with the anterior ethmoidal artery between the frontal and ethmoid bones [see Fig. 2.14]. It runs forwards on the lateral edge of the cribriform plate, and enters the nose through a small aperture at the side of the crista galli. The nerve and artery supply the mucous membrane of the upper anterior part of the nasal cavity and end as the external nasal artery and nerve.

> **DISSECTION 7.8 Anterior cranial fossa**
>
> **Objective**
>
> **I.** To expose the cribriform plate of the ethmoid and the anterior ethmoidal nerve.
>
> **Instructions**
>
> 1. Carefully remove the dura mater from the cribriform plate of the ethmoid.
> 2. Attempt to find the anterior ethmoidal nerve running anteriorly on the lateral margin of the cribriform plate.

The small **posterior ethmoidal artery** follows the same course from the orbit, but further posteriorly. Along with the anterior ethmoidal and middle meningeal arteries, it supplies the dura mater of the anterior cranial fossa.

## Middle cranial fossa

Using the instructions given in Dissection 7.9, remove the pituitary gland from the hypophysial fossa.

### Hypophysis or pituitary gland

The pituitary is an important endocrine gland with a wide range of functions, including the control of the other ductless glands and of body growth.

It is a flattened, ovoid structure lying in the hypophysial fossa and connected to the inferior surface of the hypothalamus by the **infundibulum** [Fig. 7.11]. The **posterior lobe** of the pituitary is the expanded inferior end of the infundibulum and is developed from the brain. The **anterior lobe** is much larger than the posterior lobe and partly surrounds the posterior lobe and infundibulum.

> **DISSECTION 7.9 Pituitary gland**
>
> **Objective**
>
> **I.** To remove and study the pituitary gland.
>
> **Instructions**
>
> 1. Cut the diaphragma sellae radially, and dislodge the pituitary gland from the hypophysial fossa. Examine its shape with a hand lens, and then make a median section through it.

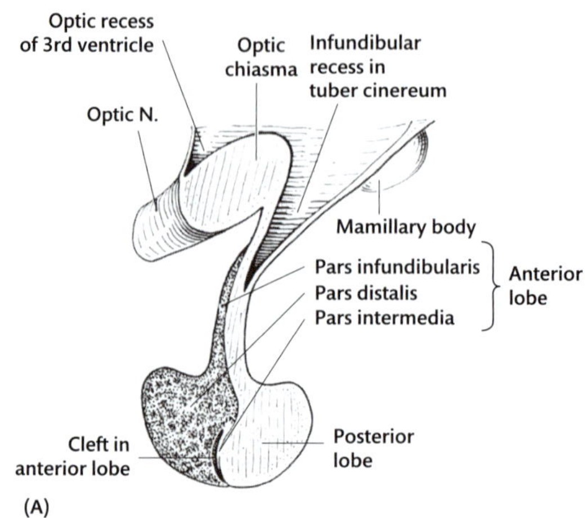


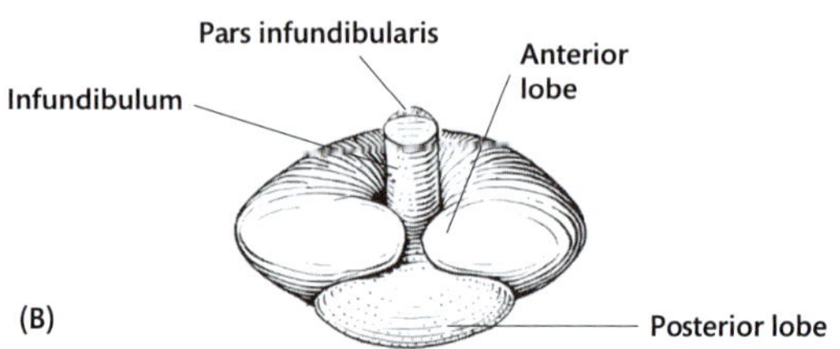


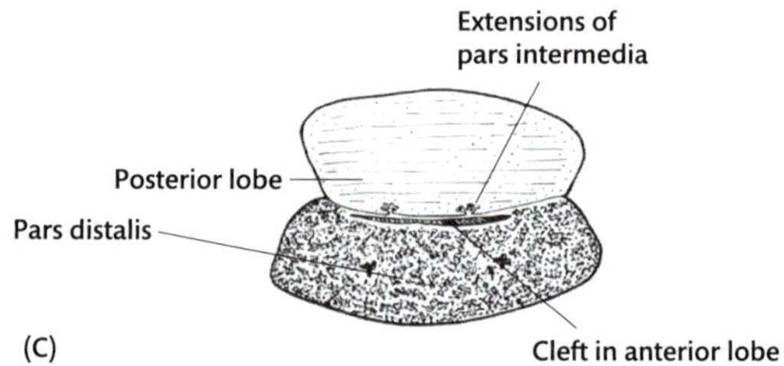


**Fig. 7.11** Diagrammatic views of the hypophysis. (A) In median section; (B) from above and behind; (C) in horizontal section.

The pituitary lies posterosuperior to the sphenoidal air sinuses, below the optic chiasma, in front of the dorsum sellae, and between the two cavernous sinuses. Several venous channels (**intercavernous sinuses**) connect the two cavernous sinuses around the pituitary [Figs. 7.5, 7.6].

### Blood supply of the pituitary

The pituitary is supplied by twigs from the internal carotid and anterior cerebral arteries. The anterior lobe also receives venous blood from the hypothalamus via the **hypothalamo-hypophysial**

**portal system** of veins. The veins of the pituitary drain into the cavernous sinuses.

➲ See Clinical Application 7.1 for presentation, types, and treatment of pituitary tumours.

## Cavernous sinus

The paired cavernous sinuses are dural venous sinuses which lie between the endosteal and meningeal layers of the dura on the lateral side of the body of the sphenoid. They consist of a large number of incompletely fused venous channels surrounding the structures which lie within them, and are important because of the structures which are in and around them.

### Position and contents

Each cavernous sinus lies lateral to the pituitary and the sphenoidal air sinus. It extends from the medial end of the superior orbital fissure anteriorly to the apex of the petrous temporal bone posteriorly. Lateral to it is the trigeminal ganglion. The following nerves lie on the lateral wall—the oculomotor, trochlear, ophthalmic, and maxillary divisions of the trigeminal nerve. Within the sinus, but separated from it by the endothelium, lie the internal carotid artery and the abducens nerve [Figs. 7.5, 7.12].

### Tributaries and communications

The cavernous sinus communicates with a number of other veins [Fig. 7.5]. Anteriorly, it communicates with the ophthalmic veins and the sphenoparietal sinus. Posteriorly, it communicates with the superior and inferior petrosal sinuses. Medially, it is connected to its fellow on the opposite side by intercavernous sinuses in the hypophysial fossa. Superiorly, the superficial middle cerebral vein and one or two small cerebral veins enter it. Inferiorly, it communicates with: (1) the pharyngeal plexus through the carotid canal; and (2) the pterygoid plexus through the foramen ovale and the sphenoidal emissary foramen.

➲ The carotid artery may be damaged within the cavernous sinus in injuries to the skull and lead to arterial bleeding within the cavernous sinus. Such a bleed would raise the pressure in the sinus and in the veins entering it. Back pressure in the ophthalmic veins may cause the eyeball to protrude and even to pulsate.

➲ **Cavernous sinus thrombosis** (CST) is clot formation in the cavernous sinus. It often results from spread of infection from the nose, paranasal air sinuses, tonsils, or tooth. Patients with CST could present with headache due to meningeal irritation, periorbital oedema due to venous congestion of the ophthalmic veins, visual impairment due to papilloedema, and retinal haemorrhage secondary to retinal congestion. Other symptoms of CST occur because of the close relationship between the cavernous sinus and the third, fourth, fifth—ophthalmic and maxillary divisions—and sixth cranial nerves in the lateral wall of the cavernous sinus. Pain and loss of sensation over the upper face are the result of stretching/pressure of the ophthalmic and maxillary divisions of the trigeminal nerve. It has high morbidity and can have residual visual impairment like diplopia (double vision) due to involvement of the sixth cranial nerve.



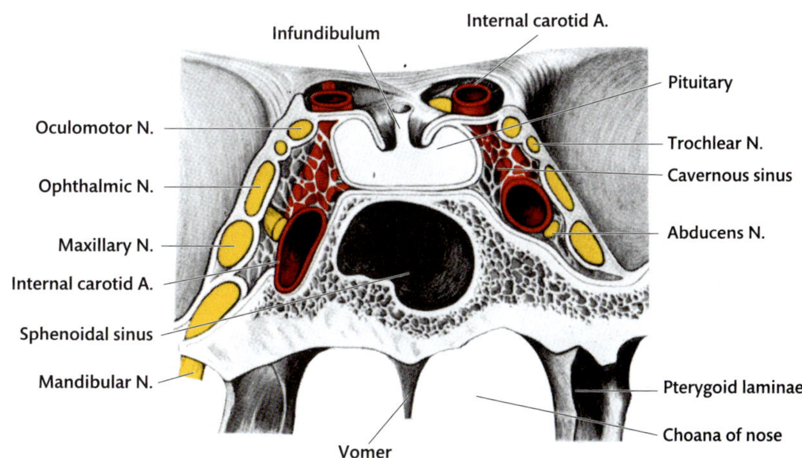


**Fig. 7.12** Coronal section through the sella turcica and cavernous sinuses.

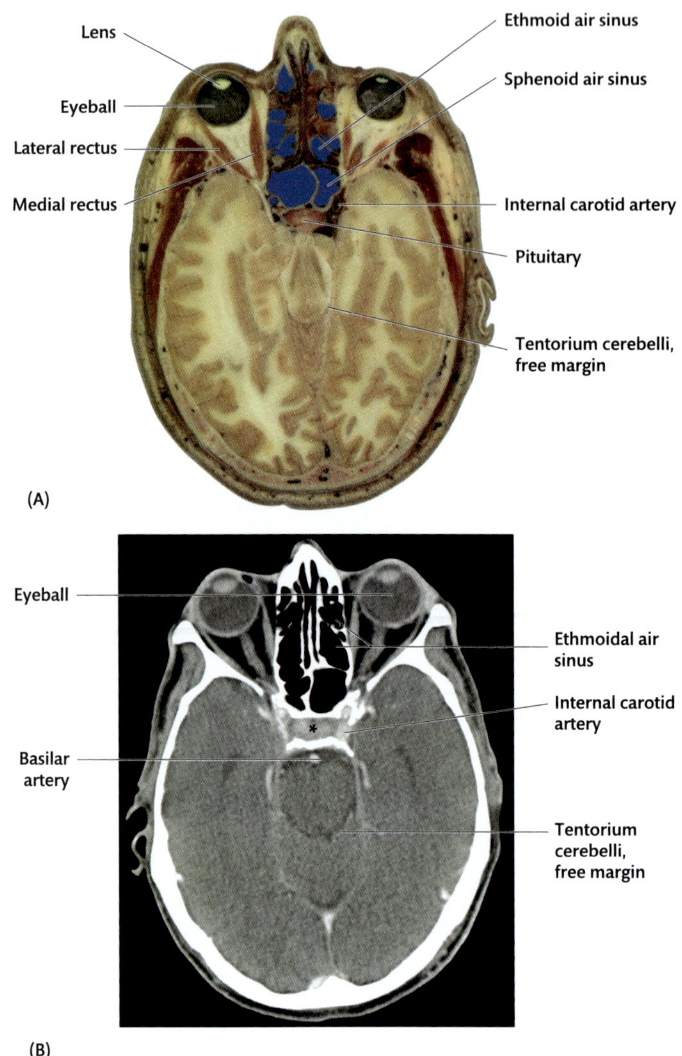


**Fig. 7.13** (A) Transverse section through the head at the level of the pituitary gland. (B) Axial contrast computerized tomography (CT) through the pituitary (asterisk) and orbit.

(A) Image courtesy of the Visible Human Project of the US National Library of Medicine.

Fig. 7.13 is an axial section through the pituitary gland.

Using the instructions given in Dissection 7.10 (and Figs. 7.14, 7.15), expose the structures on the floor of the middle cranial fossa.

## Trigeminal nerve

The trigeminal nerve is the fifth cranial nerve. It has three divisions: the **ophthalmic**, **maxillary**, and **mandibular** divisions. It is the principal sensory nerve of the head, supplying: (1) the skin of the face and anterior half of the head; (2) the mucous membrane of the nose, paranasal air sinuses, mouth, and anterior two-thirds of the tongue; (3) the teeth and temporomandibular joint; (4) the contents of the orbit, except the retina; and (5) parts of the dura mater.

The **motor fibres** arise in the pons and pass into the mandibular nerve. They supply the four muscles of mastication—the temporalis, masseter, and medial and lateral pterygoid—and the mylohyoid, anterior belly of the digastric, tensor palati, and tensor tympani.

Almost all of the **sensory fibres** in the trigeminal nerve are processes of the cells in the large trigeminal ganglion. The central processes

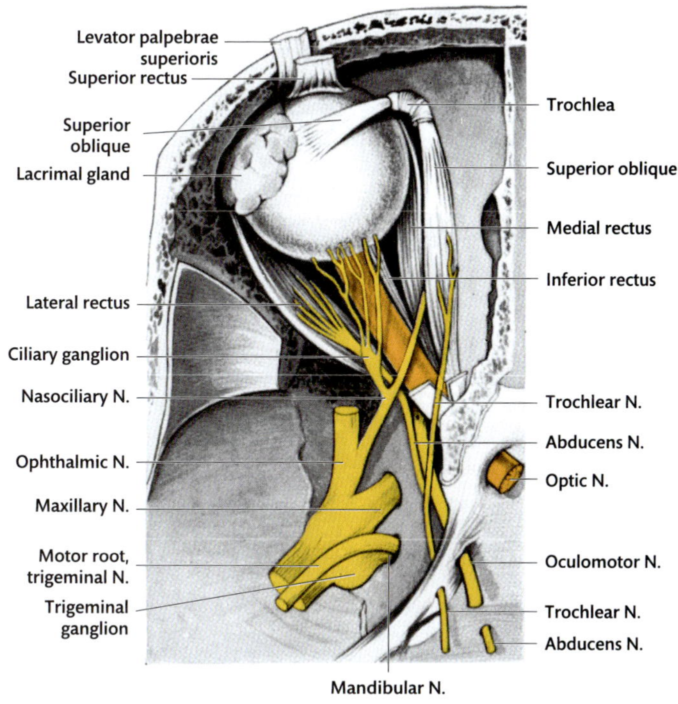


**Fig. 7.14** Orbit and middle cranial fossa. The trigeminal nerve and ganglion have been turned laterally to expose the motor root.

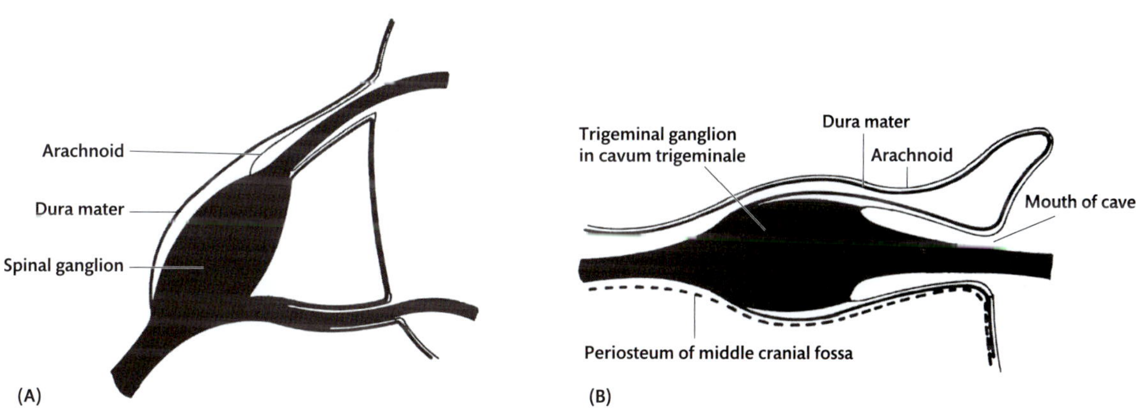


**Fig. 7.15** Diagram to show the relations of the meninges to: (A) a spinal nerve; and (B) the trigeminal ganglion in the cavum trigeminale.





converge to form the **sensory root** of the nerve which enters the pons. The peripheral processes enter the ophthalmic, maxillary, and mandibular nerves. Proprioceptive nerve fibres from the same three nerves pass through the ganglion to cells in the midbrain—a unique arrangement where primary sensory nerve cells have their cell bodies within the central nervous system. (The sensory and motor nuclei of the trigeminal nerve are described in Chapter 27.)

## Trigeminal ganglion

The trigeminal ganglion is a semilunar sensory ganglion. It lies in a shallow depression on the anterior surface of the petrous temporal bone (near the apex) and on the adjacent margin of the greater wing of the sphenoid [Fig. 7.14]. Like other sensory ganglia, it lies in a pocket of dura mater—the **cavum trigeminale**. The dura mater forming the cave is tucked forwards from the posterior cranial fossa between the meningeal and endosteal layers on the

**DISSECTION 7.10 Middle cranial fossa**

**Objectives**

**I.** To remove the dura from the cavernous sinus and the rest of the middle cranial fossa. **II.** To identify and trace the structures in the cavernous sinus. **III.** To open the cavum trigeminale and dissect the trigeminal ganglion and its branches. **IV.** To trace the greater and lesser petrosal nerves.

**Instructions**

1. Turn each half of the tentorium anterolaterally on its attachment to the petrous temporal bone.
2. Find the **trochlear nerve** [Fig. 7.9]. It pierces the inferior surface of the tentorium, close to its free border and near the apex of the petrous temporal bone.
3. Inferior to the trochlear nerve, find the large **trigeminal nerve** [Figs. 7.9, 7.14]. Pass a blunt probe forwards along the nerve. The probe enters a dural sac—the **cavum trigeminale** which surrounds the nerve—and the trigeminal ganglion underneath the dural floor of the middle cranial fossa. Elevate the probe to raise the dural floor of the middle cranial fossa, and outline the position of the nerve and ganglion [Fig. 7.15].
4. Carefully remove the dura mater from the floor of the middle cranial fossa by cutting through it on the probe in the cavum trigeminale.
5. Strip the dura forwards and laterally to uncover the trigeminal nerve, the ganglion, and the three large branches of the nerve [Fig. 7.15]. The branches arise from the convex anterior border of the ganglion. Remove the dura from the ganglion with care, because the ganglion is a loose mass of cells which is easily destroyed.
6. Trace the **mandibular nerve** inferolaterally to the foramen ovale, close to the entry of the middle meningeal artery.
7. Follow the **maxillary nerve** to the foramen rotundum.
8. Follow the **ophthalmic nerve** into the lateral wall of the cavernous sinus where it divides into three branches which can be traced to the superior orbital fissure [Fig. 7.14].
9. Find the **trochlear** and **oculomotor nerves** in the lateral wall of the cavernous sinus. Pick them up as they pierce the dura, and gently pull on them to identify their more peripheral parts.
10. Preserve the dura where the nerves enter it, but remove it in front of that point so as to follow the nerves to the superior orbital fissure.
11. Remove the remains of the lateral wall of the cavernous sinus from around the nerves, and expose the **internal carotid artery** and the **abducens nerve** within the sinus. Note that the nerve passes forwards, lateral to the artery. Follow the nerve forwards and backwards.
12. Carefully strip the remainder of the dura from the anterior surface of the petrous temporal bone, and look for the greater and lesser **petrosal nerves**. These slender nerves emerge through slits in the temporal bone and run anteromedially in shallow grooves. The lesser petrosal nerve pierces the skull near the foramen ovale; the greater petrosal nerve is larger and more medial. It disappears under the trigeminal ganglion [Fig. 7.5].
13. Lift the trigeminal ganglion, and try to identify the **motor root of the trigeminal nerve** on its inferior surface. It runs deep to the ganglion to the foramen ovale.

floor of the middle cranial fossa [Fig. 7.15]. Posteriorly, the narrow neck of the cavum contains the sensory and motor roots of the nerve enclosed in a sleeve of the pia and arachnoid. They groove the upper margin of the petrous temporal bone close to the apex. The distal part of the roots lies above the internal carotid artery in the carotid canal. The superomedial part of the ganglion lies lateral to the cavernous sinus and the internal carotid artery [Figs. 7.14, 7.15].

## Mandibular nerve

The mandibular nerve is the largest of the three branches of the trigeminal nerve. It arises from the inferolateral part of the ganglion, gives a meningeal twig to the floor of the middle cranial fossa, and immediately leaves the skull through the foramen ovale. The small motor root of the mandibular nerve leaves the pons beside the sensory root and passes under the ganglion to the foramen ovale [Fig. 7.14].

## Maxillary nerve

The maxillary nerve arises from the anterior surface of the ganglion, inferior to the ophthalmic nerve. It runs forwards between the dura and the lower border of the cavernous sinus, gives off a fine meningeal branch to the middle cranial fossa, and leaves the skull by passing through the foramen rotundum [see Fig. 2.14].

### Ophthalmic nerve

The ophthalmic nerve is the smallest of the three nerves. It arises from the ganglion, runs forwards in the lateral wall of the cavernous sinus, and divides into three branches—the **nasociliary**, **lacrimal**, and **frontal nerves**—which enter the orbit through the superior orbital fissure [Fig. 7.14]. Near its origin, the ophthalmic nerve communicates with the oculomotor, trochlear, and abducens nerves in the lateral wall of the cavernous sinus. It also gives off a small **tentorial branch** which curves back into the tentorium cerebelli.

## Oculomotor nerve

The **oculomotor nerve** is the third cranial nerve. It supplies four of the six muscles that move the eyeball, and two of the three muscles within the eyeball [Chapters 10 and 11]. It emerges through the ventral surface of the midbrain, passes anterolaterally, and pierces the dura mater in the roof of the cavernous sinus. It then runs forwards in the lateral wall of the cavernous sinus (above the other nerves) and divides into superior and inferior branches which enter the orbit through the superior orbital fissure [Figs. 7.12, 7.14].

## Trochlear nerve

The **trochlear nerve** is the fourth cranial nerve. It supplies one extraocular muscle of the eyeball [Chapter 10]. It arises from the dorsal surface of the midbrain and curves forwards on the side of the lower midbrain. It pierces the tentorium below the free margin and runs anteriorly in the lateral wall of the cavernous sinus [Fig. 7.12]. It crosses the lateral aspect of the oculomotor nerve to enter the orbit through the superior orbital fissure.

## Abducens nerve

The **abducens nerve** is the sixth cranial nerve and supplies one extraocular muscle of the eyeball [Chapter 10]. It emerges at the lower border of the pons and pierces the dura mater 1 cm below the root of the dorsum sellae [Fig. 7.8]. Outside the dura, it runs superolaterally to the apex of the petrous temporal bone and crosses the sphenopetrous suture to enter the cavernous sinus. In the sinus, it runs anteriorly, lateral to the internal carotid artery, and enters the orbit through the superior orbital fissure [Fig. 7.12].

## Intracranial part of the internal carotid artery

### Course

The **internal carotid artery** enters the skull through the carotid canal in the petrous part of the temporal bone. It passes anteromedially in the carotid canal into the upper part of the foramen lacerum and enters the cavernous sinus by piercing the dural floor. In the cavernous sinus, it turns sharply forwards and runs anteriorly. At the root of the lesser wing of the sphenoid, the artery again turns sharply upwards and backwards, and pierces the dura and arachnoid mater on the roof of the cavernous sinus, medial to the anterior clinoid process and behind the optic canal. It then divides into the anterior and middle cerebral arteries on the surface of the brain. The internal carotid artery produces a sinuous groove on the side of the body of the sphenoid [Fig. 7.16]. The internal carotid artery is surrounded by the internal carotid plexus of sympathetic nerves [see Fig. 8.13].

### Branches of the internal carotid artery

The internal carotid artery gives off the following branches at the base of the brain: (1) the **ophthalmic artery** to the orbit; (2) small twigs to the pituitary, trigeminal ganglion, and dura mater in the cavernous sinus; (3) the posterior communicating artery; (4) the anterior choroidal artery; and (5) the middle and (6) anterior cerebral arteries. Other details of the internal carotid artery are described in Chapter 26.

## Meningeal vessels of the middle cranial fossa

The meningeal vessels are embedded on the external surface of the dura mater. They protrude from its surface and groove the skull [Fig. 7.1]. They supply the bone and dura mater but do not cross the subdural space to supply the brain or the pia-arachnoid.

The **middle meningeal artery** is a branch of the maxillary artery. It enters the skull through the foramen spinosum and runs anterolaterally on the floor of the middle cranial fossa. It divides into the **frontal** and **parietal** branches on the greater wing of the sphenoid. The parietal branch turns posteriorly, and runs across the lateral wall of the cranial cavity towards the lambda. The larger frontal branch runs towards the lateral end of the lesser

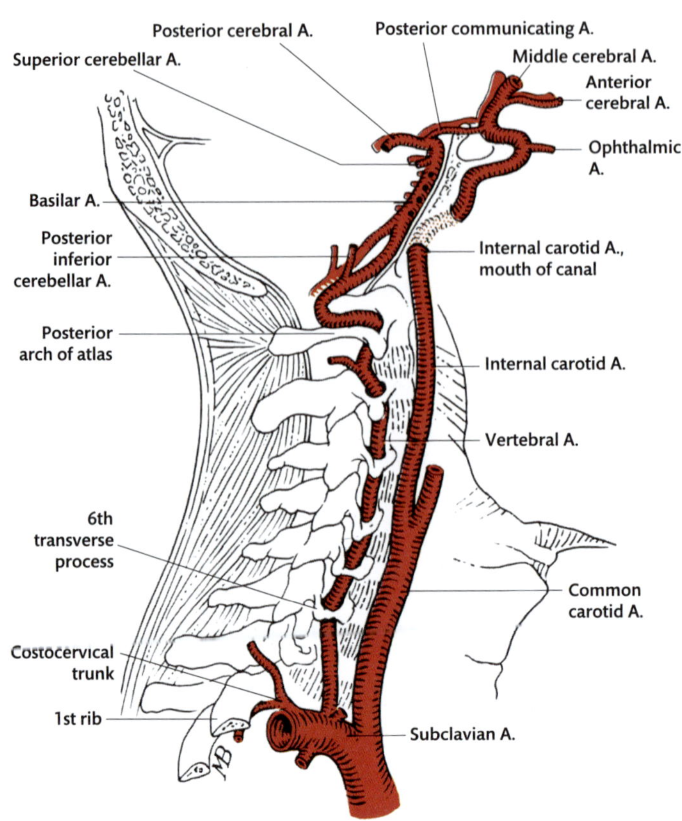


**Fig. 7.16** The course and communications of the internal carotid and vertebral arteries.

wing of the sphenoid [see Fig. 2.14]. At the pterion (area where the greater wing of the sphenoid, frontal, parietal, and temporal bones meet), the frontal branch of the middle meningeal artery grooves the skull deeply or even tunnels through the bone, increasing the probability of damage to it in fractures. It then runs obliquely upwards and backwards, parallel to, and slightly behind, the coronal suture, and frequently sends a large branch posteriorly on the deep surface of the parietal bone [Fig. 7.17]. The parietal branch is a small, but important, artery because it is a common source of extradural haemorrhage, and lies adjacent to an important area in the brain—the motor cortex.

The middle meningeal vein accompanies the artery through the foramen spinosum to the pterygoid venous plexus.

### Accessory meningeal vessels

A small branch of the maxillary or middle meningeal artery—the **accessory meningeal artery**—often traverses the foramen ovale to supply the trigeminal ganglion and adjacent dura. The **ophthalmic** and **lacrimal arteries** from the orbit also send twigs through the superior orbital fissure to the middle cranial fossa.

## Petrosal nerves

The greater and lesser petrosal nerves carry preganglionic parasympathetic secretomotor fibres to the lacrimal, nasal, palatine, nasopharyngeal, and parotid glands, and sensory (taste) fibres from the palate.

The **greater petrosal nerve** arises from the genu of the facial nerve in the petrous temporal bone. It runs on the anterior surface of the petrous bone into a narrow groove leading to the foramen lacerum, inferior to the trigeminal ganglion [see Fig. 2.14]. Its fibres synapse with the cells of the pterygopalatine ganglion.

The slender **lesser petrosal nerve** arises from the glossopharyngeal nerve. It emerges on the anterior surface of the petrous temporal bone, lateral to the greater petrosal nerve, and runs on the bony floor of the middle cranial fossa to the foramen ovale. Its fibres synapse with the cells of the

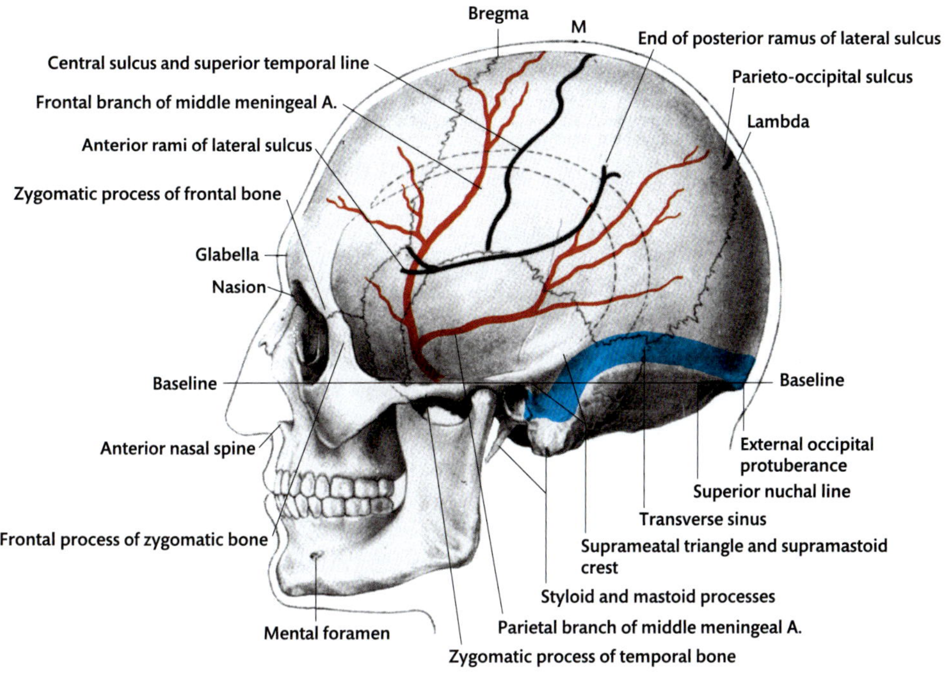


Fig. 7.17 Lateral view of the skull to show the position of certain important intracranial structures. M = midpoint between the nasion and the inion.





otic ganglion on the medial side of the mandibular nerve [see Fig. 12.8].

## Posterior cranial fossa

Using the instructions given in Dissection 7.11, identify the cut ends of the cranial nerves in the posterior cranial fossa.

## Structures seen in the posterior cranial fossa

1. The upper end of the spinal cord, attached to the margin of the foramen magnum by the first tooth of the denticulate ligament [Fig. 7.5].
2. The **vertebral artery** as it ascends through the foramen magnum, anterior to the first tooth of the

### DISSECTION 7.11 Cranial nerves in the posterior cranial fossa

#### Objective

**I.** To identify the cut ends of the trigeminal, abducens, facial, vestibulocochlear, glossopharyngeal, vagus, spinal accessory, and hypoglossal nerves.

#### Instructions

1. Using Figs. 7.5, 7.8, 7.9 and a dry skull, identify the cranial nerves in the posterior cranial fossa. (1) The **trigeminal nerve** passes into the cavum trigeminale on the superior margin of the petrous temporal bone. (2) The **abducens nerve** pierces the dura on the basilar part of the occipital bone. (3) The **facial** and **vestibulocochlear nerves** enter the internal acoustic meatus. (4) The **glossopharyngeal**, **vagus**, and **accessory nerves** pass through the jugular foramen. The **spinal part of the accessory nerve** ascends through the foramen magnum beside the spinal cord, to join the vagus. It passes out through the jugular foramen with the glossopharyngeal nerve. (5) The **hypoglossal nerve** enters the hypoglossal canal, close to the anterolateral margin of the foramen magnum.

denticulate ligament. It gives a meningeal branch to the posterior cranial fossa before piercing the dura mater, and passes superomedially between the first cervical and hypoglossal nerves [Fig. 7.9].

3. The **first cervical nerve**, in front of the vertebral artery.
4. The **hypoglossal nerve** superior to the first cervical. It pierces the dura at the hypoglossal canal [Fig. 7.9].
5. The spinal part of the **accessory nerve** ascends through the foramen magnum and turns laterally to join the cranial part of the accessory and vagus nerves. Together, they pierce the dura mater at the jugular foramen, beside the separate aperture for the glossopharyngeal nerve [Fig. 7.9].
6. The **facial nerve**, **nervus intermedius**, and **vestibulocochlear nerve** enter the internal acoustic meatus [Fig. 7.9].
7. The **falx cerebelli**, a small fold of the dura mater on the internal occipital crest. It contains the occipital sinus and fits into the posterior cerebellar notch [Fig. 7.11].

Using the instructions given in Dissection 7.12, open the sigmoid sinus and trace the abducens nerve.

## Dura mater of the base of the skull

The dura mater of the base is firmly attached to the bone and is continuous through the foramina, with the periosteum on the external surface of the skull.

**DISSECTION 7.12 Dural venous sinuses in the posterior cranial fossa**

**Objectives**

**I.** To explore the occipital and sigmoid sinuses. **II.** To find and trace the abducens nerve.

**Instructions**

1. Slit up the falx cerebelli, and look for the **occipital sinus**.
2. Open the **sigmoid sinus** by passing a knife into it at the anterior end of the transverse sinus, and cutting along it to the base of the skull and then forwards to the jugular foramen.
3. Pull gently on the cut end of the abducens nerve, and trace it to the apex of the petrous temporal bone by slitting the dura.

At the foramen magnum, the meningeal layer of the dura mater becomes continuous with the spinal dura mater.

### Venous sinuses of the posterior cranial fossa

#### Sigmoid sinus

The S-shaped **sigmoid sinus** begins as a continuation of the transverse sinus at the base of the petrous temporal bone [Fig. 7.5]. It curves downwards and grooves the mastoid and petrous parts of the temporal bone. The sinus is medial to the mastoid air cells, posterior to the mastoid antrum and the vertical part of the facial nerve, and lateral to the cerebellum.

On the base of the skull, the sigmoid sinus curves forwards on the occipital bone. It joins the inferior petrosal sinus at the jugular foramen to form the internal jugular vein.

It communicates with: (1) the **occipital veins**, through the mastoid emissary vein in the mastoid foramen; (2) the **suboccipital plexus**, by the emissary veins in the condylar canal; and (3) the beginning of the **transverse sinus**, through the occipital sinus [Fig. 7.5].

#### Occipital sinus

When present, this narrow sinus descends in the falx cerebelli from the beginning of the transverse sinus. It communicates through the foramen magnum with the internal vertebral venous plexus [Fig. 7.5].

#### Inferior petrosal sinus

The inferior petrosal sinus lies in the groove between the basilar part of the occipital bone and the petrous temporal bone. It drains the posterior end of the cavernous sinus through the jugular foramen to the internal jugular vein [Fig. 7.5].

#### Basilar plexus of veins

The basilar plexus of veins lies on the clivus of the skull and unites the inferior petrosal sinuses with the internal vertebral venous plexus through the foramen magnum [Fig. 7.5].

### Diploic veins

These are wide venous spaces of the marrow cavity between the outer and inner tables of the flat bones of the skull. They communicate with the venous sinuses of the dura mater and with the emissary veins.

## Emissary veins

Emissary veins are small veins which pass through the foramina in the skull and connect the dural venous sinuses with veins outside the skull. They do not have valves and blood flows through them in both directions. Not all named emissary veins are always present—the parietal, condylar, and sphenoidal emissary veins are frequently absent.

The superior sagittal sinus may be connected to the veins of the frontal air sinus through emissary veins in the foramen caecum, and to the veins of the scalp through the **parietal emissary foramina** in the top of the skull. The **sigmoid sinus** is connected to the occipital or posterior auricular veins through the **mastoid emissary vein** behind the auricle, and to the vertebral veins through the **condylar emissary vein**. The **cavernous sinus** has the greatest number of such communications. It is connected: (1) through the **ophthalmic veins** to the veins of the face; (2) through a plexus of veins along the internal carotid artery to the **pharyngeal veins**; and (3) through the foramen ovale to the **pterygoid venous plexus** in the infratemporal region [Fig. 7.16].

➲ The emissary veins may transmit extracranial infections into the venous sinuses.

## Meningeal veins

The meningeal veins are very thin-walled veins which lie between the meningeal arteries and the bone. They end either in the venous sinuses or in veins outside the skull by passing through foramina with the corresponding arteries.

See Clinical Applications 7.1 and 7.2 for the practical implications of the anatomy discussed in this chapter.





### CLINICAL APPLICATION 7.1 Pituitary adenoma

A 28-year-old unmarried woman presented with a history of amenorrhoea (lack of menstruation) and spontaneous secretion of milk from her breasts for the past year. She also reported recent onset of headache and visual disturbances. Testing for visual fields revealed bitemporal hemianopia—loss of temporal field of vision. Computerized tomography (CT) scans showed a large pituitary adenoma [Fig. 7.18].

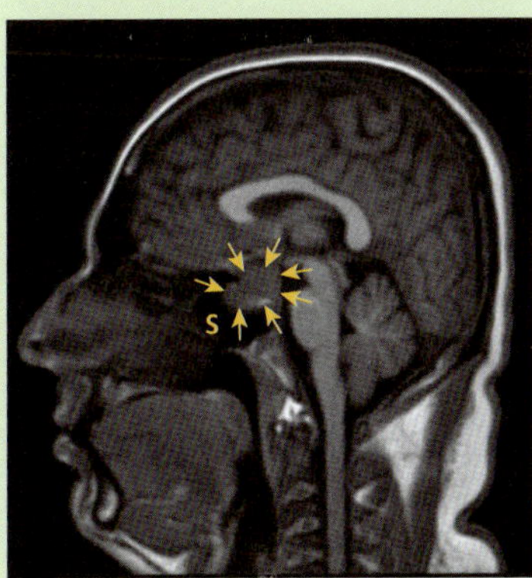


Fig. 7.18 T1-weighted sagittal magnetic resonance imaging (MRI) of a pituitary macroadenoma, sagittal view. Arrows = boundary of macroadenoma; S = sphenoid air sinus.

Study question 1: why does the patient experience visual disturbance? (Answer: a large pituitary adenoma can compress the optic chiasma above and disrupt the nasal fibres from the retina. This causes bitemporal hemianopia.)

Study question 2: what cell type could this tumour be composed of? (Answer: the history suggests a prolactin-secreting tumour called prolactinoma. This causes secretion of breast milk, even in non-lactating women (galactorrhoea). A high content of prolactin in the circulating blood can cause suppression of the menstrual cycle (amenorrhoea) and anovular cycles leading to infertility.)

Study question 3: what are the other tumours of the pituitary gland? (Answer: other common hormone-secreting tumours are somatotrophic adenomas—secrete growth hormone; corticotrophic adenomas—secrete adrenocorticotrophin; and gonadotrophic adenomas—secrete follicle-stimulating hormone (FSH) or luteinizing hormone (LH).)

Study question 4: how are these tumours treated? (Answer: most tumours resolve with medicines. Others can be treated with surgery. The endonasal trans-sphenoidal approach to the pituitary is commonly used.)

## CLINICAL APPLICATION 7.2 Intracranial haemorrhage—epidural versus subdural haematomas

A 23-year-old man sustained a head injury in a road traffic accident. He was conscious for a short while and then lapsed into a coma. He was suspected of having an intracranial haemorrhage. Intracranial haemorrhages can be classified according to location as: (1) extradural; (2) subdural; (3) subarachnoid; and (4) intracerebral.

Study question 1: use your knowledge of anatomy and Figs. 7.1 and 7.3 to determine which vessels would be the source of bleeding in: (1) extradural; (2) subdural; and (3) subarachnoid haemorrhage. (Answer: (1) extradural haemorrhage = meningeal vessels; (2) subdural haemorrhage = bridging veins as they run from the subarachnoid space to the superior sagittal sinus; and (3) subarachnoid haemorrhage = cerebral vessels.)

With time, blood from ruptured vessels collects within the confines of the space and forms a haematoma. Epidural haematomas are formed by high-pressure arterial blood rapidly filling the space between the dura mater and bone. On CT, they are shaped like a biconvex lens and are confined to the area bound by sutures (as the dura is firmly adherent to the bone at the sutures and does not separate easily). If the dura mater is torn, bleeding from extradural vessels can spread into the subdural space.

Subdural haematomas result in slowly developing brain compression and unconsciousness, and are formed by venous blood. They lie between the dura and the arachnoid mater. On CT, they are crescent-shaped and follow the contours of the brain.

# CHAPTER 8
# Deep dissection of the neck

## Introduction

This chapter deals with the description and dissection of the trachea and oesophagus, the thyroid and parathyroid glands, the large vessels of the head and neck, the lower cranial nerves, and the cervical lymph nodes [Fig. 8.1]. These important structures lie deep to the anterior and posterior triangles, and in front of the prevertebral structures described in Chapter 9.

Dissection 8.1 provides instructions on dissection of the trachea, oesophagus, thyroid gland, and related structures.



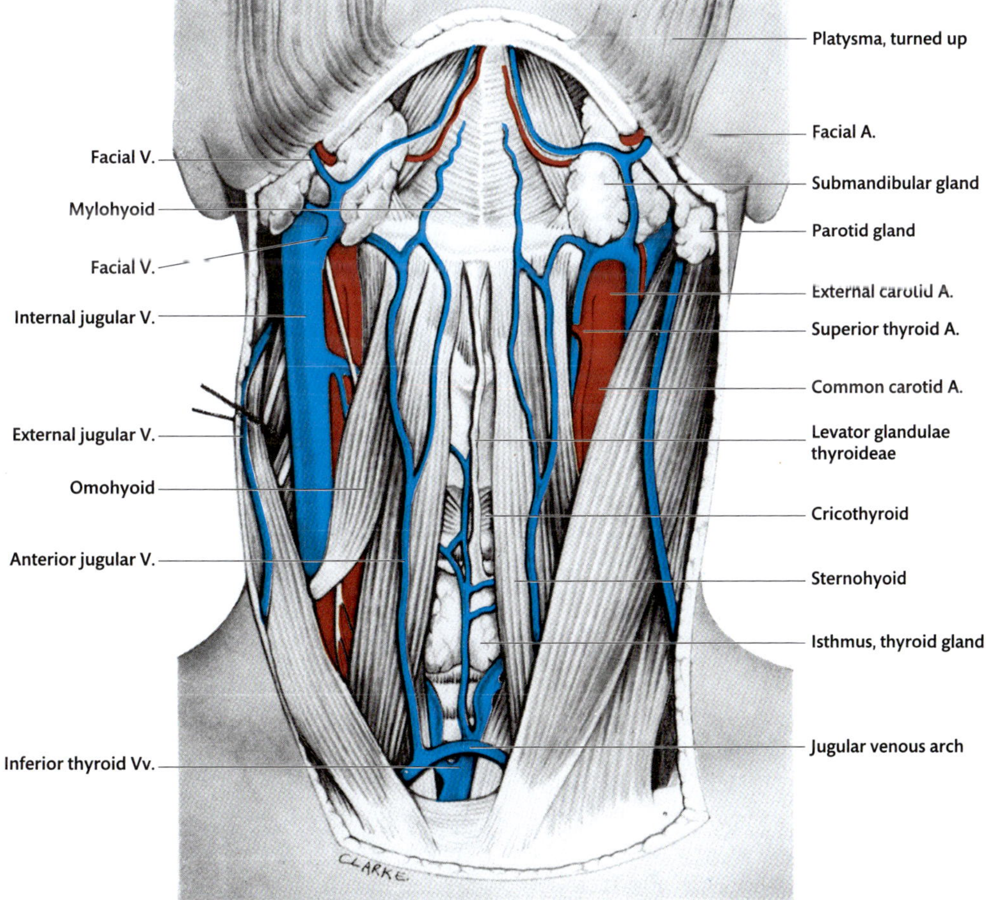


**Fig. 8.1** Dissection of the front of the neck. The right sternocleidomastoid has been retracted.

**DISSECTION 8.1 Thyroid gland, trachea, oesophagus, and related structures**

**Objectives**

**I.** To expose the thyroid gland and the blood vessels supplying it. **II.** To identify and trace the trachea, oesophagus, thoracic duct, and recurrent laryngeal nerves.

**Instructions**

Most of the structures dealt with in this dissection are under cover of the sternocleidomastoid. Others are hidden by the infrahyoid muscles or by the parotid gland and adjacent structures. Try to retain the sternocleidomastoid as far as possible during the dissection, for it is an important landmark in the neck.

1. Identify again the infrahyoid muscles—sternohyoid, sternothyroid, thyrohyoid, and omohyoid.
2. Displace the sternocleidomastoid and the superior belly of the omohyoid laterally. Cut through the sternothyroid near its lower end, and turn it upwards with the nerve which supplies it.
3. Before removing the fat from in front of the trachea, find the inferior thyroid veins in this fat. Note if any parts of the right and left lobes of the **thymus** extend up into the fat. These are difficult to differentiate from the fat but are darker and ensheathed in the fascia.
4. Remove the fascia from the lobes of the thyroid gland, and expose the arteries and veins supplying it. Lift the lower part of the gland to expose the lateral surfaces of the trachea and oesophagus, with the recurrent laryngeal nerves in the groove between them.
5. On the left side, look for the thoracic duct on the oesophagus. If the thorax has been dissected, the thoracic duct and recurrent laryngeal nerve can often be followed upwards.
6. Pull the upper part of the thyroid gland laterally, and trace the external laryngeal branch of the superior laryngeal nerve to the cricothyroid muscle.
7. Find the lower part of the inferior constrictor muscle arising from a fibrous arch crossing the cricothyroid muscle and hiding its posterior part [see Fig. 5.6].

## Thymus

This important lymphoid structure is particularly large in the child. In the adult, it consists chiefly of fat and fibrous tissue. Its two lobes are two slender, elongated, yellowish bodies that lie side by side, anterior to the pericardium and great vessels in the upper part of the thorax [see Figs. 5.20, 5.21 in Vol. 2]. The thymus develops as lateral outgrowths of the pharynx and subsequently descends into the thorax. As such, the superior parts of the thymus may be found in the neck, anterior to the trachea, and attached to the lower ends of the thyroid gland.

## Thyroid gland

The thyroid gland is a highly vascular endocrine gland which partially surrounds the upper part of the trachea. It consists of a pair of **lobes** joined across the midline by a narrow **isthmus** [Fig. 8.2]. It extends from the oblique line on the thyroid cartilage down to the fifth or sixth tracheal ring. It is enclosed in a **sheath** of pre-tracheal fascia which is attached above to the oblique line of the thyroid cartilage and to the arch of the cricoid cartilage. This attachment makes the thyroid gland move with the larynx in swallowing and speaking—a feature which helps to differentiate swellings of the thyroid gland from those of adjacent structures.

Deep to the covering formed by the pre-tracheal fascia is the **fibrous capsule** of the gland. Between the pre-tracheal fascia and the fibrous capsule are the arteries and veins. The gland varies greatly in size and is relatively larger in women and children than in men.

### Lobes of the thyroid gland

The **right** and **left lobes** of the thyroid gland are conical and have three surfaces—superficial, medial, and posterior. The convex superficial surface is covered by the sternohyoid, sternothyroid, and omohyoid muscles, and overlapped by the anterior border of the sternocleidomastoid. Inferiorly, the medial surface is related to the trachea and oesophagus, with the recurrent laryngeal nerve

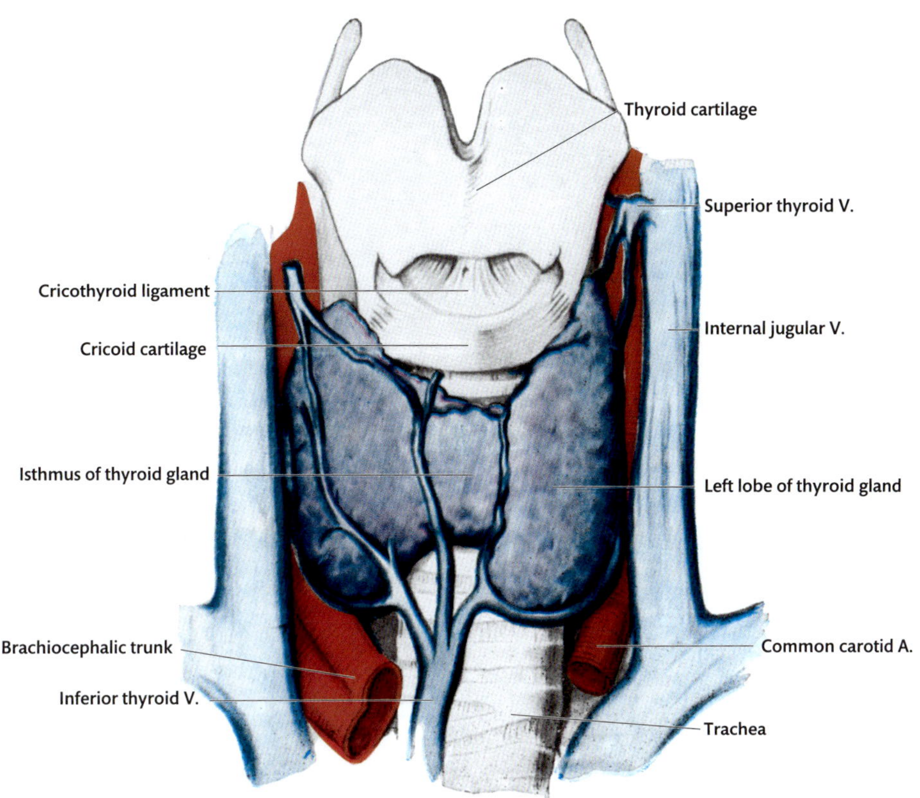


**Fig. 8.2** The thyroid gland, anterior surface.

between them. Superiorly, the medial surface is related to the cricoid and thyroid cartilages, with the cricothyroid, inferior constrictor muscle, and external branch of the superior laryngeal nerve between them. The posterior surface of the thyroid lobe lies on the prevertebral fascia, anterior to the longus colli, and overlaps the medial part of the carotid sheath. The **parathyroid glands** are embedded in the posterior surface [see Fig. 4.2; Figs. 8.3, 8.4, 8.5].

## Isthmus of the thyroid gland

The isthmus of the thyroid gland is of variable width and lies on the second to fourth tracheal rings. It is closer to the lower border of the thyroid lobes and is covered by skin and fasciae of the neck. A slender **pyramidal lobe** frequently extends superiorly from the upper border of the isthmus, usually to the left of the midline. It may be attached to the hyoid bone by a narrow slip of muscle—the **levator glandulae thyroideae**—or by a fibrous strand [Figs. 8.1, 8.2]. This strand is a remnant of the median diverticulum from which the thyroid gland developed. (The diverticulum originates in the foramen caecum of the tongue as a median epithelial downgrowth. It descends in front of the body of the hyoid, hooks up posterior to it, and continues to descend in front of the thyroid and cricoid cartilages. The lower end of the diverticulum expands to form the thyroid gland. The suprahyoid part of this structure rarely persists.)

## Arteries of the thyroid gland

The apex of each lobe receives the **superior thyroid artery** (branch of the external carotid artery) which divides into two or three branches. The base and deep surfaces of each lobe receive branches from the **inferior thyroid arteries** (branches of the thyrocervical trunk of the subclavian artery). A small **thyroidea ima** artery may arise from the brachiocephalic trunk, aortic arch, or left common carotid artery, and ascend on the anterior surface of the trachea to the isthmus. The arteries anastomose freely, especially on the posterior surface of each lobe. (The thyroid arteries are arteries of the gut tube, so they also supply the larynx, laryngeal part of the pharynx, trachea, and oesophagus [Figs. 8.1, 8.5, 8.6].)

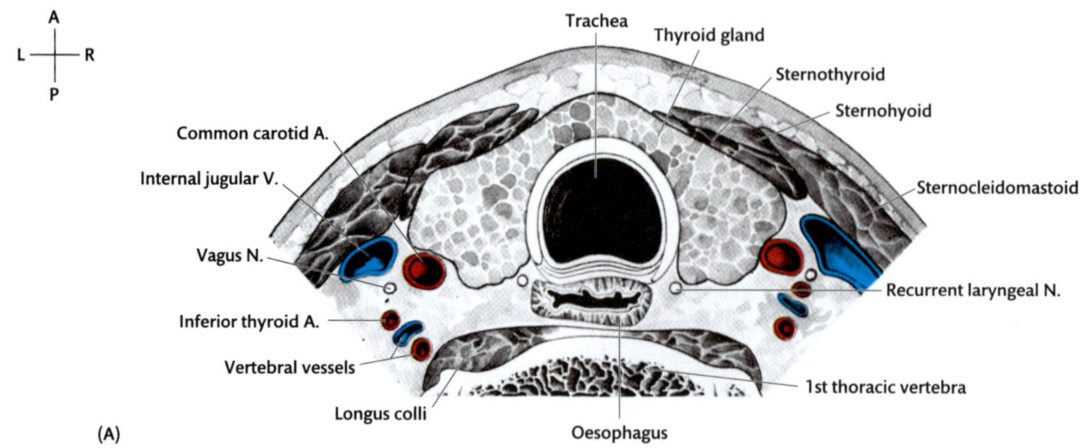


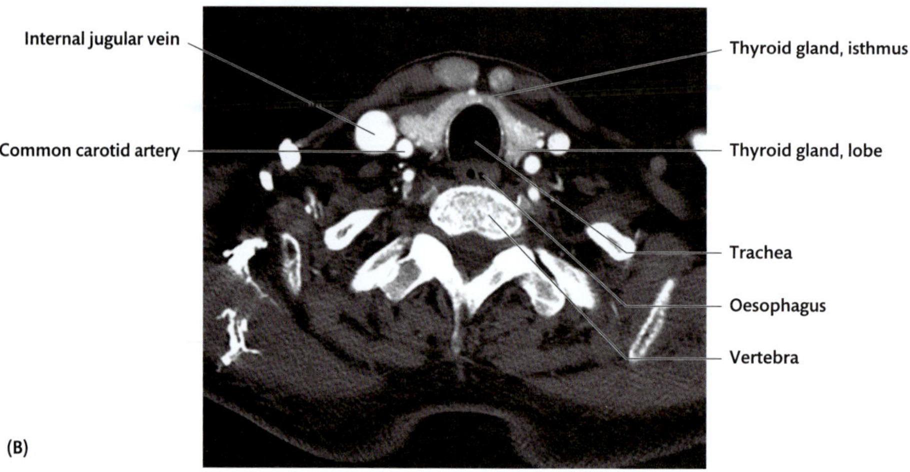


**Fig. 8.3** (A) Schematic drawing of a transverse section and (B) axial computerized tomography (CT) through the anterior part of the neck at the level of the first thoracic vertebra.

## Veins of the thyroid gland

Three pairs of veins drain the thyroid gland. A **superior thyroid vein** arises near the upper end of each lobe. It either crosses the common carotid artery and drains into the internal jugular vein or ascends with the superior thyroid artery to drain into the facial vein. A short **middle thyroid vein** arises from the lower part of each lobe and crosses the common carotid artery to drain into the internal jugular vein. The **inferior thyroid vein** descends in front of the trachea from the isthmus and lower parts of the lobes to the corresponding brachiocephalic veins. Occasionally, the inferior thyroid veins unite with each other [Fig. 8.2] and end in one or other of the brachiocephalic veins. They also receive tributaries from the trachea, larynx, and oesophagus.

## Lymph vessels of the thyroid gland

The lymph vessels of the thyroid gland drain mostly to nodes on the carotid sheath—the upper and lower deep cervical nodes.

## Clinical features of thyroid swelling

➲ The fascia covering the thyroid gland is attached to the hyoid bone, and the oblique line of the thyroid cartilage. In addition, a thickened band of fascia, called the ligament of Berry, anchors the medial surface of the thyroid gland to the cricoid cartilage. Because of these fascial attachments, the thyroid

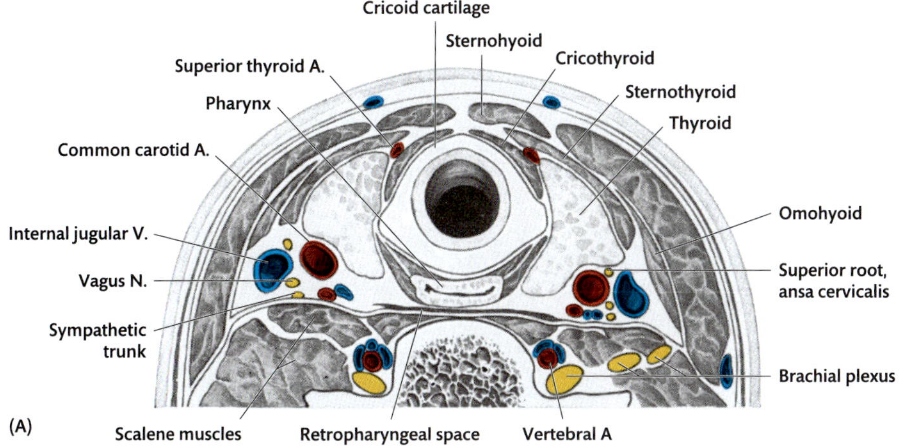


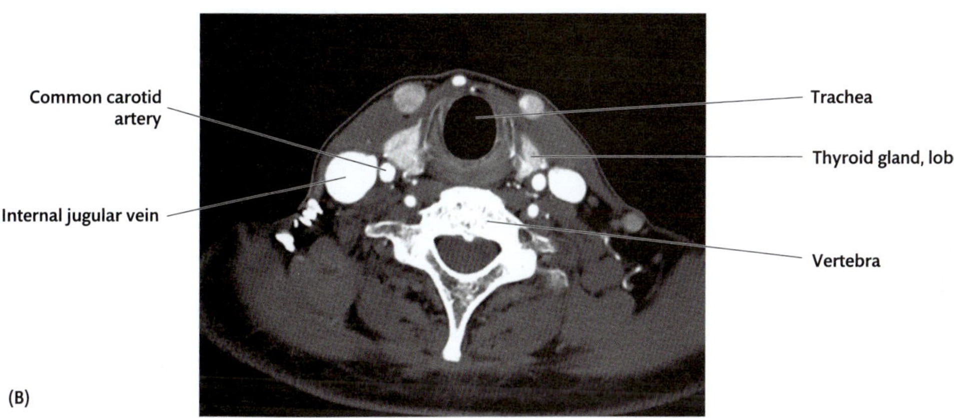


**Fig. 8.4** (A) Schematic drawing of a transverse section and (B) axial computerized tomography (CT) through the anterior part of the neck at the level of the cricoid cartilage.

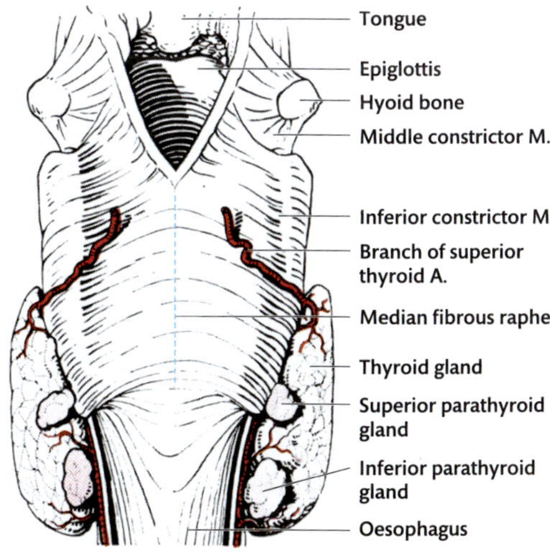


**Fig. 8.5** Posterior surface of the thyroid gland to show the parathyroid glands.

gland moves up on swallowing. While examining the front of the neck, any swelling that moves up on deglutition is likely to originate in the thyroid gland.

➲ The proximity of the thyroid gland to the trachea, oesophagus, and recurrent laryngeal nerve may lead to compression symptoms on these structures when the thyroid is enlarged. Pressure on the trachea causes dyspnoea, cough, wheeze, or tightness of the chest. Pressure on the oesophagus causes dysphagia, and pressure on the recurrent laryngeal nerve causes hoarseness of voice.

➲ The proximity of the thyroid gland to the veins of the neck may cause neck vein swelling, venous congestion and flushing of the face, and dyspnoea when the arms are raised above the head, due to increased venous return—Pemberton's sign.

Following the instructions given in Dissection 8.2, examine the posterior surface of the thyroid gland.

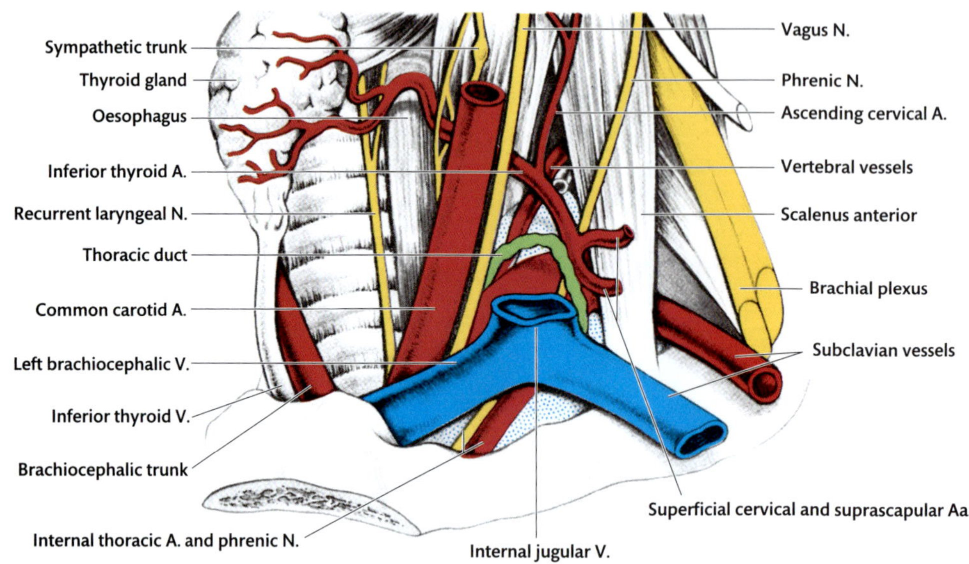


**Fig. 8.6** Deep dissection of the root of the neck on the left side. The clavicle, sternocleidomastoid, and infrahyoid muscles have been removed, and the thyroid gland is displaced anteriorly. Pleura, blue stipple.

### DISSECTION 8.2 Thyroid and parathyroid glands

**Objective**

**I.** To examine the posterior surface of a lobe of the thyroid gland and identify the blood vessels and parathyroids.

**Instructions**

1. Cut through the isthmus and the vessels of one lobe, and remove that lobe.
2. Find the anastomotic vessel between the superior and inferior thyroid arteries on the medial part of the posterior surface. Look for the yellowish-brown parathyroid glands immediately lateral to it. The best guide to the parathyroids is the small parathyroid artery which arises from the inferior thyroid artery.
3. Make a cut through the lobe of the thyroid gland, and examine the surface with a hand lens.

## Parathyroid glands

Two pairs of small yellowish-brown endocrine glands are embedded in the posterior surface of the capsule of the thyroid gland—the superior and inferior parathyroid glands. They are approximately 6×3×2 mm. Their important secretion stimulates the mobilization of calcium from the bones to maintain the normal blood calcium level.

The **superior parathyroid glands** are more constant in position than the inferior glands and lie at about the middle of the posterior surface of each lobe. Each **inferior parathyroid gland** is close to the inferior surface of the lobe [Fig. 8.5].

Using the instructions given in Dissection 8.3, study the trachea, oesophagus, and related structures.

### DISSECTION 8.3 Trachea and oesophagus

**Objective**

**I.** To re-examine the trachea, oesophagus, recurrent laryngeal nerves, and thoracic duct after the thyroid is mobilized.

**Instructions**

1. Complete the exposure of the trachea and oesophagus.
2. Identify the recurrent laryngeal nerves on either side between the trachea and the oesophagus.
3. Identify the thoracic duct on the left of the oesophagus.

## Trachea and oesophagus

The trachea and oesophagus begin at the lower border of the cricoid cartilage, anterior to the sixth cervical vertebra, and descend into the thorax.

### Trachea

The trachea is a wide tube, approximately 12 cm long. It is kept constantly patent by the U-shaped cartilaginous bars embedded in its walls. Posteriorly, where the cartilage is deficient, the flat wall of the trachea lies against the oesophagus. Superiorly, the trachea is continuous with the larynx. Laterally are the common carotid arteries and the lobes of the thyroid gland, and on the right side is the brachiocephalic trunk. The recurrent laryngeal nerves lie in the groove between the oesophagus and the trachea [Figs. 8.2, 8.3, 8.7].

### Oesophagus

The oesophagus is a thick, distensible, muscular tube, approximately 25 cm long. It extends from the pharynx to the stomach [Figs. 8.3, 8.4, 8.5, 8.6, 8.7]. It is surrounded by loose connective tissue which permits distension of the tube. In the neck, the oesophagus lies between the trachea and the prevertebral fascia overlying the prevertebral muscles. On the right, it is in contact with the thyroid gland and the cervical pleura. On the left, it is in contact with the thyroid gland, but the subclavian artery and the thoracic duct separate it from the pleura. The oesophagus inclines to the left as it descends in the neck [Figs. 8.6, 8.7]. Thus, it is more readily accessible to the surgeon on that side.

Dissection 8.4 (and Fig. 8.8) provides instructions on dissecting the vessels and nerves of the neck.

## Brachiocephalic trunk

The **brachiocephalic trunk** is a large artery which arises from the arch of the aorta and passes superiorly and to the right. For the most part, it lies in the thorax and divides into the right subclavian and right common carotid arteries behind the right sternoclavicular joint.

## Subclavian artery

The **left subclavian artery** arises from the arch of the aorta and ascends on the pleura to enter the neck behind the left sternoclavicular joint. The **right subclavian artery** arises from the brachiocephalic artery behind the right sternoclavicular joint. On both sides, the subclavian artery arches laterally across the anterior surface of the cervical pleura on to the first rib, posterior to the anterior scalenus [Figs. 8.6, 8.7, 8.8]. It becomes the axillary





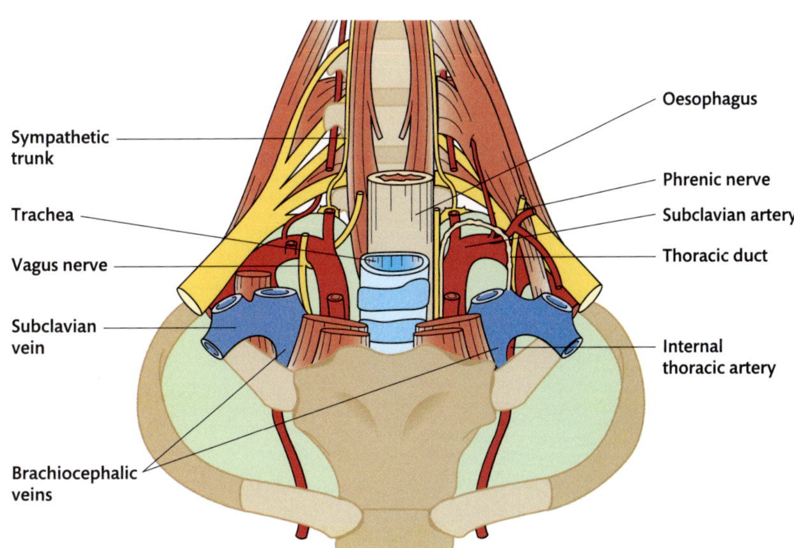


**Fig. 8.7** Dissection of the root of the neck to show the structures adjacent to the cervical pleura (green shading).

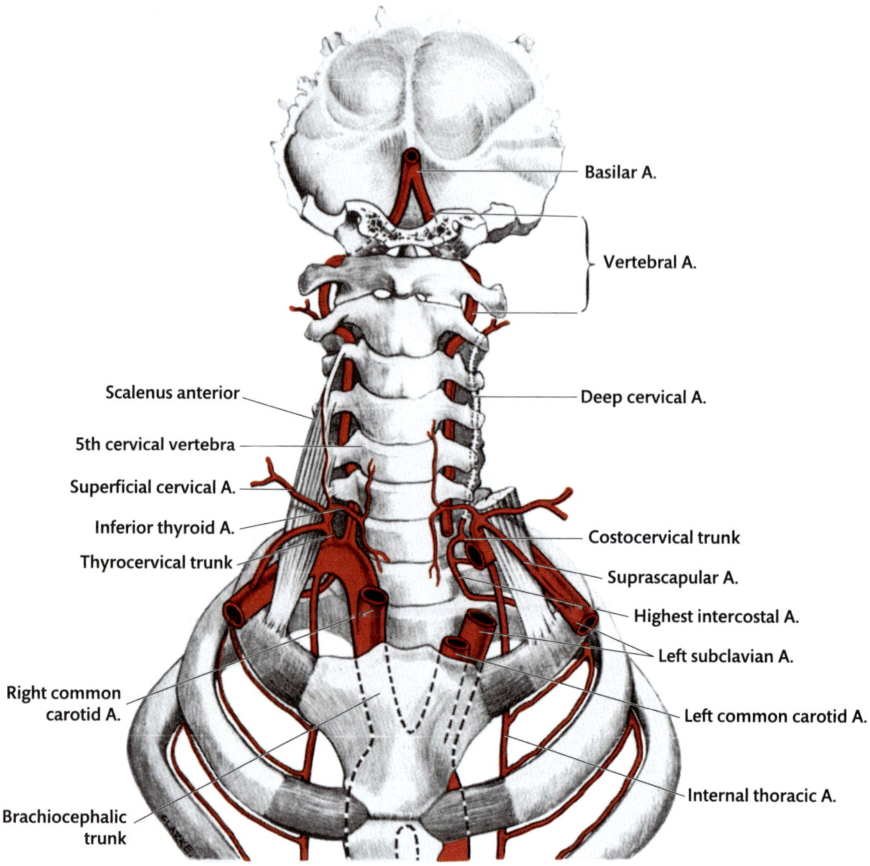


**Fig. 8.8** Diagram of the branches of the subclavian arteries. (The deep cervical artery lies deep among the muscles of the back of the neck.)

### DISSECTION 8.4 Vessels and nerves of the neck

#### Objectives

**I.** To expose the contents of the carotid sheath. **II.** To expose the vessels and nerves at the root of the neck.

#### Instructions

1. Remove the fat, lymph nodes, and the remains of the carotid sheath from the common carotid artery and internal jugular vein.
2. Separate the vessels, and find the vagus nerve between and behind the vein and the artery.
3. Expose the vagus, and find the right recurrent laryngeal nerve arising from it as it crosses the subclavian artery. Follow it to the groove between the trachea and the oesophagus.
4. On the left side, find the thoracic duct entering the junction of the internal jugular and subclavian veins [Fig. 8.6] from above and behind. Trace it backwards and downwards to where it lies behind the left common carotid artery.
5. On both sides, expose the small cervical part of the brachiocephalic vein and its tributaries.
6. On the right side, expose the small part of the brachiocephalic trunk which lies in the neck.
7. Identify the phrenic nerve behind the internal jugular vein and prevertebral fascia. Trace it to the thorax.
8. Displace the internal jugular vein medially to expose the subclavian artery and cervical pleura. Avoid injury to the thoracic duct and vertebral veins.
9. Trace the internal thoracic artery, the thyrocervical trunk, and its branches from the first part of the subclavian artery [Fig. 8.6].
10. Pull the anterior scalene laterally to expose the **costocervical trunk** arising from the subclavian artery at the medial border of the muscle. Trace the trunk over the cervical pleura to the neck of the first rib.
11. Separate the internal jugular vein and the common carotid artery. Carefully dissect deep to the vertebral veins and thoracic duct to find the **vertebral artery** posterior to them.

12. Trace the vertebral artery superiorly in front of the transverse process of the seventh cervical vertebra till it passes into the transverse foramen of the sixth cervical vertebra.
13. Remove the fat posterior to the vertebral artery to expose the ventral rami of the seventh and eighth cervical nerves, above and below the seventh cervical transverse process, respectively [Fig. 8.8].
14. Displace the common carotid artery laterally to expose the **sympathetic trunk** posteromedial to it [Fig. 8.6]. Trace the trunk superiorly and inferiorly.
15. Find the **cervicothoracic ganglion** between the seventh cervical transverse process and the neck of the first rib, posterior to the vertebral artery.
16. Find the small **middle cervical ganglion** anterior to the inferior thyroid artery, close to the sixth cervical transverse process.
17. Find the grey rami communicantes passing from these ganglia to the ventral rami of the spinal nerves.

artery at the outer border of the first rib. The subclavian artery is arbitrarily divided into three parts by the anterior scalene. The first part is medial to the muscle; the second part is posterior to it, and the third part is lateral. (The third part has been described in Chapter 5.)

## First part of the subclavian artery

On the right, the first part runs superolaterally at the medial edge of the anterior scalene. At its origin, it lies posterior to the sternocleidomastoid, sternohyoid, sternothyroid, and vagus nerve. The **right recurrent laryngeal** branch of the vagus hooks around the first part of the subclavian artery. A loop from the sympathetic trunk—the **ansa subclavia**—also loops around the subclavian artery at this point. The ansa subclavia contains fibres that unite the inferior and middle cervical sympathetic ganglia around the subclavian artery. Near the medial border of the anterior scalene, the subclavian artery lies posterior to the internal jugular and vertebral veins. It lies anterior to the suprapleural membrane covering the anterior surface of the cervical pleura [Fig. 8.7]. (If the lung has already been removed, investigate the position of the artery from the pleural cavity.)

On the left, the first part of the subclavian artery ascends vertically from the aortic arch, posterior to the vagus, phrenic, and cardiac nerves. It lies behind the left brachiocephalic vein at the sternoclavicular joint. From then onwards, the course of the left subclavian artery is the same as that of the right, except that the thoracic duct and phrenic nerve also descend anterior to it [Fig. 8.6]. The **left recurrent laryngeal nerve** is medial to the artery as it ascends from the aortic arch in the groove between the trachea and the oesophagus.

## Second part of the subclavian artery

The second part of the subclavian artery curves upwards and rises 1.5–2.5 cm above the clavicle. It lies posterior to the anterior scalene and phrenic nerve, and anterior to the suprapleural membrane [Figs. 8.6, 8.7].

### Branches of the subclavian artery

The first part gives rise to the **vertebral artery**, the **thyrocervical trunk**, and the **internal thoracic artery**. The thyrocervical trunk gives rise to the **inferior thyroid**, **superficial cervical**, and **suprascapular arteries**. The second part gives rise to the **costocervical trunk**, which gives off the **highest intercostal** and **deep cervical arteries** [Fig. 8.8].

#### Vertebral artery

The vertebral artery is the first branch of the subclavian artery *(first part)* and mainly supplies the brain. It arises at the level of the sternoclavicular joint, ascends between the longus colli and anterior scalene muscles, and enters into the foramen transversarium of the sixth cervical vertebra. It is posterior to the common carotid and inferior thyroid arteries and to its own vein, and anterior to the ventral rami of the seventh and eighth cervical nerves and the seventh cervical transverse process. The sympathetic trunk lies along its medial side, and the cervicothoracic ganglion, which is partly behind the artery, sends branches to form a plexus on it. It is crossed anteriorly by the thoracic duct on the left [see Fig. 7.15; Figs. 8.6, 8.7, 8.8].

#### Thyrocervical trunk

The short thyrocervical trunk arises from the *first part* of the subclavian artery at the medial margin of the anterior scalene, posterior to the internal jugular vein. It branches immediately into the inferior thyroid artery, and the superficial cervical and suprascapular branches.

The **inferior thyroid artery** arises from the thyrocervical trunk and ascends along the medial border of the anterior scalene. Just below the transverse process of the sixth cervical vertebra, it turns medially in front of the vertebral artery and behind the vagus, sympathetic trunk, and common carotid artery, to reach the middle of the posterior surface of the thyroid gland. It then descends to the lower pole of the gland and branches close to the recurrent laryngeal nerve. It supplies the thyroid and parathyroid glands, and anastomoses with the superior thyroid artery [Figs. 8.6, 8.8].

The **ascending cervical branch** of the inferior thyroid artery passes upwards on the cervical transverse processes. It supplies the prevertebral muscles and sends branches to the spinal cord [Fig. 8.8].

The **inferior laryngeal artery** arises from the inferior thyroid artery and accompanies the recurrent laryngeal nerve to the larynx. Other branches from the thyrocervical trunk pass to the trachea, oesophagus, pharynx, and infrahyoid muscles.

#### Internal thoracic artery

The internal thoracic artery arises from the inferior surface of the *first part* of the subclavian artery near the medial border of the anterior scalene. It passes inferomedially to the back of the first costal cartilage. In the neck, it lies anterior to the pleura behind the medial part of the clavicle [Fig. 8.7].

#### Costocervical trunk

The **costocervical trunk** arises from the posterior surface of the *second part* of the subclavian artery [Fig. 8.8]. It arches posteriorly over the pleura and divides at the neck of the first rib into the deep cervical and superior intercostal arteries.

The **deep cervical artery** passes into the back of the neck above the neck of the first rib. Together with the descending branch of the occipital artery, it is the main source of blood supply to the muscles of the back of the neck.

The **superior intercostal artery** descends anterior to the neck of the first rib and gives posterior intercostal arteries to the first and second intercostal spaces. If the lung has been removed, examine these from the interior of the thorax [Fig. 8.8].

### Third part of the subclavian artery

The third part of the subclavian lies in the posterior triangle. It gives off the dorsal scapula artery.

## Subclavian vein

The **subclavian vein** is a continuation of the axillary vein at the outer border of the first rib. It unites with the internal jugular vein behind the sternoclavicular joint to form the brachiocephalic vein. It receives the external jugular vein.

The veins corresponding to the branches of the subclavian artery do not drain into the subclavian vein. The vertebral vein and the internal thoracic vein drain into the brachiocephalic vein. The deep cervical vein joins the vertebral vein [Figs. 8.6, 8.7].

## Brachiocephalic veins

The brachiocephalic veins receive blood from the head and neck, upper limbs, walls of the thorax, and anterior abdominal wall (internal thoracic veins). They are formed behind the medial end of the clavicle by the union of the internal jugular and subclavian veins [Figs. 8.7, 8.9]. They descend into the thorax and end by uniting with each other to form the superior vena cava. They have no valves.

In the neck, the right brachiocephalic vein lies on the cervical pleura, with the phrenic nerve and internal thoracic artery intervening. It is lateral to the brachiocephalic trunk (with the vagus behind and between them) and posterior to the medial end of the clavicle. It enters the thorax behind the right first costal cartilage. On the left, the vein is first posterior to the clavicle and anterior to the pleura and internal thoracic artery. It then descends posterior to the sternoclavicular joint, anterior to the phrenic and vagus nerves, and the arteries arising from the aortic arch [Figs. 8.7, 8.10].

### Tributaries in the neck

The brachiocephalic veins receive the vertebral, highest intercostal, and frequently inferior thyroid veins, and one or two lymph trunks. In addition, the left brachiocephalic vein receives the thoracic duct and left superior intercostal vein.

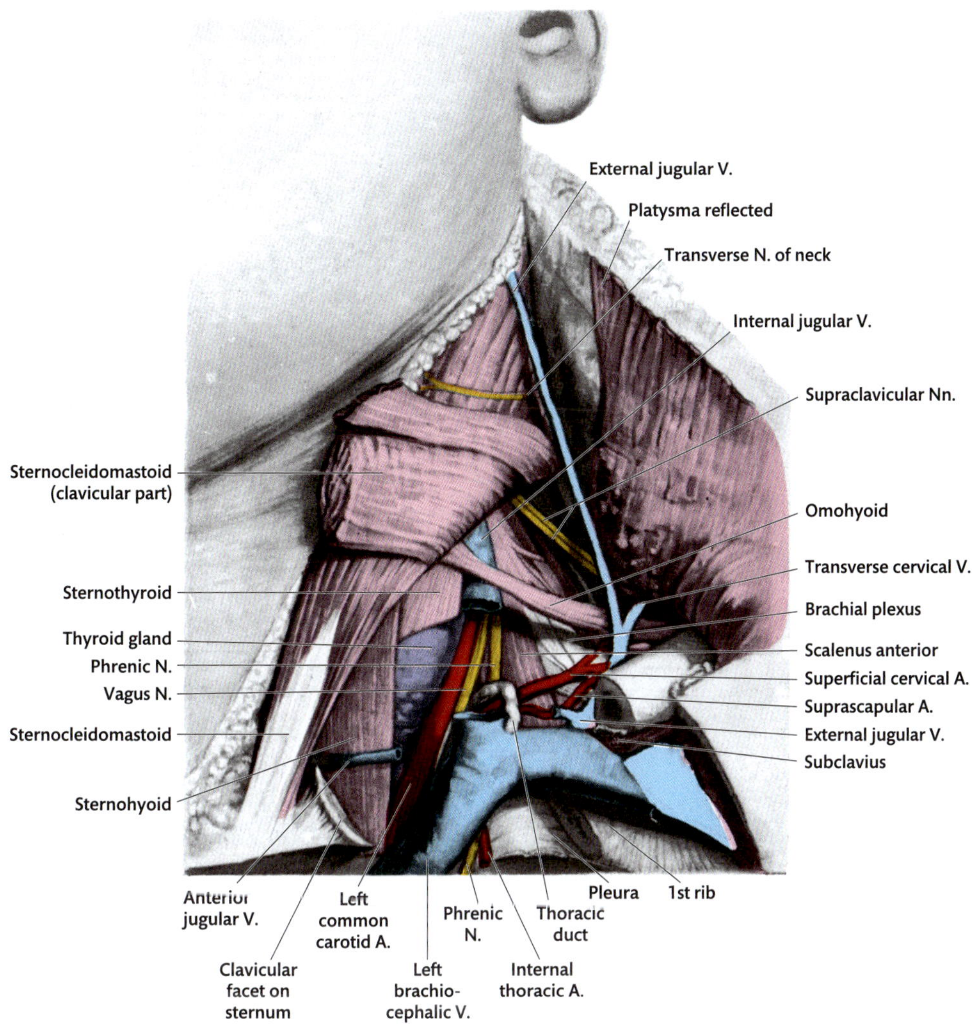


**Fig. 8.9** Deep dissection of the root of the neck to show the termination of the thoracic duct.

Fig. 8.10 is a schematic section through the neck at the level of C. 5, showing the areas supplied by branches of the external carotid and subclavian arteries.

## Thoracic duct

The thoracic duct is a large lymph vessel which drains lymph into the venous system. It drains lymph from: (1) all the regions below the diaphragm, except for the upper part of the right lobe of the liver and the upper half of the anterior abdominal wall; (2) the posterior thoracic wall on both sides; and (3) the left half of the body above the diaphragm. The lymph in the duct has a milky appearance due to the fat from the small intestine.

The thoracic duct is slender, thin-walled, and frequently mistaken for a vein. It ascends from the thorax along the left margin of the oesophagus. At the level of the seventh cervical vertebra, it arches anterolaterally between the carotid sheath and the cervical pleura, and turns inferiorly to enter the left brachiocephalic vein in the angle between the internal jugular and subclavian veins [Figs. 8.7, 8.9]. Its opening into the vein is guarded by a valve.

There are three other lymph trunks in the root of the neck on each side: (1) the **subclavian lymph trunk** which drains the upper limb; (2) the **jugular lymph trunk** which drains the head and neck; and (3) the **bronchomediastinal lymph trunk** which drains the lung, mediastinum, and part of the anterior walls of the thorax and abdomen through the **internal thoracic lymph**

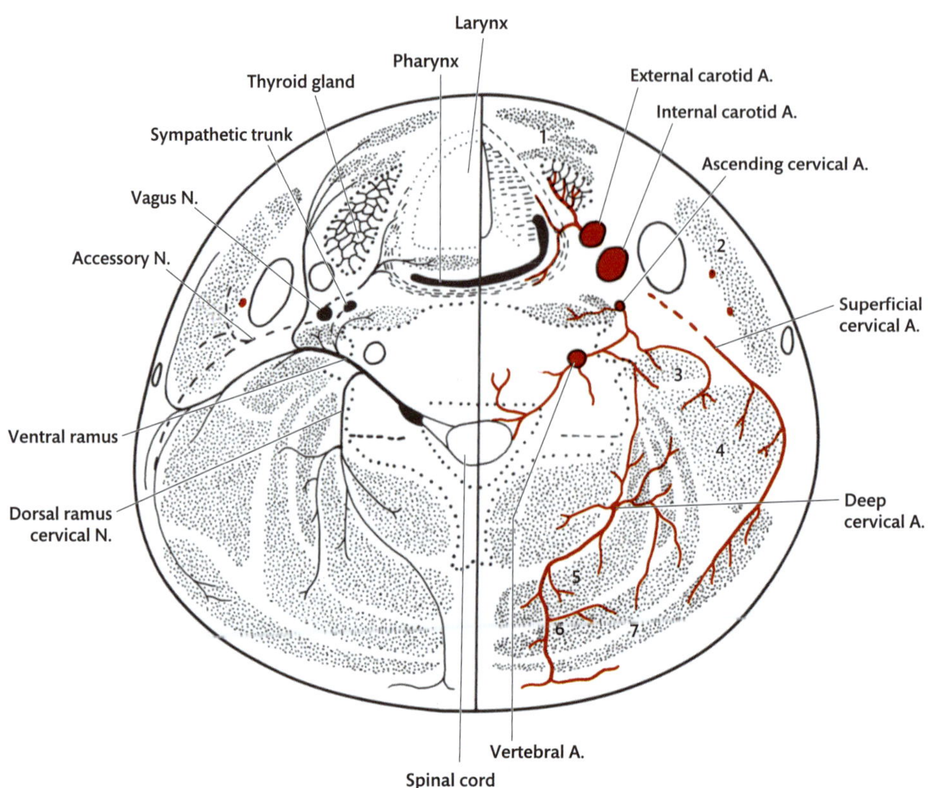


**Fig. 8.10** Diagrammatic transverse section through the neck to show the distribution of nerves (left) and arteries (right). The diagram is constructed from a number of adjacent levels. The part of the accessory nerve shown by an interrupted line is at a still higher level. 1 = infrahyoid muscles. 2 = sternocleidomastoid. 3 = middle scalene. 4 = levator scapulae. 5 = semispinalis capitis. 6 = splenius capitis. 7 = trapezius.

**vessels**. The mode of termination of these lymph trunks is variable. The bronchomediastinal trunks usually enter the corresponding brachiocephalic veins. On the left side, all three lymph trunks may end in the thoracic duct. Commonly, the subclavian lymph trunk ends in the subclavian vein. On the right side, the jugular and subclavian lymph trunks may end separately in the corresponding veins but frequently unite to form a **right lymph duct** which drains into the junction of the right internal jugular and subclavian veins. The mode of termination of the three lymph trunks alters the territory drained by the thoracic duct. These smaller vessels cannot be demonstrated by dissection.

## Cervical pleura

The parietal pleura forms the dome of the pleura and bulges upwards into the root of the neck [Fig. 8.7]. It reaches the level of the neck of the first rib, which is 2.5–5.0 cm above the sternal end of the first rib. A thickening of the fascia—the **suprapleural membrane**—stretches from the transverse process of the seventh cervical vertebra to the inner margin of the first rib and covers the cervical pleura. This membrane may contain some muscle fibres—the **scalenus minimus**.

The upper two ribs, first intercostal space, and sympathetic trunk lie posterior to the cervical pleura. The great vessels of the upper limb and head and neck lie anterior to it. The vertebral artery curves superiorly over the dome of the pleura to reach the vertebral column [Fig. 8.7].

The vertebral bodies, oesophagus, and trachea, and on the left side the thoracic duct and recurrent laryngeal nerve, lie medial to the cervical pleura. The anterior scalene, subclavian artery, and lower trunk of the brachial plexus lie lateral to it. The ascending and descending branches of the subclavian artery—the vertebral artery, inferior thyroid artery, and internal thoracic artery—also lie on the anterior surface of the cervical pleura. The costocervical trunk and its superior intercostal branch arch over the dome of the pleura from the anterior to the posterior surface.

## Vertical neurovascular bundles of the neck

A neurovascular bundle lies on each side of the trachea and oesophagus. In the lower part of the neck, the bundle consists of the **internal jugular vein** laterally, the **common carotid artery** medially, and the **vagus nerve** behind and between them. Above the level of the thyroid cartilage, the neurovascular bundle consists of the **internal carotid artery**, internal jugular vein, **glossopharyngeal**, **vagus**, **spinal accessory**, and **hypoglossal nerves**. The bundle is enclosed in a fascial sheath—the **carotid sheath** [see Fig. 4.2; Fig. 8.11]—which extends from the root of the neck to the base of the skull. It lies on the sympathetic trunk, prevertebral fascia, prevertebral muscles, and cervical transverse processes. Parts of this neurovascular bundle have been seen and described in the carotid triangle in Chapter 5.

Dissection 8.5 (and Figs. 8.12, 8.13, 8.14) provides instructions on dissection of the neurovascular structures of the neck.

Before beginning the dissection, identify the carotid canal, jugular foramen, hypoglossal canal, and foramen magnum on the base of a dried skull, and note the openings of these foramina on its internal aspect [see Fig. 2.14]. The **carotid canal** lies furthest anteriorly and transmits the internal carotid artery. Immediately posterior to it is the **jugular foramen** which transmits the sigmoid and inferior petrosal sinuses and the glossopharyngeal, vagus, and accessory nerves between the two veins. The hypoglossal nerve traverses the **hypoglossal canal**, immediately above the occipital condyle, and joins the other nerves between the internal carotid artery and the internal jugular vein close to the skull.

## Common carotid artery

The **right common carotid artery** arises from the brachiocephalic trunk behind the right sternoclavicular joint. The **left common carotid artery** arises from the arch of the aorta and ascends into the neck, posterior to the left sternoclavicular joint. Each artery ascends to the upper border of the thyroid cartilage at the level of the disc between the third and fourth cervical vertebrae, and ends by dividing into the internal and external carotid arteries [Figs. 8.2, 8.3, 8.4, 8.6, 8.12].

In the neck, the common carotid artery ascends anterior to the subclavian and vertebral arteries to lie on the prevertebral fascia on the sixth cervical transverse process—the **carotid tubercle**. (The anterior tubercle of the sixth cervical vertebra is longer than the others and is called the carotid tubercle. The carotid artery can be forcibly compressed on this bony prominence.)

The common carotid arteries lie in the carotid sheath. The lower part of both common carotid arteries is overlapped anteriorly by the sternocleidomastoid, infrahyoid muscles, and thyroid gland. Medially, they are related to the thyroid cartilage, thyroid gland, pharynx, larynx, trachea, and oesophagus [see Fig. 4.2; Fig. 8.1].



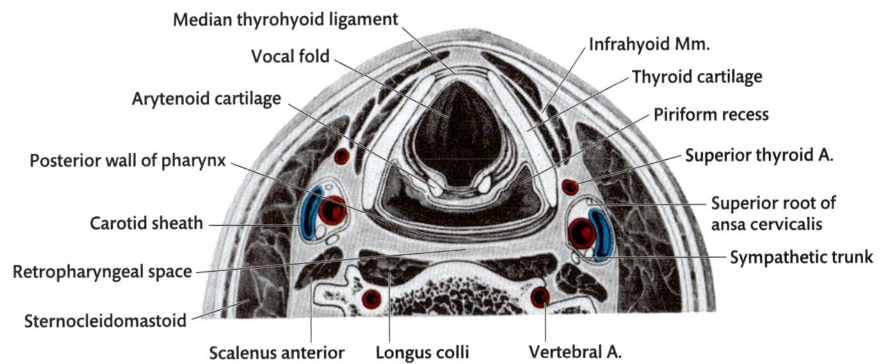


**Fig. 8.11** Transverse section through the anterior part of the neck at the level of the upper part of the thyroid cartilage.

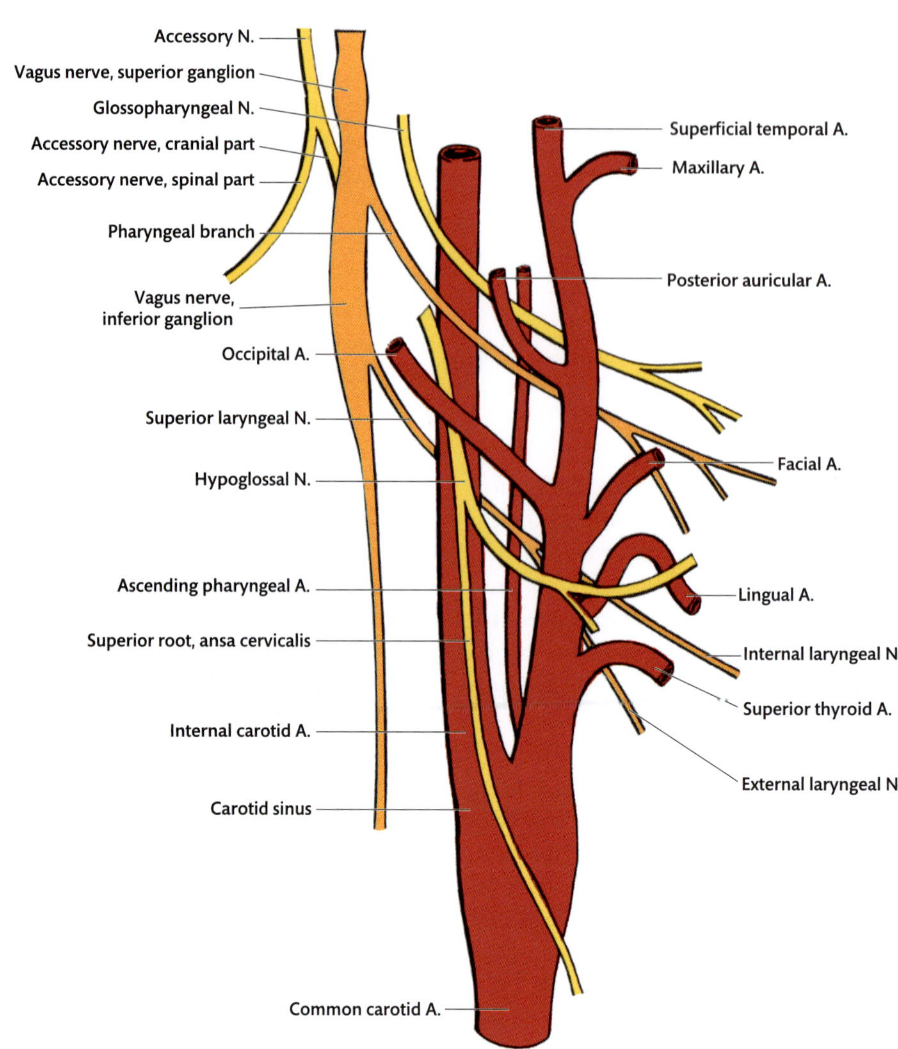


**Fig. 8.12** Diagram of the carotid arteries and the nerves associated with them.

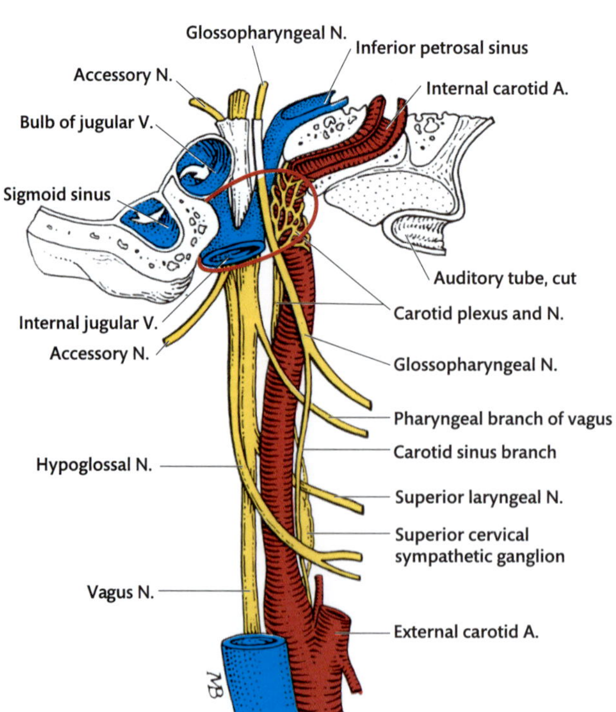


**Fig. 8.13** Diagram of structures in and below the right jugular foramen. Circle = jugular foramen.

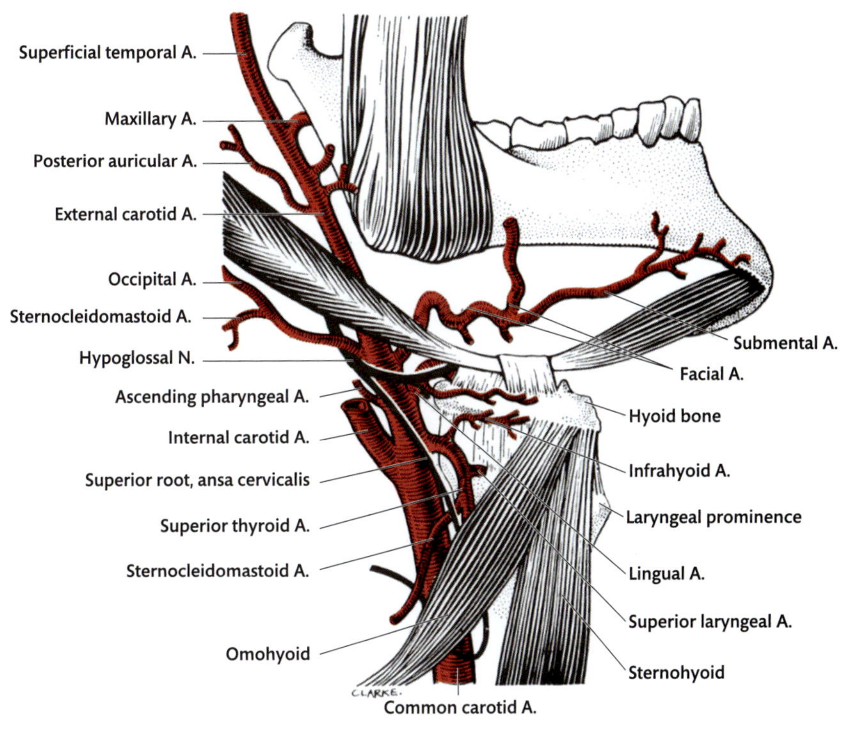


**Fig. 8.14** Diagram of the external carotid artery and its branches. The mandible has been tilted upwards.





### DISSECTION 8.5 Neurovascular structures of the neck

#### Objectives

**I.** To remove the right half of the skull and related structures, so as to gain approach to the cavities of the nose, mouth, pharynx, and larynx from the medial side.
**II.** To expose the superior parts of the internal carotid artery, the internal jugular vein, and the lower four cranial nerves in the upper part of the carotid sheath.

#### Instructions

1. On the right side, free the greater occipital nerve from the scalp, and turn it inferiorly. Cut through the great auricular, lesser occipital, and transverse nerve of the neck on the sternocleidomastoid. Leave sufficient nerve on both sides of the cuts to allow the ends to be identified subsequently.
2. In the suboccipital triangle, separate the superior oblique and rectus capitis posterior major and minor muscles from their bony attachments, and remove them. This exposes the posterior atlanto-occipital membrane [see Fig. 21.4]. Cut across this membrane close to the skull, but avoid damage to the vertebral arteries on the posterior arch of the atlas.
3. Detach the longissimus muscle from the skull [see Fig. 6.4].
4. Cut across the sternocleidomastoid 2–3 cm above the clavicle, and turn it superiorly. Clean the deep surface of the sternocleidomastoid as far as the skull, and identify the accessory nerve entering it. Cut the nerve in the posterior triangle, so that the superior part of the nerve remains with the sternocleidomastoid.
5. Pass a finger behind the carotid sheath and pharynx, and separate them from the prevertebral fascia and the sympathetic trunk as far superiorly as the superior cervical ganglion. Note how easily the loose fascia behind the pharynx is torn. (In the living, this loose areolar tissue permits the pharynx to slide on the vertebral column.)
6. Saw through the mandible in the midline, and continue this cut through the tongue and epiglottis with a knife. Cut through the hyoid bone in the midline, and extend the incision inferiorly through the larynx, pharynx, and trachea to the inferior border of the isthmus of the thyroid gland.
7. Cut transversely through the right half of the trachea, oesophagus, and neurovascular bundle. (Do not cut the sympathetic trunk, phrenic nerve, and anterior scalene.)

8. Separate the upper parts of the transected structures from those behind them.
9. Make a mid-sagittal saw cut through the anterior part of the skull up to the foramen magnum. Do not damage the atlas vertebra.
10. Within the skull, detach the dura mater and membrana tectoria [see Fig. 21.4] from the anterior margin of the foramen magnum, and turn it inferiorly to expose the alar ligaments and the longitudinal fibres of the cruciate ligament [see Fig. 21.1].
11. Cut across the right alar ligament, and flex the right half of the head on the vertebral column. Divide the tight posterior part of the capsule of the atlanto-occipital joint. Now lever the occipital condyle out of its articulation, cutting any remaining parts of the capsule of the joint as they are exposed.
12. Free the vertebral artery and the first cervical nerve from the posterior arch of the atlas, and cut across the artery where it emerges from the transverse process of the atlas. Cut through the rectus capitis lateralis, rectus capitis anterior, longus capitis [see Fig. 9.1], and anterior atlanto-occipital membrane [see Fig. 21.4].
13. Complete the median division of the soft palate and of the posterior pharyngeal wall with a knife. Gently lift away the right half of the skull and attached structures. (Leave the ganglion and sympathethic trunk on the vertebral column.)

On the right side:

14. Find the internal laryngeal nerve piercing the thyrohyoid membrane. Trace it superiorly to the superior laryngeal nerve, medial to the external and internal carotid arteries. Trace the superior laryngeal nerve to the vagus. Above its origin from the vagus, find the pharyngeal branch of the vagus, and trace it between the carotid arteries to the pharynx [see Fig. 5.6; Fig. 8.12].
15. Find the glossopharyngeal, accessory, and hypoglossal nerves in the upper part of the neurovascular bundle, and trace them distally. The nerves separate inferiorly [Figs. 8.12, 8.13]. The accessory nerve (spinal part) runs posteroinferiorly, either superficial or deep to the internal jugular vein. The glossopharyngeal nerve passes anteroinferiorly with the stylopharyngeus muscle, lateral to the internal carotid artery. The hypoglossal nerve curves anteriorly, superficial to the internal and external carotid arteries. The vagus descends vertically between the artery and the vein in the carotid sheath.
16. When following the glossopharyngeal nerve, identify the stylopharyngeus muscle on which it runs to the pharynx. Trace the muscle to its origin from the styloid process.
17. The **stylopharyngeus** enters the pharynx between the superior and middle constrictor muscles of the pharynx. The upper margin of the **middle constrictor** can be defined and followed forwards to the hyoid bone [see Fig. 5.6].
18. Trace a branch from the glossopharyngeal and vagus nerves down between the two carotid arteries to the carotid sinus [Fig. 8.12]. This branch is the **carotid sinus nerve** and may be followed to the carotid body in the bifurcation of the common carotid artery.
19. Find the branches of the sympathetic ganglion (grey rami communicantes) passing posteriorly to the upper four cervical ventral rami.
20. Trace the occipital artery from the occiput to its origin.
21. Expose the posterior belly of the digastric from behind, and find the hypoglossal nerve hooking round the origin of the occipital artery, superficial to both carotid arteries [Fig. 8.14].

On the left side:

22. Cut through the posterior belly of the digastric, close to its origin. Turn it anteroinferiorly to expose the stylopharyngeus [see Fig. 5.6], but avoid damage to the glossopharyngeal nerve which curves round the lateral aspect of the muscle.
23. Lift the neurovascular bundle from the sympathetic trunk, and trace the trunk upwards to the superior cervical ganglion. Attempt to find the branches of the ganglion to the internal carotid artery, the external carotid artery, and the cranial nerves in the bundle.

## Carotid sinus and carotid body

The **carotid sinus** is a slight dilatation of the upper part of the common carotid artery and the adjacent part of the internal carotid artery. At the sinus, the wall of the arteries is more elastic than elsewhere and is heavily innervated. The carotid sinus is a pressure receptor. Distension of the sinus wall stimulates the nerve endings and leads to a reflex slowing of the heart and a fall in blood pressure.

The **carotid body** is a small gland-like structure situated in the carotid bifurcation. It consists of clusters of epithelial-like cells arranged around capillaries. The carotid body responds to changes in blood gas tension and brings about reflex changes in respiration. The carotid body may be seen by twisting the arteries round and dissecting between them.

Both the carotid sinus and the carotid body are innervated principally by the **glossopharyngeal nerve** through the **carotid sinus nerve**, but they are also supplied by the vagus and sympathetics.

## External carotid artery

The **external carotid artery** begins as a branch of the common carotid artery in the carotid triangle [Chapter 5]. It ascends on the lateral aspect of the pharynx, anteromedial and parallel to the internal carotid artery. The transverse nerve of the neck, cervical branches of the facial nerve, facial and lingual veins, and hypoglossal nerve lie superficial to it. Branches of the superior laryngeal nerve are deep to it [see Figs. 5.4, 5.5; Fig. 8.12]. Above the carotid triangle, the external carotid artery is covered by the angle of the mandible, posterior belly of the digastric, and stylohyoid. Superior to the stylohyoid, the external carotid artery and its facial branch turn laterally, away from the internal carotid artery, and enter the deep surface of the parotid gland. Before it enters the parotid gland, the styloid process of the temporal bone, stylopharyngeus muscle, glossopharyngeal nerve, styloglossus muscle, and pharyngeal branch of the vagus lie between the internal and external carotid arteries [Fig. 8.15]. In the parotid gland, the external carotid artery ascends to the back of the neck of the mandible and divides into the **superficial temporal** and **maxillary arteries**. In the gland, it lies deep to the facial nerve and retromandibular vein.

The external carotid artery is surrounded by the **external carotid plexus** of sympathetic nerve fibres. These nerve fibres arise in the cells of the superior cervical ganglion of the sympathetic trunk. Like the internal carotid nerve on the corresponding artery, this plexus is one of the main routes of distribution of sympathetic nerves to the head. (Similar plexuses on the vertebral and subclavian arteries and sympathetic fibres from the cervical sympathetic ganglia in the spinal and cranial nerves complete the sympathetic distribution to the head and neck.)

### Branches of the external carotid artery

#### Superior thyroid artery

The **superior thyroid artery** arises from the anterior surface of the external carotid, close to its origin. It runs anteroinferiorly in the carotid triangle, deep to the infrahyoid muscles. The initial segment of the artery has been seen in the carotid triangle. It divides into anterior and posterior branches at the apex of the lobe of the thyroid gland. It gives rise to: (1) small muscular branches; (2) the small **infrahyoid artery** which runs along the lower border of the hyoid bone; (3) the larger **superior laryngeal artery** which pierces the thyrohyoid membrane with the internal laryngeal nerve; (4) the small **sternocleidomastoid branch** which runs posteroinferiorly across the carotid sheath; and (5) the **cricothyroid branch** which arises deep to the sternothyroid muscle and runs anteriorly across the cricothyroid muscle to anastomose with its fellow on the cricothyroid membrane [see Fig. 5.7].

#### Occipital artery

The **occipital artery** arises from the posterior surface of the external carotid artery, opposite the origin of the facial branch [Figs. 8.12, 8.14]. It runs along the lower border of the posterior belly of the digastric, deep to the sternocleidomastoid, to reach and groove the base of the skull, medial to the mastoid notch. Its further course and branches are described in Chapter 3. In the neck, it lies superficial to the internal carotid artery, hypoglossal nerve (which hooks anteriorly round its origin), internal jugular vein, and accessory nerve [Fig. 8.15]. It gives off several muscular branches, one of which accompanies the accessory nerve to the sternocleidomastoid, and a meningeal branch which enters the skull through the jugular foramen.

#### Posterior auricular artery

The **posterior auricular artery** is a small branch which lies along the upper border of the posterior belly of the digastric [Fig. 8.14]. It passes superficial to the mastoid process with the posterior auricular nerve. It supplies the adjacent muscles and the parotid gland, and sends a stylomastoid branch superiorly into the stylomastoid foramen to supply the facial nerve and other structures within the temporal bone.

#### Ascending pharyngeal artery

The **ascending pharyngeal artery** is the first and smallest branch of the external carotid artery. It ascends on the pharynx, medial to the carotid arteries [Fig. 8.12].

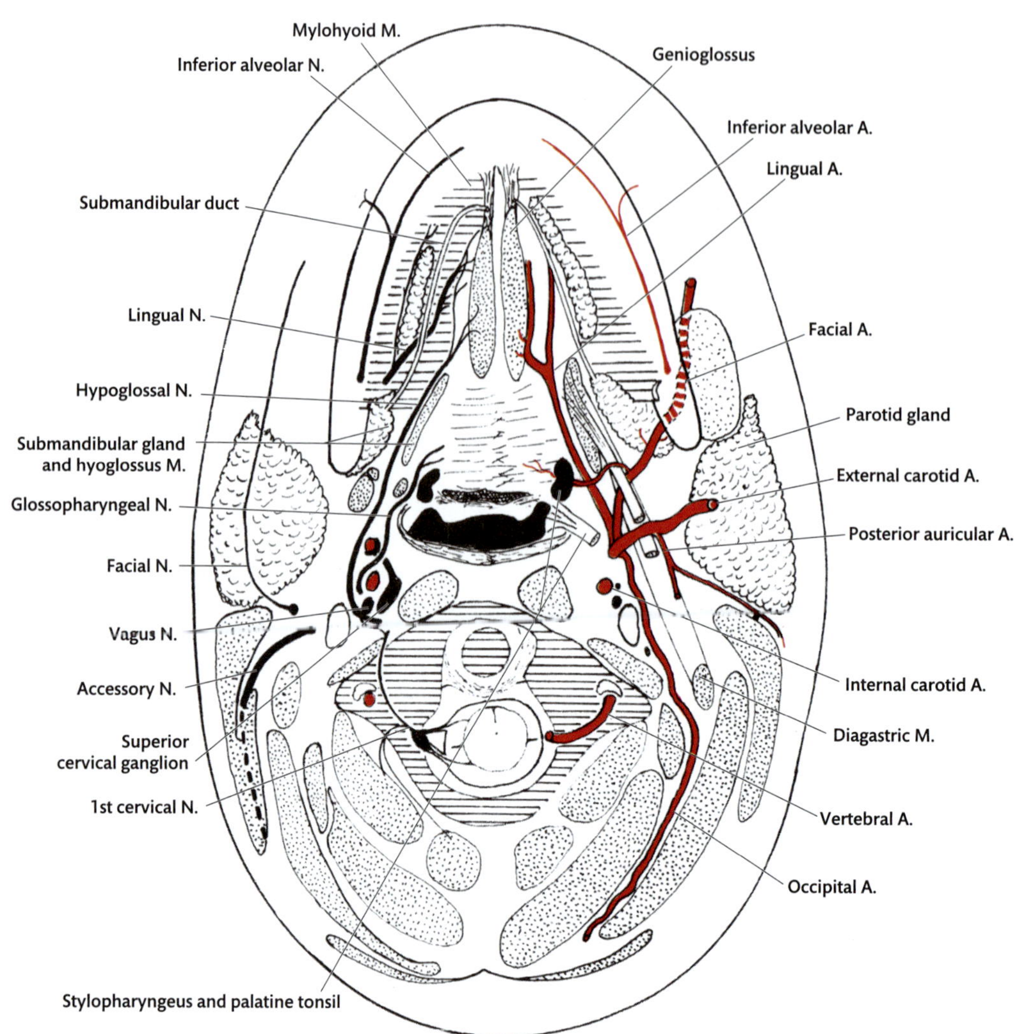


**Fig. 8.15** A diagrammatic section through the first cervical vertebra and the floor of the mouth to show the course of nerves (left) and arteries (right). The diagram is constructed from a number of adjacent levels. The muscle immediately superior to the facial artery is the styloglossus; that inferior to it is the stylohyoid.





### Facial artery

The **facial artery** is the main artery of the face. It enters the face at the lower border of the mandible and runs anterosuperiorly to a point 1.5 cm lateral to the angle of the mouth. It then ascends more vertically to end near the medial angle of the eye [see Fig. 3.6]. It has a sinuous course on the face. The facial artery gives large branches to the chin, lips (inferior labial and superior labial), and nose (lateral nasal), and smaller branches to the adjacent muscles.

### Superficial temporal artery

The **superficial temporal artery** is a large terminal branch of the external carotid artery, best seen in the temple. It begins behind the neck of the mandible and runs upwards into the scalp. It divides into anterior and posterior branches which run towards the frontal and parietal eminences. Small branches of the superficial temporal artery supply the temple and scalp (middle temporal branch), and face (transverse facial and zygomatico-orbital branches).

### Maxillary artery

The maxillary artery is a branch of the external carotid artery which arises posterior to the neck of the mandible. It is arbitrarily divided into three parts. The first part runs horizontally on the lower border of the lateral pterygoid muscle (a muscle of mastication). The second part runs anterosuperiorly, superficial to the lower head of the lateral pterygoid muscle and, the third part turns medially between the two heads of the lateral pterygoid. The artery ends in a number of branches in the pterygopalatine fossa. These details are better appreciated when the infratemporal fossa is dissected.

## Internal carotid artery

The cervical part of the internal carotid artery lies on the longus capitis and the sympathetic trunk [see Fig. 4.2]. The vagus lies posterolateral to it in the neck, with the glossopharyngeal, accessory, and hypoglossal nerves also posterior at the base of the skull. The artery lies between the internal jugular vein and the pharynx.

Inferiorly, the artery lies deep to the sternocleidomastoid, lingual and facial veins, hypoglossal nerve, and occipital artery [Fig. 8.13]. The superior root of the ansa cervicalis is anterior, and the external carotid is anteromedial to it. The internal carotid artery ascends deep to the posterior belly of the digastric, the styloid process, and the muscles attached to it. These structures separate it from the parotid gland. It then passes anterior to the internal jugular vein and enters the carotid canal. It is accompanied by the **internal carotid nerve** from the superior cervical ganglion of the sympathetic trunk.

Of the three carotid arteries in the neck—the common carotid, internal carotid, and external carotid—only the external carotid artery gives branches in the neck. The internal carotid arteries supply a considerable part of the brain, the orbital contents, the forehead, the anterior part of the scalp, and parts of the external nose and walls of the nasal cavities. The remainder of the structures in the head is supplied by the external carotid arteries.

## Internal jugular vein

The **internal jugular vein** is usually the largest vein in the neck. It begins at the jugular foramen by the union of the sigmoid and inferior petrosal sinuses [Fig. 8.13]. The right internal jugular vein is larger than the left because it usually drains the superior sagittal sinus.

It descends vertically on the lateral side of the internal and common carotid arteries, enclosed with them and the vagus nerve in the carotid sheath [Fig. 8.11]. It ends behind the medial part of the clavicle by uniting with the subclavian vein to form the brachiocephalic vein [see Fig. 5.7; Fig. 8.9].

The upper end of the internal jugular vein is dilated to form the **superior bulb**. At the lower end of the vein, there is a smaller dilatation—the **inferior bulb**—with a valve just above it [Fig. 8.13].

At the base of the skull, the internal jugular vein lies posterolateral to the internal carotid artery, with the last four cranial nerves between them. Along its course, the longus capitis, sympathetic trunk, roots of the cervical plexus, anterior scalene, and phrenic nerve lie posterior to the vein. The internal carotid artery, common carotid artery, glossopharyngeal nerve, pharyngeal branch of the vagus, hypoglossal nerve, and superior root of the ansa cervicalis lie medial to it. The spinal part of the accessory nerve may run anterior to the upper part of the vein, and the inferior root of the ansa cervicalis may be lateral or medial to its lower part [Fig. 8.13]. In the lower part of the neck, the left internal jugular vein overlaps the left common carotid artery, whereas on the right, the right internal jugular vein remains lateral to the common carotid artery.

### Tributaries of the internal jugular vein

1. The **pharyngeal plexus** drains into the upper part by two or more veins.
2. The **facial**, **lingual**, and **superior thyroid veins** enter the internal jugular vein in the carotid triangle.
3. The **middle thyroid vein** and sometimes the **jugular lymph trunk** enter it at the root of the neck.

## Nerves of the neck

The structures in the neck are derived from one of two embryological sources, each with its own source of nerve supply. The vertebral column and its associated muscles, the muscles of the tongue, and the infrahyoid muscles are derived from the occipital and upper cervical somites (somatic in origin). They are supplied by the **hypoglossal** and **upper cervical spinal nerves**.

The walls of the respiratory and digestive systems—nasal cavities, oral cavity, pharynx, larynx, trachea, oesophagus, and their associated glands—are derived from the pharyngeal or branchial arches (visceral in origin). They are supplied by cranial nerves of **branchiomeric origin**—the

**Table 8.1** Distribution of branchiomeric nerves in the neck

| Nerve | Area supplied in head and neck | | |
|---|---|---|---|
| | Sensory | Striated muscle | Parasympathetic |
| Trigeminal (V) | Skin and mucous membrane of oronasal region, face, forehead, scalp, dura mater | Muscles of mastication, anterior belly of digastric, mylohyoid, tensor tympani, tensor palati | - |
| Facial (VII) | Anterior two-thirds of tongue and palate—taste | Muscles of facial expression, posterior belly of digastric, stylohyoid, stapedius | Submandibular, sublingual, nasal, lacrimal, palatine, oral glands |
| Glossopharyngeal (IX) | Posterior one-third of tongue, epiglottis, palate—taste and general sensation, middle ear, auditory tube, mastoid antrum, carotid sinus, carotid body | Stylopharyngeus | Parotid and glands in posterior one-third of tongue |
| Vagus (X) | Pharynx, larynx, oesophagus, trachea, dura mater, external acoustic meatus | Muscles of pharynx, larynx, and soft palate, except tensor palati | Glands and smooth muscle of pharynx, larynx, trachea, oesophagus (also many thoracic and abdominal viscera) |
| Accessory, cranial part (XI) | Larynx, pharynx, oesophagus, trachea | Muscles of pharynx and larynx | - |
| Accessory, spinal part (XI) | - | Sternocleidomastoid and trapezius | - |

**trigeminal** (V), **facial** (VII), **glossopharyngeal** (IX), **vagus** (X), and **accessory** (XI) nerves. (The territory supplied by the branchiomeric nerves extends from the oral and nasal orifices to the upper part of the gut tube in the abdomen.) The muscles of facial expression (VII) and the sternocleidomastoid and trapezius muscles (XI) are also innervated by cranial nerves of branchiomeric origin, as they originate from the wall of the gut tube. Table 8.1 gives the distribution of the branchiomeric cranial nerves supplying the head and neck.

The glossopharyngeal, vagus, and spinal accessory nerves enter the neurovascular bundle through the jugular foramen. They descend between the internal carotid artery and the internal jugular vein, and either leave the bundle (IX and spinal part of XI) or send branches from it (X and cranial part of XI). The hypoglossal nerve also enters the bundle but leaves it shortly to supply the muscles of the tongue.

## Glossopharyngeal nerve

The glossopharyngeal (ninth) cranial nerve arises from the side of the medulla oblongata and passes through the jugular foramen in its own dural sheath, between the sigmoid and inferior petrosal sinuses. At the base of the skull, it has two small sensory ganglia—the **superior** and **inferior glossopharyngeal ganglia**. It descends between the internal jugular vein and the internal carotid artery, curves around the lateral surface of the stylopharyngeus, between the internal and external carotid arteries, and passes with that muscle into the pharynx [see Fig. 5.6; Figs. 8.12, 8.13]. In the wall of the pharynx, it lies external to the mucous membrane of the lower part of the tonsillar fossa and runs forwards into the tongue, deep to the hyoglossus. It receives taste and general sensation from the posterior third of the tongue, vallate papillae [see Fig. 17.1], palatine tonsil, part of the soft palate and adjacent pharynx, and anterior surface of the epiglottis.

## Branches of the glossopharyngeal nerve

1. The slender **tympanic branch** of the glossopharyngeal nerve enters a minute canal on the ridge of the bone between the jugular foramen and the carotid canal. It ascends to the middle ear and forms the **tympanic plexus** on the medial wall of the middle ear cavity, with minute

**caroticotympanic nerves** from the sympathetic plexus on the internal carotid artery [see Fig. 12.8]. The tympanic plexus supplies the mucous membrane of the middle ear, auditory tube, mastoid antrum, and mastoid air cells, and sends preganglionic parasympathetic (secretomotor) nerves through the **lesser petrosal nerve** to the otic ganglion. (The otic ganglion innervates the parotid gland.)
2. The **nerve to the stylopharyngeus** supplies the stylopharyngeus and passes through it to the pharyngeal mucous membrane.
3. The **pharyngeal branches** supply the pharyngeal mucous membrane and run with the pharyngeal branch of the vagus to the pharyngeal plexus.
4. One branch from the glossopharyngeal nerve joins a branch of the vagus to form the **carotid sinus nerve** to the carotid sinus and body.

## Vagus nerve

The vagus arises by a row of rootlets from the side of the medulla oblongata [see Fig. 24.2], immediately inferior to the glossopharyngeal nerve. It leaves the skull with the accessory nerve through the middle compartment of the jugular foramen. Like the glossopharyngeal nerve, it has two sensory ganglia—superior and inferior vagal ganglia—at the base of the skull. The vagus descends vertically in the carotid sheath, posteromedial to the internal jugular vein and posterolateral to the internal and common carotid arteries [Figs. 8.12, 8.13].

At the root of the neck, each vagus crosses the anterior surface of the corresponding subclavian artery. The right vagus then descends, posterior to the brachiocephalic vein, to the right side of the trachea in the thorax. The left vagus descends between the subclavian and common carotid arteries, posterior to the left brachiocephalic vein [Figs. 8.7, 8.9].

### Branches of the vagus nerve

1. The vagus communicates with the other nerves in the jugular foramen.
2. It is joined by the cranial part of the accessory nerve and gives branches to the larynx.
3. A small **meningeal branch** passes back through the jugular foramen to the dura mater of the posterior cranial fossa.
4. The slender **auricular branch** runs through a minute canal in the lateral wall of the jugular fossa to the tympanomastoid fissure. It pierces the cartilage of the external acoustic meatus and supplies the skin lining of the lower half of the meatus and the tympanic membrane. ➲ Irritation of the skin in this region may give rise to an intractable cough or cause other vagal reflexes.
5. The **pharyngeal branch** of the vagus arises immediately below the skull. It runs anteroinferiorly between the internal and external carotid arteries, to form a large part of the **pharyngeal plexus** in the fascia covering the middle constrictor muscle of the pharynx. The plexus also receives branches from the glossopharyngeal nerve and superior cervical sympathetic ganglion. It supplies the pharyngeal wall [Figs. 8.12, 8.13].
6. The **superior laryngeal nerve** is larger than the pharyngeal branch and arises inferior to it. It descends deep to both carotid arteries and divides into two branches—the **internal** and **external** laryngeal nerves [Figs. 8.12, 8.13]. The internal laryngeal nerve descends on the lateral wall of the pharynx and pierces the thyrohyoid membrane. It descends deep to the mucous lining of the piriform recess of the pharynx and supplies the mucous membrane of the pharynx and the upper part of the larynx. The thin **external branch** descends on the side of the pharynx, deep to the carotid and superior thyroid arteries, sternothyroid muscle, and thyroid gland. It supplies the cricothyroid muscle [see Fig. 5.6] (the only intrinsic laryngeal muscle not supplied by the recurrent laryngeal nerve) and the inferior constrictor muscle [see Fig. 5.6].
7. Two slender **cardiac branches** arise from each vagus, one in the upper and the other in the lower part of the neck. They descend with the vagus into the thorax and join the superficial and deep cardiac plexuses.
8. The right **recurrent laryngeal nerve** arises as the vagus crosses the first part of the subclavian artery (the left as it crosses the arch of the aorta). Each nerve hooks below the artery and ascends in the groove between the oesophagus and the trachea. It passes deep to the lobe of the thyroid gland and the inferior border of the inferior constrictor muscle to enter the larynx [Figs. 8.6, 8.7]. Within the larynx, it communicates with the internal branch of the superior laryngeal nerve and supplies the mucous membrane below the level of the vocal folds and all the intrinsic muscles, except the cricothyroid. The recurrent laryn-

geal nerve also gives off cardiac branches near its origin, and supplies the trachea, oesophagus, and inferior part of the pharynx.

## Accessory nerve

The eleventh cranial nerve—the spinal accessory—is mainly motor. The **cranial roots** emerge from the side of the medulla oblongata as a vertical row in series with those of the vagus. The **spinal roots** arise from the upper five cervical segments of the spinal cord and ascend through the foramen magnum. The spinal roots join the cranial rootlets within the skull [see Fig. 7.10].

The accessory nerve leaves the skull through the jugular foramen in the same dural sheath as the vagus. At the jugular foramen, the cranial part continues with the vagus and enters its laryngeal branches. The spinal part turns posteroinferiorly, and crosses the tip of the transverse process of the atlas and the upper part of the carotid triangle to enter and supply the sternocleidomastoid [Fig. 8.12]. The nerve then runs through the sternocleidomastoid and emerges in the posterior triangle from its posterior border. It continues posteroinferiorly in the investing layer of the deep fascia of the posterior triangle, enters the deep surface of the trapezius, and supplies it [see Fig. 4.4]. It receives sensory branches from the second to fourth cervical ventral rami.

## Hypoglossal nerve

The **hypoglossal nerve** arises as a row of rootlets from the anterior surface of the medulla oblongata [see Fig. 24.2]. The rootlets unite to form the nerve which leaves the skull through the hypoglossal canal. At the base of the skull, the hypoglossal nerve lies medial to the structures in the carotid sheath. The nerve then enters the neurovascular bundle, adheres briefly to the lateral surface of the vagus, and receives a branch from the first cervical ventral ramus [Figs. 8.12, 8.13, 8.14]. It descends with the vagus, deep to the posterior belly of the digastric, curves anteriorly on the root of the occipital artery, and enters the anterior triangle, lateral to the external carotid artery.

### Branches of the hypoglossal nerve

1. A **meningeal branch**, composed of nerve fibres of the first cervical nerve, runs back through the hypoglossal canal to supply the dura mater near the foramen magnum.
2. A descending branch—the **superior root of the ansa cervicalis** (C. 1).
3. Nerves to the **thyrohyoid** and **geniohyoid** (C. 1).
4. Branches to all intrinsic and extrinsic **muscles of the tongue**, except the palatoglossus [Figs. 8.15, 8.16].

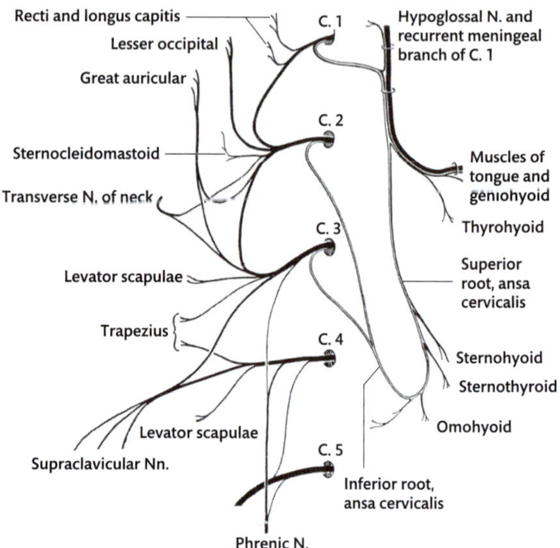


**Fig. 8.16** A diagram of the cervical plexus and ansa cervicalis. C. 1 to C. 5 = ventral rami of the upper five cervical nerves. Note that the nerves to the geniohyoid and thyrohyoid muscles and the superior root of the ansa cervicalis are derived from the first cervical ventral ramus, although they appear to arise from the hypoglossal nerve.

**DISSECTION 8.6 Cervical sympathetic ganglion**

**Objective**

**I.** To identify the cervical sympathetic ganglion and trace its branches.

**Instructions**

1. Identify the cervicothoracic (inferior cervical) ganglion of the sympathetic trunk, and expose it completely by displacing the vertebral artery laterally.
2. Find the branches of this ganglion and of the middle and superior cervical ganglia, including the grey rami communicantes to the cervical nerves. These are most easily demonstrated on the right side.

## Cervical sympathethic trunk

The dissection of the cervical sympathetic ganglion is described in Dissection 8.6.

Start by reviewing the general features of the sympathetic trunk [Vol. 2, p. 9]. In the neck, the sympathetic trunk consists of **preganglionic sympathetic fibres** which ascend from the upper thoracic segments to the cervical ganglia. The trunk runs almost vertically, anterior to the longus colli and longus capitis muscles on the roots of the transverse processes, posterior to the common and internal carotid arteries. Inferiorly, it is medial to the vertebral artery and is crossed by the inferior thyroid artery posteriorly. (The thoracic duct lies anteriorly on the left.)

Superiorly, the trunk ends in the superior cervical ganglion. Nerve fibres from the ganglion extend into the skull as the **internal carotid nerve** on the internal carotid artery [Fig. 8.13]. Inferiorly, the sympathetic trunk enters the thorax by passing in front of the neck of the first rib.

### Sympathetic ganglia and rami communicantes

There are three cervical ganglia—superior, middle, and inferior cervical ganglia. The inferior cervical ganglion is often fused with the first thoracic ganglion to form the **cervicothoracic ganglion**. **Preganglionic sympathetic fibres** from the upper thoracic segments enter the ganglion and synapse in it. **Post-ganglionic sympathetic fibres** from the ganglia pass in the **grey rami communicantes** to the ventral rami of the cervical nerves. The post-ganglionic sympathetic fibres are distributed to the head, neck, and upper limbs through: (1) the grey rami communicantes; (2) communications with the cranial nerves; and (3) plexuses around the branches of the major arteries.

#### Superior cervical ganglion

The superior cervical ganglion is the largest (2.5 cm long) ganglion of the sympathetic trunk. It lies between the internal carotid artery and the longus capitis, at the level of the second and third cervical vertebrae.

It gives a number of branches: (1) communicating branches to the ninth, tenth, and twelfth cranial nerves; (2) the **grey rami communicantes** to the upper four cervical ventral rami; (3) the **internal carotid nerve** which runs on the internal carotid artery; (4) the **laryngopharyngeal branches** to the pharyngeal plexus; (5) the **external carotid nerves** which form the external carotid plexus on the external carotid artery and its branches; and (6) the **superior cervical cardiac nerve** to the cardiac plexus. On the left, the superior cervical cardiac branch ends in the superficial cardiac plexus. On the right, it crosses the subclavian artery and descends behind the brachiocephalic trunk to end in the deep cardiac plexus.

#### Middle cervical ganglion

This small ganglion lies on the inferior thyroid artery at the level of the cricoid cartilage. It gives rise to: (1) the **grey rami communicantes** to the fifth and sixth cervical nerves; (2) the **thyroid branches** which form a plexus on the inferior thyroid artery and communicate with the recurrent and external laryngeal nerves; (3) the **middle cervical cardiac nerves** to the deep cardiac plexus; and (4) the **ansa subclavia**, a slender branch which loops round the subclavian artery and sends nerve fibres to the phrenic nerve.

#### Inferior cervical or cervicothoracic ganglion

The cervicothoracic ganglion represents the fused inferior cervical and first thoracic ganglia. It lies across the neck of the first rib. It receives a **white ramus** from the first thoracic ventral ramus and sends a grey ramus to the first, and sometimes to the second thoracic ventral ramus. When the inferior cervical ganglion is not fused with the first thoracic ganglion, it is small and lies behind the common carotid and vertebral arteries, anterior to the eighth cervical ventral ramus. The inferior cervical ganglion has the following branches, which arise from the cervicothoracic ganglion when they are fused: (1) the **grey rami communicantes** to the seventh and eighth cervical ventral rami; (2) fine filaments from the ansa subclavia to form the **subclavian plexus** on the subclavian artery; (3) larger filaments to form the **vertebral plexus** on the vertebral artery; and (4) the **inferior cervical cardiac nerves** which pass with the middle cervical nerve to the deep cardiac plexus.

All the sympathetic ganglia send post-ganglionic nerve fibres to structures in the head, neck, and upper limbs. They receive preganglionic fibres through the white rami communicantes of the upper thoracic ventral rami. The preganglionic fibres ascend in the trunk to the ganglia.

➲ **Horner's syndrome**: destruction of the sympathetic trunk at the root of the neck, as a result of surgery (cervical sympathectomy) or of some pathological condition, isolates these sympathetic ganglion cells from the central nervous system and eliminates reflex responses to sympathetic stimuli. Thus, sweating from heat or fear, vasoconstriction from cold or fright, and dilation of the pupils as a result of darkness or terror are lost on the side of the injury. In addition, there is loss of cutaneous vasodilation in response to heat and drooping of the upper eyelid (ptosis) due to paralysis of the smooth muscle in the upper eyelid. **Horner's syndrome** is the combination of anhidrosis, miosis, and ptosis seen in patients with damage to the sympathetic nerve pathway.

Using the instructions given in Dissection 8.7, trace the ventral rami of the cervical spinal nerves.

### DISSECTION 8.7 Ventral rami of cervical spinal nerves

#### Objective

**I.** To identify and trace the ventral rami of the cervical spinal nerves.

#### Instructions

1. Expose the prevertebral muscles and the cervical plexus on the right side.
2. Follow the ventral rami of the cervical nerves and their branches, noting the communications between the upper five.
3. Define the attachments of the scalene muscles [see Fig. 9.1], and trace the lower cervical and first thoracic ventral rami as far medially as possible, detaching the anterior scalene if necessary.

## Cervical plexus

The cervical plexus is formed by communications between the ventral rami of the upper four cervical nerves. These nerves emerge from the vertebral canal, superior to the corresponding vertebrae. The **ventral rami of the first cervical nerve** emerge between the rectus capitis anterior and the rectus capitis lateralis. The **ventral rami of the second to fourth cervical nerves** emerge anterior to the middle scalene. They communicate serially with each other. The communication between the fourth and fifth ventral rami unites the cervical and brachial plexuses. When C. 4 makes a large contribution to the brachial plexus, the brachial plexus is said to be **prefixed**. The cervical plexus lies posterior to the internal jugular vein and the prevertebral fascia [Fig. 8.16].

### Branches of the cervical plexus

(a) **Communicating branches**: (1) the superior cervical ganglion gives a grey **ramus communicans** to the first four cervical ventral rami; (2) a branch from the first cervical ventral ramus descends to join the **hypoglossal nerve**. This branch usually supplies the geniohyoid and thyrohyoid, and forms the **superior root of the ansa cervicalis**; (3) sensory branches from the second, third, and fourth cervical ventral rami join the **accessory nerve** and supply the sternocleidomastoid (C. 2, 3) and trapezius (C. 3, 4).

(b) **Cutaneous branches**: lesser occipital, great auricular, transverse cervical, and supraclavicular nerves [Chapter 4].

(c) **Muscular branches** to the diaphragm (**phrenic nerve**—C. 3, 4, 5), infrahyoid muscles, prevertebral muscles, scalene, intertransverse, and levator scapulae [Fig. 8.16].

## Phrenic nerve (C. 3, 4, 5)

The phrenic nerve arises mainly from the fourth cervical ventral ramus, with a contribution from C. 3 and C. 5 [Fig. 8.16]. At its origin, it is at the lateral border of the anterior scalene and posterolateral to the internal jugular vein. On both sides, the nerve descends with the internal jugular vein obliquely across the anterior scalene, to reach the medial border of the anterior scalene, just inferior to the subclavian artery [Figs. 8.6, 8.7, 8.9]. The right phrenic nerve enters the thorax, posterolateral to the right brachiocephalic vein and the superior vena cava. The left phrenic nerve enters the thorax between the common carotid artery and the pleura.

## Scalene muscles

The three scalene muscles—**anterior scalene**, **middle scalene**, and **posterior scalene**—form a thick muscular mass behind the prevertebral fascia. They extend inferolaterally from the cervical transverse processes to the first two ribs. **Nerve supply**: twigs from the ventral rami of the lower five or six cervical ventral rami. **Actions**: they elevate the first two ribs on inspiration and produce lateral flexion of the cervical vertebrae when acting unilaterally [Fig. 8.7].

## Anterior scalene

The anterior scalene takes origin from the anterior tubercles of the transverse processes of the third to sixth cervical vertebrae. It descends between the subclavian artery and vein, to be inserted into the scalene tubercle on the first rib [Figs. 8.7, 8.17].

It is separated from the middle scalene posteriorly by the roots of the brachial plexus and the subclavian artery. Anteriorly, it is crossed obliquely by the internal jugular vein and the phrenic nerve. More superficially, it is crossed by the inferior belly of the omohyoid and the superficial cervical and suprascapular arteries. The anterior scalene lies lateral to the thyrocervical trunk [Fig. 8.8], suprapleural membrane, pleura, and vertebral artery [Figs. 8.6, 8.7, 8.8].

## Middle scalene

The middle scalene is larger than the anterior scalene. It takes origin from the posterior tubercles of all the cervical transverse processes and is inserted into a rough area on the superior surface of the first rib, posterior to the groove for the subclavian artery [Fig. 8.17]. It lies deep to the prevertebral fascia in the posterior triangle of the neck, immediately posterior to the ventral rami of the spinal nerves and the third part of the subclavian artery. It lies anterior to the levator scapulae muscle. The middle scalene is pierced by the **dorsal scapular nerve** and by the upper two roots of the **long thoracic nerve** [see Figs. 4.4, 4.7]. Inferiorly, it is in contact with the cervical pleura.

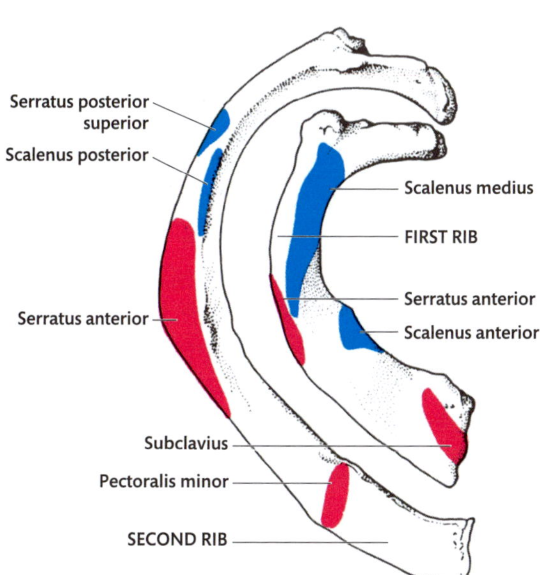


**Fig. 8.17** Attachments of the scalene muscles to the first and second ribs.

## Posterior scalene

This small muscle is a part of the middle scalene which is inserted into the external surface of the second rib [Fig. 8.17].

# Cervical fascia

The three layers of the deep fascia—the **investing layer**, **pre-tracheal layer**, and **prevertebral layer**—enclose the structures in the neck, and are adherent to them and to the surrounding structures by loose areolar tissue. The presence of the cervical fascia permits movement between and within the layers. The layers also form planes which tend to direct the spread of infection in the neck. The layers of the cervical fascia are difficult to dissect.

## Investing fascia

The investing layer of the deep fascia encircles the neck and splits to enclose the sternocleidomastoid and trapezius muscles. It forms the roof of the posterior triangle. It is attached to the body and greater horn of the hyoid bone. Above the hyoid, it splits into two layers to enclose the submandibular gland. The thin, deeper layer passes deep to the gland and gets attached to the mylohyoid line of the mandible [see Figs. 4.2, 5.3]. The thick, superficial layer passes to the inferior border of the body and ramus of the mandible. Posterior to the submandibular gland, the superficial layer is partially disrupted by the parotid gland. Its deepest part extends inwards to the styloid process and forms the **stylomandibular ligament**.

Inferiorly, the investing fascia splits to enclose the **suprasternal space** above the manubrium sternum [see Fig. 5.3], and is attached to the sternum, clavicle, acromion, and spine of the scapula. The fascia of the infrahyoid muscles is in contact with the deep surface of the investing layer. It also forms a sling around the intermediate tendon of the omohyoid and binds it down to the clavicle.

## Pre-tracheal fascia

The pre-tracheal fascia covers the front and sides of the trachea and splits to enclose the **thyroid gland**. It is attached to the oblique line on the thyroid cartilage and to the arch of the cricoid cartilage superiorly. These attachments cause the thyroid gland to rise and fall with the larynx in swallowing. Inferiorly, the pre-tracheal fascia surrounds the inferior thyroid veins and fuses with the pericardium [see Fig. 5.3].

## Carotid sheath

The carotid sheath is a tubular condensation of the fascia which extends from the base of the skull to the root of the neck. It encloses the common and internal carotid arteries, internal jugular vein, vagus nerve, and ansa cervicalis [Fig. 8.11]. It is wedged between the investing, pre-tracheal, and prevertebral fasciae [see Fig. 4.2].

## Prevertebral fascia

The prevertebral layer encloses the vertebral column and its muscles. Anteriorly, it extends from the base of the skull to the level of the third thoracic vertebra where it fuses with the anterior longitudinal ligament [see Fig. 5.3]. Laterally, it covers the scalene muscles, levator scapulae, and splenius capitis, and forms the fascial floor of the posterior triangle. It descends on the scalene muscles to the outer border of the first rib. An extension of the prevertebral fascia—the **axillary sheath**—is carried outwards from the outer border of the first rib around the brachial plexus and the subclavian artery as they emerge through the cervico-axillary canal between the scalene muscles [see Fig. 4.8]. Medial to the anterior scalene, the prevertebral fascia is continuous with the **suprapleural membrane**. The prevertebral fascia is separated from the pharynx and oesophagus by loose areolar tissue—the **retropharyngeal space** [Fig. 8.11]. This space allows the pharynx and oesophagus to be distended with food and to slide on the prevertebral fascia during swallowing and speaking.

The **alar fascia** lies anterior to the prevertebral fascia on the anterior surface of the vertebrae, behind the pharynx and oesophagus. Laterally, it is attached to the transverse process of the cervical vertebra. It extends from the base of the skull to the seventh cervical vertebra.

## Buccopharyngeal fascia

The buccopharyngeal fascia is a delicate, distensible fascial layer covering the constrictor muscles of the pharynx and buccinator. It extends from the base of the skull to the oesophagus.

# Lymph nodes and lymph vessels of the head and neck

Some of the lymph nodes along the carotid sheath and in the root of the neck may have been seen already, but the nodes and vessels cannot be demonstrated satisfactorily by routine dissection. The following account gives a brief description of the lymphatic system in the head and neck [Fig. 8.18].

The lymph nodes of the head and neck are numerous and may be divided into superficial and deep groups. The **superficial groups** are situated around the junction of the head with the neck. They drain all the superficial structures and some deep tissue of the head. Most of the efferent lymph vessels from the superficial nodes pass to the deep group. The **deep group** consists of a chain of lymph nodes—the **deep cervical lymph nodes**—arranged along the internal jugular vein, from the level of the digastric to the root of the neck. They are arbitrarily divided into the upper deep cervical and lower deep cervical nodes by the omohyoid. A few scattered, superficial nodes are found along the external and anterior jugular veins. These drain to the deep cervical nodes.

## Superficial lymph nodes of the head

### Occipital lymph nodes

The few, small occipital lymph nodes lie on the upper end of the trapezius and on the fascia at the apex of the posterior triangle. They drain the occipital part of the scalp and the upper part of the back of the neck to the upper deep cervical lymph nodes.

### Retro-auricular lymph nodes

The retro-auricular nodes lie on the superior part of the sternocleidomastoid, posterior to the auricle. They drain the posterior side of the head and the

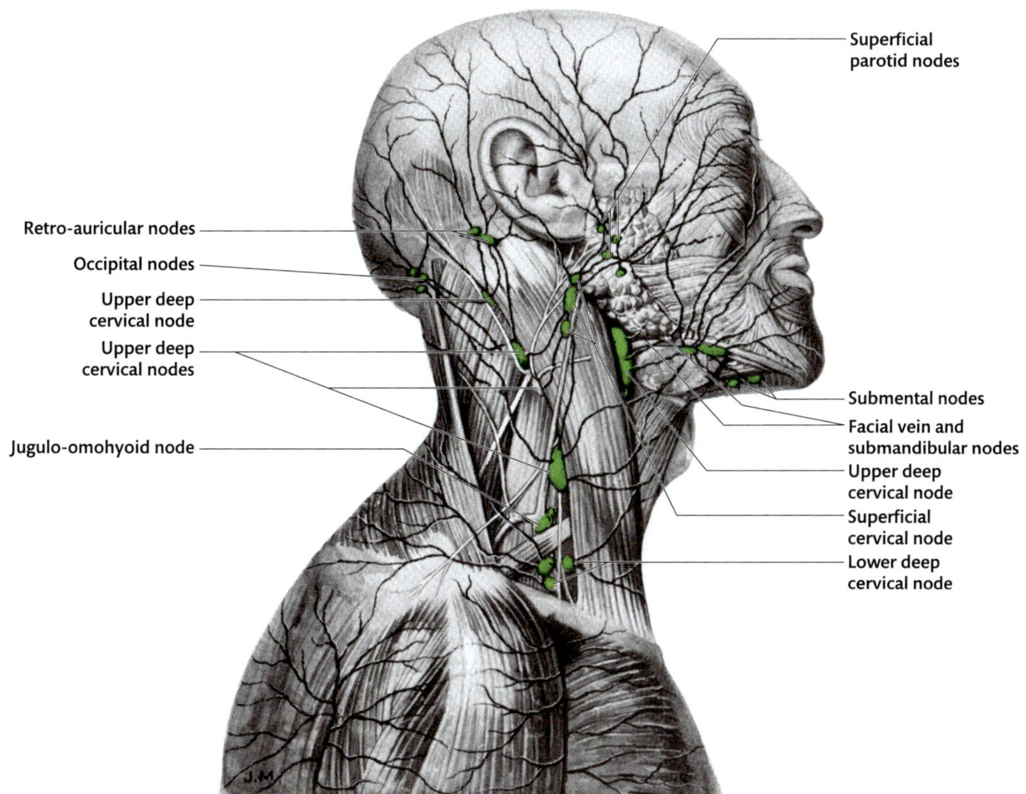


**Fig. 8.18** Lymph nodes of the head and neck, shown with the sternocleidomastoid in position.

posterior surface of the auricle, to the deep nodes under the sternocleidomastoid.

## Parotid lymph nodes

Several small lymph nodes are scattered through the parotid gland. The superficial nodes drain the area between a vertical line through the auricle and an oblique line joining the medial angle of the eye to the angle of the mandible. This area includes most of the auricle and the external acoustic meatus. Deeper nodes in this region drain the temporal and infratemporal fossae, the middle ear, the auditory tube, and the upper molar teeth and gums. Efferent vessels from these nodes drain either to nodes on the external jugular vein or to the upper deep cervical lymph nodes.

## Submandibular lymph nodes

The submandibular lymph nodes lie along the submandibular gland, mainly under cover of the mandible. They receive superficial lymph vessels from the area below the line joining the medial angle of the eye and the angle of the mandible. They also receive lymph from the submandibular and sublingual salivary glands, the side of the tongue and posterior part of the floor of the mouth, most of the teeth and gums, part of the palate, and the anterior parts of the walls of the nasal cavity. They drain to the deep cervical nodes under the sternocleidomastoid. Some small nodes lie along the course of the facial vein. One of these—the mandibular node—lies at the anterior border of the masseter and drains the cheek and lateral parts of the lips to the submandibular nodes.

## Submental lymph nodes

The submental nodes lie on the fascia covering the mylohyoid, between the anterior bellies of the digastric muscles [see Fig. 5.1]. They receive lymph from a wedge-shaped area, including the lower incisor teeth, gums, and anterior part of the floor of the mouth. They drain to the deep cervical lymph nodes. Though small, some of these nodes may be palpable, even in healthy individuals.

## Retropharyngeal lymph nodes

A few nodes lie in the fascia of the posterior wall of the upper pharynx, at the level of the mastoid process. They receive lymph from the oropharynx, nasopharynx, palate, nose, paranasal sinuses, auditory tube, and middle ear. These nodes drain posteroinferiorly to the nodes in the posterior triangle.

### Other superficial lymph nodes

Three or four superficial cervical nodes lie along the *external jugular vein*. They drain the parotid nodes and the adjoining skin to the deep nodes in the carotid triangle or at the root of the neck. A few small nodes lie on the *anterior jugular vein* and drain the skin and muscles along the vein to the lower deep cervical nodes. Small anterior cervical lymph nodes lie on the *front and sides of the trachea*. They are continuous with the tracheobronchial nodes in the thorax. They drain lymph from the larynx, trachea, and thyroid gland to the lower deep cervical lymph nodes.

## Deep cervical lymph nodes

The deep cervical lymph nodes form a broad strip of nodes extending from the digastric muscles to the root of the neck. Most of them lie under cover of the sternocleidomastoid. The deep cervical nodes receive lymph from all the other groups. Two of the nodes are particularly large—the **jugulodigastric nodes** which drain the palatine tonsil and tongue, and the **jugulo-omohyoid nodes**. Both are named after their relation to the corresponding muscles.

**Table 8.2** Movements of the hyoid bone

| Movement | Muscles | Nerve supply |
|---|---|---|
| Elevation | Digastric | Trigeminal and facial |
| | Stylohyoid | Facial |
| | Mylohyoid | Trigeminal |
| Depression | Sternohyoid | Ansa cervicalis |
| | Omohyoid | Ansa cervicalis |
| | Thyrohyoid and sternothyroid | C. 1 and ansa cervicalis |
| Protraction | Geniohyoid | C. 1 ventral ramus |
| Retraction | Middle constrictor of pharynx | Pharyngeal plexus |
| | Stylohyoid | Facial |

Some of the deep nodes extend into the posterior triangle: (1) along the accessory nerve (draining the retropharyngeal nodes); and (2) on the superficial cervical artery across the upper part of the brachial plexus. The final efferent pathway for all the lymph of the head and neck is the **jugular lymph trunk** at the root of the neck. This trunk enters the thoracic duct on the left side and the internal jugular vein on the right.

See Clinical Applications 8.1, 8.2, and 8.3 for the practical implications of the anatomy discussed in this chapter.

Table 8.2 provides an overview of the movements of the hyoid bone.

**CLINICAL APPLICATION 8.1 Tracheostomy**

A 53-year-old male was rescued from a burning building by the fire rescue team. He suffered burn injuries to his face, trunk, and upper limbs. He was breathless, partially conscious, and in severe pain. Examination revealed severe laryngeal oedema and possible inhalational injury to the lungs due to inhaled smoke. At the hospital, his condition deteriorated and a tracheostomy was done.

Study question 1: what is laryngeal oedema? (Answer: laryngeal oedema is inflammation and damage to the mucosa of the larynx.)

Study question 2: what is tracheostomy? (Answer: tracheostomy is an emergency procedure done to create a passage into the trachea in someone with an impending airway obstruction. A surgical incision is made in the anterior neck into the cervical trachea. A cuffed tube is introduced into the incision and connected to a ventilator machine.)

Study question 3: what are the important anatomical structures that one must be careful to avoid while doing a tracheostomy? (Answer: important structures in close relation to the cervical trachea include the thyroid gland and its isthmus lying in front of the trachea, carotid vessels and the internal jugular vein on either side, and the recurrent laryngeal nerve in the tracheo-oesophageal groove.)

Study question 4: what are the common indications for a tracheostomy? (Answer: common indications include upper airway obstruction by a foreign body or cancerous growth, laryngeal oedema following burns and anaphylaxis, bilateral paralysis of the vocal cord, and severe fractures of the midface and mandible making orotracheal or nasotracheal intubation impossible.)

## CLINICAL APPLICATION 8.2 Thyromegaly

A 35-year-old woman presented with a history of weight gain, intolerance to cold, tiredness, excessive sleepiness, lethargy, and constipation. On examination, she has a swelling in front of the neck that moves up on deglutition.

Study question 1: what is the likely diagnosis? (Answer: thyroid swelling, based on the evidence that the swelling moved on deglutition; and hypothyroidism, based on the history.)

Study question 2: what is an enlargement of the thyroid gland called? (Answer: an enlargement of the thyroid is called thyromegaly or goitre. It may be associated with excess or decreased secretion of T3 and T4 hormones, leading to hyperthyroidism or hypothyroidism, respectively. Features of hyperthyroidism include weight loss, tachycardia, palpitations, anxiety, tremor, easy muscle fatigue, increased bowel movements, and heat intolerance.)

Study question 3: why does the thyroid gland move up on deglutition? (Answer: the thyroid gland is enveloped by the pre-tracheal fascia that is attached in the midline to the hyoid bone, and laterally to the oblique line of the thyroid cartilage. Further, a thickened band of fascia, called the ligament of Berry, anchors the medial surface of the thyroid gland to the cricoid cartilage. Elevation of the hyoid bone and thyroid and cricoid cartilages during deglutition causes elevation of the thyroid gland.)

Study question 4: what anatomical structures should the surgeon be careful of during thyroidectomy? (Answer: (1) the external laryngeal branch of the superior laryngeal nerve; (2) the recurrent laryngeal nerve; and (3) accidental removal of the parathyroid glands which can lead to hypoparathyroidism.) See Clinical Application 8.3 for neurological complications of thyroid surgery.





## CLINICAL APPLICATION 8.3 Neurological complications of thyroid surgery

The superior and inferior laryngeal nerves are cervical branches of the vagus nerve that are pertinent to thyroid surgery because of their intimate relation to the thyroid gland. The external branch of the superior laryngeal nerve runs with the superior thyroid vessels to the superior pole of the thyroid gland. Injury to the nerve causes paralysis of the cricothyroid muscle and an inability to produce high-pitched sounds. Identifying the nerve during surgery helps to avoid accidental transection and excessive stretching. When the nerve is not identified, the superior thyroid artery branches should be ligated close to the thyroid gland.

The recurrent laryngeal nerve runs in the tracheo-oesophageal groove towards the larynx, close to the posterior aspect of the thyroid and the inferior thyroid artery. Injury to this nerve causes paralysis of the vocal cord and sensory loss below the level of the glottis. The patient could experience mild to severe hoarseness of the voice, acute airway obstruction, and difficulty in swallowing [Fig. 8.6].

CHAPTER 9

# The prevertebral region

## Introduction

This chapter describes the muscles and vessels which lie immediately in front of the cervical vertebrae. These muscles are enclosed in the prevertebral fascia [see Fig. 4.2].

## Muscles

The four muscles seen anterior to the vertebral bodies are the **longus colli**, **longus capitis**, **rectus capitis anterior**, and **rectus capitis lateralis**. They are most easily seen on the right in the dissected specimen, though the longus capitis, rectus capitis lateralis, and rectus capitis anterior have been cut across. The cut ends of these can be seen on the base of the skull, or the entire muscles can be exposed on the left by displacing the left half of the pharynx. The muscles are covered anteriorly by the prevertebral fascia and are supplied by the ventral rami of the cervical nerves. As a group, they flex the neck and the head on the neck.

### Longus colli

This is the longest and most medial of the muscles. A detailed account of the bony attachments is beyond the scope of this book. **Attachments**: the student should know that it extends from the anterior tubercle of the atlas to the third thoracic vertebra. It is attached to the bodies of the intervening vertebrae and to the transverse processes of the third to sixth cervical vertebrae [Figs. 9.1, 9.2]. **Nerve supply**: ventral rami of the cervical nerves. **Action**: flexion of the neck.

### Longus capitis

The longus capitis is anterolateral to the longus colli. **Attachments**: it takes origin from the anterior tubercles of the third to sixth cervical transverse processes and is inserted into the base of the skull in front of the rectus capitis anterior [see Fig. 6.2; Fig. 9.1]. **Nerve supply**: ventral rami of the cervical nerves. **Action**: flexion of the head on the neck.

### Rectus capitis anterior

**Attachment**: the rectus capitis anterior extends from the anterior surface of the lateral mass of the atlas to the base of the skull, immediately anterior to the occipital condyle [see Fig. 6.2; Fig. 9.1]. **Nerve supply**: ventral rami of the cervical nerves. **Action**: acting with the rectus capitis lateralis and the suboccipital muscles, the rectus capitis anterior stabilizes the skull on the vertebral column.

### Rectus capitis lateralis

**Attachments**: the rectus capitis lateralis extends from the superior surface of the transverse process of the atlas to the jugular process of the occipital bone. It is immediately posterior to the jugular foramen and is separated from the rectus capitis anterior by the ventral ramus of the **first cervical nerve**, which supplies both muscles [see Fig. 6.2; Fig. 9.1]. **Action**: it acts with the rectus capitis anterior and the suboccipital muscles to stabilize the skull on the vertebral column.

Using the instructions given in Dissection 9.1, find and trace the initial segments of the vertebral artery.

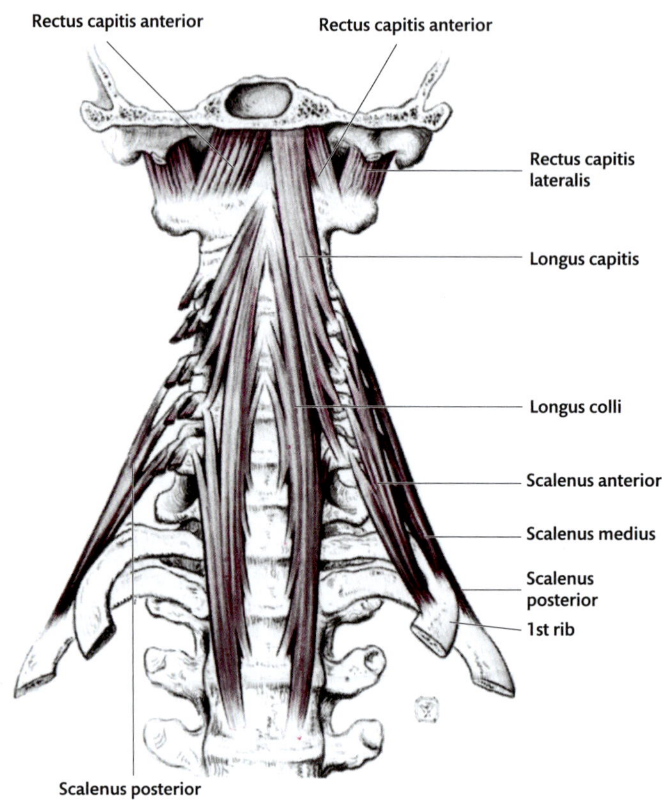


**Fig. 9.1** The prevertebral muscles of the neck.

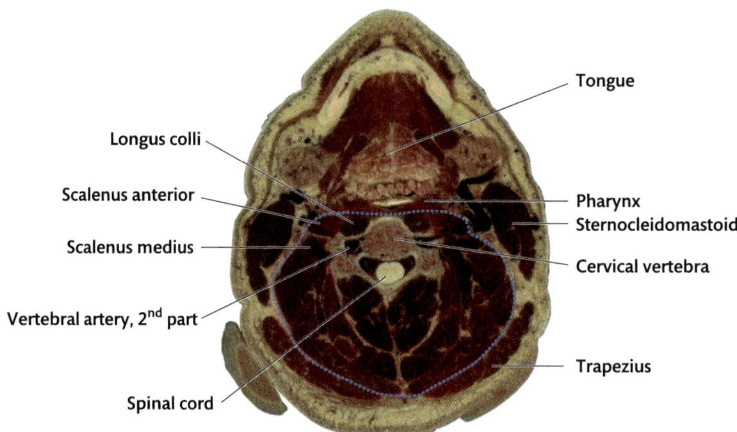


**Fig. 9.2** Transverse section at the level of the oropharynx. The position of the prevertebral fascia is shown by the dotted blue line.

Image courtesy of the Visible Human Project of the US National Library of Medicine.

## DISSECTION 9.1 Vertebral artery

### Objective

**I.** To trace the first and second parts of the vertebral artery.

### Instructions

1. Redefine the attachments of the scalene muscles on both sides.
2. Remove the scalenus anterior to expose the anterior and posterior **intertransverse muscles**, which unite the corresponding tubercles of adjacent cervical transverse processes. They are separated from each other by the ventral rami of the cervical nerves. The dorsal rami pass posteriorly, medial to the posterior intertransverse muscles.
3. The vertebral artery may now be exposed in the intertransverse spaces by removing the anterior intertransverse muscles.

## Vertebral artery

The vertebral artery is an important branch of the first part of the subclavian artery. The two vertebral arteries join to form the basilar artery within the cranial cavity. Together, they supply the upper part of the spinal cord, medulla oblongata, pons, cerebellum, midbrain, and posterior part of the cerebrum.

### First part of the vertebral artery

The vertebral artery begins as a branch of the first part of the subclavian artery and ascends behind the common carotid artery to the sixth cervical transverse process [Fig. 9.3].

### Second part of the vertebral artery

The second part of the vertebral artery ascends through the transverse foramen of the upper six cervical vertebrae, accompanied by the **vertebral veins** and a **sympathetic nerve plexus** derived from the cervicothoracic ganglion. Between the transverse processes, it is anterior to the ventral rami of the cervical nerves. The artery runs vertically upwards through the foramen transversaria of the sixth to second cervical vertebrae. In the transverse foramen of the axis, the artery turns laterally under the superior articular facet, bends upwards, and enters the transverse foramen of the atlas, which is placed further laterally than the others [see Fig. 8.8; Fig. 9.3].

### Third part of the vertebral artery

The third part of the vertebral artery emerges on the superior surface of the atlas between the rectus capitis lateralis and the superior articular process of the atlas. It curves horizontally over the lateral and posterior surfaces of the superior articular process with the ventral ramus of the first cervical nerve. It grooves the superior articular process and the root of the posterior arch of the atlas. It passes medially in front of the posterior atlanto-occipital membrane to enter the vertebral canal [see Figs. 6.4, 6.6; Fig. 9.3].

### Fourth part of the vertebral artery

The fourth part of the vertebral artery lies in the vertebral canal and cranial cavity. In the vertebral canal, the artery turns superiorly, pierces the dura mater and arachnoid, and enters the cranial cavity through the foramen magnum, anterior to the uppermost tooth of the denticulate ligament. It then runs anterosuperiorly on the medulla





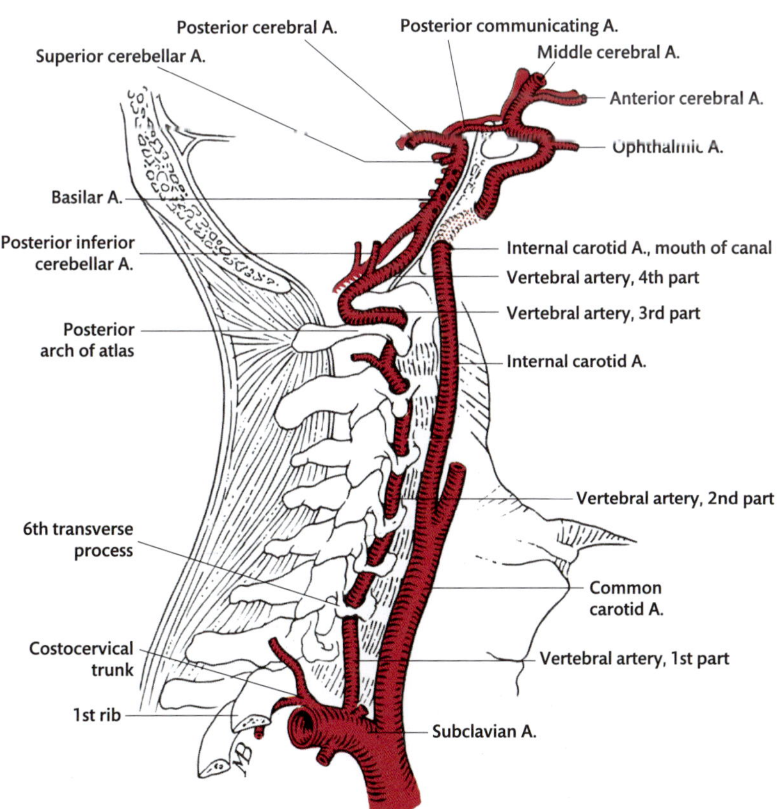


**Fig. 9.3** The course and communications of the internal carotid and vertebral arteries.

oblongata between the rootlets of the first cervical and hypoglossal nerves. At the lower border of the pons, it unites with the vertebral artery of the opposite side to form the basilar artery [see Fig. 7.10; Fig. 9.3].

## Branches of vertebral artery

There are no branches from the first part of the artery. The second and third parts of the artery give rise to **spinal** and **muscular** branches, which anastomose with branches of the occipital and deep cervical arteries. The fourth part gives off the **meningeal branch**, **anterior** and **posterior spinal arteries**, and **posterior inferior cerebellar artery** to the brain and spinal cord.

## Vertebral vein

A plexus of veins is formed around the beginning of the third part of the vertebral artery by the union of veins from the internal vertebral venous plexus and the suboccipital triangle. This plexus runs with the second part of the artery through the transverse foramen. It anastomoses with the **internal vertebral venous plexus** and the **deep cervical veins**. It ends as one or two vertebral veins, which descend with the artery from the sixth cervical transverse process, and enters the posterior surface of the brachiocephalic vein near its origin. One or two veins pass through the transverse foramen of the seventh cervical vertebra.

See Clinical Application 9.1 for the practical implications of the anatomy discussed in this chapter.

Table 9.1 provides an overview of the movements of the neck and of the head on the neck.

**Table 9.1** Movements of the neck and of the head on the neck

| Movement | Muscles | Nerve supply |
|---|---|---|
| Flexion | Sternocleidomastoid | Accessory |
| | Longus colli (both muscles acting) | Cervical ventral rami |
| | Longus capitis | Cervical ventral rami |
| | Rectus capitis anterior* | C. 1 ventral ramus |
| Extension | Splenius cervicis and capitis | Cervical dorsal rami |
| | Erector spinae | Cervical dorsal rami |
| | Rectus capitis posterior major and minor* | C. 1 dorsal ramus |
| | Obliquus capitis superior* | C. 1 dorsal ramus |
| | Trapezius | Accessory |
| Lateral flexion and rotation | Sternocleidomastoid† | Accessory |
| | Scalenes | Cervical ventral rami |
| | Longus colli | Cervical ventral rami |
| | Rectus capitis lateralis* | C. 1 ventral ramus |
| | Levator scapulae (shoulder fixed) | Cervical ventral rami |
| | Splenius† | Cervical dorsal rami |
| | Longissimus | Cervical dorsal rami |
| | Obliquus capitis superior‡ and inferior | C. 1 dorsal ramus |

* These muscles act mainly as ligaments of adjustable length and tension.

† In rotation (one muscle acting), turns the face towards the opposite side.

‡ In rotation, turns the face to the same side.

**CLINICAL APPLICATION 9.1 Prevertebral, retropharyngeal, and danger spaces in the neck**

The fascia of the neck limits the fascial spaces (or potential spaces) to form closed compartments. Infections tend to remain and spread within these compartments. A thin prevertebral tissue space exists between the vertebral column and the prevertebral fascia. It extends from the skull to the coccyx and encloses the prevertebral muscles. Between the prevertebral and alar fasciae is a space known as the danger space. It is a closed space and infections can reach it only through penetrating injury. It extends downwards into the posterior mediastinum. (It forms a ready path through which infection can spread to the thorax.) The retropharyngeal space lies between the alar fascia and the pharynx. (The alar fascia lies anterior to the prevertebral fascia on the anterior surface of the vertebra and behind the pharynx and oesophagus [Chapter 9].)

# CHAPTER 10
# The orbit

## Introduction

The orbit contains the eyeball, optic nerve, extraocular muscles which move the eye, associated vessels and nerves, orbital fat, and fascia. It also contains the lacrimal gland and the levator palpebrae superioris, the muscle which raises the upper eyelid. (The lacrimal apparatus and the eyeball are described Chapter 3 and Chapter 11.)

## Bony orbit

The bony orbit is pyramidal in shape. The base lies anteriorly at the orbital margin; the apex is directed posteriorly. Review the details of the bone orbit described in Chapter 2. The relations of the orbit are the anterior cranial fossa superiorly, the ethmoidal air sinuses medially, and the maxillary sinus inferiorly [Fig. 10.1].

Using the instructions given in Dissection 10.1, remove the roof of the orbit and explore the frontal and ethmoidal air sinuses.

## Ethmoidal sinuses

The ethmoidal air cells, or sinuses, are multiple, thin-walled cavities, which occupy the part of the ethmoid between the orbit and the upper part of the nasal cavity [see Figs. 7.13A, 2.3B; Fig. 10.1]. They are in three groups: the anterior, middle, and posterior ethmoidal sinuses. Explore them with a blunt probe, and attempt to find their openings into the nasal cavity.

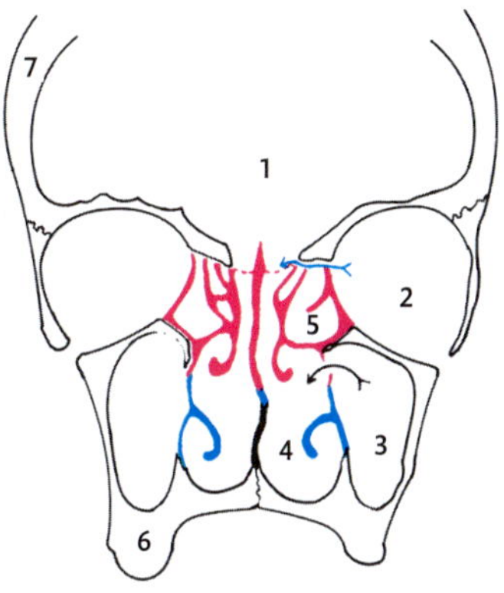


**Fig. 10.1** Drawing of a coronal section through the skull to show the relative positions of the orbit, maxillary sinus, nasal cavity, and ethmoidal air cells. Blue arrow shows the route of the anterior ethmoidal vessels and nerve; black arrow is in the opening of the maxillary sinus. Blue = inferior concha and septal cartilage; red = ethmoid bone; solid black = vomer. 1 = anterior cranial fossa. 2 = orbit. 3 = maxillary sinus. 4 = nasal cavity. 5 = ethmoidal air cell. 6 = alveolar process of the maxilla. 7 = frontal bone. [See also Fig. 2.1B.]

## Orbital periosteum

The orbital periosteum lines the bony orbit and encloses all the contents of the orbit, except the zygomatic nerve and the infraorbital nerve and vessels. It forms a funnel-shaped sheath which is loosely attached to the bony walls of the orbit. Posteriorly, it is continuous with the middle cranial fossa through the optic canal and the superior orbital fissure.

**DISSECTION 10.1 Roof of the orbit**

**Objectives**

**I.** To remove the roof of the orbit. **II.** To explore the frontal and ethmoidal air sinuses.

**Instructions**

1. Strip the periosteum from the floor of the anterior cranial fossa, except over the cribriform plate of the ethmoid. With a gentle tap of the hammer on a chisel, crack the orbital roof and remove the broken pieces of bone from the underlying orbital periosteum. Extend the opening with bone forceps, keeping outside the orbital periosteum, until all but the anterior margin of the orbital roof is removed.
2. Occasionally, the **frontal air sinus** extends into the roof of the orbit; in this case, two layers of bone and the contained sinus must be removed.
3. The **orbital part of the frontal bone** forms most of the roof of the orbit and extends medially over the ethmoidal air cells.
4. Chip away the frontal bone overlying the ethmoidal air cells. Avoid injury to the vessels and nerves beneath, and expose the mucoperiosteal lining of the **ethmoidal sinuses**. Open some of them.
5. Remove the remains of the lesser wing of the sphenoid, but leave the margin of the optic canal intact. The superior orbital fissure is now opened, and the nerves from the wall of the cavernous sinus can be traced into the orbit.

Using the instructions given in Dissection 10.2 (and Figs. 10.2, 10.3), dissect the muscles and nerves that lie immediately inferior to the orbital periosteum on the roof of the orbit.

## Frontal nerve

The **frontal nerve** is a direct continuation of the ophthalmic nerve. It enters the orbit through the superior orbital fissure and runs forwards, under the orbital periosteum, on the levator palpebrae superioris. It ends by dividing into the supraorbital and supratrochlear nerves [Fig. 10.2].

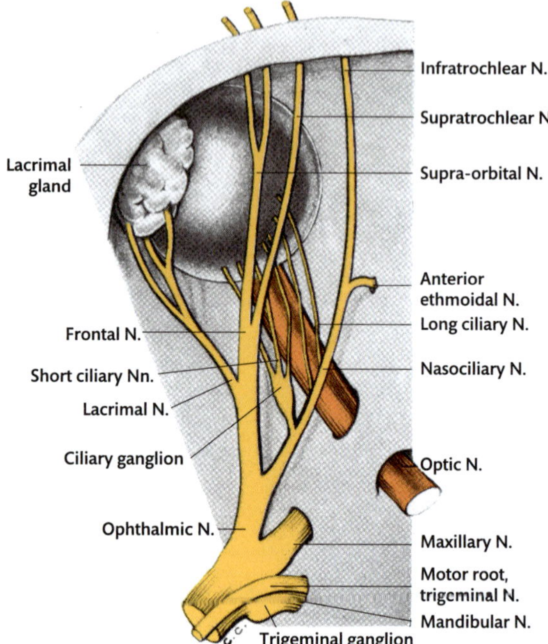


Fig. 10.2 The left ophthalmic nerve. The trigeminal nerve and ganglion have been turned laterally.

### Supratrochlear nerve

The supratrochlear nerve is the small medial branch of the frontal nerve. It runs towards the pulley of the superior oblique muscle, pierces the palpebral fascia above it, and leaves the orbit to run upwards into the forehead to supply the scalp [Chapter 3]. In the orbit, it communicates with the infratrochlear nerve.

### Supraorbital nerve

The supraorbital branch runs forwards, in line with the parent stem. It passes through the supraorbital notch or foramen and turns upwards into the forehead to supply the scalp [Chapter 3].

## Lacrimal nerve

The lacrimal nerve is the smallest branch of the ophthalmic nerve. It passes through the lateral

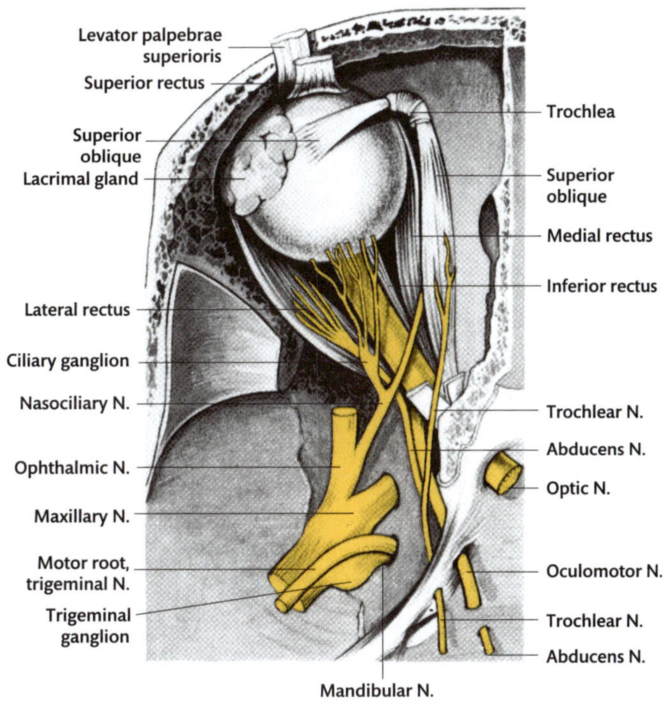






**Fig. 10.3** Dissection of the orbit and middle cranial fossa. The cut ends of the levator palpebrae superioris and superior rectus have been turned anteriorly. The trigeminal nerve and ganglion have been turned laterally.

### DISSECTION 10.2 Orbit

#### Objectives

**I.** To identify the levator palpebrae superioris, superior rectus, and superior oblique muscles. **II.** To identify and trace the frontal, trochlear, and lacrimal nerves and the corresponding arteries.

#### Instructions

1. Cut through the orbital periosteum transversely, close to the anterior margin of the orbit, and then anteroposteriorly along the midline of the orbit.
2. Take care not to injure the nerves which pass through the superior orbital fissure. Find the trochlear nerve, and trace it forwards and medially to the superior oblique muscle in the upper medial part of the orbit. The **trochlear nerve** lies immediately beneath the periosteum and is easily damaged when the periosteum is cut.
3. In the midline of the orbit, find the frontal nerve lying on the levator palpebrae superioris. Trace it forwards to its division into the supraorbital and supratrochlear nerves, each of which runs with the corresponding artery [Fig. 10.2].
4. Follow the supratrochlear nerve to the medial angle of the orbit where it passes above the pulley (trochlea) of the superior oblique muscle.
5. Identify the levator palpebrae superioris and superior oblique muscles.
6. Expose the superior oblique muscle, and follow its tendon to the pulley at the superomedial angle of the orbit [Fig. 10.3]. The tendon passes through the pulley and then turns posterolaterally to its insertion. It disappears from view beneath the levator palpebrae superioris and the superior rectus.
7. Raise the levator palpebrae superioris, and identify the superior rectus muscle beneath it. Find the branch of the oculomotor nerve which pierces that muscle to enter the levator.
8. Find the lacrimal nerve and artery which lie in the fat along the superolateral part of the orbit. Trace them to the lacrimal gland [Fig. 10.2].
9. Define the extent of the lacrimal gland.

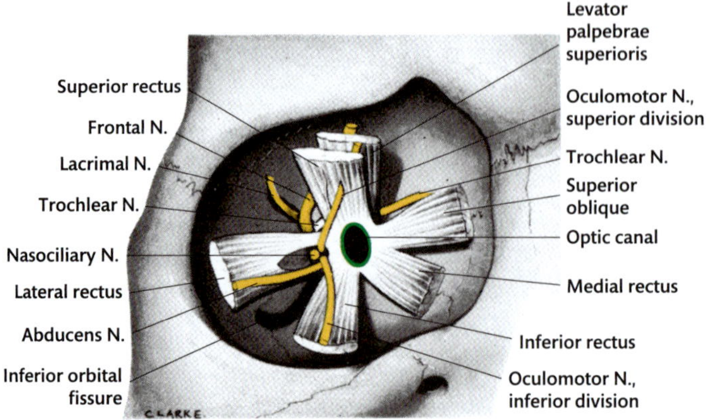


**Fig. 10.4** Diagram showing the origin of the ocular muscles and the routes of entry of nerves into the right orbit. Green = common tendinous ring.



part of the superior orbital fissure [Fig. 10.4] and runs forwards and laterally above the lateral rectus muscle. At the anterior part of the orbit, it receives post-ganglionic parasympathetic fibres from the **zygomatic nerve**. It gives branches to the lacrimal gland, and the **palpebral branch** to the skin of the upper eyelid [see Fig. 13.5].

## Trochlear nerve

The trochlear nerve is the fourth cranial nerve. It supplies only the superior oblique muscle. It enters the orbit through the superior orbital fissure, and passes forwards and medially to the superior oblique [Fig. 10.3]. (The remaining nerves of the orbit are seen later.)

## Lacrimal gland

The lacrimal gland is a lobulated gland situated at the superolateral angle of the orbit. It lies in a depression on the medial side of the zygomatic process of the frontal bone, mostly hidden by the orbital margin [Fig. 10.2]. The concave medial surface of the gland rests on the levator palpebrae superioris and the lateral rectus. These muscles separate it from the eyeball. The small **palpebral part of the lacrimal gland** projects down into the upper lid between the palpebral fascia and the conjunctiva. Nine to ten thin ducts from the gland open on the deep surface of the upper eyelid near the superior conjunctival fornix [see Fig. 3.13]. Parasympathetic secretomotor nerve fibres to the gland arise in the **pterygopalatine ganglion** and reach the gland through a branch of the zygomatic nerve.

## Levator palpebrae superioris

The levator palpebrae superioris lies superior to the superior rectus [Fig. 10.4]. It takes origin from the roof of the orbit, immediately anterior to the optic canal. It passes forwards above the rectus superior. Anteriorly, it widens into a broad membranous tendon which is inserted into the: (1) skin of the upper eyelid; (2) anterior surface of the superior tarsus; and (3) superior conjunctival fornix [see Fig. 3.11]. A layer of **involuntary** (smooth) **muscle** arises from the aponeurosis and is attached to the superior tarsus.

**Nerve supply**: the skeletal muscle is supplied by the oculomotor nerve, superior division. The smooth muscle is supplied by the cervical sympathetics through the carotid plexus. ➲ Denervation of the muscle by injury to the cervical sympathetics or the oculomotor nerve leads to drooping of the eyelid (**ptosis**). **Action**: it opens the eye by raising the upper eyelid and the superior conjunctival fornix.

Using the instructions given in Dissection 10.3, define the fascial sheath of the eyeball.

**DISSECTION 10.3 Fascial sheath of the eyeball**

**Objective**

**I.** To try and define the fascial sheath of the eyeball.

**Instructions**

1. Divide the frontal nerve and the levator palpebrae superioris, and turn them out of the way. If possible, inflate the eyeball through a small cut in the sclera (the white part of the eye).
2. Cut through the superior rectus, and reflect it.
3. Note the amount of loose tissue, posterior to the eyeball. This is the fascial sheath of the eyeball. Insert a blunt seeker between it and the eyeball, and gauge the extent of the sheath.

## Extraocular muscles of the eyeball

Six muscles move the eyeball—the medial, lateral, superior, and inferior recti, and the superior and inferior obliques. The superior rectus and superior oblique have been exposed already and will be described here. The other muscles will be seen after the vessels and nerves are dissected.

### Superior rectus

**Origin**: the superior rectus takes origin from the upper margin of the common tendinous ring which surrounds the orbital end of the optic canal and the medial part of the superior orbital fissure [Fig. 10.4]. **Insertion**: it passes anterolaterally above the optic nerve and is inserted into the sclera, about 6 mm behind the sclerocorneal junction [Fig. 10.5].

**Nerve supply**: superior division of the oculomotor nerve. **Action**: elevation of the eye when the eye is turned laterally.

### Superior oblique

**Origin**: the superior oblique takes origin from the roof of the orbit, immediately anteromedial to the optic canal, and passes anteriorly along the upper part of the medial wall of the orbit. Anteriorly, it forms a thin tendon which enters the trochlea. The **trochlea** is a small fibrocartilaginous ring attached by fibrous tissue to the trochlear fossa on the frontal bone. It is lined with a synovial sheath which allows the tendon to slide freely in it. **Insertion**: at the trochlea, the tendon of the superior oblique turns posterolaterally and passes backwards between the superior rectus and the eyeball [Figs. 10.3, 10.5]. Lateral to the superior rectus, the tendon flattens out and is inserted into the sclera, midway between the attachment of the optic nerve and the cornea. **Nerve supply**: the trochlear nerve. **Action**: it turns the cornea downwards when it is already turned medially, a position in which the inferior rectus is ineffective as a depressor of the cornea.

Using the instructions given in Dissection 10.4 (and Fig. 10.6), dissect the optic nerve and ciliary ganglion.

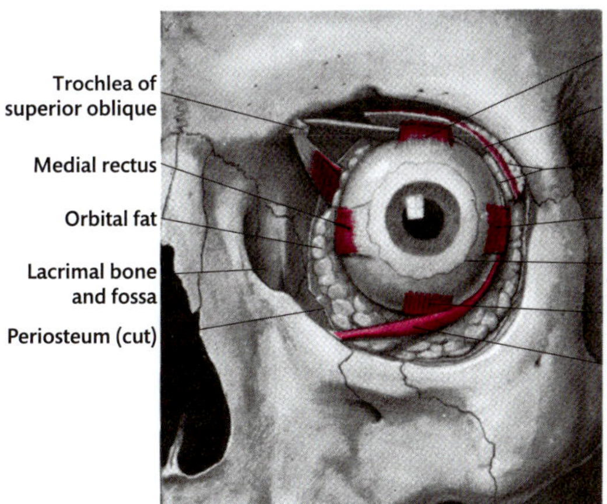


**Fig. 10.5** Dissection of the left orbit to show the insertions of the muscles of the eyeball.

**DISSECTION 10.4 Optic nerve and ciliary ganglion**

**Objectives**

**I.** To identify and trace the optic nerve. **II.** To identify the ciliary ganglion, and the long and short ciliary nerves. **III.** To identify and trace the nasociliary nerve.

**Instructions**

1. Remove the fat beneath the superior rectus, and expose the optic nerve.
2. Look for the structures which cross the optic nerve posteriorly. They are the nasociliary nerve, the ophthalmic artery, and the superior ophthalmic vein. Trace these structures and their branches forwards [Fig. 10.6].
3. Two thread-like branches from the nasociliary nerve—the long ciliary nerves—run along the optic nerve to the eyeball [Fig. 10.2]. Find them.
4. Numerous short ciliary nerves run forwards in the fat around the optic nerve. Find them [Fig. 10.2]. They are branches from the ciliary ganglion.
5. Follow the short ciliary nerve posterior to the ciliary ganglion, a small collection of nerve cells between the optic nerve and the lateral rectus.
6. With care, find the branches to the ciliary ganglion from the nasociliary and inferior divisions of the oculomotor nerve.
7. Remove the fat lateral to the ganglion, and expose the abducens nerve on the medial side of the lateral rectus muscle [Fig. 10.3].
8. Expose the optic nerve in its sheaths.

## Optic nerve

The **optic nerve** is the second cranial nerve. It is a sensory nerve, made up mainly of fibres which originate in the retina (the light-sensitive layer of the eye). It leaves the orbit through the optic canal. It is surrounded by sheaths of the dura mater, arachnoid, and pia mater, which enclose extensions of the subdural and subarachnoid spaces between them. From the optic canal, the nerve runs anterolaterally to pierce the sclera, a short distance medial to the centre of the posterior surface. The nasociliary nerve, ophthalmic artery, and superior ophthalmic vein cross above. The ciliary nerves and vessels surround it near the eyeball [Figs. 10.3, 10.6]. The nerve is slightly longer than the distance it has to run, so as to allow for the movements of the eyeball.

## Nasociliary nerve

The **nasociliary nerve** arises from the ophthalmic nerve in the anterior part of the cavernous sinus [Fig. 10.2]. It passes through the superior orbital fissure within the common tendinous ring [Fig. 10.4] and runs anteromedially above the optic nerve to the medial wall of the orbit. It continues forwards between the superior oblique and the medial rectus muscles, and ends by dividing into the infratrochlear and anterior ethmoidal nerves.

**Branches**: it gives off: (1) the **communicating branch to the ciliary ganglion** which runs along the lateral side of the optic nerve to reach the ganglion; (2) two **long ciliary nerves** which run along the medial side of the optic nerve and pierce the sclera in this position. The long ciliary nerves are sensory to all of the eyeball, except the retina, and also carry post-ganglionic sympathetic nerves from the internal carotid plexus to the dilator pupillae; (3) the **posterior ethmoidal nerve** which arises at the medial wall of the orbit. It runs through the posterior ethmoidal foramen and supplies the mucous membrane of the ethmoid and sphenoid air sinuses; (4) the **infratrochlear nerve** which is the smaller terminal branch of the nasociliary nerve—it runs forwards and leaves the orbit below the trochlea; it appears on the face, above the medial angle of the eye, and supplies the skin of the eyelids and the upper half of the external nose [see Fig. 3.7; Fig. 10.2]; and (5) the **anterior ethmoidal nerve** which leaves the orbit through the anterior ethmoidal foramen, crosses above the ethmoidal sinuses [Fig. 10.6], and appears at the lateral margin of the cribriform plate of the ethmoid [Fig. 10.1]. It turns forwards under the dura mater and descends into the wall of the nasal cavity through a slit-like aperture at the side of the crista galli. It gives **internal nasal branches** to the adjacent mucous

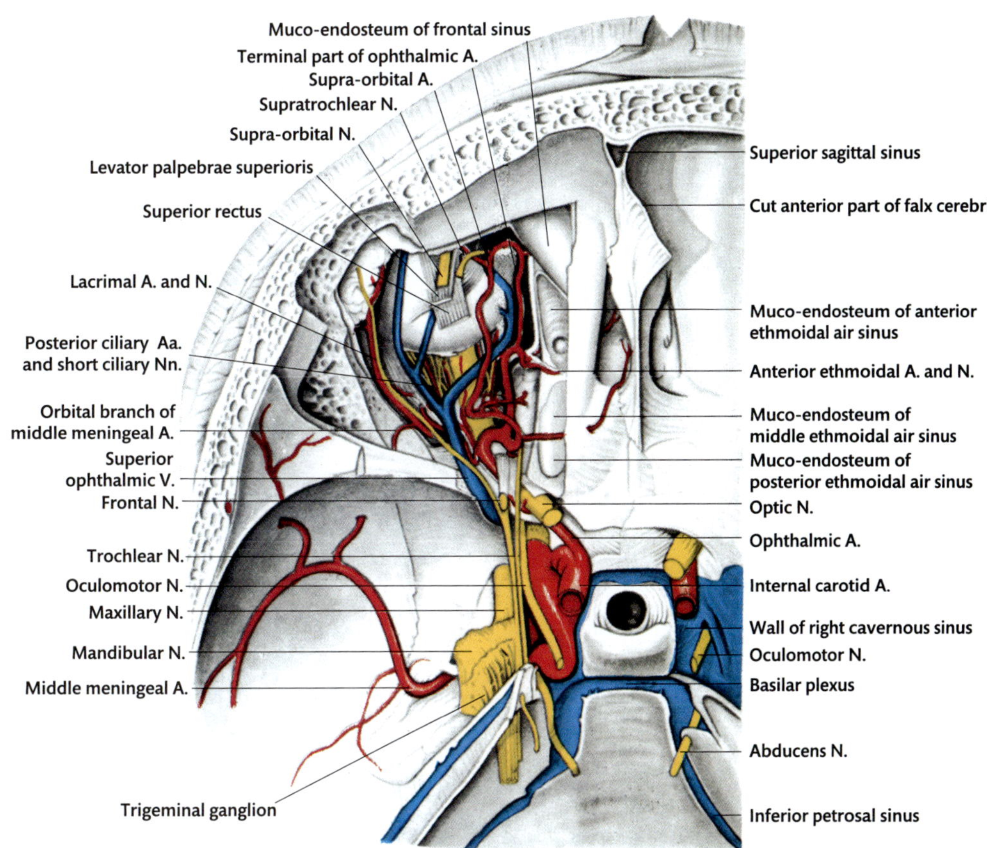


**Fig. 10.6** Dissection of the orbit and middle cranial fossa.





membrane of the lateral and septal walls, runs on the deep surface of the nasal bone, and emerges between the nasal bone and the lateral nasal cartilage [see Fig. 3.7] as the **external nasal** nerve. It supplies the skin of the lower half of the nose.

## Parasympathetic ganglia

The four small parasympathetic ganglia—ciliary, pterygopalatine, otic, and submandibular ganglion—are associated with the branches of the trigeminal nerve. They belong to the parasympathetic part of the autonomic nervous system. Although only the ciliary ganglion lies in the orbit, the general features to these ganglia are mentioned here.

The parasympathetic ganglia lie closer to the structures they supply than the cervical sympathetic ganglia which send sympathetic nerves to the same structures. The ganglia receive **preganglionic fibres** from either the oculomotor, facial, or glossopharyngeal nerves and give rise to **post-ganglionic nerve fibres**. Post-ganglionic fibres are distributed mainly through the branches of the trigeminal nerve to glands of the orbit, nose, nasopharynx, and mouth [see Table 8.1], and to the sphincter of the pupil and ciliary muscle of the eyeball.

Post-ganglionic sympathetic and sensory fibres of the trigeminal nerve frequently run through these ganglia but have no functional connection with them. The post-ganglionic sympathetic nerves reach the ganglia through plexuses on the arteries which supply them.

## Ciliary ganglion

The **ciliary ganglion** consists of a small collection of parasympathetic nerve cells, about the size of a large pinhead. It lies in the fatty tissue between the optic nerve and the lateral rectus muscle.

The ganglion cells receive preganglionic parasympathetic fibres from the oculomotor nerve, and send post-ganglionic parasympathetic fibres to the sphincter pupillae through the short ciliary nerves.

## Connections of the ciliary ganglion

Parasympathetic, sympathetic, and sensory nerves pass through the ciliary ganglion, though only the parasympathetic nerves synapse in it. (1) Preganglionic parasympathetic nerves enter the ganglion, synapse in it, and give rise to post-ganglionic parasympathetic nerves. (2) Post-ganglionic sympathetic nerves to the dilator pupillae pass through the ganglion without synapsing in it. They enter the ganglion through branches of the nasociliary nerve and exit through the short ciliary nerves. (3) Sensory fibres from the eyeball pass through the ganglion without synapsing in it. They enter through the short ciliary nerves and exit through the branch of the nasociliary nerve.

The nerves connected to the ciliary ganglion are: (1) the long, thin branches of the nasociliary nerve carrying branches of sensory and sympathetic nerves which enter the ganglion; (2) a short, thick branch from the nerve to the inferior oblique muscle (oculomotor nerve) which enters the ganglion from below. It carries preganglionic **parasympathetic** fibres which synapse with the cells of the ganglion; (3) approximately six **short ciliary nerves** which divide into 12–20 nerves and pierce the sclera around the attachment of the optic nerve. They carry the post-ganglionic parasympathetic, sympathetic, and sensory fibres. (Details of the intraocular muscles of the eyeball are described in Chapter 11.)

# Ophthalmic artery

The ophthalmic artery arises from the internal carotid artery as it pierces the arachnoid mater [Figs. 10.6, 10.7].

## Course of ophthalmic artery

It enters the orbit through the optic canal, in the subarachnoid space around the optic nerve, and pierces the arachnoid and dura mater. In its course, the ophthalmic artery moves from its position below the optic nerve to the lateral side and then above it to reach the medial wall of the orbit [Fig. 10.7]. It runs forwards on the medial wall

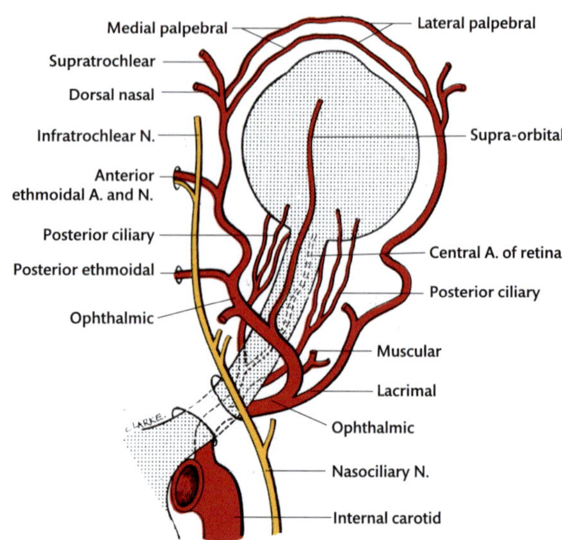


**Fig. 10.7** The ophthalmic artery and its branches.

below the superior oblique muscle, and ends by dividing into the supratrochlear and dorsal nasal arteries near the front of the orbit.

## Branches of the ophthalmic artery

The branches of the ophthalmic artery are numerous and difficult to display but correspond to the nerves in the orbit [Fig. 10.7]. They supply the contents of the orbit through **muscular branches**, the **central artery of the retina** and the **posterior ciliary** and **lacrimal arteries**. Branches of the ophthalmic artery also extend beyond the orbit to the eyelids—**palpebral arteries**; forehead and scalp—**supraorbital and supratrochlear arteries**; ethmoidal air cells and walls of the upper nasal cavity—**anterior** and **posterior ethmoidal arteries**; and skin of the nose—**dorsal** and **external nasal arteries**. The most important branch is the central artery of the retina. It enters the optic nerve in the orbit and runs in it to the retina. ➲ It is the only artery to the retina, and its occlusion results in blindness of that eye.

The lacrimal artery communicates with the middle meningeal artery through the superior orbital fissure [Fig. 10.6].

# Ophthalmic veins

The orbit is drained by the superior and inferior ophthalmic veins. The **superior ophthalmic**

**vein** begins in the anterior part of the orbit, close to the ophthalmic artery, and runs with the ophthalmic artery in the orbit. It communicates with the supraorbital and supratrochlear tributaries of the facial vein.

The **inferior ophthalmic vein** is smaller and lies below the optic nerve. Both superior and inferior ophthalmic veins receive numerous tributaries in the orbit, pass through the superior orbital fissure, and drain into the cavernous sinus, either separately or by a common trunk.

## Extraocular muscles of the eyeball (*continued*)

### Origin of the extraocular muscles

Using the instructions given in Dissection 10.5, expose the origin of the extraocular muscles.

**Origin of recti**: the four recti arise from a **common tendinous ring** which surrounds the orbital end of the optic canal and the medial part of the superior orbital fissure. The superior, inferior, and medial recti arise from the ring above, below, and medial to the optic canal, respectively. The lateral rectus arises by two heads from the lateral part of the ring and the adjoining margins of the orbital fissure. The two divisions of the oculomotor nerve, nasociliary nerve, abducens nerve, and ophthalmic veins pass between the two heads of the lateral rectus [Fig. 10.4].

**Origin of the obliques**: the superior oblique arises from the body of the sphenoid between the superior and medial recti. The inferior oblique is entirely separate from the others. It takes origin from a small area of the floor of the orbit, just lateral to the opening of the nasolacrimal canal. It passes laterally and backwards below the inferior rectus [Figs. 10.5, 10.8].

### Insertion of the extraocular muscles

The recti are inserted into the sclera about 6 mm behind the corneoscleral junction. The oblique muscles are inserted into the sclera much further back. The superior oblique is inserted into the upper lateral quadrant of the eyeball behind the equator, and the inferior oblique into the lower lateral quadrant also behind the equator [Fig. 10.5].

### Actions of the extraocular muscles

The **medial** and **lateral recti** have the simple function of moving the eye around a vertical axis. The medial rectus turns the cornea medially—adduction of the eye; and the lateral rectus turns it laterally—abduction of the eye.

Elevation and depression of the cornea are brought about by different sets of muscles when the eye is abducted or adducted. When the eye is abducted, the **superior** and **inferior recti** produce simple elevation and depression of the cornea. In this position, the **visual axis** corresponds to the axis of these muscles [Fig. 10.9A]. As the cornea is turned medially, the superior and inferior recti become progressively less effective in elevating and depressing the cornea, but tend to turn it further medially [Figs. 10.9B, 10.9C]. When the eye is adducted, the visual axis lies nearer the axis of the **oblique muscles**. In the medially turned eye, the

**DISSECTION 10.5 Origin of the extraocular muscles**

**Objectives**

**I.** To expose the origin of the muscles that arise from the common tendinous ring and the origin of the superior oblique. **II.** To display the inferior oblique muscle.

**Instructions**

1. Divide the optic nerve close to the canal, and turn it forwards with the eyeball. Expose the origin of the recti and the superior oblique.
2. Replace the eyeball. Make an incision through the lower eyelid. Raise the eyeball slightly, and dissect away the fat and loose connective tissue to expose the inferior oblique muscle.
3. Expose the recti muscles, and trace the nerves into the inferior oblique, and the inferior and medial recti from the inferior division of the oculomotor nerve.
4. Once again, trace the nerves forwards from the cavernous sinus into the orbit, and note the relative positions in the superior orbital fissure [Fig. 10.4].

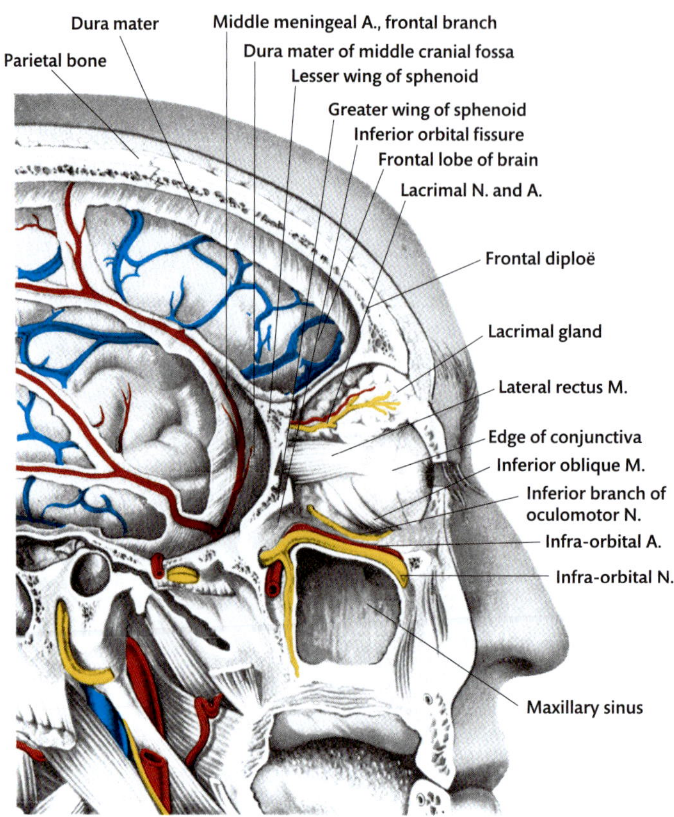


**Fig. 10.8** Dissection of the orbit and maxillary sinus from the lateral side.

inferior oblique produces elevation, and the superior oblique produces depression. Apart from the four primary movements of adduction, abduction, elevation, and depression of the eyeball, the eyeball is also rotated around an anteroposterior axis. Movement of the 12 o'clock position of the cornea inwards or nasally is called **intorsion**. It is brought about by the superior rectus and superior oblique. Movement of the 12 o'clock position of the cornea outwards is called **extorsion**. It is brought about by the inferior rectus and inferior oblique.

## Nerve supply of the extraocular muscles

The superior oblique is supplied by the trochlear nerve. The lateral rectus is supplied by the abducens nerve. The other extraocular muscles—superior rectus, medial rectus, inferior rectus, and inferior oblique—are supplied by the oculomotor nerve.

## Conjugate eye movements

Conjugate eye movements refer to coordinated movements of both eyes in the same direction to maintain binocular vision. It is the motor coordination of the eyes which allows both eyes to fix on a single object. Yoked muscles are contralaterally paired extraocular muscles which work together to direct the gaze in a particular direction. The movement of the two eyes should be matched accurately to avoid diplopia—double vision.

Table 10.1 shows the yoked muscles for each direction of gaze. It must be remembered that when one set of muscles contract to act, the antagonists of those muscles will relax to allow movement.

**Table 10.1** Yoked muscles

| Direction of gaze | Muscle acting in left eye | Muscle acting in right eye |
|---|---|---|
| To the left | Lateral rectus | Medial rectus |
| To the right | Medial rectus | Lateral rectus |
| To the left and up | Superior rectus | Inferior oblique |
| To the right and up | Inferior oblique | Superior rectus |
| To the left and down | Inferior rectus | Superior oblique |
| To the right and down | Superior oblique | Inferior rectus |

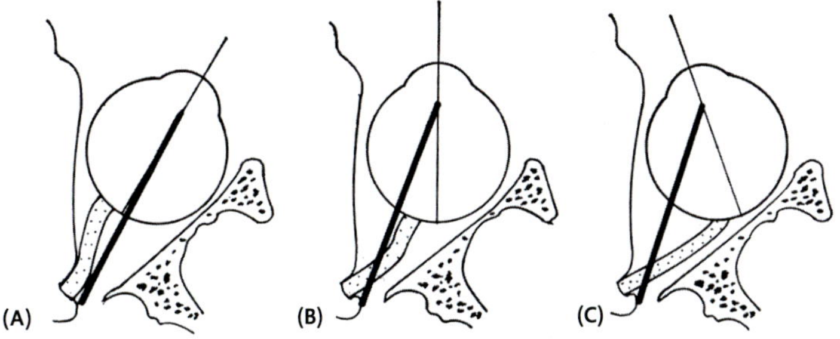


**Fig. 10.9** Three diagrams to show the changing relationship and actions of the superior and inferior rectus muscles (thick line) as the cornea is turned from lateral to medial. (A) When the cornea is turned laterally, the two muscles elevate and depress the cornea, respectively. (B) and (C) As the cornea is turned further medially, they become progressively less effective in this action but turn the cornea further medially. It is in this position that the oblique muscles become effective elevators (inferior oblique) and depressors (superior oblique) of the cornea.

The eye muscles may be used in any combination to produce intermediate movements, and delicate control of eye movements is essential for normal vision.

## Oculomotor nerve

The oculomotor (third cranial nerve) divides into two—the superior and inferior divisions. Both divisions enter the orbit between the two heads of the lateral rectus [Fig. 10.4]. The superior division passes to the superior rectus and, through it, to the levator palpebrae superioris. The larger inferior division supplies the medial rectus, inferior rectus, and inferior oblique, and gives the parasympathetic root to the ciliary ganglion.

## Abducens nerve

The abducens (sixth cranial nerve) enters the orbit between the two heads of the lateral rectus and continues forwards, closely applied to the medial surface of that muscle and supplies it [Figs. 10.3, 10.4]. It supplies only the lateral rectus.

## Nerve palsies and strabismus

➲ Strabismus, or malalignment of the eyes, is a condition where both eyes are turned in different directions. It could be due to nerve palsy, muscle weakness, or muscle incoordination.

➲ Paralysis of the extraocular muscles can result from brainstem or nerve injuries and can be due to trauma, compression by a tumour, or ischaemia. Typically, the patient would present with diplopia (double vision) and strabismus.

➲ Trochlear nerve palsy results in paralyses of the superior oblique. To test the function of the superior oblique muscle, the subject is asked to adduct the eye and look down. In the adducted position, the axis of the eyeball is in line with the oblique muscles and downward gaze is achieved solely by the superior oblique. (The inferior rectus cannot depress the adducted eye.) Inability to look down when the eye is adducted is a sign of trochlear nerve palsy.

➲ Abducens nerve palsy results in paralyses of the lateral rectus. To test the function of the lateral rectus, the subject is asked to abduct the eye. Inability to abduct the eye is a sign of abducens nerve palsy.

➲ Oculomotor nerve palsy results in paralyses of the superior rectus, medial rectus, inferior rectus, and inferior oblique. To test the function of the medial rectus, the subject is asked to adduct the eye. Inability to adduct the eye is a sign of medial rectus paralysis. To test the function of the superior rectus, the subject is asked to elevate the eye with the eye abducted. Inability to elevate the abducted eye is a sign of superior rectus paralysis. To test the function of the inferior rectus, the subject is asked to depress the eye with the eye abducted. Inability to depress the abducted eye is a sign of inferior rectus paralysis.

➲ Oculomotor nerve palsy results in the paralysed eye being turned down and out, due to unopposed action of the lateral rectus and superior oblique. The patient would also have ptosis due to paralysis of the levator palpebrae superioris, and a dilated pupil due to paralysis of the sphincter pupillae.

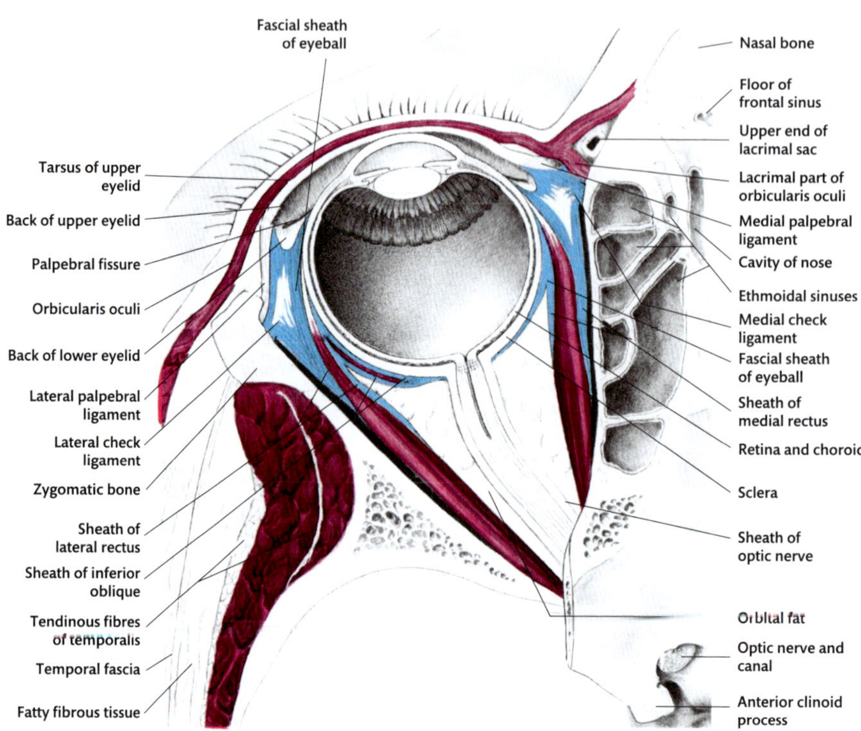


**Fig. 10.10** Horizontal section through the left orbit to show arrangement of the fascial sheath of the eyeball (blue) and check ligaments. [See also Fig. 7.13A.]

## Fascial sheath of the eyeball

The fascial sheath of the eyeball is a membranous socket for the eyeball. It is deficient in front over the cornea. It is separated from the eyeball by soft, semi-fluid areolar tissue which allows the eyeball to slide freely in the sheath. The free anterior margin of the sheath fuses with the ocular conjunctiva close to the margin of the cornea. Posteriorly, the sheath is adherent to the dural sheath of the optic nerve. The sheath is loosely attached to orbital fat [Fig. 10.10].

Each of the extrinsic muscles of the eyeball pierces the fascial sheath at the equator of the eyeball and receives a covering sleeve from it. The sleeve over the recti extends posteriorly and merge with the epimysium. Note the position of the sheath over the medial and lateral recti in Fig. 10.10. Each of these sleeves is attached by fibrous tissue to the bony wall of the orbit and acts as a pulley which prevents the muscle from compressing the eyeball when it contracts. The sheath of the superior oblique passes to the trochlea and fuses with it. The sheath of the inferior oblique reaches the floor of the orbit.

## Ligaments in the orbit

(1) The **suspensory ligament** is a hammock-shaped sling stretched below the eyeball in the anterior part of the orbit. It extends between the lacrimal and zygomatic bones. It is broadest beneath the eyeball where it is attached to the fascial sheath and helps to support the eyeball and steady the fascial sheath. (2) The **check ligaments** are strong bands which pass from the sheaths around the lateral and medial rectus muscles to the zygomatic and lacrimal bones, respectively, close to the attachments of the suspensory ligament [Fig. 10.10]. These ligaments limit the movement of the lateral and medial recti. Similar checks are present on the superior and inferior rectus muscles.

The zygomatic and infraorbital nerves, though contents of the orbit, lie outside the orbital periosteum. They are most conveniently dissected later with the maxillary sinus.

CHAPTER 11

# The eyeball

The eyeball lies in the anterior part of the orbit, enclosed in a fascial sheath which separates it from the orbital muscles and fat. It is about 2.5 cm in diameter but is not perfectly spherical. The anterior clear part—the cornea—has a smaller radius of curvature than the rest of the globe and protrudes from the anterior surface of the eyeball.

For a satisfactory dissection of the eyeball, use one which has been hardened for a few days in formaldehyde. You will need four of these to do all the dissections described here.

## General structure of the eyeball

The eyeball consists of three concentric coats or layers, which enclose a cavity.

The coats are: (1) an external fibrous coat made up of the cornea and sclera. The posterior five-sixths of this layer is the white, opaque **sclera**. The anterior one-sixth is the more highly curved, transparent **cornea**; (2) a middle coat which is vascular and muscular; it consists of the **iris** anteriorly, the **choroid** posteriorly, and the thickest part—the **ciliary body**—in between the iris and choroid; and (3) the internal coat—the **retina**; it contains the light-sensitive elements (rods and cones) and gives rise to the nerve fibres of the optic nerve.

The lens is suspended in the eyeball by the suspensory ligament. Together, the lens and suspensory ligament divide the cavity of the eyeball into an aqueous chamber in front and a vitreous chamber behind. The aqueous chamber is further divided by the iris into an **anterior chamber** between the cornea and the iris, and a **posterior chamber** between the iris and the lens. The anterior and posterior chambers are continuous with each other through the aperture in the middle of the iris—the **pupil** [Fig. 11.1].

The middle of the cornea is referred to as the **anterior pole**. A point on the back of the eyeball opposite the anterior pole is the **posterior pole**.

Using the instructions given in Dissection 11.1 (and Fig. 11.2), clean the surface of the eyeball and section it.

The light rays which enter the eye travel through the following **refracting media**: (1) the cornea; (2) the aqueous humour, a watery medium which fills the **anterior** and **posterior chambers**; (3) the lens; and (4) the vitreous body, which occupies the **vitreous chamber**. Because the greatest change in refractive index is between the air and the cornea, its curved surface plays a very important part in the optical system. ➲ Pathological changes in the shape of the cornea markedly interfere with the ability of the eye to bring an image to focus on the retina.

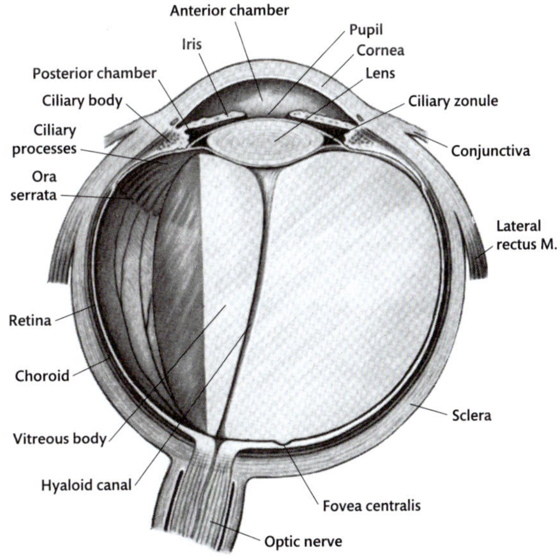


**Fig. 11.1** Diagrammatic section of the eyeball.

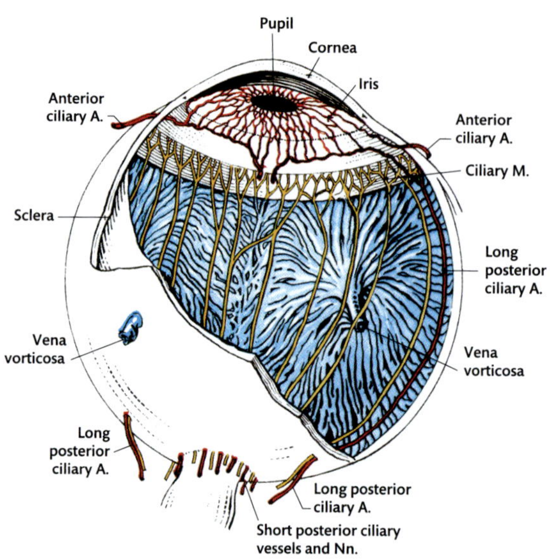


**Fig. 11.2** Dissection of the eyeball. Part of the sclera has been removed to show the vascular coat and the arrangement of ciliary nerves and vessels.

**DISSECTION 11.1 Sectioning of the eyeball**

**Objectives**

**I.** To clean the surface of the eyeball. **II.** To section the eyeball for study of the interior.

**Instructions**

1. Remove the loose tissue from the surface of the eyeball.
2. Pick up the conjunctiva and fascial sheath close to the corneal margin, and cut through these layers around the margin of the cornea. Proceed to strip these soft parts from the surface of the white part of the eye (the sclera), working steadily backwards towards the entry of the optic nerve.
3. Identify the vorticose veins which pierce the sclera a little posterior to the equator, in the coronal plane [Fig. 11.2].
4. Identify the posterior ciliary arteries and ciliary nerves, as they enter the sclera around the attachment of the optic nerve [Fig. 11.2].
5. To obtain a general idea of the parts of the eyeball, make sections through hardened specimens in different planes: (1) through the equator; and (2) in a horizontal section. Remove the vitreous body from one-half cut horizontally, and retain it in the other [Fig. 11.1].
6. Place the sections in formaldehyde solution for reference during dissection.

## Fibrous coat

The outer fibrous coat is made up of the cornea and sclera which are continuous with each other at the corneoscleral junction.

### Sclera

The sclera is a dense, collagenous coat which covers the posterior five-sixths of the eyeball [Figs. 11.1, 11.2]. It is loosely attached to the choroid by delicate, pigmented areolar tissue, but firmly adherent to the ciliary body. The sclera is continuous anteriorly with the cornea [Fig. 11.1].

A number of nerves and vessels pierce the sclera. The optic nerve and blood vessels to the retina pierce the sclera approximately 3 mm nasal to the posterior pole. The optic nerve is covered by the meninges of the brain which fuse with the sclera at this point. The subdural and subarachnoid spaces also end at this point [see Fig. 10.10].

The sclera is also pierced by numerous blood vessels and nerves, which supply the fibrous and vascular coats. They are: (1) the long and short **posterior ciliary arteries** and **ciliary nerves** which pierce the sclera around the optic nerve; (2) 4–5 veins—the **vorticose veins**—which emerge a short distance posterior to the equator and are spaced equally around the eyeball; and (3) the **anterior ciliary arteries** which pierce the sclera near the corneal margin [Fig. 11.2].

### Cornea

The cornea is the transparent one-sixth of the fibrous coat of the eyeball. The anterior surface of the cornea is covered with a layer of epithelium which is firmly bound to it and is continuous with the conjunctiva at the margin of the cornea. On the posterior surface is the **posterior limiting lamina**, an elastic glassy layer. The iris lies behind the cornea and is separated from it by the aqueous humour [Fig. 11.1].

## Middle (vascular) coat

The middle or vascular coat of the eye consists of the iris, the ciliary body, and the choroid.

## Iris

The iris is a thin, circular structure that lies between the cornea anteriorly and the lens posteriorly. It surrounds a central circular aperture—the **pupil**. Its anterior surface shows faint radial striations, and its posterior surface is deeply pigmented [see Fig. 3.2].

It is separated from the cornea by the anterior chamber and is bathed by the aqueous humour on both surfaces. At its circumference, the iris is continuous with the ciliary body behind and is connected to the cornea by the pectinate ligament of the iris [Fig. 11.1].

The iris is the coloured part of the eye and varies greatly in colour in light-skinned races. The diameter of the pupil is constantly changing to control the amount of light reaching the retina. These changes in the size of the pupil are brought about by two sets of involuntary muscles—the sphincter pupillae and the dilator pupillae.

### Sphincter pupillae

The **sphincter pupillae** is made up of circularly placed smooth muscle fibres that lie in the pupillary margin of the iris and constrict the pupil. **Nerve supply**: it is supplied by post-ganglionic parasympathetic fibres from the ciliary ganglion which reach it through the short ciliary nerves.

### Dilator pupillae

The **dilator pupillae** is made up of smooth muscle fibres which run radially towards the periphery of the iris and dilate the pupil. **Nerve supply**: it is supplied by post-ganglionic sympathetic fibres from the carotid plexus, which reach it through the nasociliary and long ciliary nerves [see Fig. 10.2].

## Iridocorneal angle

At the junction of the cornea and iris is a small, circular venous channel—the **sinus venosus sclerae**. At the margin of the cornea, the posterior limiting lamina of the cornea breaks up into bundles of fibres, some of which pass posteriorly into the choroid and sclera. Others arch medially into the iris, crossing the angle between the cornea and the iris in the form of a number of separate bundles, known as the **pectinate ligament of the iris** [Figs. 11.3, 11.4]. Between the bundles are the minute **spaces of the iridocorneal angle** which drain aqueous fluid from the anterior chamber into the sinus venosus sclerae.

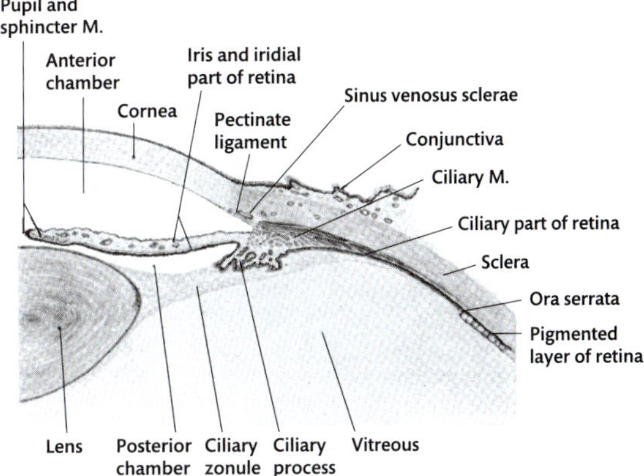


**Fig. 11.3** Section through the anterior part of the eyeball.

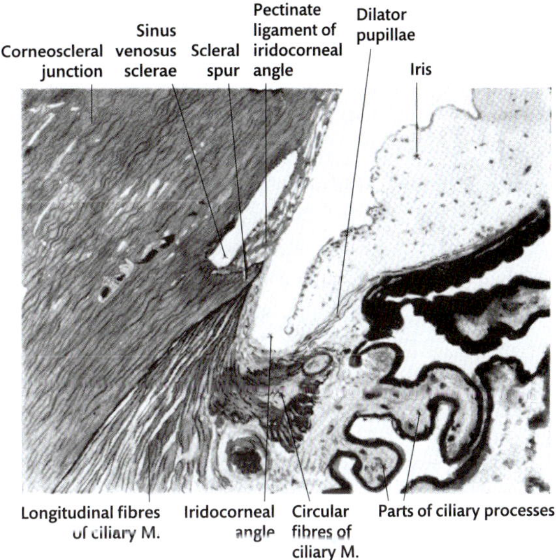


**Fig. 11.4** The iridocorneal angle.

➲ Blockage of this system leads to build-up of aqueous fluid and raised intraocular tension, a serious condition called **glaucoma**.

## Ciliary body

The ciliary body is that part of the middle coat that lies between the iris anteriorly and the choroid posteriorly. It is divisible into: (1) an external part—the **ciliary muscle**; and (2) an internal part—the **ciliary processes** [Figs. 11.1, 11.3, 11.4, 11.5].

### Ciliary muscle

The ciliary muscle is composed of involuntary muscle fibres arranged in two groups—radiating or longitudinal and circular [Fig. 11.4]. The **radiating fibres** arise from the deep surface of the sclera,

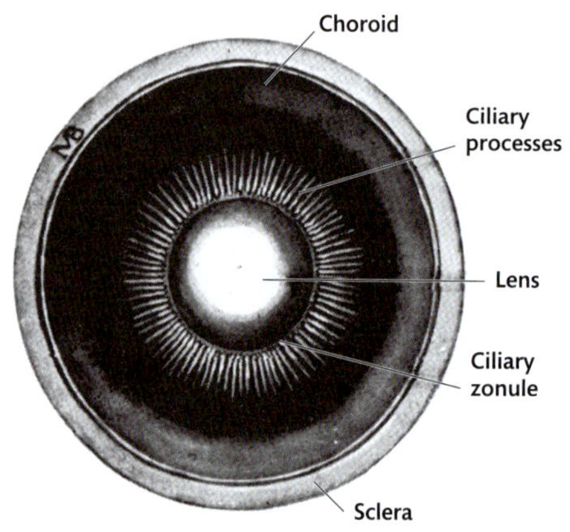


**Fig. 11.5** Anterior half of the interior of the eyeball viewed from behind after removal of the vitreous.





close to the cornea, and radiate posteriorly into the ciliary processes. The **circular fibres** form a muscular ring close to the peripheral margin of the iris and are arranged in two or three bundles that lie on the deep surface of the radiating fibres. **Nerve supply**: parasympathetic fibres from the ciliary ganglion through the short ciliary nerves. **Action**: accommodation of the eye to focus on near objects. Contraction of the ciliary muscles relaxes the suspensory ligament of the lens and increases the curvature of the lens to enable the eye to focus on near objects.

Using the instructions given in Dissection 11.2, dissect the iris and the ciliary processes.

**DISSECTION 11.2 Iris and ciliary processes**

**Objective**

**I.** To study the iris and ciliary processes.

**Instructions**

1. To expose the ciliary processes, make a coronal section through an eyeball anterior to the equator [Fig. 11.5]. Remove the vitreous body from the anterior segment. Then wash out the pigment from the anterior part of the middle coat to expose the ciliary processes more fully.
2. Alternatively, remove the cornea by cutting around the corneoscleral junction, and examine the exposed iris.
3. Make a number of radial cuts into the anterior part of the sclera, and fold each segment of the sclera outwards, stripping it from the ciliary body.
4. Remove the iris.

### Ciliary processes

Ciliary processes are radial folds which extend from the anterior margin of the choroid inwards towards the margin of the lens. They end behind the margin of the iris. They are approximately 70 in number and extend across the posterior surface of the ciliary body. The posterior surface of the ciliary processes is applied to the vitreous membrane—the outer condensed part of the vitreous body—and to the peripheral part of the ciliary zonule [Figs. 11.3, 11.5].

## Choroid

The choroid is the largest part of the middle coat. It lies between the sclera and the retina. It is thickest posteriorly where it is pierced by the optic nerve, and becomes thinner as it approaches the ciliary body. The choroid is connected to the sclera by delicate, pigmented areolar tissue, and also by the blood vessels and nerves which pass between them. The deep surface of the choroid is adherent to the outer layer of the retina.

The choroid consists mainly of blood vessels which are arranged in two layers: (1) a deep, close-meshed capillary net; and (2) a more superficial venous layer from which the vorticose veins arise. The short posterior ciliary arteries run between these layers [Figs. 11.2, 11.6].

Using the instructions given in Dissection 11.3, remove the sclera from one eyeball.

## Ciliary nerves

Twelve or more fine **short ciliary nerves** arise from the ciliary ganglion and pierce the sclera around the optic nerve. On the inner aspect of the sclera, they run anteriorly and break up into fine plexiform branches to the ciliary muscle, iris, and cornea [Fig. 11.2]. The short ciliary nerves contain: (1) **post-ganglionic parasympathetic fibres** from the ciliary ganglion to the ciliary muscle and the sphincter pupillae; (2) **post-ganglionic sympathetic fibres** from the internal carotid plexus to the vessels of the eyeball; and (3) **sensory fibres** from the eyeball to the nasociliary nerve. (The sympathetic and sensory fibres have no connection with the cells of the ciliary ganglion.)

The **long ciliary branches** of the nasociliary nerve transmit sensory and sympathetic nerve fibres to the eyeball. They pierce the sclera close to the optic nerve. The sympathetic fibres come from

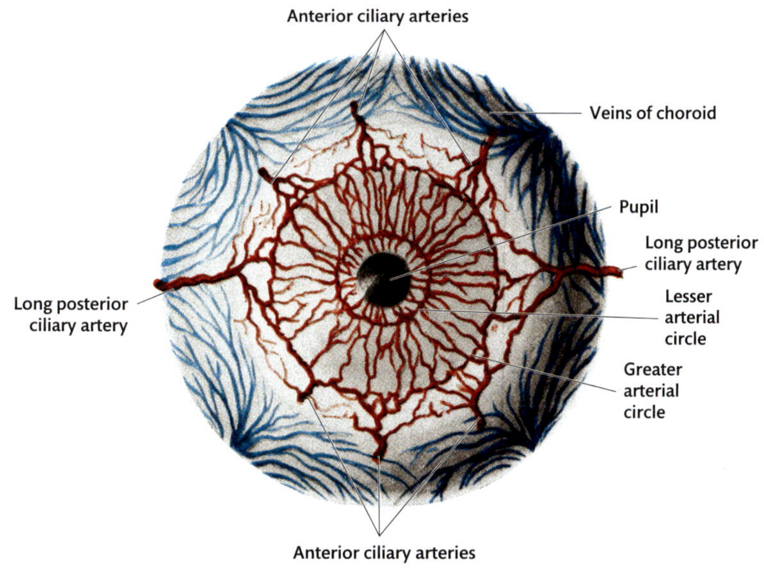


**Fig. 11.6** Blood vessels of the iris and the anterior part of the choroid viewed from the front.



**DISSECTION 11.3 Choroid**

**Objective**

**I.** To remove the sclera and expose the choroid.

**Instructions**

1. Start with an undissected eye. Using a sharp knife, make an incision through the sclera at the equator, stopping as soon as the black choroid appears. Introduce one blade of blunt-ended scissors through the cut, and extend the incision through the sclera around the equator. Take care to separate the choroid from its deep surface as you proceed.
2. Raise the anterior and posterior parts of the divided sclera from the choroid, and by careful blunt dissection, turn these parts anteriorly and posteriorly, stripping them from the choroid. Some resistance will be encountered with the anterior part close to the cornea, due to the attachment of the ciliary muscle to the deep surface of the sclera. As this attachment is broken down by continued blunt dissection, the aqueous humour will escape.
3. Remove the posterior part of the sclera by dividing the optic nerve fibres where they enter the deep surface.
4. The eyeball, denuded of its fibrous coat, should be placed in water for further investigation.
5. Gently brush the eyeball under water with a brush. This removes the pigment and exposes the curved tributaries of the vorticose veins, which appear as white lines [Fig. 11.2].

the internal carotid plexus, and some of them supply the dilator pupillae.

## Ciliary arteries

The **short posterior ciliary arteries** are branches of the ophthalmic artery. They pierce the sclera close to the optic nerve and end in the choroid [Figs. 11.2, 11.6].

The **long posterior ciliary arteries** are two branches of the ophthalmic artery which pierce the sclera some distance from the optic nerve. They run anteriorly, between the sclera and the choroid, on opposite sides of the eyeball. In the region of the ciliary body, they branch and anastomose with the anterior ciliary arteries to form the **greater arterial circle** at the periphery of the iris [Fig. 11.6]. This circle supplies the iris, the ciliary muscle, and the ciliary processes.

The **anterior ciliary arteries** are minute twigs which arise from the arteries to the recti muscles. They pierce the sclera close to the cornea and take part in the formation of the greater arterial circle. The **lesser arterial circle** is a small anastomotic ring in the iris at the margin of the pupil [Fig. 11.6].

## Vorticose veins

Four to five large veins arise from the venous plexus in the choroid and pierce the sclera immediately posterior to the equator. These are the vorticose veins. They drain into the ophthalmic veins [Fig. 11.2].

Using the instructions given in Dissection 11.4, identify the layers of the retina.

### DISSECTION 11.4 Retina

**Objective**

**I.** To study the layers of the retina.

**Instructions**

1. Remove the vitreous body from the posterior segment of the specimen used to show the ciliary processes.
2. Study the white nervous layer of the retina which has been exposed.
3. Gently lift the inner nervous layer of the retina, and appreciate the outer pigmented layer.

# Inner coat–retina

The retina consists of two layers: (1) an outer **pigment layer** which is adherent to the choroid; and (2) a thicker inner **nervous layer**. A potential space (the remnant of the optic cavity in the embryo) exists between the pigment layer of the retina and the nervous layer. The nervous layer is attached to the vitreous and pigment layers only where the optic nerve pierces the sclera. It is readily detached from the pigment layer, even during life. ➲ Such a retinal detachment makes it impossible to focus an image on the nervous layer and leads to blurring of vision. It may also interfere with nutrition to the retina.

The pigment layer absorbs the light which has passed through the nervous layer and prevents it from being reflected back and interfering with the sharpness of the image. (In many nocturnal animals, the choroid forms a reflecting layer known as the tapetum. The presence of the tapetum ensures the passage of low intensities of light twice through the retina to increase its sensitivity.)

The nervous layer is the light-sensitive part of the retina. It ends anteriorly, at a wavy margin—the **ora serrata**—close to the posterior margin of the ciliary body [Fig. 11.1]. The two layers—the pigment and nervous layers—are continued, anterior to the ora serrata, as a very thin layer on the posterior aspect of the ciliary processes and the posterior surface of the iris. This continuation of the retina on the ciliary processes and the iris is known as the **pars ciliaris retinae** and the **pars iridica retinae**, respectively.

The nervous layer of the retina consists of multiple layers of cells. The outermost are the light-sensitive **rods** and **cones**. The innermost are the **ganglion** cells that give rise to the fibres in the optic nerve [Fig. 11.7]. The nerve fibres originating in the ganglion cell run over the inner surface of the retina and converge on the optic nerve.

## Optic disc

At the commencement of the optic nerve is the **optic disc**, a circular elevation, with a slight central depression on it [Fig. 11.8]. The optic disc is situated approximately 3 mm to the nasal side of the posterior pole of the eyeball and is the site where the fibres from the ganglion cells enter the optic nerve. There are no sensory elements at the optic disc, resulting in a blind spot in the visual field. The central artery of the retina enters the retina at the optic disc.

## Macula lutea

In the centre of the visual axis is a small yellowish spot on the retina—the **macula lutea**. In it is a slight depression at the centre—the **fovea centralis** [Fig. 11.8]. The fovea is the site of maximum visual acuity. At the fovea, the inner layers of the nervous layer of the retina are swept aside to expose the cones. This allows light to fall directly on the cones and improves the quality of the image on them [Fig. 11.7]. The nerve fibres and blood vessels which pass to and from the optic disc do not cross the macula but go around it, so as not to obstruct the light rays.

## Central retinal arteries and veins

The **central artery of the retina** is a branch of the ophthalmic artery [see Fig. 10.7]. It is the only source of blood supply to the inner layers of the retina. (The outer retinal layers are nourished to some extent by diffusion from the choroidal

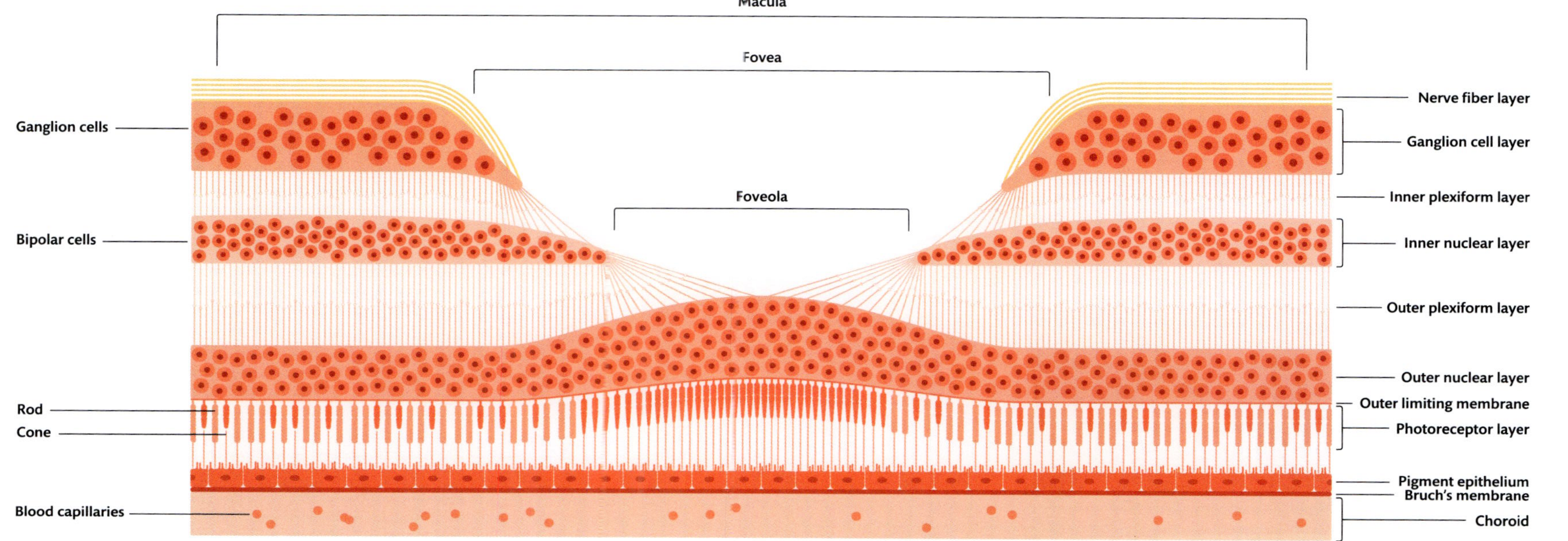


**Fig. 11.7** Arrangement of cells in the peripheral and central parts of the retina. © Pikovit/Shutterstock.com

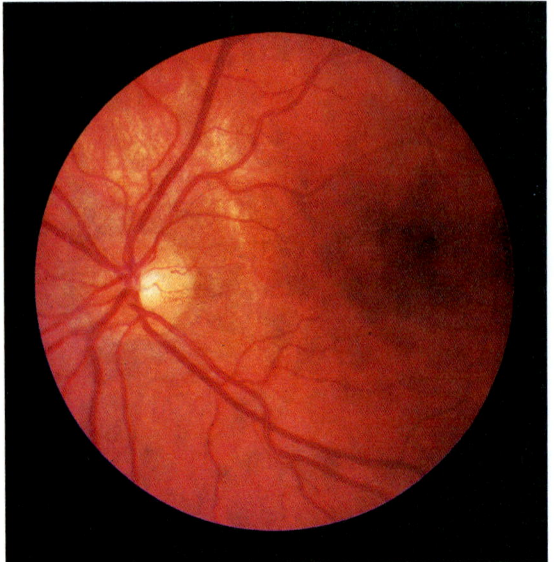

(A)

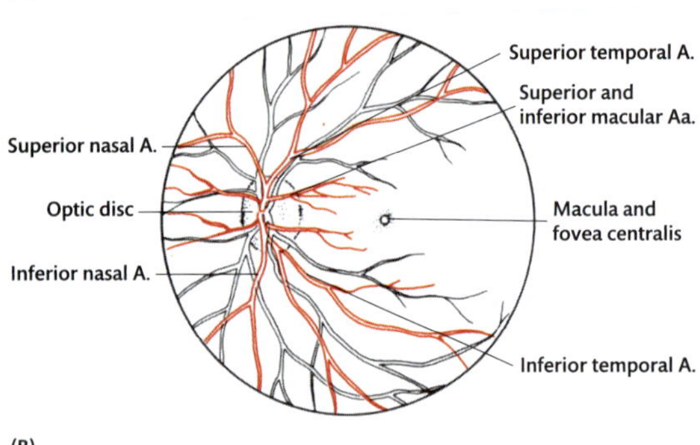


(B)

**Fig. 11.8** (A) Retinal blood vessels, as seen through the ophthalmoscope. (B) Diagrammatic representation of (A).

vessels.) It pierces the sheath of the optic nerve and enters the optic nerve in the orbit. It runs in the optic nerve with the central vein of the retina, and reaches the retina at the optic disc. At the optic disc, the artery divides into superior and inferior branches, each of which divides into a large temporal, and a smaller nasal, arteriole [Fig. 11.8]. These branches run on the internal surface of the retina to the ora serrata. They do not anastomose with each other or with any of the other arteries of the eyeball.

The **retinal veins** converge on the optic disc and enter the optic nerve as two small trunks which soon unite to form the **central vein of the retina**. The central vein of the retina drains into the superior ophthalmic vein, after piercing the meningeal sheaths of the optic nerve.

➲ The central artery of the retina and its branches are blood vessels which can be examined in the living by using an ophthalmoscope.

➲ The central retinal artery is an end artery. Obstruction of the artery results in acute-onset loss of vision due to ischaemia of the retina. If only a branch of the vessel is occluded, it will result in deprivation of blood to the area supplied by it and patchy loss of vision.

➲ Increased pressure in the subarachnoid space can compress the central vein of the retina and cause distension of its tributaries in the retina. These distended veins can be seen with the ophthalmoscope.

Using the instructions given in Dissection 11.5, examine the ciliary zonule and the lens.

## Vitreous body

The vitreous body is a soft, transparent, jelly-like substance which fills the posterior four-fifths of the eyeball. It lies in contact with the retina, the ciliary processes, the ciliary zonule, and the lens. The lens forms a deep depression—the **hyaloid fossa**—on the anterior surface of the vitreous body [Fig. 11.3].

The outer surface of the vitreous body is condensed to form a transparent envelope—the **vitreous membrane**. A minute canal—the **hyaloid canal**—runs through the vitreous body from the optic disc to the posterior surface of the lens [Fig. 11.1]. It represents the remains of a branch of the central artery of the retina—the **hyaloid artery**—which supplied the developing lens in the fetus. The hyaloid canal cannot be seen in an ordinary

### DISSECTION 11.5 Ciliary zonule and lens

#### Objective

**I.** To examine the ciliary zonule, capsule of the lens, and lens.

#### Instructions

1. In the anterior segment of a freshly dissected eye, examine the vitreous membrane, the capsule of the lens, and the ciliary zonule.
2. Remove the lens (which is now hardened), and examine it.

dissection but may be visualized in the living with a slit-lamp. The minute remnant of the hyaloid artery attaches the vitreous body to the optic disc, though elsewhere the vitreous body is entirely free from the retina.

## Ciliary zonule and suspensory ligament of the lens

The **ciliary zonule** is a thickened part of the vitreous membrane which is in contact with the posterior surface of the ciliary process [Figs. 11.1, 11.3, 11.5]. At the inner margin of the ciliary processes, it splits into two layers. The posterior layer is extremely thin and lines the hyaloid fossa. The anterior layer is thicker and forms the **suspensory ligament of the lens**. It is attached principally to: (1) the anterior surface of the capsule of the lens, a short distance from its margin; (2) the margin of the lens; and (3) the posterior surface close to the margin [Figs. 11.1, 11.3]. The multiple attachments of the suspensory ligament to the lens result in the formation of a multilocular, fluid-filled space around the margin of the lens—the zonular space.

The suspensory ligament holds the lens firmly in the hyaloid fossa. When the eye is at rest, the suspensory ligament maintains a certain degree of tension on the lens. The lens is drawn out radially and flattens, so as to maintain a long focal length When the eye focuses on near objects, the ciliary muscle contracts and pulls the ciliary processes and zonule anteriorly. This movement relaxes the suspensory ligament and allows the elastic lens to round up and shorten its focal length.

## Lens

The lens is a biconvex, transparent, solid, elastic structure which lies between the iris and the vitreous body. It is enclosed in a glassy, elastic capsule. It contains no blood vessels.

The **anterior surface** of the lens is less curved than the posterior. Its central part is opposite the pupil, and lateral to this, the margin of the iris is in contact with the lens. Further laterally, the lens and iris are separated from each other by the aqueous humour in the posterior chamber. The **posterior surface** of the lens fits into the hyaloid fossa. The equator of the lens is a blunt margin that forms one boundary of the zonular spaces.

➲ The lens becomes tougher and less elastic with age. This accounts for the decreased ability to focus on near objects. **Cataract** is a clinical condition where the lens becomes less transparent and more opaque with age. Cataract surgery is a procedure where the clouded natural lens is removed and replaced with a clear artificial lens to improve vision.

Dissection 11.6 provides instructions on how to study the capsule of the lens and the lens.

See Clinical Applications 11.1, 11.2, and 11.3 for the practical implications of the anatomy discussed in this chapter.

**DISSECTION 11.6 Lens**

**Objective**

**I.** To study the lens and the capsule of the lens.

**Instructions**

1. Incise the anterior surface of the lens with a sharp knife, and apply a little pressure to the margin with the finger and thumb. This will extrude the body of the lens and allow the capsule to be studied separately.
2. Compress the body of the lens between the finger and the thumb, and note that the central part (nucleus) is firmer than the remainder. The lens is made up of a number of concentric laminae, which can be easily peeled off after the lens has been hardened in alcohol.

**CLINICAL APPLICATION 11.1 Corneal reflex**

Testing for the corneal or blink reflex is part of the neurological examination. It is especially useful in patients with head injury to assess the integrity of the brainstem. Stimulation of the cornea of one eye with a wisp of cotton causes both eyelids to blink. This reflex blink protects the eye from foreign bodies. Stimulus of the cornea of one side causes a direct (same side) and consensual (opposite side) blink response.

The afferent (sensory) limb of the reflex arc is mediated through the nasociliary branch of the ophthalmic division of the trigeminal nerve, which supplies the cornea. The efferent (motor) limb is through the temporal and zygomatic branches of the facial nerve which supply the orbicularis oculi. An absent corneal reflex may be due to sensory neuropathy affecting the trigeminal nerve, a lesion in the seventh cranial nerve, or a brainstem injury. Failure to blink on one side indicates seventh nerve palsy on that side. Failure to blink on both sides usually indicates a sensory loss on the tested side.

**CLINICAL APPLICATION 11.2 Corneal transplant**

Corneal transplant, or keratoplasty, is a procedure where diseased corneal tissue is surgically removed and replaced by healthy donor corneal tissue harvested from a recently deceased individual. Corneal transplants can be 'penetrating' when the whole thickness of the cornea is replaced, or 'lamellar' when the graft involves only a few layers of the cornea. The fact that the cornea is avascular and devoid of lymphatics, and has relatively few antigen-presenting cells, makes it immunologically privileged and less likely to be rejected than other organ transplants.

**CLINICAL APPLICATION 11.3 Convergence-accommodation reflex**

Failure to bring both eyes to focus on an object leads to double vision. To test this, hold up your finger about 30 cm from your nose and look past it at a distant object (do not focus on the finger). In this situation, the finger appears double and out of focus. Now slowly bring your eyes to focus on the finger. The two images move together and come into focus as a single object.

The ability to change focus from distant objects to near objects is dependent on convergence and accommodation. Convergence occurs when the two medial recti work together and ensure that the image of the finger falls on corresponding parts of the two retinae. Accommodation occurs when the ciliary muscles contract, the ciliary zonule and lens are brought forward, the suspensory ligament of the lens is relaxed, and the lens becomes more spherical, bringing the near object to focus on the retina.

The two actions are linked together in the convergence-accommodation reflex and are associated with constriction of the pupil.

CHAPTER 12

# Organs of hearing and equilibrium



## Introduction

The ear contains the auditory apparatus and the organs for balance and equilibrium. It is readily divisible into three parts: the external ear, the middle ear, and the internal ear [Fig. 12.1]. The **external ear** consists of the auricle and the external acoustic meatus. The auricle collects the sound waves, and the external acoustic meatus transmits them medially to the tympanic membrane. The tympanic membrane separates the external ear from the middle ear. The **middle ear** is a narrow air-filled chamber, also known as the **tympanic cavity**. It lies between the tympanic membrane and the lateral wall of the internal ear. The pressure in the tympanic cavity is maintained at atmospheric pressure by the communication of the cavity with the nasal part of the pharynx through the auditory tube. Three small auditory ossicles—the **malleus**, **incus**, and **stapes**—lie in the middle ear and stretch across it from the tympanic membrane to the lateral wall of the internal ear. They transmit the vibrations of the tympanic membrane

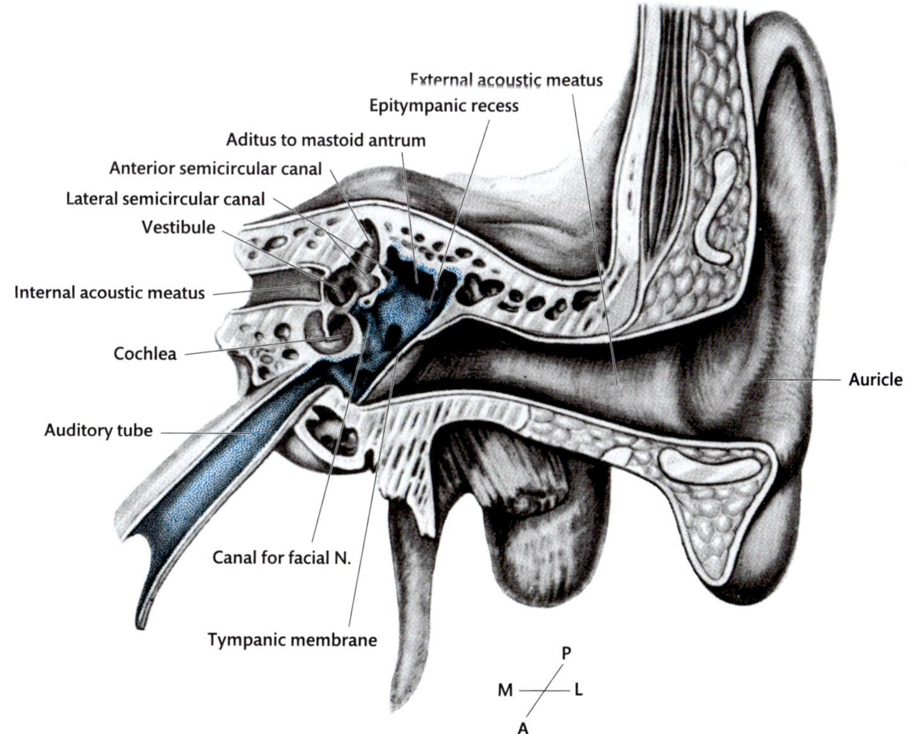


**Fig. 12.1** The parts of the ear (semi-diagrammatic). The mucous membrane lining the middle ear cavity and auditory tube is shown in blue. M = medial; L = lateral; A = anterior; P = posterior.

to the internal ear. The **internal ear** consists of a complex system of communicating cavities—the **bony labyrinth**—situated in the dense part of the petrous temporal bone. Suspended in the bony labyrinth is a similarly shaped, but narrower, complex of membranous tubes and sacs—the **membranous labyrinth**—on which the sensory nerve fibres of the vestibulocochlear nerve end [Fig. 12.1].

## The external ear

Review the parts of the auricle described in Chapter 3.

Dissection 12.1 provides instructions on how to dissect the external acoustic meatus.

**DISSECTION 12.1 External acoustic meatus**

**Objective**

**I.** To study the external acoustic meatus.

**Instructions**

1. Remove the anterior wall of the cartilaginous part of the external acoustic meatus with a knife or scissors.
2. Pass a probe into the bony part of the meatus to determine its length, and using the probe as a guide, cut away the anterior wall of the bony part of the meatus (tympanic bone). Take care not to injure the tympanic membrane.

### External acoustic meatus

The external acoustic meatus runs medially and slightly forwards. It is almost exactly in line with the internal acoustic meatus, and their shadows are superimposed in a true lateral radiograph of the skull. The external acoustic meatus is approximately 24 mm long. The lateral one-third of it is cartilaginous, and the medial two-thirds is bony. The tympanic membrane lies obliquely, so that the anterior wall and floor are longer than the posterior wall and roof. The diameter of the external acoustic meatus is not uniform; the narrowest point—the **isthmus**—is about 5 mm from the tympanic membrane. The vertical diameter is greatest at the lateral end, and the anteroposterior diameter is greatest at the medial end. The meatus is slightly curved with an upward convexity [Fig. 12.1].

➲ The direction and the narrowing of the external acoustic meatus should be kept in mind when attempting to remove a foreign body from the meatus.

➲ The bony part of the meatus is absent in the newborn, and the tympanic membrane is much nearer the surface and more oblique than in the adult.

The skin of the cartilaginous portion contains many **ceruminous glands** and hair follicles. The hairs are directed laterally and prevent the entry of small objects into the meatus. In the bony part of the canal, the skin is thin and tightly adherent to the periosteum. It has no hairs and few, if any, glands and continues as a very delicate layer over the lateral surface of the tympanic membrane.

➲ **Otitis externa** is an inflammation or infection of the outer ear canal. It is characterized by ear pain, itching, and discharge.

### Tympanic membrane

The tympanic membrane is shaped like an elliptical disc. It is stretched across the medial end of the external acoustic meatus and forms the greater part of the lateral wall of the middle ear cavity. It slopes obliquely downwards, forwards, and medially, and its lateral surface is deeply concave. The point of maximum convexity on the medial surface is called the **umbo** [Figs. 12.2, 12.3]. The tympanic membrane is made up of a taut fibrous layer with a thickened margin. The thickened membrane is inserted into the tympanic groove on a ring-like ridge of the tympanic bone at the medial end of the meatus [Fig. 12.4]. The **handle of the malleus** is attached to the medial surface of the tympanic membrane, and the lower end reaches the umbo. Close to the upper edge of the membrane, the lateral process of the malleus projects laterally, causing the membrane to bulge into the meatus.

Above the lateral process of the malleus, the ring and groove are replaced by a shallow depression—the **tympanic notch**. At the tympanic notch, the thickened edge of the tympanic membrane leaves the bone and passes to the lateral process of the malleus, forming the anterior and posterior **malleolar folds** [Fig. 12.2B]. Between these folds and the margin of the tympanic notch lies the less tense, **flaccid part** of the membrane, which differs from the rest in not having a well-defined fibrous layer.

➲ When the tympanic membrane is examined in the living, its surface appears highly polished,

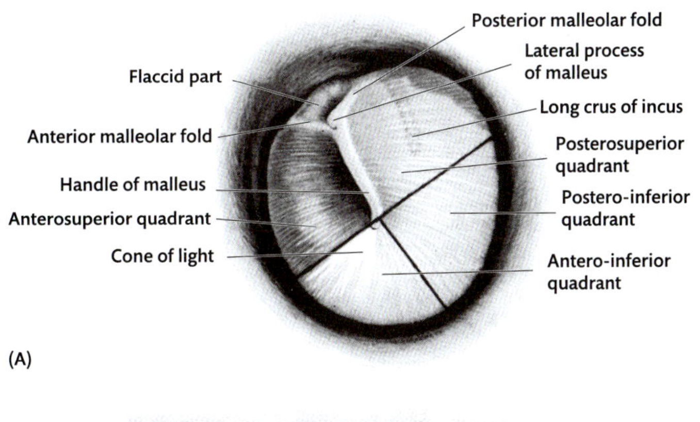


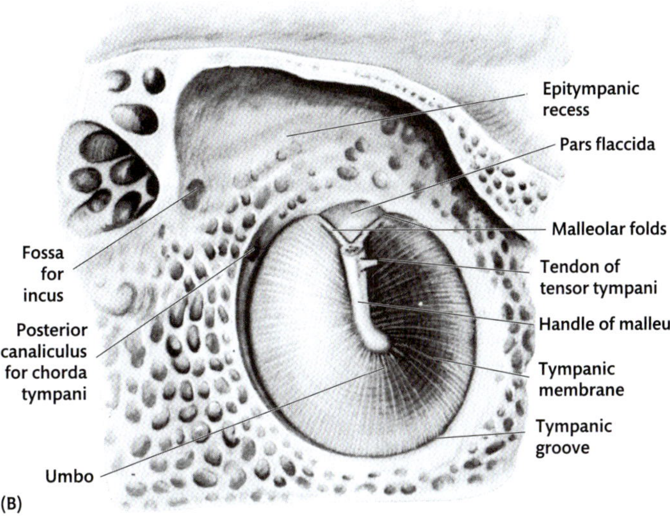


**Fig. 12.2** (A) Left tympanic membrane seen from the lateral side. The four arbitrary quadrants are indicated by solid lines and the handle of the malleus. (B) The left tympanic membrane and epitympanic recess seen from the medial side. The head and neck of the malleus have been removed.

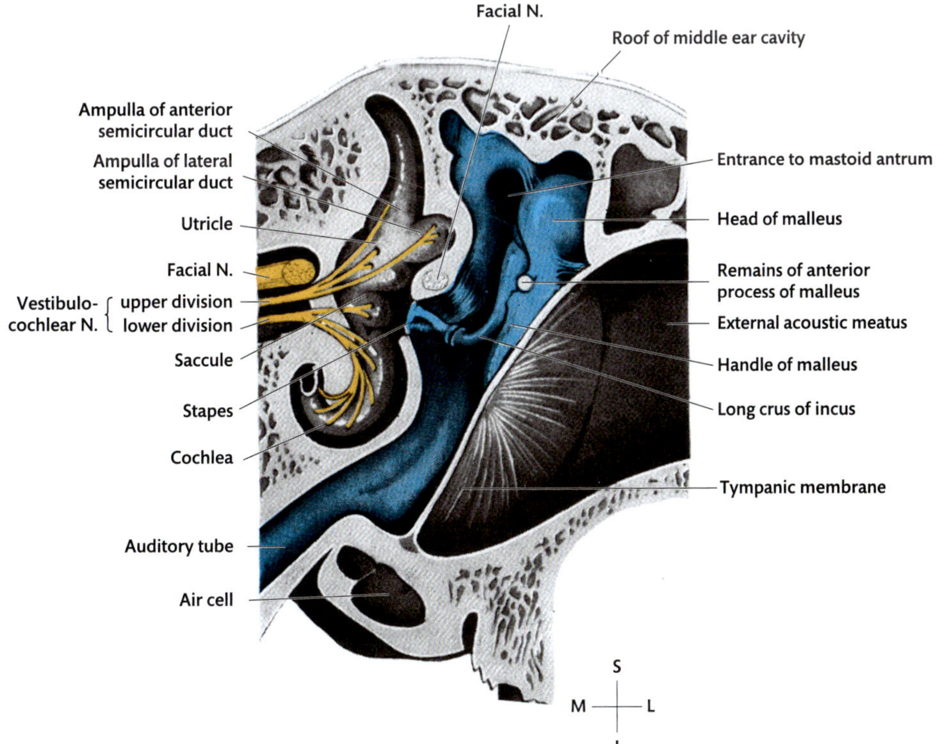


**Fig. 12.3** Coronal section through the left tympanic cavity, viewed from the front (semi-diagrammatic). L = lateral; M = medial; S = superior; I = inferior.

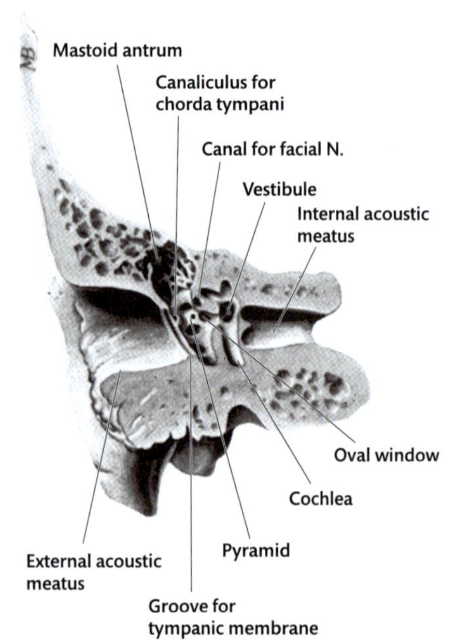


**Fig. 12.4** Coronal section through the right temporal bone, seen from in front. The posterior wall of the middle ear cavity is seen.

and a cone of reflected light extends anteroinferiorly from the tip of the handle of the malleus. The malleolar folds can be seen as two lines outlining the flaccid part, and the **long process of the incus** (the intermediate auditory ossicle) can be seen dimly through the membrane, parallel and posterior to the handle of the malleus.

➲ Perforation of the tympanic membrane can occur as a result of trauma or even spontaneously when there is infection in the middle ear cavity (otitis media). Most often, these perforations heal spontaneously. However, large perforations may require surgical repair.

➲ In some instances, it may be necessary to surgically incise the tympanic membrane, a procedure called **myringotomy**, to relieve pressure built up within the middle ear cavity. While performing a myringotomy, care should be taken to stay away from the upper third of the tympanic membrane to avoid injury to the chorda tympani nerve.

Dissection 12.2 (and Fig. 12.5) provides instructions on dissection of the middle ear cavity.

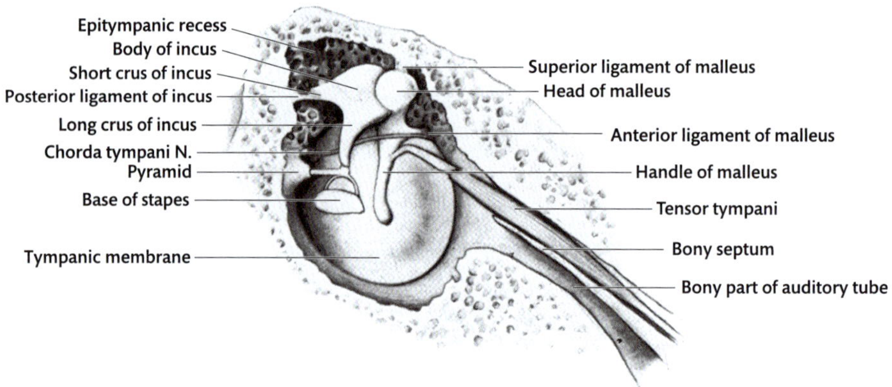


**Fig. 12.5** Left tympanic membrane and auditory ossicles, seen from the medial side. Note the auditory tube and the tensor tympani in its semicanal.

## DISSECTION 12.2 Middle ear cavity

### Objectives

**I.** To open into the middle ear cavity. **II.** To identify the parts of the ossicles seen after removing the roof. **III.** To identify the openings of the auditory tube, the aditus of the mastoid antrum, and the semicanal for the tensor tympani.

### Instructions

1. Strip the dura mater from the floor of the middle cranial fossa as far anteriorly as the mandibular nerve. The greater petrosal nerve will be found emerging from the anterior surface of the petrous temporal bone and running anteromedially, inferior to the trigeminal ganglion.
2. The cavity of the middle ear is separated from the middle cranial fossa by a thin layer of bone—the **tegmen tympani**. It lies parallel and slightly lateral to the greater petrosal nerve.
3. Force a small aperture in the tegmen tympani with the point of a rigid knife or seeker. Slip a strong probe through the aperture under the tegmen,

and lever it up. Break it away, first in an anteromedial, and then in a posterolateral, direction towards the junction of the transverse and sigmoid sinuses. Keep the probe close to the tegmen to avoid damage to the contents of the middle ear cavity.

4. Remove the broken edges of the tegmen, and expose the cavity of the middle ear. Avoid injury to the parts of the auditory ossicles which extend superiorly.
5. Attempt to pass a blunt seeker into the anteromedial part of the cavity, and slide it anteromedially till it appears through the pharyngeal opening of the auditory tube.
6. Explore the middle ear cavity.
7. The upper part of the posterior wall of the middle ear cavity has an opening—the **aditus**. This opening links the middle ear with the mastoid antrum and the mastoid air cells. Make an attempt to find the aditus [Fig. 12.3].
8. Identify the rounded head of the malleus articulating with the incus, and the short crus of the incus which passes posteriorly towards the posterior wall of the cavity [Fig. 12.5].
9. Inferior to the head of the malleus, note the sloping tympanic membrane and the handle of the malleus lying in it.
10. Identify the thin tendon which passes from the malleus to the medial wall of the middle ear. This is the tendon of the **tensor tympani** which turns nearly 90 degrees at the medial wall to become continuous with the muscle belly.
11. The tensor tympani lies in a semicanal, superomedial to the auditory tube. Break through the thin wall of this canal, and expose the muscle [Fig. 12.5].
12. Immediately superior to the attachment of the tendon to the malleus, the chorda tympani nerve [Fig. 12.3] runs across the medial surface of the tympanic membrane and the malleus, forming a narrow ridge. Identify it.
13. Look for the long crus of the incus which passes inferiorly to the stapes, which is not visible at this stage.



## Middle ear

### Introduction to middle ear cavity

The narrow middle ear cavity, together with the tympanic membrane, is known as the tympanum. It is lined with mucous membrane and is filled with air. It communicates anteriorly with the nasopharynx through the auditory tube [Fig. 12.6], and posteriorly through the mastoid antrum [Fig. 12.7] with the mastoid air cells—small air-filled cavities in the mastoid process.

**Dimensions**: the vertical and anteroposterior diameters of the middle ear cavity are each approximately 15 mm; the width varies from 6 mm above to 4 mm below, and is even less in the middle where the medial and lateral walls bulge into the cavity [Fig. 12.3]. The part of the cavity superior to the tympanic membrane is called the **epitympanic recess** [Figs. 12.1, 12.2B, 12.5].

### Boundaries of the middle ear cavity

The middle ear cavity has a roof, floor, and posterior, anterior, medial, and lateral walls. The **roof** or **tegmental wall** of the tympanic cavity is the thin bone **tegmen tympani** which separates the cavity from the middle cranial fossa [Fig. 12.3]. The **floor** or **jugular wall** is narrow. It is formed by a thin plate of bone which separates the cavity from the jugular fossa which contains the superior bulb of the jugular vein. ➲ Chronic inflammation of the middle ear may spread through the tegmen to the meninges of the brain, or through the floor to the jugular vein, and lead to thrombosis (clotting) of the blood in the vein and spread of infection through the bloodstream.

The **posterior** or **mastoid wall** [Figs. 12.4, 12.7] has a series of openings in it: (1) above is the opening, or **aditus**, which leads from the epitympanic recess into the mastoid antrum; (2) inferiorly, close to the medial wall, is a small conical projection called the **pyramid** [Fig. 12.4] with an opening on the apex. The pyramid contains the **stapedius muscle**, and the stapedius tendon exits through the opening on the apex to reach the stapes; (3) lateral to the pyramid, there is an opening through which the **chorda tympani branch** of the facial nerve enters the middle ear [Fig. 12.4].

The **anterior** or **carotid wall** is narrow, because the medial and lateral walls converge anteriorly. Three features are present on the anterior wall: (1) superiorly, the opening of the semicanal for the tensor tympani; (2) the orifice of the auditory tube

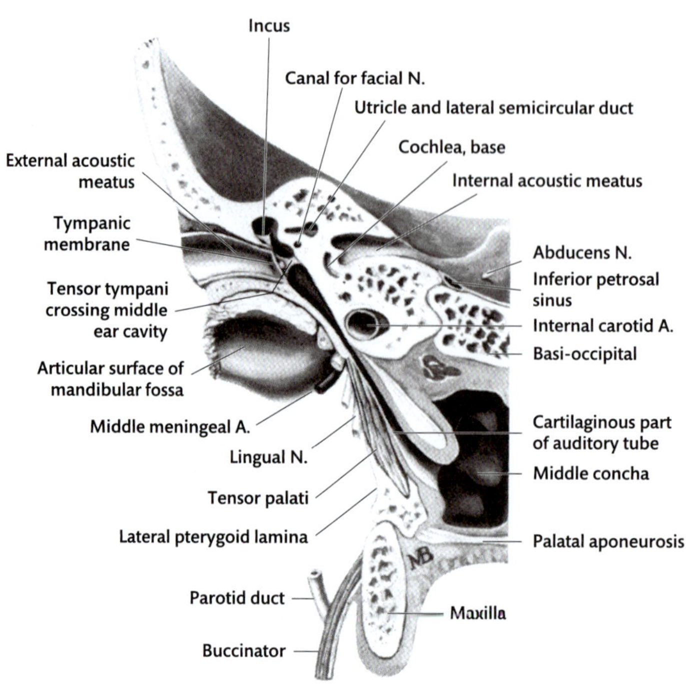


Fig. 12.6 An oblique coronal section passing downwards and forwards along the line of the auditory tube, viewed from behind. The mandible and muscles of mastication have been removed, leaving the branches of the mandibular nerve on the lateral aspect of the tensor palati.

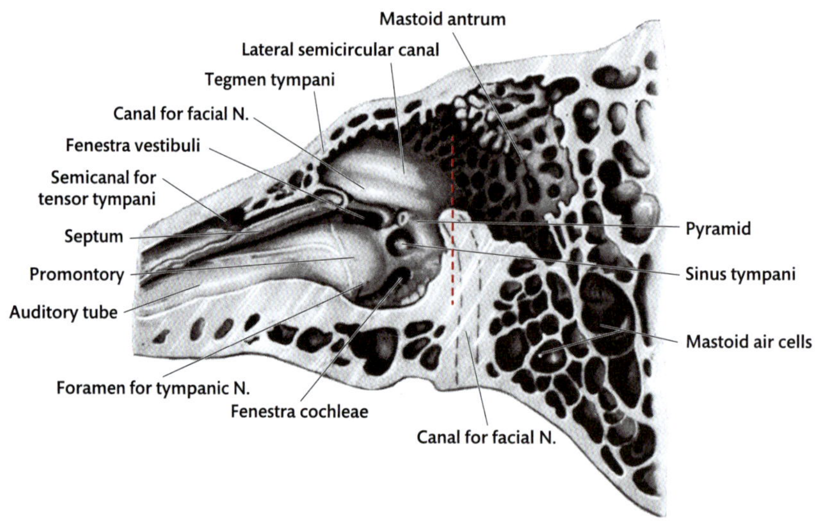


Fig. 12.7 Vertical section through the left middle ear cavity and auditory tube to show the medial wall of the middle ear cavity. The auditory ossicles have been removed. The position of the posterior wall of the middle ear cavity is shown by the red line.

in an intermediate position [Fig. 12.5]; and (3) inferiorly, a plate of bone which separates the middle ear cavity from the carotid canal [Fig. 12.6]. The semicanals for the tensor tympani and the auditory tube are separated by a bony septum. This septum is continued posteriorly on the medial wall of the middle ear as a shelf-like projection—the **processus cochleariformis**. The posterior end of this projection forms a pulley, around which the tendon of the tensor tympani turns laterally to run to the malleus [Fig. 12.5].

The **medial** or **labyrinthine wall** separates the middle ear from the internal ear. It is almost entirely bony [Fig. 12.7]. The cochlea of the internal ear forms a bulge—the **promontory**—on the medial wall. Two small apertures are seen in relation to the promontory: (1) the **fenestra vestibuli**, or oval window, lies above the promontory and is filled by the base of the stapes [Fig. 12.3]; and (2) the **fenestra cochleae**, or round window, lies below the promontory and is closed by the delicate **secondary tympanic membrane**. These two apertures lead into the cavity of the bony labyrinth. The **sinus tympani** is a depression between and behind the two windows. The facial nerve and the lateral semicircular canal, enclosed in the bone, produce parallel ridges on the superior aspect of the medial wall. These bony ridges extend posteriorly into the aditus and the mastoid antrum [Fig. 12.7].

The **lateral wall** of the middle ear cavity is formed by the tympanic membrane.

## Mucous membrane of the middle ear cavity

The thin delicate lining of the walls of the tympanic cavity also covers the auditory ossicles and is continuous with the lining of the auditory tube, mastoid antrum, and mastoid air cells. The tendon of the stapedius and tensor tympani muscles, and the chorda tympani and tympanic plexus of nerves are all covered by the mucous membrane.

➲ Blocked auditory tube: the auditory tube forms a route through which infections can pass from the nasopharynx to the middle ear cavity. It is readily blocked by infections, because the walls of its cartilaginous part lie in apposition. When the auditory tube is blocked, the residual air in the middle ear is absorbed into the blood vessels, causing a fall in pressure inside the middle ear cavity. When the block is associated with infection of the middle ear, there is an outpouring of fluid from the damaged mucous membrane, with an increase in pressure within the cavity. When the pressure in the middle ear cavity is either raised or lowered, free movement of the tympanic membrane is impeded and hearing is affected. With raised pressure, the normally concave tympanic membrane bulges into the external acoustic meatus—a feature readily confirmed with an otoscope.

## Auditory ossicles

These three small bones form a bony chain which extends from the tympanic membrane on the lateral wall of the middle ear cavity to the oval window on the medial wall. The malleus is attached to the tympanic membrane, the stapes to the oval window, and the incus is slung between the two [Fig. 12.5].

### Malleus

The **head of the malleus** is the rounded upper part of the bone which lies in the epitympanic recess. The slender **manubrium**, or handle, is attached to the tympanic membrane. The **lateral process** projects onto the tympanic membrane and the **anterior process** projects anteriorly.

### Incus

The **body of the incus** lies in the epitympanic recess and articulates with the head of the malleus. It has a **long crus** which projects inferiorly and articulates with the head of the stapes, and a **short crus** which extends posteriorly and is attached to the wall of the epitympanic recess by a ligament.

### Stapes

The stapes is shaped like a stirrup. It has a head which articulates with the long crus of the incus, and an oval foot piece, or **base**, which is attached to the oval window (fenestra vestibuli) by an elastic **annular ligament**.

### Movements of the ear ossicles

Movement of the ear ossicles is responsible for transmitting sound waves across the middle ear cavity. Vibration of the tympanic membrane and the handle of the malleus produce movement of the head of the malleus which imparts a rotatory movement to the body of the incus, which, in turn, is transmitted to the stapes through the long crus of the incus. Movement of the stapes is transmitted to the perilymph in the bony labyrinth through the oval window.

Tympanic membrane > handle of malleus > head of malleus > body of incus > long crus of incus > head of stapes > foot plate of stapes > oval window.

## Tympanic muscles

There are two muscles in the tympanic cavity—the stapedius and the tensor tympani.

### Stapedius

The **stapedius** lies in the pyramid and the canal which curves inferiorly from it on the posterior wall of the tympanic cavity. Its tendon enters the middle ear through an opening on the apex of the pyramid. It is inserted into the posterior surface of the neck of the stapes [Fig. 12.5]. **Nerve supply**: the facial nerve. **Action**: it prevents excessive movements of the stapes. ➲ Paralysis of the stapedius leads to uninhibited movement of the stapes and increased sensitivity to sounds (hyperacusis).

### Tensor tympani

The tensor tympani takes origin from the superior surface of the cartilaginous part of the auditory tube and the adjacent parts of the greater wing of the sphenoid and petrous temporal bone [see Fig. 2.11]. It passes posterolaterally in the semicanal, superior to the bony part of the auditory tube. In the middle ear cavity, it turns laterally through 90 degrees on the processus cochleariformis and is inserted on the superior part of the handle of the malleus [Fig. 12.5]. **Nerve supply**: the mandibular nerve, through fibres which traverse the otic ganglion. **Actions**: it tenses the tympanic membrane, increases its medial convexity, and restricts its movement. It prevents wide excursions of the ear ossicles and damage to the inner ear from loud sounds.

## Chorda tympani nerve

The chorda tympani branch of the facial nerve arises in the temporal bone, a short distance above the stylomastoid foramen [Fig. 12.8]. It ascends in a bony canaliculus to the posterior wall of the middle ear cavity and enters the cavity through the posterior wall. In the tympanic cavity, the chorda tympani runs forwards across the medial surface of the upper part of the tympanic membrane and the neck of the malleus [Fig. 12.5]. It leaves the middle ear through the petrotympanic fissure [see Fig. 14.7] and joins the lingual nerve a short distance below the skull [Fig. 12.8].

The chorda tympani carries taste fibres from the anterior two-thirds of the tongue, and preganglionic parasympathetic fibres to the submandibular ganglion. The parasympathetic fibres innervate the submandibular and sublingual salivary glands and the glands in the anterior two-thirds of the tongue.

➲ Otitis media is inflammation within the middle ear cavity. It could be the result of an acute infection and could resolve spontaneously or with antibiotics. It presents with fever and severe earache, often leading to rupture of the tympanic membrane and ear discharge. Acute otitis media is common in children and is often due to a spread of infection from the pharynx

Chronic otitis media refers to long-term damage of the middle ear mucosa due to repeated infection and inflammation. It is invariably associated with a perforated tympanic membrane, repeated episodes of ear discharge, and conductive hearing loss.

➲ An invasive, non-cancerous epithelial growth can occur within the middle ear—**cholesteatoma**—and cause extensive bone damage.

## Mastoid antrum and mastoid air cells

The mastoid antrum is an air-filled extension from the middle ear cavity. It lies posterior to the

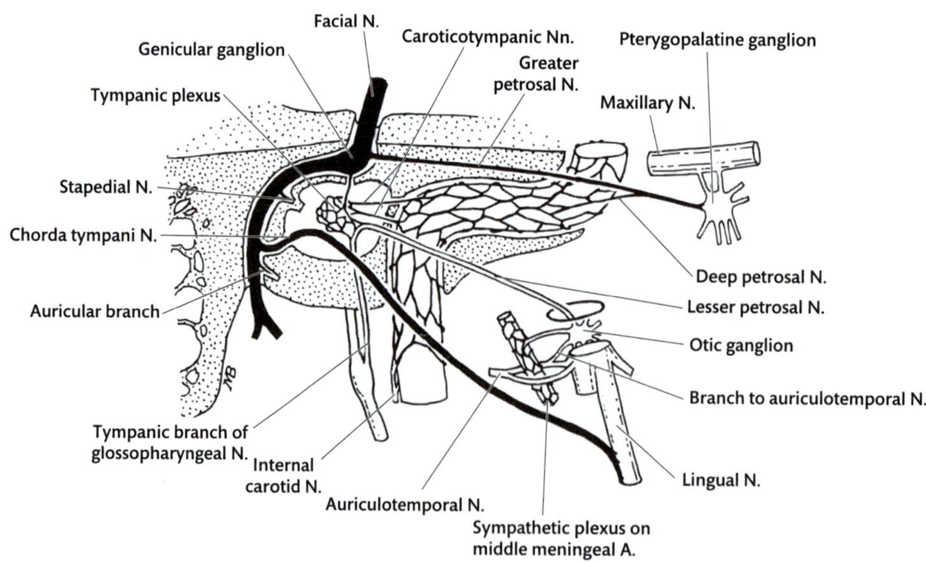


**Fig. 12.8** The intrapetrous course of the facial nerve and its branches.

epitympanic recess and communicates with it through an opening—the **aditus ad antrum**—on the posterior wall of the middle ear [Fig. 12.7]. Mastoid air cells are numerous small cavities lined with mucous membrane, located in the petromastoid part of the temporal bone. They are interconnected and open into the posterior wall of the mastoid antrum. In the adult, the mastoid antrum is 1.5 cm medial to the **suprameatal triangle** (the small triangular area on the surface of the skull, immediately posterosuperior to the bony external acoustic meatus). In the child, the mastoid antrum is more superficial.

The walls of the antrum are formed by parts of the temporal bone. The tegmen tympani forms the **roof**. The **floor** and **posterior wall** are formed by the mastoid process and have the openings of the mastoid air cells in them. The sigmoid venous sinus lies close to the posterior wall and may be separated from it only by a thin plate of bone [Figs. 12.9, 12.10, 12.11]. The jugular bulb may have the same close relation to the floor. ➲ Infections of the antrum may involve both the sigmoid sinus and the internal jugular vein in septic thrombosis, and may spread along their tributaries to form an abscess in the adjacent part (cerebellum) of the brain. The **medial wall** of the antrum is the petrous temporal bone. The bony ridge produced by the lateral semicircular canal in the medial wall of the tympanic cavity extends posteriorly into the medial wall of the mastoid antrum [Fig. 12.9].

The ridge produced on the medial wall of the middle ear cavity by the **facial nerve** in its bony canal does not reach the antrum but turns inferiorly (at the aditus) into the bone which separates the middle ear cavity from the mastoid air cells and the inferior part of the antrum [Fig. 12.9]. The facial nerve descends vertically in this bone to emerge at the stylomastoid foramen [Fig. 12.7].

## Auditory tube

The auditory, or pharyngotympanic, tube consists of bony and cartilaginous parts. The cartilaginous part is approximately 2.5 cm long and is described with the pharynx.

The **bony part** is approximately 1.5 cm long. It is widest at its junction with the middle ear cavity, and narrowest where it joins the cartilaginous part, posteromedial to the spine of the sphenoid. The bony part lies between the petrous and tympanic parts of the temporal bone, below the semicanal for the tensor tympani, lateral to the internal carotid artery in the carotid canal [Figs. 12.1, 12.5, 12.6, 12.7, 12.10, 12.11].

Using the instructions given in Dissection 12.3, dissect the mastoid antrum, mastoid air cells, and middle ear cavity.



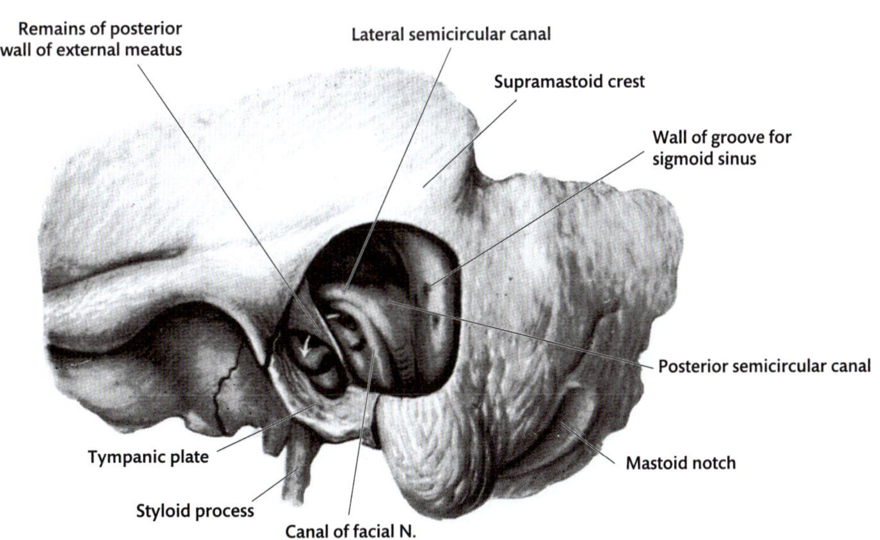


**Fig. 12.9** Dissection of the mastoid antrum and petromastoid part of the temporal bone from the lateral side. The arrow passes from the mastoid antrum into the tympanic cavity through the aditus.

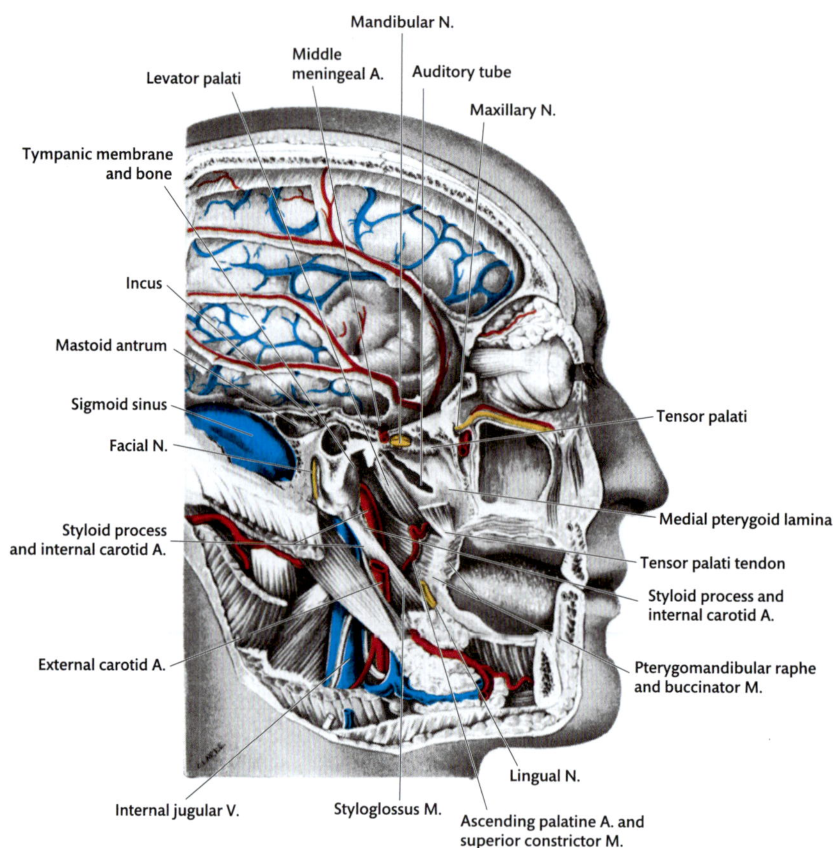


**Fig. 12.10** Dissection of the auditory tube and mastoid antrum from the lateral side. Note the continuity of the mastoid antrum, middle ear cavity, and auditory tube.

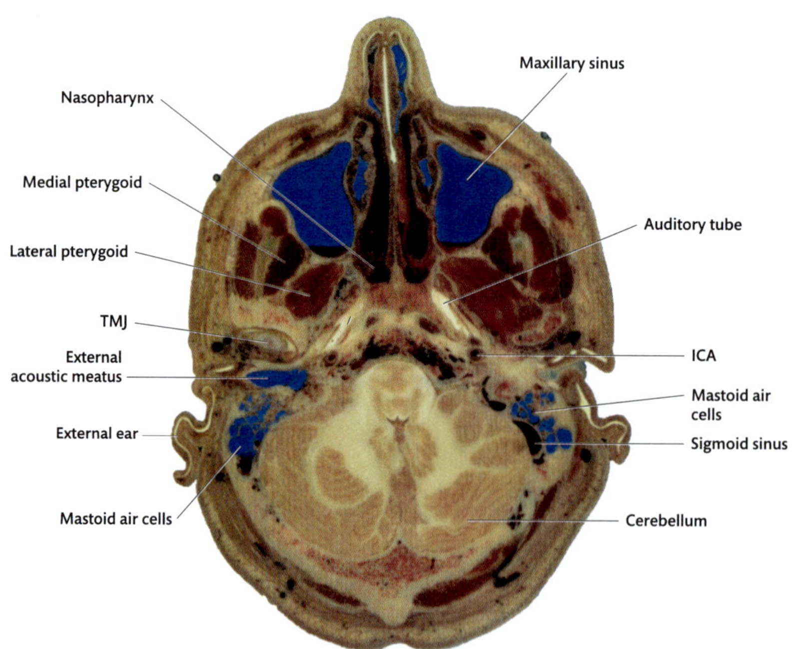


**Fig. 12.11** Transverse section of the head at the level of the external acoustic meatus. ICA = internal carotid artery; TMJ = temporomandibular joint.

Image courtesy of the Visible Human Project of the US National Library of Medicine.

**DISSECTION 12.3 Mastoid antrum, mastoid air cells, and middle ear cavity**

**Objectives**

**I.** To open the mastoid antrum and mastoid air cells.
**II.** To remove the tympanic membrane and study the middle ear cavity from the lateral aspect.

**Instructions**

1. Remove all the soft parts, including the periosteum, from the lateral surface of the mastoid temporal bone, and identify the suprameatal triangle and the supramastoid crest. With a fine chisel, remove the cortical bone from the suprameatal triangle. Extend the bone removal anteromedially, parallel to the posterior wall of the external acoustic meatus, until the mastoid antrum is opened.
2. Remove the spongy bone from the mastoid area until the compact bone, posterior and medial to it, is exposed. This process exposes the **mastoid air cells** and mastoid antrum. The extent of the mastoid air cells and antrum is variable.
3. Identify the structures which cause projections on the bony walls of the aditus and antrum, particularly the canal for the facial nerve, the sigmoid sinus, and the ridge produced by the lateral semicircular canal [Fig. 12.9].
4. Cut away the posterior and superior walls of the external acoustic meatus up to the level of the roof of the mastoid antrum.
5. Remove the tympanic membrane. Try to identify the chorda tympani nerve at its posterosuperior margin and the handle of the malleus.
6. Examine the long crus of the incus, the position of the stapes, and the stapedius tendon.
7. Review the medial wall of the middle ear cavity [Figs. 12.3, 12.7].

## Intrapetrous parts of the facial and vestibulocochlear nerves

The **facial** and **vestibulocochlear nerves** have already been traced to the internal acoustic meatus [Chapter 7]. These nerves should now be followed into the petrous temporal bone. The vestibulocochlear nerve ends in the internal ear. The facial nerve follows an angulated course through the petrous bone to emerge at the stylomastoid foramen on the inferior surface of the temporal bone.

Dissection 12.4 provides instructions on dissecting the intrapetrous part of the facial nerve.

**DISSECTION 12.4 Facial nerve**

**Objective**

**I.** To expose the intrapetrous part of the facial nerve.

**Instructions**

1. Identify the **arcuate eminence** on the anterior surface of the petrous temporal bone (in the middle cranial fossa). It marks the position of the **anterior semicircular canal**.
2. On the posterior surface of the petrous temporal bone (posterior cranial fossa), identify the internal acoustic meatus and the nerves entering it.
3. Place a chisel horizontally across the upper part of the internal acoustic meatus and, with a sharp tap from a hammer, attempt to break off the superior part of the petrous temporal bone. Frequently, the bone breaks along the canal for the facial nerve, through parts of the anterior and lateral semicircular canals, and removes the roof of the internal acoustic meatus.
4. Chip away any extra pieces of bone to expose the facial nerve as far as the aditus.
5. Note the sharp bend—the **genu**—of the facial nerve and the swelling on it at the point of the bend—the **genicular ganglion**.
6. Identify the greater petrosal nerve which arises from the genicular ganglion.
7. Trace the facial nerve, as it turns posteriorly into the medial wall of the middle ear cavity. Follow it posteriorly above the fenestra vestibuli, till it turns inferiorly in the medial wall of the aditus.

8. Turn to the inferior surface of the skull, and identify the facial nerve as it emerges at the stylomastoid foramen.
9. Place the edge of a chisel across the lateral margin of the foramen, and attempt to split the bone along the line of the vertical part of the facial nerve with a sharp tap. If it splits satisfactorily, the posterior canaliculus for the chorda tympani and the entire length of the canal for the facial nerve will be exposed. If not, complete the exposure with bone forceps.
10. Note the position of the vertical part of the facial nerve in relation to the middle ear cavity, mastoid air cells, and antrum.
11. Finally, break away one wall of the pyramid and expose the stapedius.

## Facial nerve

The **facial nerve** runs laterally through the internal acoustic meatus, anterosuperior to the vestibulocochlear nerve. Here it is joined by the **nervus intermedius**. At the lateral end of the meatus, it enters the facial canal in the bone and continues laterally for a short distance to the **genicular ganglion** [Figs. 12.8, 12.12]. At the genicular ganglion, the facial nerve gives off the **greater petrosal nerve** [Fig. 12.8] and turns abruptly backwards to run posteriorly in the medial wall of the middle ear, immediately superior to the oval window and the pyramid. It turns inferolaterally below the aditus to descend through the bone between the middle ear cavity anteriorly and the mastoid antrum and air cells posteriorly. In the vertical part of its course, the facial nerve gives off: (1) the nerve to the stapedius; (2) the chorda tympani; and (3) small branches to the auricular branch of the vagus [Figs. 12.7, 12.8, 12.9].

## Vestibulocochlear nerve

The **vestibulocochlear nerve** is posteroinferior to the facial nerve in the internal acoustic meatus. At the lateral end of the meatus, it splits into the **cochlear** and **vestibular nerves**. Each of these nerves divides into a number of small branches which pass through foramina in the lateral part of the meatus, to supply the membranous labyrinth of the internal ear [Figs. 12.3, 12.12].

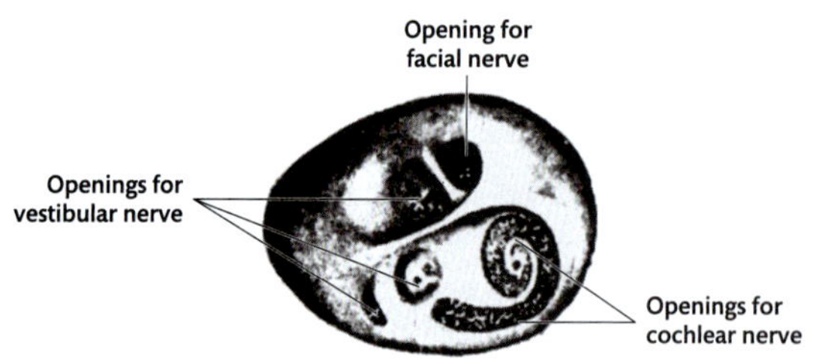


**Fig. 12.12** Lateral end of the left internal acoustic meatus showing the openings in the bone for passage of facial, vestibular, and cochlear nerves.

# The internal ear

The internal ear consists of a series of communicating bony spaces (the **bony labyrinth**) in the petrous temporal bone [Fig. 12.13], and a series of smaller membranous tubes and sacs—the **membranous labyrinth**—within the bony labyrinth [Fig. 12.14]. The membranous labyrinth is filled

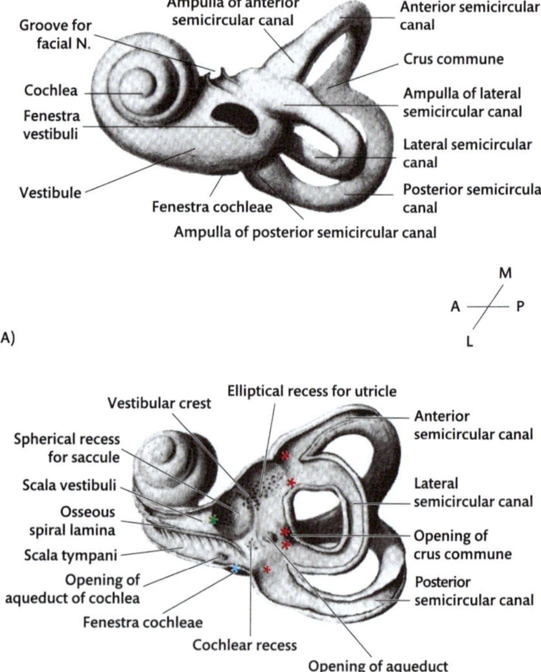


**Fig. 12.13** Left bony labyrinth, viewed from the lateral side. (A) External surface. (B) Inner aspect. Red asterisks = opening of the semicircular canals into the vestibule. Green asterisk = opening of the scala vestibuli into the vestibule. Blue asterisk = opening of the scala tympani into the round window.

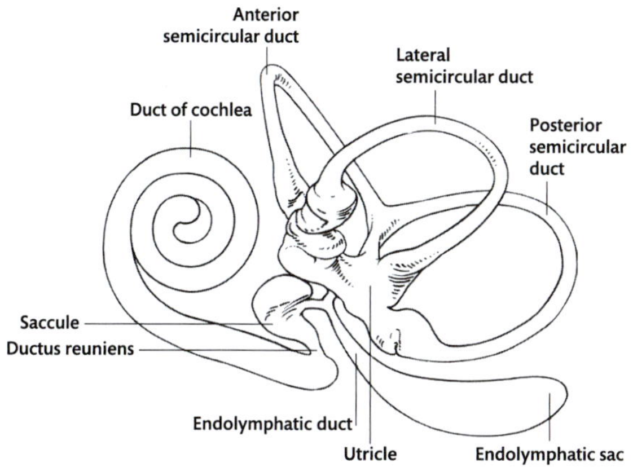


**Fig. 12.14** Diagrammatic representation of the right membranous labyrinth.

with a clear fluid—the **endolymph**. It is separated from the walls of the bony labyrinth by a space which contains a similar fluid—the **perilymph**—and some delicate connective tissue. The cochlear portion of the inner ear is concerned with hearing. The vestibular portion is concerned with maintaining equilibrium. It records the direction of gravity acting on the head, and rotational movements of the head.

Using the instructions given in Dissection 12.5 (and Fig. 12.13), expose the bony and membranous labyrinths.

## Bony labyrinth

The bony labyrinth is divided into three parts: (1) a small chamber called the **vestibule**; (2) a coiled tube—the **cochlea**—anterior to the vestibule; and (3) three **semicircular canals**, superior and posterior to the vestibule [Fig. 12.13A]. The vestibule, cochlea, and semicircular canals communicate freely with each other and are lined by a delicate endosteum [Fig. 12.13B].

### Vestibule

The vestibule is a small, ovoid bony chamber about 5 mm long, placed between the lateral end of the internal acoustic meatus and the medial wall of the middle ear. The three semicircular canals open into its superior and posterior aspects through five openings [Fig. 12.13B, red asterisks]. Two tubes within the cochlea—the **scala vestibuli** and **scala tympani**—open into the anterior aspect of the vestibule [Fig. 12.13B, green and blue asterisks]. The **oval window**, or **fenestra vestibuli**, lies on the lateral wall of the vestibule and is closed by the base of the stapes. The round window, or fenestra cochleae, lies on the inferior aspect of the vestibule and is closed by the secondary tympanic membrane [Figs. 12.13A, 12.13B]. In the posterior part of the medial wall of the vestibule is the mouth of a small canal—the **aqueduct of the vestibule**—which





### DISSECTION 12.5 Internal ear

#### Objective

**I.** To expose the bony and membranous labyrinths.

#### Instructions

1. Free the facial nerve from its canal as far as the aditus, but retain its continuity with the greater petrosal nerve.
2. Using the chisel and hammer, cut more bone from the superior surface of the petrous temporal bone, till the level of the middle of the internal acoustic meatus is reached. (The bone should be cracked by sharp taps from a hammer, so as to avoid driving the chisel into the middle ear cavity and the ear ossicles.) As each flake of bone is removed, examine the holes in the bone produced by the semicircular canals, and try to see the semicircular ducts of the membranous labyrinth lying free within them.
3. Note also the branches of the vestibulocochlear nerve entering the bone at the lateral end of the meatus.
4. Identify the vestibule and cochlea [Fig. 12.13]. The vestibule is the cavity lying immediately lateral to the internal acoustic meatus, between it and the medial wall of the middle ear. The cochlea lies anterolateral to the lateral end of the meatus.
5. The main features of the bony labyrinth are now exposed. It is desirable at each stage to establish the continuity of its various parts by passing a fine wire through each foramen that is exposed.
6. If time permits, a better dissection may be obtained by decalcifying an intact temporal bone in dilute acid for several weeks, and then dissecting it carefully with a sharp knife.

passes to the posterior surface of the petrous temporal bone and opens between the bone and the dura mater [Figs. 12.13A, 12.13B, 12.4].

### Semicircular canals

The three semicircular canals—anterior, posterior, and lateral—open into the vestibule. Each of the three canals forms more than half a circle and has a swelling—the **ampulla**—at one end. The canals are oriented such that each canal forms one of three adjacent sides of an obliquely set cube. The anterior and posterior canals lie in approximately vertical planes, and their adjoining ends meet in a common limb—the **crus commune** [Fig. 12.13B]. The crus commune opens into the vestibule (note that the presence of the common limb means that there are five—not six—points of communication between the semicircular canals and the vestibule). The **ampullae** of the anterior and lateral semicircular canals lie at the anterior ends.

The **anterior canal** is at right angles to the long axis of the petrous temporal bone and produces the **arcuate eminence** on the anterior surface of that bone. The **posterior canal** is posteroinferior to the anterior canal and lies almost parallel to the posterior surface of the petrous temporal bone (deep to the slit for the aqueduct of the vestibule). The **lateral canal** is nearly horizontal. Its most lateral part produces a bulge in the medial wall of the tympanic cavity, the aditus, and the mastoid antrum.

The semicircular canals of one ear are mirror images of those in the other ear. The two lateral canals lie in the same plane, and the anterior canal of one side is parallel to the posterior canal of the other.

### Cochlea

The cochlea is shaped like a tube coiled around a central pillar—the **modiolus**. The modiolus points anterolaterally. The cochlea has two-and-a-half turns and rapidly diminishes in diameter towards its apex. It has the appearance of a spiral lying on its side [Figs. 12.13A, 12.13B]. It lies anterior to the vestibule, with its base directed towards the lateral end of the internal acoustic meatus. The large first turn produces the bulge of the **promontory** on the medial wall of the middle ear cavity [Figs. 12.7, 12.13A].

The **modiolus** is thick at its base where it abuts on the internal meatus, but rapidly tapers towards the apex, forming the internal wall of the cochlear tube. Winding spirally round the modiolus, like the thread of a screw, is a thin, narrow plate of bone—the **spiral lamina**—which partially divides the cochlear tube into two canals—the **scala vestibuli** and the **scala tympani** [Fig. 12.13B]. The **spiral canal** runs in the base of the spiral lamina and lodges the sensory **spiral ganglion** of the cochlea.

The scala vestibuli and scala tympani run parallel to each other on either side of the cochlear duct (a part of the membranous labyrinth), and are continuous with each other at the apex of the cochlea around the blind end of the cochlear duct—the **helicotrema**. At the base of the cochlea, the scala vestibuli is continuous with the vestibule and the scala tympani ends on the round window (fenestra cochleae) [Fig. 12.13B, blue asterisk]. Pressure waves generated in the scala vestibuli, by movements of the stapes, are transferred through the scala vestibuli and the scala tympani. The scala tympani is also continuous with the **aqueduct of the cochlea**, which passes through a canal in the bone—the **cochlear canaliculus** [Fig. 12.13B].

## Membranous labyrinth

The membranous labyrinth consists of: (1) the duct of the cochlea which lies in the bony cochlea; (2) the utricle and saccule—two small membranous sacs which lie in the vestibule; and (3) three membranous tubes—the semicircular ducts—which lie in the semicircular canals [Figs. 12.3, 12.14]. The saccule and utricle are joined to each other by a narrow tube through the root of the **endolymphatic duct**. The saccule is continuous with the base of the cochlear duct through the **ductus reuniens**. The utricle has the membranous semicircular ducts opening into it.

### Cochlear duct

The **cochlear duct** lies in the cochlear part of the bony labyrinth between the scala vestibuli and the scala tympani. It contains the sensory organ—the **organ of Corti**—which respond to pressure changes in the scala vestibuli. **Function**: the cochlear duct is innervated by the cochlear division of the vestibulocochlear nerve and functions as the organ of hearing.

### Semicircular ducts

The **semicircular ducts** lie in the semicircular canals of the bony labyrinth. They are considerably narrower than the canals and are situated against the peripheral bony walls of the canals. They open into the utricle and have ampullae in the same position as the ampullae of the canals. The **ampullae** of the ducts contain specialized folds of lining epithelium—the **crista ampullaris**. The crista is surmounted by hair cells embedded in a gelatinous **cupula** and is the sensory organ of the duct. **Function**: the crista ampullaris are innervated by the vestibular part of the vestibulocochlear nerve. They record movements which result from rotation of the head in the plane of the duct. The ampullae are so arranged that, in any parallel pair of semicircular ducts, rotation of the head causes the endolymph to flow in the same direction. It moves towards the ampulla in one canal, and away from the ampulla in the other opposite canal.

### Utricle and saccule

The **utricle** occupies a depression in the superior wall of the vestibule, and the smaller **saccule** lies anteroinferior to it [Fig. 12.13B]. The endolymphatic duct unites the utricle and saccule, and passes through the aqueduct of the vestibule to end as a dilated **endolymphatic sac**, external to the dura mater. The utricle and saccule each have an area of thickened epithelium in their walls known as the **macula**. The macula has hair cells on which are a number of concretions of calcium salts—the **statoconia**. The macula of the utricle lies in a horizontal plane, and that of the saccule lies in a vertical plane. **Function**: the maculae of the utricle and saccule are innervated by the vestibular part of the vestibulocochlear nerve and record the direction of the gravitational field relative to the head.

See Clinical Applications 12.1 and 12.2 for the practical implications of the anatomy discussed in this chapter.





**CLINICAL APPLICATION 12.1 Mastoiditis**

Mastoiditis is inflammation of the mucosa lining the mastoid antrum and air cells. The mucosa of the middle ear is continuous with the mucosa of the mastoid antrum, and infections can spread from one cavity to the other. Surgery for chronic otitis media with mastoiditis aims to remove diseased tissue and repair the tympanic membrane to restore hearing. The common approach to the mastoid antrum is through its lateral wall—the suprameatal triangle.

Study question 1: discuss the important relations of the mastoid antrum. (Answer: the vertical course of the facial nerve lies along the anterior wall of the mastoid antrum. The cranial cavity lies just above the roof. The sigmoid venous sinus lies posterior to the antrum at a variable distance, depending on the pneumatization of the mastoid process.)

**CLINICAL APPLICATION 12.2 Facial nerve lesions**

Clinically, it is possible to differentiate injuries to the facial nerve at different sites along its course. (1) When the facial nerve is affected at, or distal to, the stylomastoid foramen, the patient will show only signs of paralysis of the facial muscles on that side. (2) When the facial nerve is affected in the brain, in the internal acoustic meatus, or at the level of the genicular ganglion, in addition to paralysis of the facial muscles, the patient will also have loss of taste on the anterior two-thirds of the corresponding half of the tongue (due to destruction of fibres in the chorda tympani) and hyperacusis (due to destruction of the nerve to the stapedius). Secretions of the submandibular and sublingual glands and lacrimal, nasal, palatine, and oral glands will be diminished (due to damage to the secretomotor fibres in the greater petrosal and chorda tympani nerves). An injury in the internal acoustic meatus is also likely to involve the vestibulocochlear nerve.

# CHAPTER 13
# The parotid region

## Parotid gland

The parotid gland lies below the external acoustic meatus, between the mandible in front and the sternocleidomastoid behind. It is the largest salivary gland and produces serous secretions. It has a very irregular shape because during development, it does not grow within a well-defined capsule, as does the submandibular gland, but invades the fascia of this region. It becomes disseminated through the fascia and encloses the structures which traverse the fascia.

### Shape and position of the parotid gland

The parotid gland is shaped like an inverted pyramid, with the base directed superiorly and the apex directed inferiorly. It has lateral or superficial, anteromedial, and posterolateral surfaces [Figs. 13.1, 13.2, 13.3, 13.4].

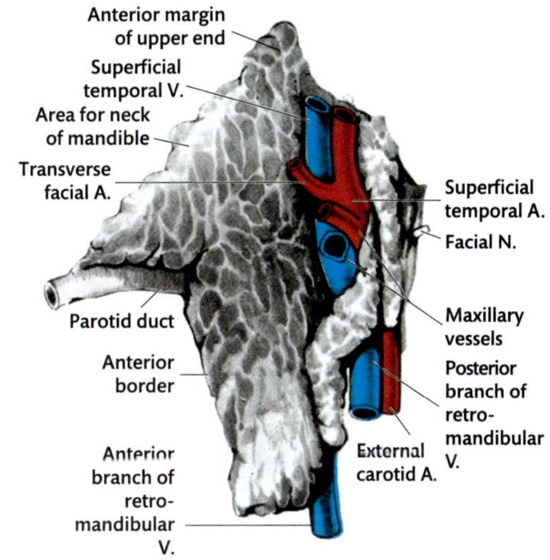


**Fig. 13.2** Parotid gland, anteromedial surface.

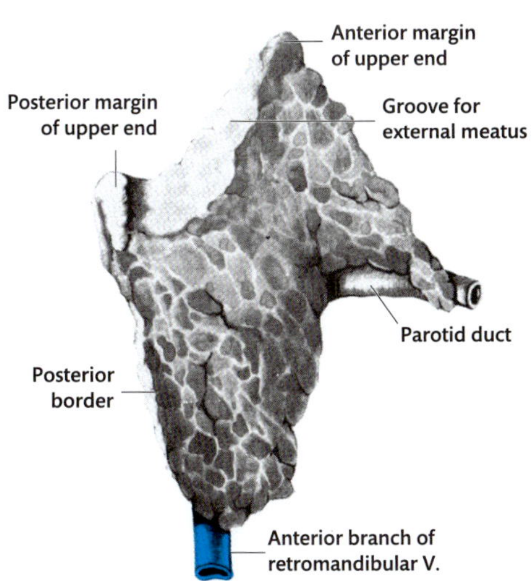


**Fig. 13.1** Parotid gland, lateral surface.

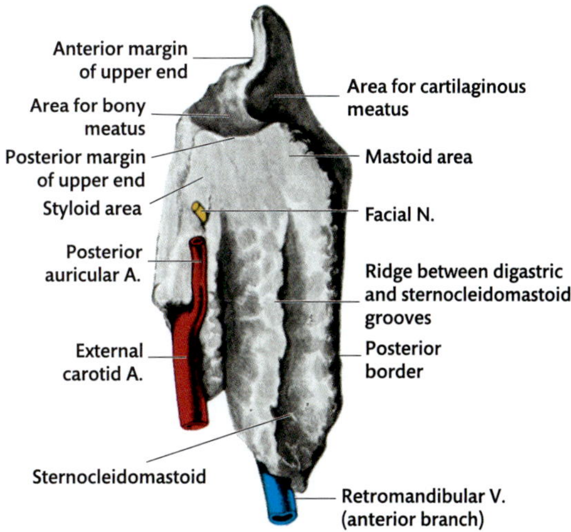


**Fig. 13.3** Parotid gland, posteromedial surface.

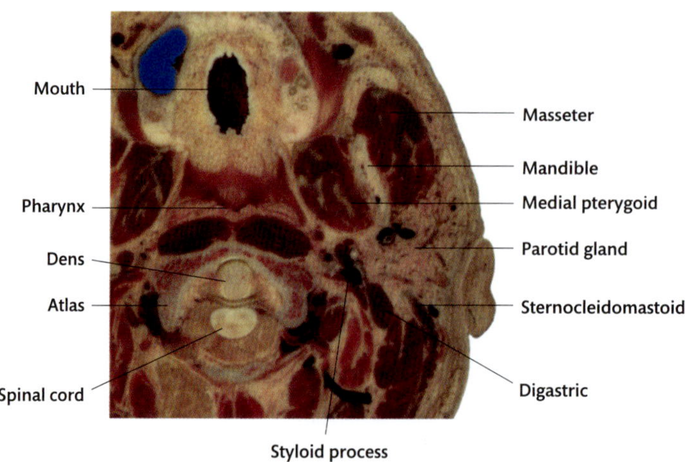


**Fig. 13.4** Horizontal section through the head, showing the parotid gland.

Image courtesy of the Visible Human Project of the US National Library of Medicine.





The **upper end** of the parotid gland is grooved by the external acoustic meatus and is wedged between it and the back of the temporomandibular joint. The auriculotemporal nerve and the superficial temporal vessels pierce the gland just behind the joint [see Fig. 3.6].

The **lower end** of the gland, or **apex** of the gland, lies between the sternocleidomastoid and the angle of the mandible, on the posterior belly of the digastric [see Fig. 5.5]. It extends into the carotid triangle. It is pierced by the cervical branch of the facial nerve and the two branches of the retromandibular vein. It is separated from the submandibular gland by the stylomandibular ligament. Note the close proximity of the parotid and submandibular glands in Fig. 5.1.

The **lateral** or **superficial surface** of the gland is covered by skin, superficial fascia, branches of the great auricular nerve, and the platysma. The **deep surface** of the parotid is very irregular and is divided into anteromedial and posteromedial surfaces. The **anteromedial surface** is related to the posterior margin of the ramus of the mandible, the masseter, and the medial pterygoid [Fig. 13.2]. The part of the gland deep to the ramus of the mandible is the **deep lobe**. The **posteromedial surface** of the parotid gland is related to, and grooved by, the mastoid process, the sternocleidomastoid muscle, and the posterior belly of the digastric. The stylohyoid muscle and styloid process lie medial to the parotid [Fig. 13.5].

A part of the cervical fascia is thickened, deep to the gland, to form the **stylomandibular ligament**. This ligament passes from the styloid process of the temporal bone to the posterior border of the ramus of the mandible and separates the parotid from the submandibular gland.

## Accessory parotid gland

A portion of this superficial part of the gland is often detached from the rest of the gland and forms the **accessory parotid gland** [see Fig. 3.6].

➲ **Parotitis** is inflammation of the parotid glands. It is commonly caused by mumps, a viral infection.

## Parotid duct

The parotid duct is a thick-walled tube formed within the gland by the union of the ductules which drain its lobules. It appears at the anterior border of the gland on the surface of the masseter, approximately a finger-breadth below the zygomatic arch. It runs anteriorly across the masseter, below the accessory parotid gland, accompanying the zygomatic branches of the facial nerve. The duct hooks medially over the anterior border of the masseter and can be felt there by rolling it against the muscle, with the jaw clenched. The duct pierces the buccal pad of fat, the buccopharyngeal fascia, and the buccinator muscle to open into the vestibule of the mouth, opposite the second upper molar tooth [see Figs. 3.6, 3.8; Figs. 13.1, 13.2].

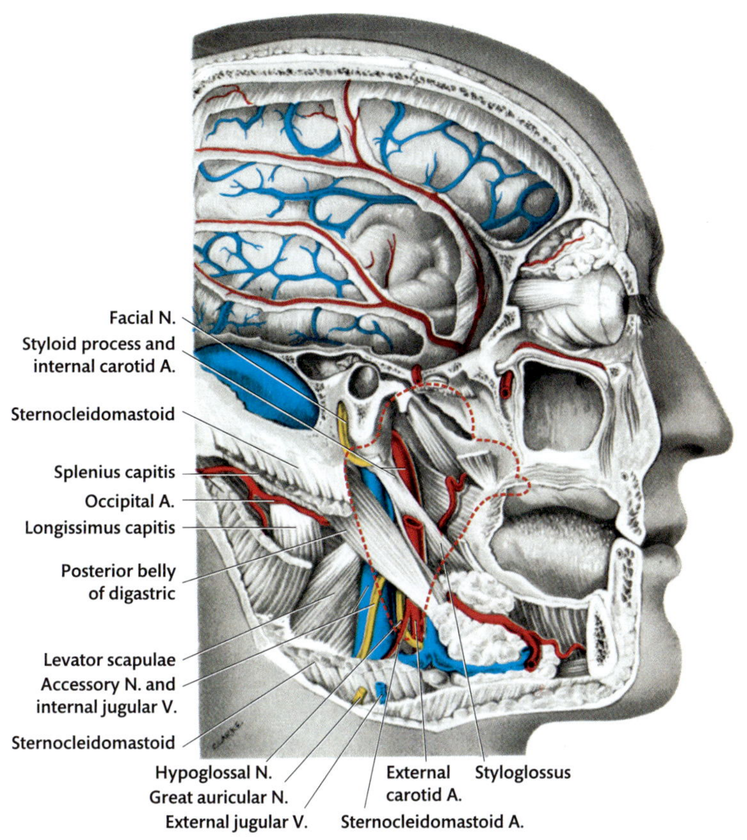


**Fig. 13.5** Dissection of the head to show the structures deep to the parotid gland. The outline of the parotid gland is shown by the red dotted line.



## Structures within the parotid gland

Branches of the facial, great auricular, and auriculotemporal nerves; the external carotid, superficial temporal, and transverse facial arteries; and the retromandibular vein traverse the substance of the parotid gland.

### External carotid artery

The **external carotid artery** enters and leaves the gland on its deep surface. It gives off the **posterior auricular artery** immediately before entering the gland, and divides into the **maxillary** and **superficial temporal arteries** behind the neck of the mandible. Within the gland, the superficial temporal artery gives off the **transverse facial** and **middle temporal arteries** [Figs. 13.2, 13.3].

### Retromandibular vein

The **retromandibular vein** is formed in the parotid by the union of the **superficial temporal** and **maxillary veins**. It is joined by the middle temporal and transverse facial veins. It divides into anterior and posterior branches at the lower end of the gland [Fig. 13.2].

### Facial nerve

The **facial nerve** enters the posteromedial surface of the gland, close to the stylomastoid foramen [Fig. 13.3], and divides into five terminal branches in the gland—**temporal**, **zygomatic**, **buccal**, **mandibular**, and **cervical**. The branches radiate forwards, superficial to the artery and the vein, and emerge from the anteromedial surface close to the anterior border of the gland. Within the gland, branches of the facial nerve receive communicating branches from the great auricular and auriculotemporal nerves.

➲ Care should be taken to identify and preserve branches of the facial nerve during parotid gland surgery to minimize the risk of facial paralysis.

### Parotid lymph nodes

The **parotid lymph nodes** are embedded in the gland, especially near its superficial surface. The superficial nodes drain the auricle, the anterior part of the scalp, and the upper part of the face. The deeper nodes drain the external acoustic meatus, middle ear, auditory tube, nose, palate, and deeper parts of the cheek. Both groups drain to the cervical lymph nodes [see Fig. 8.18].

Using the instructions given in Dissection 13.1, identify and clean the structures within the parotid gland.

**DISSECTION 13.1 Structures in the parotid gland**

**Objectives**

**I.** To identify and trace the facial nerve and its branches in the parotid gland. **II.** To expose the external carotid artery and retromandibular vein in the gland.

**Instructions**

1. Expose the surface of the parotid gland, and follow its duct to the buccinator muscle.
2. Follow one of the branches of the facial nerve back through the gland to the trunk of the nerve, and then trace the other branches forwards through it. Look for communicating branches from the auriculotemporal nerve which are relatively large.
3. Trace the trunk of the facial nerve to the stylomastoid foramen, and find the posterior auricular branch and the branch to the posterior belly of the digastric and the stylohyoid. These branches are given off deep to the gland.
4. Find and trace the posterior auricular artery.
5. Expose the retromandibular vein and the external carotid artery by removing more of the gland.
6. Remove the remainder of the gland piecemeal, and expose the structures which surround it, retaining as far as possible the structures which pass through it.

## Vessels and nerves of the parotid gland

The blood supply to the parotid gland is from the adjoining vessels. Sensory fibres to the gland are carried in the **great auricular** and **auriculotemporal** nerves. **Parasympathetic nerves**: post-ganglionic secretomotor fibres come from the otic ganglion through the auriculotemporal nerve. (The preganglionic parasympathetic fibres to the otic ganglion are carried in the lesser petrosal branch of the glossopharyngeal nerve [see Fig. 12.8].) **Sympathetic nerves**: post-ganglionic sympathetic fibres to the parotid gland come from the superior cervical ganglion. They reach the gland through the plexus on the external carotid or middle meningeal arteries [see Fig. 14.6].

## Auriculotemporal or Frey's syndrome

➲ Auriculotemporal syndrome, or gustatory sweating, is redness and sweating of the side of the face in response to a salivatory stimulus of either smell or taste of food. It could follow parotid gland surgery (or other surgery involving the capsule of the parotid gland). It results from aberrant connections being formed in the post-operative period between secretomotor fibres destined for the parotid gland and the sweat glands of the face.

## Facial nerve

The seventh cranial nerve—the facial nerve—leaves the brain at the lower border of the pons [see Fig. 24.2], passes with the vestibulocochlear (eighth cranial) nerve into the internal acoustic meatus, and emerges from the temporal bone at the stylomastoid foramen [see Figs. 2.10, 2.14]. It runs a complicated course through the petrous part of the temporal bone [see Fig. 12.8]. After emerging through the stylomastoid foramen, the facial nerve curves anteriorly and enters the posteromedial surface of the parotid gland. Before entering the gland, it gives off the posterior auricular nerve (to the occipital belly of the occipitofrontalis and the auricular muscles) and small branches to the posterior belly of the digastric and the stylohyoid muscles. In the gland, it divides into its main branches—temporal, zygomatic, upper and lower buccal, marginal mandibular, and cervical [see Fig. 3.7]. The temporal and zygomatic can sometimes be felt on the zygomatic arch.

See Clinical Application 13.1 (and Fig. 13.6) for the practical implications of the anatomy discussed in this chapter.

**CLINICAL APPLICATION 13.1 Parotid tumour**

A 45-year-old woman presented with a complaint of a mass below the lobule of her right ear. The mass was not painful, and she had noticed it inadvertently while washing her face about a week ago. On examination, the mass was mobile, non-tender, firm, and solitary. The overlying skin, oral cavity, oropharynx, and neck revealed no changes. Further tests were done, and T2-weighted axial magnetic resonance imaging (MRI) showed a neoplastic mass lesion in the right parotid gland [Fig. 13.6].

The mass was found to be a benign pleomorphic adenoma, and a superficial parotidectomy was planned to remove the lesion.

Study question 1: which one structure within the parotid gland requires special attention to ensure that it is not damaged during surgical removal of the mass? (Answer: the facial nerve.)

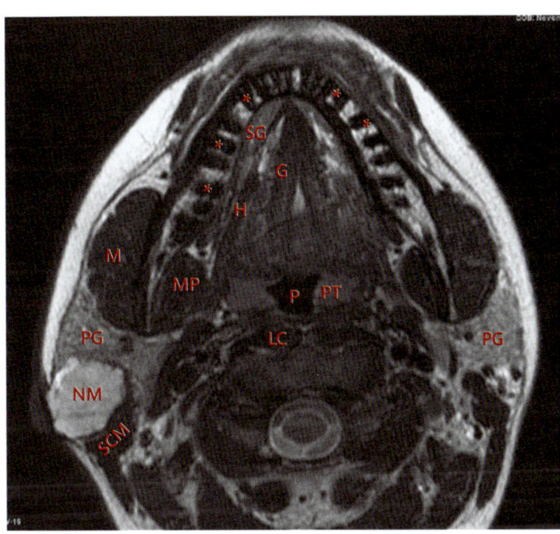


**Fig. 13.6** T2-weighted axial image at the level of the parotid gland. Asterisks = mandibular alveolus; G = genioglossus; H = hyoglossus; P = pharynx; PG = parotid gland; PT = palatine tonsils; LC = longus colli; M = masseter; MP = medial pterygoid; SCM = sternocleidomastoid; SG = sublingual gland. A neoplastic mass lesion (NM) is seen in the right parotid gland.

## CHAPTER 14

# The temporal and infratemporal regions

## Introduction to the temporal region

The main content of the temporal fossa is the temporalis muscle and its vessels and nerves. Begin your study of the temporal region by revising the details given in Chapter 3. The temporal region is bound superiorly and posteriorly by the superior temporal line, anteriorly by the zygomatic bone, and inferiorly and laterally by the zygomatic arch [see Fig. 3.4]. It is separated inferiorly from the infratemporal fossa by the infratemporal crest on the sphenoid.

### Temporal fascia

The temporal fascia is a strong, glistening membrane stretched over the temporal fossa and the temporalis muscle. Superiorly, it is attached to the superior temporal line on the lateral aspect of the skull. Inferiorly, it splits into two. The superficial layer is attached to the upper margin of the zygomatic arch. The deep layer passes medial to the arch to become continuous with the fascia deep to the masseter. The two layers are separated from each other by a little fat.

## Muscles of mastication

The masseter, temporalis, and medial and lateral pterygoids are the muscles of mastication. They share a common embryological origin—the first pharyngeal arch—and are supplied by the mandibular division of the trigeminal nerve.

Prior to studying the temporal and infratemporal fossae, examine the masseter muscle on the side of the jaw.



### Masseter

The masseter is a thick quadrate muscle of mastication which covers the lateral aspect of the ramus and coronoid process of the mandible [Fig. 14.1]. **Origin**: it takes origin from the inferior margin and deep surface of the zygomatic arch between the tubercle of the zygoma to the junction of the zygomatic arch with the zygomatic process of the maxilla. **Insertion**: it is inserted into the lateral surface of the ramus and coronoid process of the mandible [see Fig. 2.16A]. The deep fibres run vertically, and the superficial fibres run posteroinferiorly [see Figs. 3.8, 2.9].

**Nerve supply**: the mandibular division of the trigeminal nerve. The nerve enters the deep surface of the masseter by passing through the mandibular notch, immediately anterior to the capsule of the temporomandibular joint. **Actions**: it raises the mandible and clenches the teeth. Its superficial fibres help to protract the mandible. Acting alternately, the two muscles (right and left) move the chin from side to side, producing a grinding movement of the teeth.

Dissection 14.1 provides instructions on dissection of the temporalis.

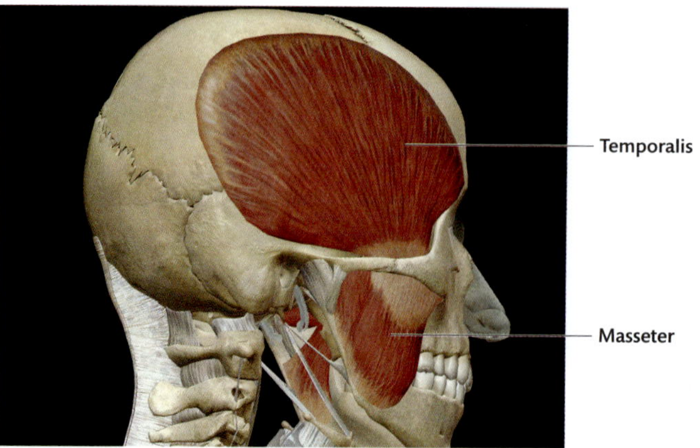


**Fig. 14.1** The temporalis and masseter muscles.



**DISSECTION 14.1 Temporalis**

**Objective**

**I.** To expose the temporalis by turning down the zygomatic arch.

**Instructions**

1. Divide the zygomatic arch anterior and posterior to the attachment of the masseter, and turn it down with that muscle. Divide the neurovascular bundle which enters the deep surface of the muscle, immediately anterior to the temporomandibular joint, and any fibres of the temporalis that may join the masseter.
2. Strip the masseter from the surface of the mandible as far as the angle, but leave it attached there.
3. Expose the temporalis.

## Temporalis

The temporalis is a fan-shaped muscle. **Origin**: it takes origin from the lateral side of the skull below the inferior temporal line and from the temporal fascia [see Fig. 2.9]. **Insertion**: it converges towards the coronoid process of the mandible, with the anterior fibres descending vertically and the posterior fibres running horizontally forwards. It forms a tendon on its superficial surface, which is inserted into the apex and anterior margin of the coronoid process and the anterior margin of the ramus. The deeper muscular fibres are attached to the medial side of the coronoid process and extend down to the junction of the anterior border of the ramus and the body of the mandible, behind the third mandibular molar tooth [see Figs. Fig. 2.16A, 2.16B]. Some of the superficial fibres may join the masseter and pass with it to the ramus of the mandible.

**Nerve supply**: deep temporal branches of the mandibular nerve. **Actions**: the temporalis raises the mandible, and its horizontal posterior fibres retract the mandible after protraction [Fig. 14.1].

## Introduction to the infratemporal region

The infratemporal fossa lies inferior to the zygomatic arch and the infratemporal surface of the greater wing of the sphenoid [see Fig. 2.10]. It is bound by the ramus and angle of the mandible laterally, the lateral pterygoid plate medially, the posterior aspect of the maxilla anteriorly, and the tympanic plate, mastoid, and styloid process of the temporal bone posteriorly [Fig. 14.2].

### Superficial contents of the infratemporal fossa

Using the instructions given in Dissection 14.2 (and Figs. 14.2, 14.3), expose the superficial contents of the infratemporal fossa.

### Lateral pterygoid muscle

**Origin**: the lateral pterygoid muscle arises by two heads. The smaller **upper head** takes origin from

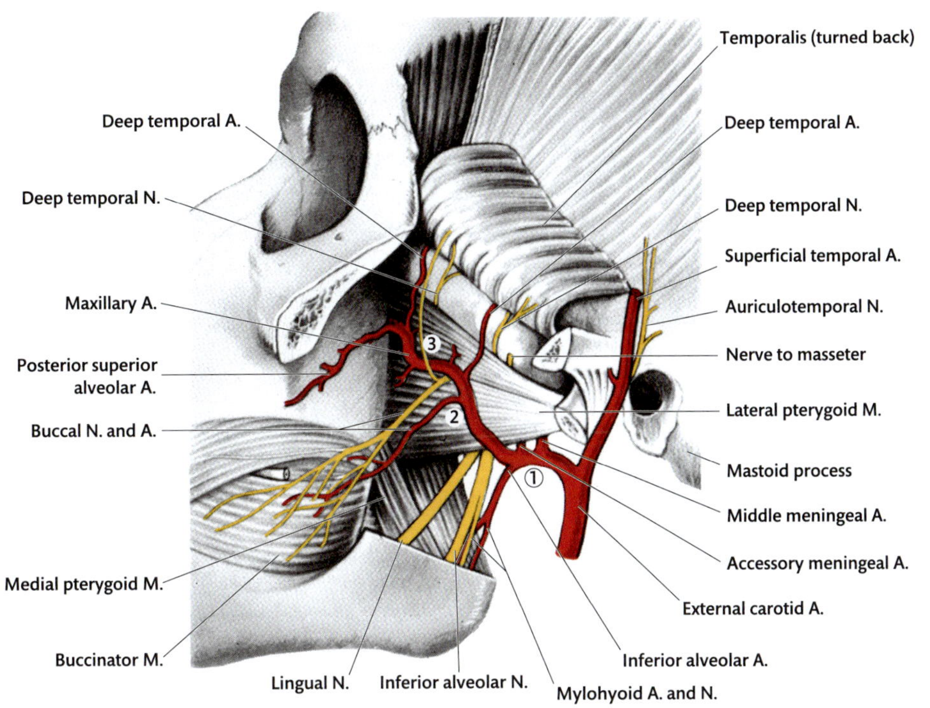


**Fig. 14.2** Dissection of the infratemporal fossa. 1 = first part of maxillary artery; 2 = second part of maxillary artery; 3 = third part of maxillary artery.

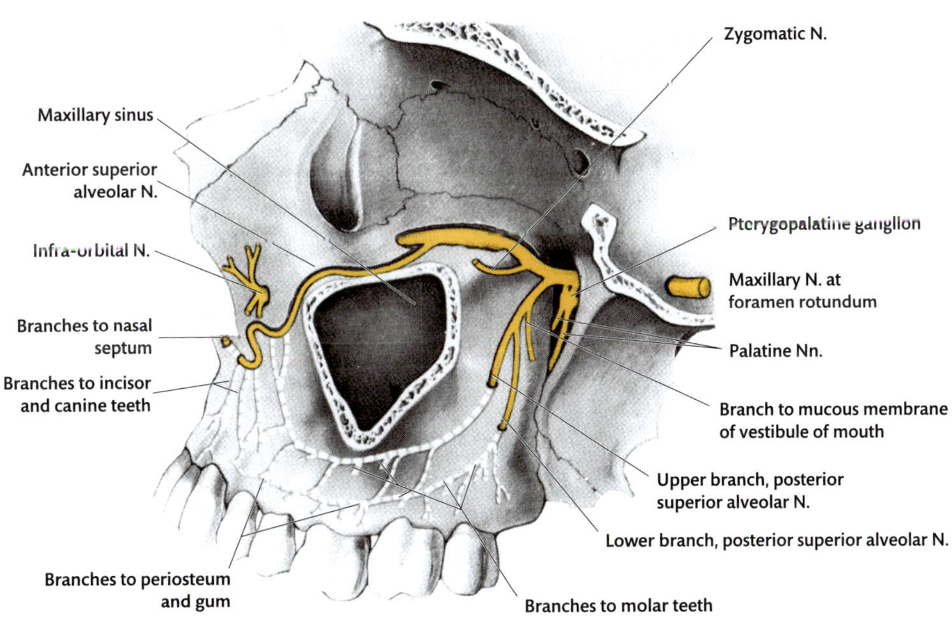


**Fig. 14.3** The maxillary nerve and its branches.

the infratemporal ridge and infratemporal surface of the greater wing of the sphenoid medial to it. The **lower head** takes origin from the lateral surface of the lateral pterygoid plate. **Insertion**: the muscle narrows, as it passes posteriorly, and is inserted into the front of the neck of the mandible and the articular disc of the temporomandibular joint through its capsule [Fig. 14.2; see Figs. 2.16A, B].

**Nerve supply**: the mandibular nerve. **Actions**: acting together, the two muscles protrude the

**DISSECTION 14.2 Superficial dissection of the infratemporal fossa**

**Objectives**

**I.** To expose the contents of the infratemporal fossa. **II.** To identify and trace the first two parts of the maxillary artery. **III.** To identify branches of the maxillary nerve.

**Instructions**

1. Using a hammer and chisel, make an oblique cut on the mandible from the mandibular notch to the point where the anterior margin of the ramus meets the body of the mandible. Separate the coronoid process from the mandible. Take care not to injure the **buccal nerve** and artery which lie close to the lowest tendinous fibres of the temporalis.
2. Turn the coronoid process and the temporalis upwards, and separate the muscle fibres from the lower part of the temporal fossa by blunt dissection [Fig. 14.2].
3. Find the deep temporal vessels and nerves which ascend between the muscle and the skull.
4. Make a horizontal cut through the neck of the mandible, and another immediately above the mandibular foramen [see Fig. 2.15B, 2.16B]. The position of the mandibular foramen can be determined by sliding the handle of a knife between the ramus of the mandible and the subjacent soft parts, and pressing down till it is arrested by the inferior alveolar nerve and vessels entering the foramen. (While making the second cut, cut halfway through the bone with a saw and complete the division with bone forceps. Remove the pieces of bone, and expose the underlying muscles, vessels, and nerves.)
5. Remove the fat and parts of the pterygoid plexus of veins which obscure your view.
6. Identify the pterygoid muscles and parts of the maxillary vessels [Fig. 14.2].
7. Identify the maxillary artery, and follow it anterosuperiorly till it disappears medially. Carefully remove the fat from the region just superior to this.
8. The maxillary nerve may be seen passing towards the inferior orbital fissure to continue as the infraorbital nerve [Fig. 14.3].
9. Find the two branches of the maxillary nerve in this region: (1) the **zygomatic nerve** which passes through the inferior orbital fissure; and (2) the **posterior superior alveolar nerve**, which divides into branches that descend and disappear into small holes in the posterior surface of the maxilla.

mandible and depress the chin, by drawing the head of the mandible and the disc forwards onto the articular tubercle. When one muscle acts alone, the head of the mandible on that side is drawn forwards, and the mandible pivots around the opposite joint so that the chin is swung towards the opposite side.

## Medial pterygoid

**Origin**: the medial pterygoid muscle also has two heads of origin which embrace the lower head of the lateral pterygoid [Fig. 14.2]. The **superficial head** is small and takes origin from the maxillary tuberosity. The **deep head** forms nearly the whole muscle and takes origin from the medial surface of the lateral pterygoid plate. **Insertion**: the two heads unite, inferior to the anterior part of the lateral pterygoid, and pass downwards, backwards, and laterally, to be inserted into the ramus of the mandible between the mandibular foramen and the angle of the mandible [see Fig. 2.16B]. Its fibres are nearly parallel to the superficial fibres of the masseter.

**Nerve supply**: the mandibular nerve. **Actions**: it (1) raises the mandible; (2) helps in protraction; and (3) moves the chin to the opposite side. The two medial pterygoid muscles acting alternatively produce a grinding movement, similar to the action of the superficial fibres of the masseter.

## Maxillary artery

The maxillary artery is a branch of the external carotid artery. It arises posterior to the neck of the mandible [Fig. 14.2]. The first part of the maxillary artery runs horizontally forwards between the neck of the mandible and the sphenomandibular ligament on the lower border of the lateral pterygoid muscle. The second part runs anterosuperiorly, superficial to the lower head of the lateral pterygoid muscle and deep to the insertion of the temporalis. The third part turns medially, between the two heads of the lateral pterygoid, enters the pterygomaxillary fissure, and ends in the pterygopalatine fossa in a number of branches. The second part of the artery often lies between the two pterygoid muscles and bends laterally between the heads of the lateral pterygoid muscle before entering the pterygopalatine fossa [see Fig. 2.8; Fig. 14.2].

### Branches of the maxillary artery

During its course, the artery gives branches to the external acoustic meatus, middle ear, muscles of the infratemporal fossa, skull bones, and dura mater, and arteries which accompany the nerves in the infratemporal and pterygopalatine fossae.

The **inferior alveolar** branch of the maxillary artery descends with the inferior alveolar nerve, enters the mandibular foramen, and runs through the mandibular canal to supply the lower teeth, gums, and mandible. It gives off the **mental artery** which supplies the skin over the chin and lower lip. It also gives off the mylohyoid artery which runs with the mylohyoid nerve in the mylohyoid groove [see Figs. 5.5, 15.2B]. The corresponding veins drain into the pterygoid venous plexus.

## Pterygoid venous plexus and maxillary vein

The numerous veins of the infratemporal fossa are difficult to dissect, since they form a dense plexus—the **pterygoid venous plexus**—around the lateral pterygoid muscle. Veins corresponding to the branches of the maxillary artery open into this network. The pterygoid plexus is drained posteriorly by one or two short, wide maxillary veins into the retromandibular vein, posterior to the neck of the mandible [see Fig. 13.2].

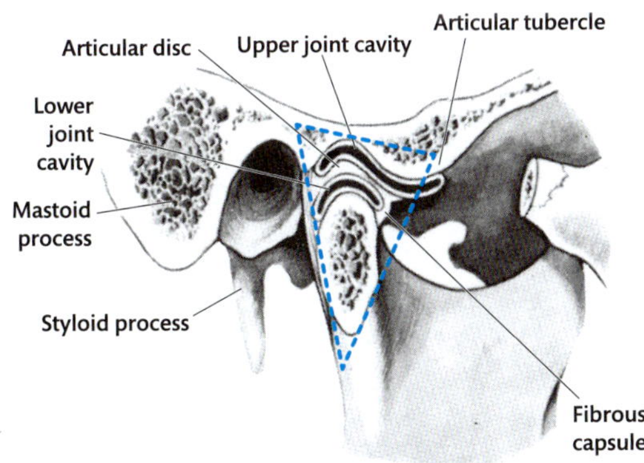


Fig. 14.4 Section through the temporomandibular joint. Dotted lines represent the position of the lateral ligament.

### Communications of the pterygoid venous plexus

The pterygoid venous plexus has widespread communications with all the surrounding veins, but particularly with: (1) the **cavernous sinus** by an emissary vein which runs through the foramen ovale or the sphenoidal emissary foramen; and (2) the **facial vein**, through the deep facial vein which runs posteriorly on the buccinator muscle, deep to the masseter and the ramus of the mandible. ➲ Infectious material from the face can reach the cavernous sinus through these communications.

## Temporomandibular joint

The temporomandibular joint is a synovial joint formed by the articulation between the head of the mandible and the mandibular fossa and the articular tubercle of the temporal bone. These two articular surfaces are separated by an articular disc which completely divides the joint cavity into upper and lower parts [Fig. 14.4].

The **fibrous capsule** of the joint is attached to the margins of the articular area on the temporal bone and around the neck of the mandible. Laterally, it is thickened to form a triangular band—the **lateral ligament**. The base of the lateral ligament is attached to the zygomatic process of the temporal bone and the zygomatic tubercle, and the apex is attached to the lateral side of the neck of the mandible. The **articular disc** is an oval plate of dense fibrous tissue which is fused with the fibrous capsule around its periphery. It is more tightly bound to the mandible than to the temporal bone. The upper surface of the disc is concavo-convex to fit the articular tubercle and the mandibular fossa. Its lower surface is concave and fits the head of the mandible [Fig. 14.4].

Using the instructions given in Dissection 14.3, open the temporomandibular joint.

**DISSECTION 14.3 The temporomandibular joint**

**Objective**

**I.** To open the temporomandibular joint and study its interior.

**Instructions**

1. Remove the lateral ligament, and expose the disc and the two separate synovial cavities within the joint.

The fibrous capsule and the lateral ligament are the only proper ligaments of the joint. The sphenomandibular and stylomandibular ligaments also connect the mandible to the skull but add little, if anything, to the strength of the joint. The integrity of the joint is maintained principally by the muscles of mastication. As with any joint maintained mainly by muscles, the temporomandibular joint is easily dislocated.

The **sphenomandibular ligament** is a long, membranous band which passes from the spine of the sphenoid to the lingula and lower margin of the mandibular foramen. It lies superficial to the medial pterygoid muscle. At the lower part, it is pierced by the mylohyoid vessels and nerve. (This ligament is a remnant of the first branchial arch cartilage, the superior part of which gives rise to the malleus.)

## Movements of the temporomandibular joint

Movements at the temporomandibular joint are elevation, depression, protraction, retraction, and side-to-side grinding movements of the jaw.

When the jaw is **depressed** to open the mouth wide, two separate movements—a sliding and a rotatory movement—take place. (1) The articular disc and the head of the mandible slide forwards on the articular surface of the temporal bone, and the head of the mandible comes to lie inferior to the articular tubercle. (2) At the same time, the head of the mandible rotates on the lower surface of the articular disc in the lower joint cavity [Fig. 14.5]. The latter movement alone is capable of permitting simple chewing movements over a small range, without separating the lips. (The rotatory movement can be confirmed by placing a forefinger on the head of the mandible, immediately in front of the tragus, while making chewing movements.) When the mouth is opened wide, the head of the mandible swings forwards and downwards. (Confirm that the finger on the head of the mandible slips into the mandibular fossa vacated by the head, and that the mouth cannot be closed while the finger remains in the fossa.) The axes for the small and wide rotatory movements are different. In small movements, the axis is through the head of the mandible; in wider range movements, the axis is through the mandibular foramen. By being on the axis, the vessels and nerves entering the mandible are not stretched when the mouth is opened wide. Muscles causing depression of the jaw are the lateral pterygoid and the digastric acting on a fixed hyoid bone.

**Elevation** of the jaw closes the mouth. It is brought about by the temporalis, masseter, and medial pterygoid.

**Protraction** of the jaw is the movement of pulling the jaw forwards. In protraction, the head of the mandible and the articular disc slide forwards on the temporal articular surface on both sides, but the mouth is not opened. The lateral pterygoid protracts the jaw. The medial pterygoid and the superficial fibres of the masseter also protract the jaw, but less effectively.

The reverse movement to protraction is **retraction** which is brought about by the posterior fibres of the temporalis. When these movements alternate on the two sides by the muscles of opposite sides acting alternately, a grinding movement is produced as the chin swings from side to side. Table 14.1 provides an overview of the movements of the mandible.

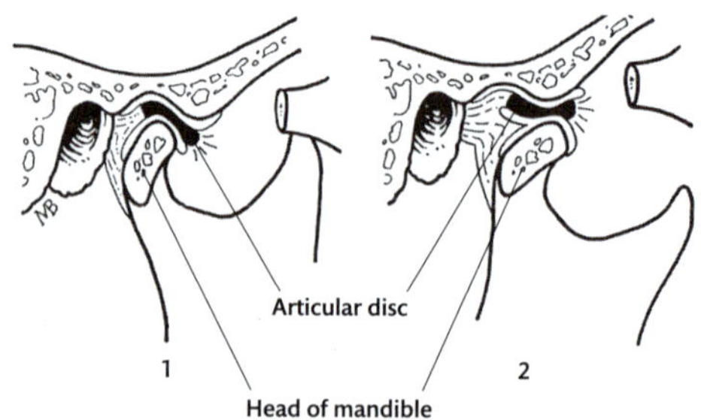


**Fig. 14.5** Diagrams to show the changing relationship between the head of the mandible and the temporal bone when the mouth is being opened. (1) The mouth is closed. (2) When the mouth is opened: (i) the head of the mandible and the articular disc slide forwards onto the articular tubercle; and (ii) the head of the mandible rotates on the disc.

**Table 14.1** Movements of the mandible

| Movement | Muscles producing the movement | Nerves supplying the muscles |
|---|---|---|
| Elevation of chin (closing the mouth) | Masseter<br>Medial pterygoid<br>Temporalis (anterior part) | Mandibular<br>Mandibular<br>Mandibular |
| Depression of chin (opening the mouth)* | Lateral pterygoid | Mandibular |
| | Digastric (hyoid fixed) | Mandibular and facial |
| | Geniohyoid (hyoid fixed) | C. 1 ventral ramus |
| | Mylohyoid (hyoid fixed) | Mandibular |
| Protraction | Lateral pterygoid | Mandibular |
| | Medial pterygoid | Mandibular |
| | Masseter (superficial part) | Mandibular |
| Retraction* | Temporalis (posterior part) | Mandibular |
| | Digastric (hyoid fixed) | Mandibular and facial |
| Chewing—a side-to-side grinding movement | Medial and lateral pterygoids and masseter | Mandibular |
| | Temporalis (all parts), masseter (deep part) | Mandibular |

* During depression and retraction of the jaw, the hyoid is fixed by the action of the infrahyoid muscles. Nerve supply: ansa cervicalis.

### Dislocation of the temporomandibular joint

➲ The temporomandibular joint may be dislocated by a side blow to the chin when the mouth is open or in fractures of the mandible. Sometimes it is dislocated with excessive stretching of the lateral pterygoid in yawning or when opening the mouth to take a big bite. The head of the mandible slips anteriorly out of the mandibular fossa—anterior dislocation—and the person is unable to close the mouth. It is reduced with downward and backward pressure on the lower molars, to disengage the head of the mandible and slip it back in place.

Posterior dislocation is rare and usually results from a frontal blow to the chin.

## Deeper contents of the infratemporal fossa

Using the instructions given in Dissection 14.4 (and Fig. 14.6), complete the deep dissection of the infratemporal fossa.

## Middle meningeal artery

The **middle meningeal artery** arises from the maxillary artery at the lower border of the lateral pterygoid muscle. It ascends between the two roots of the auriculotemporal nerve and enters the skull through the foramen spinosum [Figs. 14.2, 14.6]. It is posterolateral to the mandibular nerve and lies on the lateral surface of the tensor palati muscle and the auditory tube. Its intracranial course is described in Chapter 7.

The **accessory meningeal** and **anterior tympanic arteries** arise either from the middle meningeal artery or from the maxillary artery. The accessory meningeal artery enters the skull through the foramen ovale, and the anterior tympanic artery enters the middle ear through the petrotympanic fissure, close to the chorda tympani nerve.

## Mandibular nerve

The mandibular branch of the trigeminal nerve arises from the trigeminal ganglion in the cranium and leaves the skull through the foramen ovale. In the foramen ovale, it is joined by the motor root of the trigeminal nerve.

Immediately below the skull, it lies between the lateral pterygoid muscle and the tensor palati which separates it from the auditory tube [see Fig. 2.11]. It divides almost immediately into anterior (predominantly motor) and posterior (predominantly sensory) divisions [Figs. 14.6, 14.7].

### Branches of the trunk

The **meningeal branch** arises from the trunk of the nerve and enters the skull through the foramen spinosum. It supplies the dura mater and skull, and sends a filament to the middle ear.

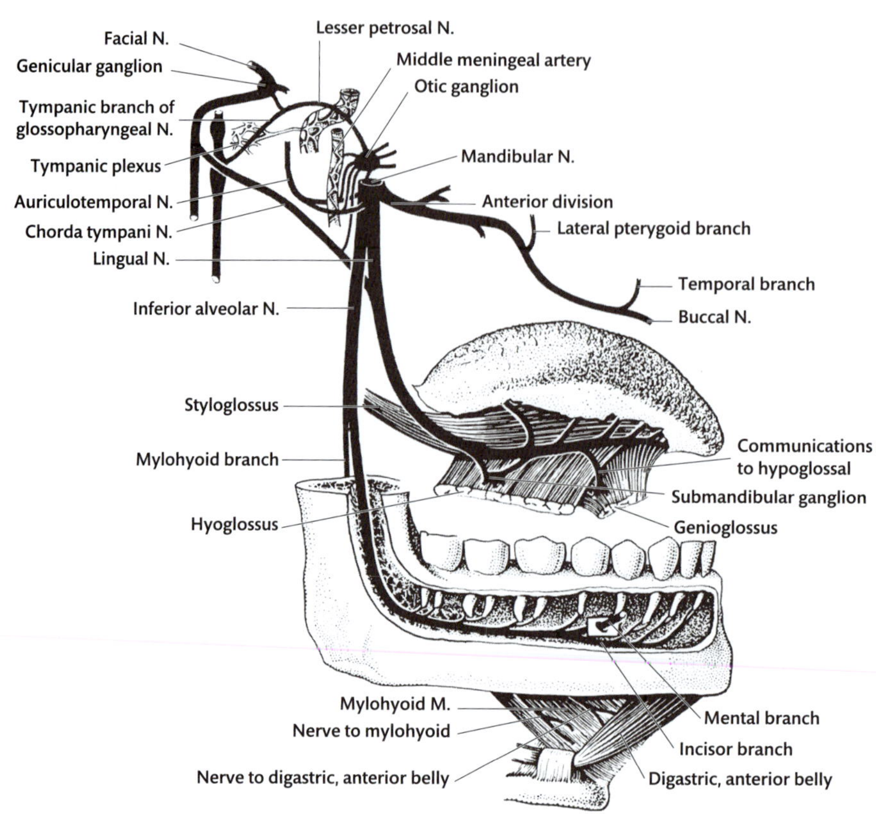


**Fig. 14.6** Distribution of the mandibular nerve. Note the sympathetic filaments to the otic ganglion and the tympanic plexus from the middle meningeal and internal carotid arteries.

### DISSECTION 14.4 Deep dissection of the infratemporal fossa

#### Objectives

**I.** To identify and trace the auriculotemporal nerve. **II.** To identify and trace the middle meningeal artery.

#### Instructions

1. Separate the two heads of the lateral pterygoid muscle, avoiding injury to the buccal nerve between them.
2. Carefully detach the upper head from the capsule of the temporomandibular joint and remove it piecemeal from the infratemporal fossa. Take care not to damage the deep temporal nerves which pass between the lateral pterygoid and the skull.
3. Separate the lower head of the lateral pterygoid from the lateral pterygoid lamina, and strip it posteriorly from the underlying structures, leaving the buccal nerve intact.
4. Disarticulate the head of the mandible from the articular disc, and remove it with the lower head of the lateral pterygoid. Take care not to damage the **auriculotemporal nerve** which curves round the medial and posterior surfaces of the joint capsule.
5. Expose the underlying structures.
6. Identify the middle meningeal artery, and trace it to the foramen spinosum. Note the two roots of the auriculotemporal nerve which surround the artery close to the skull.
7. Identify the origin of the auriculotemporal nerve from the mandibular nerve, and trace it posteriorly.
8. Expose the other branches of the mandibular nerve—inferior alveolar, lingual, and buccal [Fig. 14.6]. Identify the chorda tympani nerve joining the lingual nerve. Trace the chorda tympani towards the spine of the sphenoid.

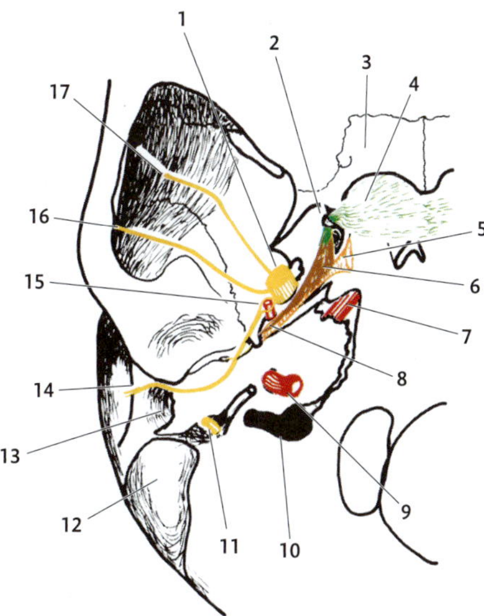


Fig. 14.7 A diagrammatic representation of the external surface of the base of the skull to show the position of some of the nerves and blood vessels and of the tensor veli palatini. Red = arteries and muscle. Green = tendon and auditory tube. 1 = mandibular nerve; 2 = pterygoid hamulus; 3 = horizontal plate of palatine bone; 4 = palatine aponeurosis (tendon of tensor veli palatini); 5 = pharyngeal opening of auditory tube; 6 = tensor veli palatini; 7 = internal carotid artery in upper part of foramen lacerum; 8 = chorda tympani nerve; 9 = internal carotid artery; 10 = jugular foramen; 11 = facial nerve; 12 = mastoid process; 13 = external acoustic meatus; 14 = auriculotemporal nerve; 15 = middle meningeal artery; 16 = nerve to masseter; 17 = deep temporal nerve to temporalis.

The **nerve to the medial pterygoid** arises from the trunk and runs forwards into the deep surface of the muscle. At its origin, it lies close to the otic ganglion.

## Branches of the anterior division

### Buccal nerve

The large sensory branch—the **buccal nerve**—passes between the two heads of the lateral pterygoid and runs anteroinferiorly to the surface of the buccinator muscle, often piercing the lowest fibres of insertion of the temporalis on the deep surface of the ramus of the mandible [Fig. 14.2]. On the buccinator, it forms a plexus with the buccal branch of the facial nerve (motor to the buccinator) and is sensory to the entire thickness of the cheek—from the skin to the mucous membrane.

### Nerve to the lateral pterygoid

The nerve to the lateral pterygoid runs with the buccal nerve and enters the muscle as it passes between the heads of the lateral pterygoid.

### Deep temporal nerves

The two deep temporal nerves—anterior and posterior—pass into the temporal fossa between the skull and the lateral pterygoid, grooving the bone to enter the deep surface of the temporalis [Figs. 14.2, 14.6, 14.7].

### Nerve to the masseter

The nerve to the masseter arises with the posterior deep temporal nerve. It runs laterally between the skull and the lateral pterygoid muscle (immediately anterior to the capsule of the temporomandibular joint), and enters the deep surface of the masseter by passing through the mandibular notch. It gives one or two twigs to the temporomandibular joint [Fig. 14.7].

## Branches of the posterior division

### Auriculotemporal nerve

The **auriculotemporal nerve** arises by two roots which surround the middle meningeal artery. They unite posterior to the artery, run backwards lateral to the spine of the sphenoid, and hook around the posterior surface of the neck of the mandible. Here the nerve turns superiorly in contact with the parotid gland and crosses the root of the zygomatic process of the temporal bone with the superficial temporal artery [Figs. 14.6, 14.7]. The nerve carries post-ganglionic parasympathetic secretomotor fibres from the otic ganglion to the parotid gland. (Preganglionic fibres reach the otic ganglion through the lesser petrosal branch of the glossopharyngeal nerve.)

The auriculotemporal nerve gives the following **branches**: (1) slender filaments to the posterior part of the capsule of the temporomandibular joint; (2) one or two thick sensory branches to the parotid gland—these nerves mingle with branches of the facial nerve in the substance of the gland; and (3) cutaneous branches to the auricle and temple [see Fig. 3.7].

### Inferior alveolar nerve

The inferior alveolar nerve is the largest branch of the posterior division. It runs vertically downwards with the inferior alveolar artery between the medial and lateral pterygoid muscles. The nerve and artery each give off a mylohyoid branch and then enter the mandibular foramen. In the body of the mandible, the inferior alveolar nerve and artery give branches to the teeth and gums, and send a branch (the **mental nerve** and **artery**) through the mental foramen to supply the skin of the chin and the mucous membrane of the lower lip [see Fig. 3.7; Figs. 14.2, 14.6, 14.7].

The **mylohyoid nerve** contains the only motor fibres present in the posterior division. It pierces the sphenomandibular ligament and runs anteroinferiorly in a groove on the medial aspect of the mandible to the digastric triangle, inferior to the mylohyoid muscle. In the triangle, it is joined by the submental artery and supplies the mylohyoid muscle and the anterior belly of the digastric [see Fig. 5.5].

#### Lingual nerve

The lingual nerve arises from the posterior division of the mandibular nerve and curves anteroinferiorly on the medial pterygoid muscle to reach the medial surface of the mandible, in front of the inferior alveolar nerve. It passes between the mandible and the mucous membrane covering it, just inferior to the last molar tooth and above the posterior fibres of the mylohyoid muscle [Figs. 14.2, 14.6; see Fig. 2.15B]. Its further course will be described in Chapter 15. The lingual nerve is sensory to the mucous membrane of the anterior two-thirds of the tongue and to the adjacent part of the floor of the mouth and gum.

The lingual nerve gives no branches in the infratemporal fossa but is joined by the chorda tympani branch of the facial nerve, deep to the lateral pterygoid muscle [Fig. 14.6]. It may send a communicating branch to the inferior alveolar nerve.

## Chorda tympani

The chorda tympani is a slender branch of the facial nerve. It arises from the facial nerve on the posterior wall of the middle ear cavity, runs anteriorly across the lateral wall of that cavity (on the tympanic membrane), and leaves the tympanic cavity through the petrotympanic fissure. It then grooves the medial side of the spine of the sphenoid, running anteroinferiorly to join the posterior surface of the lingual nerve [see Figs. 12.5, 12.8; Fig. 14.6]. It contains sensory and preganglionic parasympathetic fibres. The sensory fibres arise from the taste buds on the anterior two-thirds of the tongue. The preganglionic fibres synapse in the submandibular ganglion and supply the submandibular and sublingual glands.

Using the instructions given in Dissection 14.5, dissect the otic ganglion and tensor palati muscles.

**DISSECTION 14.5 Otic ganglion and tensor palati muscle**

**Objective**

**I.** To expose the otic ganglion and tensor palati muscle.

**Instructions**

1. Lift the mandibular nerve laterally, and attempt to find the otic ganglion medial to it. (If it cannot be found easily, do not dissect further as it can be seen more readily later from the medial side.)
2. Expose as much of the tensor palati as possible, medial to the middle meningeal artery and the mandibular nerve. (The muscle also will be seen more clearly from the medial aspect later.)

## Otic ganglion

The otic ganglion is a minute collection of parasympathetic nerve cells which lies between the mandibular nerve and the tensor palati, immediately below the foramen ovale [Fig. 14.6]. It is one of the four parasympathetic ganglia of the head.

### Connections of the otic ganglion

The preganglionic parasympathetic fibres to the otic ganglion run in the lesser petrosal nerve, a branch of the glossopharyngeal nerve [Fig. 14.6]. Post-ganglionic parasympathetic fibres (secretomotor fibres) arise from the cells of the ganglion and pass to the parotid gland in the auriculotemporal nerve.

Other nerves traverse the ganglion but have no functional connection with it. They are: (1) motor fibres to the tensor palati and tensor tympani muscles from the nerve to the medial pterygoid muscle; (2) sympathetic fibres from the plexus on the middle meningeal artery, for distribution through the branches of the ganglion; and (3) sensory fibres from the parotid gland.

## Maxillary nerve

The maxillary nerve has a very short course in the infratemporal fossa [Fig. 14.3]. It will be dissected more completely at a later stage, but its course and some of its branches can be seen now.

Dissection 14.6 provides instructions on dissecting the branches of the maxillary nerve in the orbit.

The maxillary nerve is the second of the three divisions of the trigeminal nerve. It arises from

> **DISSECTION 14.6 Branches of the maxillary nerve in the orbit**
>
> **Objective**
>
> **I.** To identify and trace the zygomatic and infraorbital vessels and nerves.
>
> **Instructions**
>
> 1. Lift the contents of the orbit upwards and medially. Find the **zygomatic nerve** in the angle between the floor and the lateral wall of the orbit, and trace the nerve forwards till it enters the bone.
> 2. Remove the periosteum from the orbital floor, and identify the infraorbital groove and infraorbital vessels and nerve lying in it.

the trigeminal ganglion in the cranium and passes forwards on the side of the body of the sphenoid, at the lower border of the cavernous sinus, to the **foramen rotundum** [see Fig. 7.14]. It emerges from the foramen rotundum into the upper part of the pterygopalatine fossa and curves laterally through the pterygomaxillary fissure to enter the infratemporal fossa. In the infratemporal fossa, it turns sharply forwards into the infraorbital groove as the **infraorbital nerve** [Fig. 14.3; see Fig. 18.5]. Confirm this course in a dried skull by passing a bristle through the foramen rotundum into the infraorbital groove.

## Branches of the maxillary nerve

The maxillary nerve gives off the following branches: (1) a **meningeal** branch which arises near the origin of the nerve; (2) in the pterygopalatine fossa, two **ganglionic** branches which pass inferiorly to join the pterygopalatine ganglion [Fig. 14.3]; (3) the **posterior superior alveolar nerve** which arises in the infratemporal fossa and divides into two branches which descend over the posterior surface of the maxilla. They supply the gum and the mucous membrane of the cheek and then enter the canals in the bone. In the canals, they run forwards above the tooth sockets and form a plexus with the superior alveolar branches of the infraorbital nerve. They give dental branches to the molar teeth. Within the bone, these nerves run with corresponding branches of the maxillary artery; (4) the **zygomatic nerve** which arises close to the foramen rotundum and enters the orbit through the inferior orbital fissure. It gives a delicate branch to the lacrimal nerve, pierces the periosteum, and divides into **zygomaticotemporal** and **zygomaticofacial** branches. These pass forwards in the periosteum of the lateral wall of the orbit and pierce the zygomatic bone to reach the skin of the temple (zygomaticotemporal nerve) and face (zygomaticofacial nerve) [see Fig. 3.7; Fig. 14.3]; and (5) the **infraorbital nerve** which is a continuation of the maxillary nerve in the infraorbital groove and canal. It emerges through the infraorbital foramen onto the face, deep to the orbicularis oculi. It divides into sensory branches to the upper lip, nose, and lower eyelid. The infraorbital nerve is accompanied by the corresponding vessels [see Fig. 3.7].

About the middle of the floor of the orbit, the infraorbital nerve gives off the **anterior superior alveolar nerve**, which descends through the anterior wall of the maxilla and joins the plexus formed by the posterior superior alveolar nerves. The anterior superior alveolar nerves supply branches to the upper first molar, premolars, canine, and incisor teeth. They also supply the adjacent gum and send branches to the maxillary sinus and to the mucous membrane of the anteroinferior part of the nose [Fig. 14.3].

A middle superior alveolar nerve is described in 30 per cent of individuals.

# Structures within the mandibular canal

Dissection 14.7 provides instructions on exposing the contents of the mandibular canal.

> **DISSECTION 14.7 Mandibular canal**
>
> **Objective**
>
> **I.** To expose the inferior alveolar nerve and vessels in the mandibular canal.
>
> **Instructions**
>
> 1. Expose the mandibular canal by removing the outer table of the mandible with a chisel and bone forceps.
> 2. Identify the inferior alveolar vessels and nerve.

The mandibular canal is traversed by the **inferior alveolar vessels and nerve**, which give dental branches to the roots of the lower teeth and gingival branches of the adjacent gum. The mental nerve and artery arise from the inferior alveolar nerve and artery in the canal, and emerge through the mental foramen.

See Clinical Application 14.1 for the practical implications of the anatomy discussed in this chapter.

**CLINICAL APPLICATION 14.1 Clinical testing of the trigeminal nerve**

There are several ways to test the integrity of the trigeminal nerve clinically.

1. Testing sensations of pain, temperature, and touch over the forehead, prominence of the cheek, and chin.

   Study question 1: using your knowledge of the nerve supply of the face, explain why, while testing the integrity of the trigeminal nerve, one must be careful not to include the skin over the angle of the mandible. (Answer: the skin over the angle of the mandible is not supplied by the trigeminal nerve. It is supplied by the great auricular nerve from the cervical plexus. The trigeminal nerve is distributed through its three divisions to the skin of the rest of the face and anterior scalp.)
2. Testing the corneal reflex.

   Study question 2: explain why in facial palsy, the corneal reflex is impaired. (Answer: the corneal reflex is impaired in facial palsy because the efferent limb of the reflex is through the branches of the facial nerve that supply the orbicularis oculi.)
3. Inspection of jaw movement. Look for deviation of the jaw when the mouth is opened.

   Study question 3: to which side does the mandible deviate if the trigeminal nerve is paralysed, and why? (Answer: deviation of the jaw is to the affected side because of the unopposed action of the pterygoid muscles of the normal side.)
4. Testing the jaw jerk. The jaw jerk is elicited by tapping the chin while the mouth is held loosely open. A positive response is jerking of the jaw upwards by the masseter muscle.

   Study question 4: which part of the trigeminal nerve carries proprioceptive impulses from the muscles of mastication? (Answer: the mandibular division.)

# CHAPTER 15
# The submandibular region

## Introduction

The submandibular region lies between the body of the mandible and the hyoid bone. The superficial part includes the submental and digastric triangles which have been dissected already. Its deeper parts, now to be dissected, include the root of the tongue and the floor of the mouth [Fig. 15.1].

Dissection 15.1 provides instructions on exposing the submandibular region.



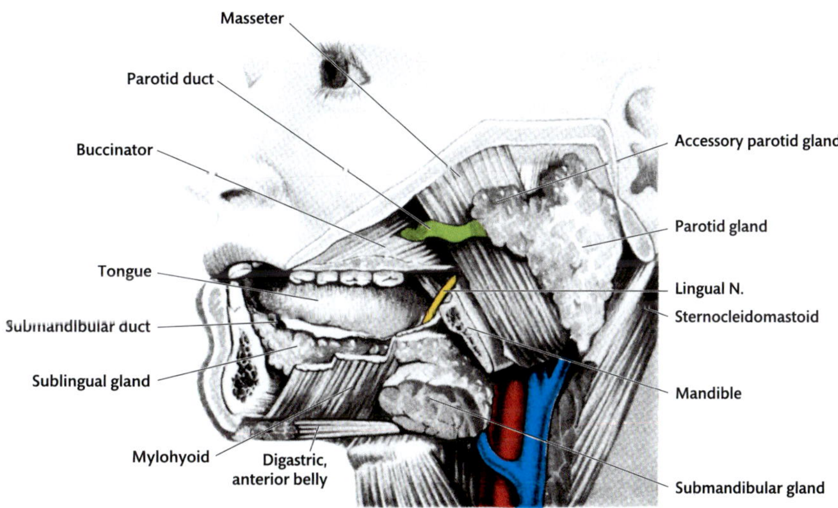


**Fig. 15.1** Dissection of the parotid, submandibular, and sublingual glands.

### DISSECTION 15.1 Exposure of the submandibular region

**Objective**

**I.** To mobilize the mandible and open into the submandibular region.

**Instructions**

1. Turn the trachea and oesophagus medially on the right. On the left, extend the neck and flex the head to the right.
2. Cut across the facial artery and vein at the lower border of the mandible, and detach the anterior belly of the digastric from the mandible. Turn the mandible upwards, and fix it with hooks.
3. Complete the exposure of the posterior belly of the digastric and of the stylohyoid muscles.

## Digastric muscle

The digastric muscle has two bellies—the **anterior** and **posterior** bellies [Chapter 5]. **Origin**: the anterior belly of the digastric takes origin from the lower border of the mandible, close to the mandibular symphysis. The posterior belly arises from the floor of the mastoid notch on the medial side of the mastoid process. **Insertion**: the two bellies are united by an intermediate tendon at the upper border of the hyoid bone. The tendon passes through a short, strong loop of fibrous tissue which binds it down to the hyoid bone at the junction of the body with the greater horn. It allows the hyoid bone to slide backwards and forwards on the tendon [see Figs. 5.2A, 5.4, 5.7, 2.16B, 17.2].

The anterior belly is covered by deep fascia and is overlapped by the submandibular gland [see Fig. 5.1]. The posterior belly is deep to the mastoid process, the lower part of the parotid gland, the angle of the mandible, the facial vein, and the submandibular gland. It runs obliquely, superficial to the neurovascular bundle of the neck—the internal jugular vein, internal and external carotid arteries, spinal accessory, and hypoglossal nerve. The occipital artery runs posterosuperiorly on its deep surface and grooves the temporal bone, just medial to the origin of the muscle [see Figs. 5.4, 5.5].

**Nerve supply**: the posterior belly of the digastric is supplied by the facial nerve, and the anterior belly by the mylohyoid nerve. **Actions**: if the hyoid bone is fixed, the digastric helps to depress the mandible. The chief action of both bellies, acting together, is to raise the hyoid bone (and hence the tongue) in swallowing. (It is not possible to swallow with the mouth open, because the digastric is already shortened.) Acting with the infrahyoid muscles, the digastric fixes the hyoid bone and forms a stable platform on which the tongue can move.

## Stylohyoid muscle

The stylohyoid is a small slip of muscle. **Origin**: it arises from the styloid process and descends along the upper border of the posterior belly of the digastric. **Insertion**: inferiorly, the tendon splits to surround the intermediate tendon of the digastric and is inserted into the hyoid bone at the junction of the body and greater horn [see Fig. 5.2]. **Nerve supply**: the facial nerve. **Action**: it helps to pull the hyoid upwards and backwards during swallowing [see Fig. 17.2].

Using the instructions given in Dissection 15.2, dissect the submandibular region.

### DISSECTION 15.2 The submandibular region

#### Objectives

**I.** To study the submandibular gland and duct. **II.** To identify and trace the facial artery in the submandibular region. **III.** To expose the posterior border of the mylohyoid and hyoglossus. **IV.** To identify and trace the hypoglossal and lingual nerves. **V.** To identify the submandibular ganglion.

#### Instructions

1. Turn the submandibular gland posteriorly, and expose the mylohyoid muscle.
2. Note the deep part of the gland which hooks round the free posterior border of the mylohyoid muscle and runs forwards on its superior surface.
3. Dissect out the facial artery from the deep surface of the gland, and trace its branches in this region.
4. Identify the mylohyoid nerve on the mylohyoid muscle.
5. Turn the submandibular gland anteriorly, and identify the hypoglossal nerve lying on the hyoglossus muscle immediately superior to the greater horn of the hyoid bone.
6. At a higher level, identify the lingual nerve as it crosses the hyoglossus.
7. Identify the submandibular ganglion, which is suspended from the lingual nerve.
8. Identify the submandibular duct, which passes forwards from the deep part of the gland.

## Submandibular gland

The **submandibular salivary gland** is about half the size of the parotid gland. It has a superficial and deep part. The **superficial part** is wedged between the body of the mandible and the mylohyoid muscle [see Fig. 8.1]. Anteriorly,

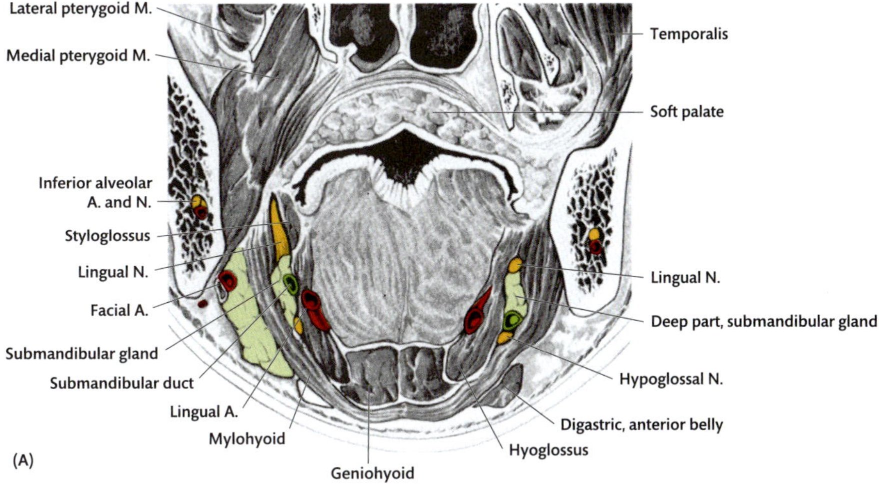


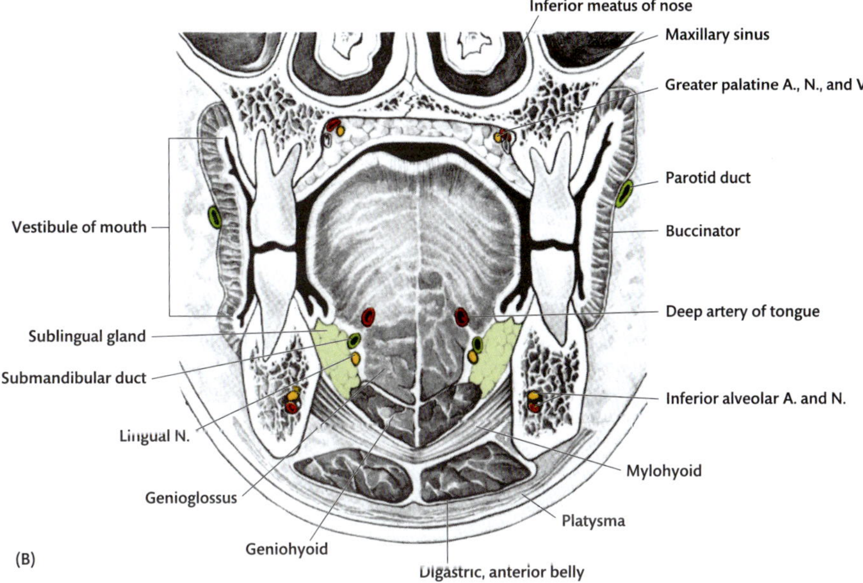


**Fig. 15.2** (A) Coronal section through the mouth, posterior to the molar teeth. (B) Coronal section through the mouth at the level of the second molar teeth.

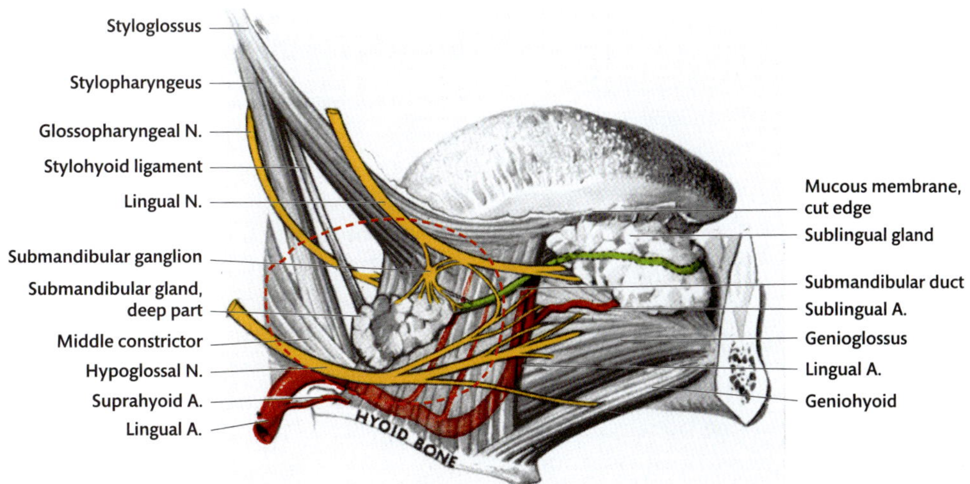


**Fig. 15.3** Dissection of the submandibular region. Dotted red line = position of the superficial part of the submandibular gland.

the superficial part reaches the level of the mental foramen, and superiorly it reaches up to the mylohyoid line on the medial surface of the mandible. Posterior to the free margin of the mylohyoid, the **deep part** of the gland extends forwards, deep to the mucous membrane of the mouth [Figs. 15.2A, 15.3].

The gland is loosely covered by the investing layer of the deep cervical fascia which ascends from the hyoid bone and splits to enclose it. The superficial layer of this fascia is attached to the inferior border of the mandible, and the thinner deep layer is attached to the mylohyoid line [see Fig. 2.15B]. Posteriorly, these layers fuse and form the stylomandibular ligament which separates the submandibular gland from the parotid gland.

## Superficial part of submandibular gland

The **superficial part** of the submandibular gland has three surfaces—inferolateral, lateral, and medial. The **inferolateral** surface is covered by: (1) the superficial fascia containing the platysma and the cervical branch of the facial nerve; (2) the deep fascia; and deep to this (3) the facial vein and a few **submandibular lymph nodes**. (Most of the lymph nodes lie in the groove between the submandibular gland and the mandible.) The **facial artery** grooves the posterosuperior part of this surface, then loops anteroinferiorly between the gland and the medial pterygoid muscle, and appears at the inferior margin of the mandible.

The **lateral** surface is related to the medial pterygoid, facial artery, and mandible [see Fig. 8.15]. The **medial** surface extends from the mylohyoid line inferiorly to the bellies of the digastric muscle. It is related to the mylohyoid, hyoglossus, hypoglossal, and lingual nerves and to the submandibular ganglion. The posterior part of the medial surface is in contact with the pharynx. This surface is grooved by the facial artery. The submandibular duct arises from the medial surface of the gland and passes anteriorly in the angle between the side of the tongue and the mylohyoid.

## Deep part of submandibular gland

The **deep part** of the gland is a thin, flat process which extends anteriorly on the lateral side of the duct [see Fig. 8.15; Figs. 15.2A, 15.3], superior to the mylohyoid. Figs. 15.4A and 15.4B are transverse sections through the head at the level of the submandibular glands.

## Nerves and vessels of the submandibular gland

(1) The sensory nerves to the gland are carried by the lingual nerve. (2) The parasympathetic secretomotor supply is from the nerve cells in the **submandibular ganglion**. The preganglionic parasympathetic fibres to the ganglion come through the chorda tympani branch of the facial nerve and the lingual nerve. The postganglionic fibres travel in the lingual nerve. (3) The sympathetics are carried by a plexus on the facial artery.

The arterial supply to the submandibular gland is from several small branches of the facial and submental arteries.

# Facial artery

The facial artery arises from the external carotid in the carotid triangle, immediately superior to the tip of the greater horn of the hyoid bone. It passes vertically upwards on the middle and superior constrictor muscles of the pharynx, under cover of the angle of the mandible and the digastric and stylohyoid muscles. It then turns forwards above these muscles and hooks round the posterosuperior part of the submandibular gland and the lower border of the mandible, to appear on the face at the anteroinferior angle of the masseter [see Figs. 3.6, 8.14, 8.15; Fig. 15.2A].

## Branches in the neck

The branches of the facial artery in the neck include: (1) the **ascending palatine artery**; (2) the **tonsillar artery**, which ascends superficial to the styloglossus and pierces the superior constrictor to reach the palatine tonsil [see Fig. 8.15]; (3) small **glandular branches**, which pass to the submandibular gland; and (4) the **submental artery**, which arises between the submandibular gland and the mandible and runs forwards on the inferior surface of the mylohyoid muscle [see Fig. 5.1]. It supplies the submandibular and sublingual glands and the adjacent muscles and skin.

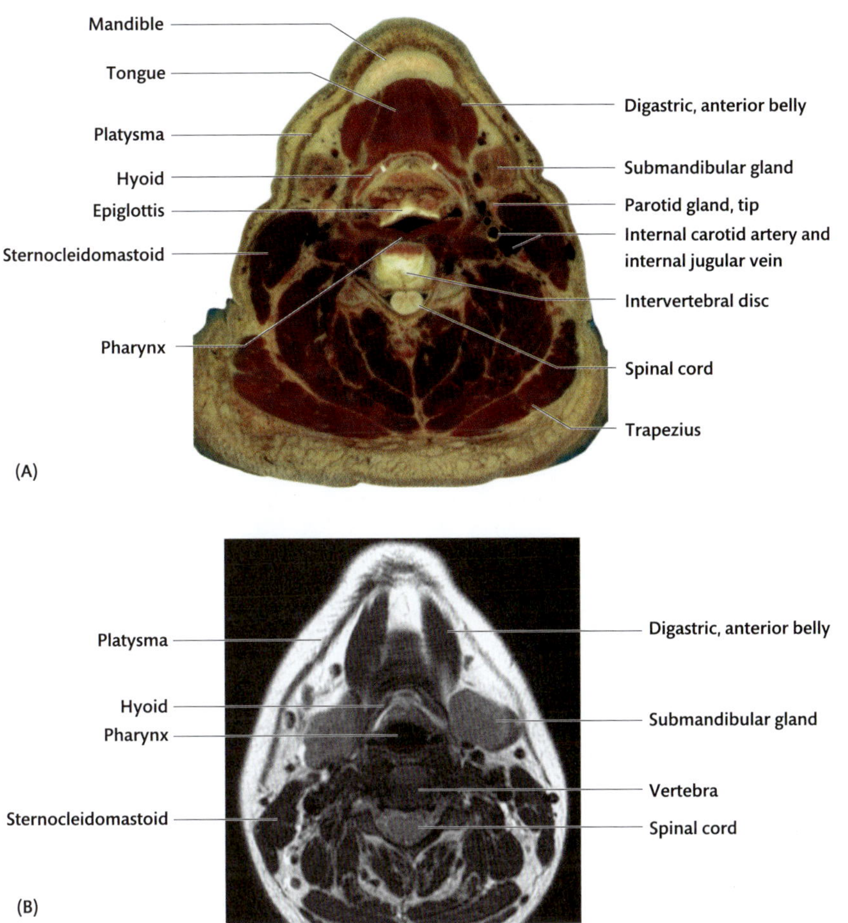


**Fig. 15.4** (A) Transverse section through the head at the level of the submandibular gland. (B) Axial T1-weighted magnetic resonance imaging (MRI) section at the level of the submandibular glands (SM).

(A) Image courtesy of the Visible Human Project of the US National Library of Medicine.

Using the instructions given in Dissection 15.3, expose the mylohyoid muscle.

### DISSECTION 15.3 Mylohyoid

**Objective**

**I.** To expose the mylohyoid muscle.

**Instructions**

1. Push the submandibular gland and the submental vessels posteriorly.
2. Cut the mylohyoid nerve, and turn the anterior belly of the digastric downwards.
3. Examine the attachments of the mylohyoid muscle.

## Mylohyoid muscle

**Origin**: the mylohyoid is a thin sheet of muscle which takes origin from the mylohyoid line on the mandible. **Insertion**: the fibres of the right and left muscles pass downwards, medially, and forwards and are inserted into a median fibrous raphe which extends from the mandible to the body of the hyoid bone. The most posterior fibres of the mylohyoid are inserted into the hyoid bone [see Fig. 5.1]. The two muscles together form a supporting sling under the tongue and separate the tongue from the submandibular region [Figs. 15.2A, 15.2B]. Each muscle has a free posterior border, around which the superficial and deep parts of the submandibular gland are continuous [see Fig. 5.5].

**Nerve supply**: the mylohyoid nerve. **Action**: it helps to raise the hyoid bone and tongue in swallowing and forms the muscular floor of the mouth.

Dissection 15.4 (and Fig. 15.5) provides instructions on further dissection of the submandibular region.





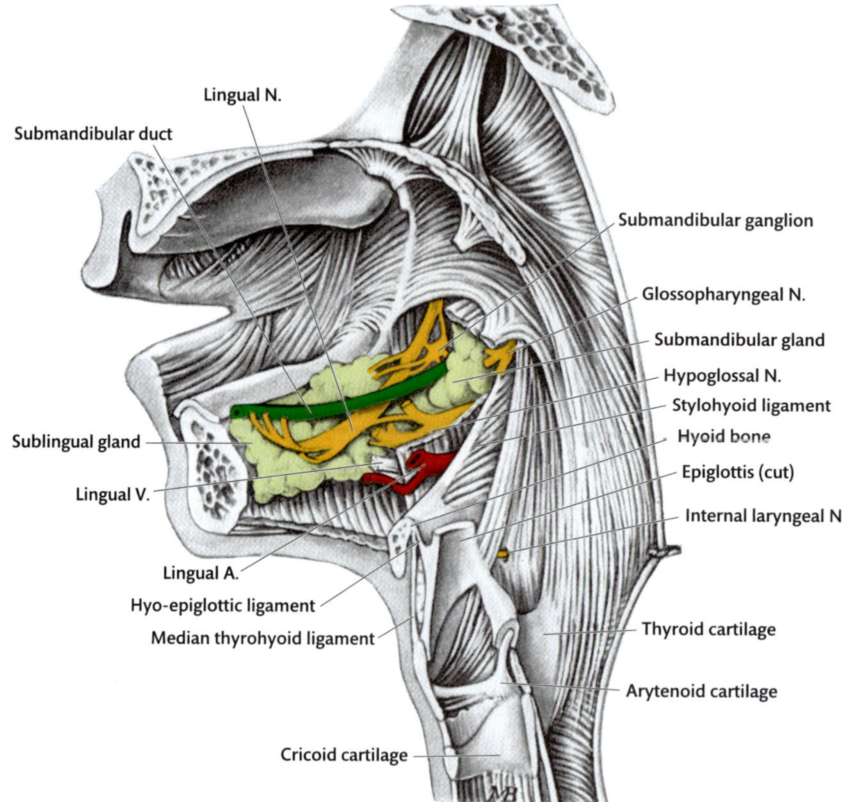


**Fig. 15.5** Dissection of the mouth and pharynx. The tongue has been removed to expose the structures which lie between it and the mylohyoid muscle.

**DISSECTION 15.4 Further dissection of the submandibular region**

**Objectives**

**I.** To identify the geniohyoid, genioglossus, styloglossus, and stylopharyngeus. **II.** To identify and trace the vessels and nerves on the floor of the mouth.

**Instructions**

1. From the medial side, identify the cut edge of the mylohyoid muscle [see Fig. 16.3], and separate it from the overlying geniohyoid by sliding a blunt instrument backwards and forwards between them.
2. Find the plane of separation between the geniohyoid and the genioglossus in the same way, and note that the fibres of the genioglossus radiate from the upper mental spine.
3. Pull the tongue away from the mandible, and cut carefully through the mucous membrane between it and the mandible. Strip the mucous membrane from the floor of the mouth and the mandible to expose the sublingual gland, the submandibular duct, the lingual nerve, the submandibular ganglion, the hypoglossal nerve [Fig. 15.3], and the deep lingual vein.
4. Make an opening into the submandibular duct, and pass a fine probe along it into the mouth.
5. Follow the lingual nerve posteriorly, and find its branches to the submandibular ganglion and the sublingual gland.
6. Note the proximity of the lingual nerve to the last molar tooth [Fig. 15.5].
7. Medial to the lingual nerve, hypoglossal nerve, and submandibular ganglion, clean the lateral surface

of the hyoglossus muscle, with the styloglossus mingling with it posteriorly.

8. The **lingual artery** is deep to the hyoglossus but appears at its anterior margin. Identify the artery.
9. Confirm the continuity of the hypoglossal nerve and lingual artery and vein with the same structures in the neck.
10. Trace the styloglossus back to the styloid process. Find the stylohyoid ligament and the stylopharyngeus attached to it. Try to trace the ligament towards the lesser horn of the hyoid bone, and follow the stylopharyngeus downwards.
11. Find the **glossopharyngeal nerve** as it curves round the **stylopharyngeus** and passes forwards deep to the hyoglossus.
12. Below the glossopharyngeal nerve, confirm the superior border of the middle constrictor muscle, and follow it to the hyoid bone and the stylohyoid ligament, lateral to the stylopharyngeus.

## Hyoglossus

**Origin**: the hyoglossus is a flat, quadrate muscle which takes origin from the greater horn and body of the hyoid bone. **Insertion**: its fibres pass superiorly into the posterior half of the side of the tongue, interdigitating with the fibres of the styloglossus [Fig. 15.3; see Fig. 2.17].

**Nerve supply**: the hypoglossal nerve. **Actions**: it depresses the side of the tongue and assists the genioglossus to enlarge the oral cavity in sucking, when the hyoid bone is fixed by the infrahyoid muscles.

## Styloglossus

**Origin**: the styloglossus is a long muscle which takes origin from the tip of the styloid process and the adjacent part of the stylohyoid ligament. **Insertion**: it passes anteroinferiorly and is inserted into the whole length of the side of the tongue, intermingling with the fibres of the hyoglossus [see Fig. 5.5; Fig. 15.3].

**Nerve supply**: the hypoglossal nerve. **Action**: it pulls the tongue posterosuperiorly in swallowing.

## Geniohyoid

**Origin**: the geniohyoid muscle takes origin from the lower mental spine on the mandible. **Insertion**: it is inserted into the body of the hyoid bone [see Figs. 2.16B, 2.17]. The two muscles lie side by side on the superior surface of the mylohyoid and are almost horizontal in the resting position [Fig. 15.2].

**Nerve supply**: the first cervical ventral ramus through the hypoglossal nerve. **Action**: it pulls the elevated hyoid bone directly forwards, sliding the pulley on the taut intermediate tendon of the digastric. This increases the anteroposterior diameter of the pharynx to receive the bolus of food during swallowing.

## Genioglossus

The genioglossus is a flat, fan-shaped muscle in contact with its fellow in the median plane. **Origin**: it arises from the upper mental spine of the mandible and spreads out into the tongue in a vertical plane. **Insertion**: it is inserted into the paramedian part of the dorsum of the tongue from the tip of the tongue almost to the hyoid bone [see Fig. 17.2; Fig. 15.3].

**Nerve supply**: the hypoglossal nerve. **Actions**: the posteroinferior fibres of the two muscles, acting together, protrude the tongue. The muscles also depress the central part of the tongue and increase the volume of the mouth (e.g. in sucking). The anterior fibres depress the tip of the tongue and retract it. ➲ If one muscle is active and the other is paralysed, the tip of the tongue deviates towards the paralysed side when protruded.

## Submandibular duct

The submandibular duct emerges from the medial surface of the submandibular gland. It runs anterosuperiorly in the angle between the mylohyoid and the side of the tongue. It opens on the floor of the mouth beneath the anterior part of the tongue, on the sublingual papilla [see Fig. 16.2; Figs. 15.3, 15.5]. Examine these structures in the floor of your mouth. The wall of the duct is much thinner than that of the parotid gland and is not easily palpated.

At first, the submandibular duct lies on the hyoglossus, between the lingual nerve above and the hypoglossal nerve below, separated from the mylohoid muscle by the deep part of the submandibular gland. Further anteriorly, it passes on to the genioglossus and has the sublingual gland between it and the mylohyoid. The **lingual nerve** hooks round the inferior surface of the duct and runs upwards into the tongue, medial to the duct [Fig. 15.3].

➲ **Sialolithiasis** is the formation of calculi (stones) within the salivary gland. If the calculus forms in a duct, then saliva will be trapped in the gland. This may cause painful swelling and inflammation of the gland.

## Sublingual gland

The sublingual gland is the smallest of the large salivary glands (3 cm long). It lies on the mylohyoid between the mandible and the genioglossus muscle, and forms the sublingual fold on the floor of the mouth [Figs. 15.1, 15.2B, 15.3, 15.5]. The lingual nerve and submandibular duct lie medial to it.

## Ducts of the sublingual gland

Numerous small ducts (8–20) open into the mouth on the sublingual fold.

➲ When the duct of a salivary gland is obstructed, the secretions remaining in the gland may develop into a retention cyst, with the gland itself becoming swollen. Such a retention cyst can be the result of minor trauma to the oral mucosa, resulting in fibrosis and scarring around the duct. A **ranula** is a large, tense, bluish swelling in the floor of the mouth, to one side of the midline. It results from obstruction to drainage of the sublingual gland.

### Vessels and nerves of the sublingual gland

The arterial supply to the sublingual gland is from the sublingual branch of the lingual artery. The nerve supply is from branches of the lingual nerve. The lingual nerve contains post-ganglionic parasympathetic fibres from the cells of the submandibular ganglion. It also contains sensory and post-ganglionic sympathetic fibres [Fig. 15.5].

## Lingual nerve

The lingual nerve is a branch of the posterior division of the mandibular nerve. It descends between the ramus of the mandible and the medial pterygoid muscle [see Fig. 14.2]. It then turns forwards and enters the mouth by passing inferior to the lower border of the superior constrictor muscle of the pharynx [see Fig. 2.16B; Fig. 15.5]. It continues anteroinferiorly between the mucous membrane of the mouth and the body of the mandible, postero-inferior to the last molar tooth [Fig. 15.1]. In the submandibular region, the nerve lies close to the side of the tongue, crosses the styloglossus and the upper part of the hyoglossus, and hooks beneath the submandibular duct [Fig. 15.3]. ➲ The lingual nerve is liable to be injured by clumsy extraction of the last molar tooth. It is also accessible to local anaesthetics at this point.

### Branches of the lingual nerve

The lingual nerve: (1) communicates with the submandibular ganglion through two or more branches; and (2) sends one or two branches to the hypoglossal nerve. These branches descend along the anterior border of the hyoglossus [Fig. 15.3]. It gives: (3) thin branches to the mucous membrane of the mouth and gums; (4) a few small branches to the sublingual gland; and (5) branches which pierce the substance of the tongue and run superiorly to supply the mucous membrane of the anterior two-thirds of the tongue.

## Submandibular ganglion

The submandibular ganglion is one of the four parasympathetic ganglia in the head. It lies on the upper part of the hyoglossus muscle, inferior to the lingual nerve and superior to the submandibular duct. It is suspended from the lingual nerve by two short branches [Fig. 15.3]. The posterior of these branches carries preganglionic **parasympathetic nerve fibres** from the chorda tympani branch of the facial nerve. These nerves synapse on the cells of the ganglion. The anterior branch carries axons from the ganglion cells (post-ganglionic fibres) to the lingual nerve for distribution to the sublingual gland and to the glands in the anterior two-thirds of the tongue. From the inferior border of the submandibular ganglion, several small branches carry post-ganglionic fibres to the submandibular gland and duct and to the mucous membrane of the mouth.

Post-ganglionic **sympathetic fibres** reach the ganglion from the plexuses on the facial and lingual arteries, and supply the glands [Figs. 15.3, 15.5]. **Sensory fibres** from the lingual nerve also traverse the ganglion and are distributed through its branches.

**DISSECTION 15.5 Structures deep to the hyoglossus**

**Objectives**

**I.** To identify and trace the lingual vessels deep to the hyoglossus. **II.** To expose the genioglossus, middle constrictor, and stylohyoid ligament.

**Instructions**

1. Detach the hyoglossus carefully from the hyoid bone, and turn it upwards without dividing the structures on its lateral surface.
2. Identify: (1) the lingual artery and its dorsal branches; (2) the lingual veins; (3) the posterior part of the genioglossus and the origin of the middle constrictor muscle of the pharynx; and (4) the attachment of the stylohyoid ligament.

## Hypoglossal nerve

The **hypoglossal nerve** has been traced to the posterior margin of the mylohyoid muscle [Chapter 5]. It can now be followed anteriorly with the deep lingual vein across the hyoglossus, between the hyoid bone and the submandibular duct. Anterior to the hyoglossus, the hypoglossal nerve pierces the genioglossus muscle and breaks up into branches to the muscles of the tongue [Fig. 15.3].

### Branches of the hypoglossal nerve

The hypoglossal nerve supplies the styloglossus, hyoglossus, genioglossus, geniohyoid (C. 1 fibres), and intrinsic muscles of the tongue (all the tongue muscles, except the palatoglossus which is supplied by the vagus).

It communicates freely with the lingual nerve on the lateral surface of the hyoglossus and in the substance of the tongue. These communications transmit sensory nerve fibres from the muscles to the brainstem. For distribution of the first cervical nerve with the hypoglossal nerve, see ansa cervicalis [Chapter 5].

Using the instructions given in Dissection 15.5, dissect the structures deep to the hyoglossus.

## Lingual artery

The lingual artery arises from the front of the external carotid artery, opposite the tip of the greater horn of the hyoid bone. It loops on the hyoid bone, runs anteriorly under cover of the hyoglossus, and ends by becoming the deep artery of the tongue [see Fig. 8.15; Fig. 15.3].

The initial segment lies deep to the skin, fasciae, and hypoglossal nerve, before passing deep to the hyoglossus. It gives off the **suprahyoid artery** which runs along the superior border of the hyoid bone, lateral to the hyoglossus. Deep to the hyoglossus, the artery gives off two or more **dorsal lingual branches**, which run posterosuperiorly to supply the substance of the tongue and end in the mucous membrane [Fig. 15.3].

At the anterior border of the hyoglossus, the lingual artery is crossed by branches of the hypoglossal nerve, the submandibular duct, and the lingual nerve. It gives off the **sublingual artery**, which runs anterosuperiorly to supply the sublingual gland and the neighbouring muscles [Fig. 15.3].

The lingual artery continues as the **deep artery of the tongue**, which enters the tongue about its middle and runs forwards to the tip, lying close to the mucous membrane of the ventral surface of the tongue. It is tortuous to allow for elongation of the tongue when protruded. It sends numerous branches into the substance of the tongue [Fig. 15.3].

## Veins of the tongue

The arrangement of the veins of the tongue is variable. The **deep lingual vein** is the principal vein of the tongue. It begins at the tip of the tongue and runs posteriorly near the median plane. It lies immediately deep to the mucous membrane on the inferior surface of the tongue and can be seen through it in life [see Fig. 16.1]. It descends along the anterior margin of the hyoglossus and crosses the superficial surface of that muscle below the hypoglossal nerve. Two venae commitantes run with the lingual artery and are joined by the dorsal lingual veins. All the veins unite at the posterior border of the hyoglossus to form the **lingual vein**. The lingual vein either joins the facial vein or crosses the external and internal carotid arteries to drain into the internal jugular vein [see Fig. 5.1].

## Stylohyoid ligament

The stylohyoid ligament passes from the tip of the styloid process of the temporal bone to the lesser horn of the hyoid bone. It may be partly cartilaginous or ossified. Occasionally, it may contain muscle fibres [Figs. 15.3, 15.5].

It is of embryological interest as it represents the remnant of the cartilage of the second pharyngeal arch of the embryo. The remainder of the cartilage forms the stapes, the styloid process of the temporal bone, the lesser horn, and the upper part of the body of the hyoid bone. It corresponds to the sphenomandibular ligament of the first pharyngeal arch.

CHAPTER 16

# The mouth and pharynx

## The mouth

The mouth is the first part of the digestive tube. It is subdivided by the teeth and gums into the smaller external vestibule, which is immediately deep to the lips and cheeks, and the larger mouth proper within the dental arch.

### Vestibule of the mouth

The vestibule receives the ducts of the parotid glands and the mucous glands of the lips and cheeks. Superiorly and inferiorly, it is bound to the maxillae and mandible by the reflection of the mucous membrane from the lips and cheeks. Posteriorly, the vestibule communicates with the cavity of the mouth proper through the interval between the last molar teeth and the rami of the mandible. ➲ In paralysis of the facial muscles, the lips and cheeks fall away from the teeth and gums, and food tends to lodge in the vestibule.

## Lips

The superficial structures in the lips have been examined [Chapter 3]. Each lip consists of a sheet of muscle covered externally by skin and internally by mucous membrane and connective tissue. The muscle layer is formed by the orbicularis oris and the facial muscles which converge on it. The mucous membrane is continuous with the skin at the margins of the lips. In the midline, the mucous membrane forms a raised fold—the **frenulum**—between the lip and the jaw. Deep to the mucous layer are numerous mucous **labial glands** with ducts which open into the vestibule of the mouth. Each lip has an **arterial arch** formed by the labial branches of the facial arteries [see Fig. 3.6].

The **lymph vessels** of the lower lip pass to the submandibular nodes; those of the upper lip pass to the submandibular and superficial parotid nodes.



## Cheeks

The cheeks are directly continuous with the lips and have the same general structure. The principal muscle in the cheek is the **buccinator**. Posteriorly, the buccinator lies edge to edge with the superior constrictor muscle of the pharynx at the pterygomandibular raphe [see Fig. 5.6]. It is covered externally by the **buccopharyngeal fascia** and internally by the **pharyngobasilar fascia**.

There is a considerable amount of subcutaneous fat in the cheek—the **buccal pad of fat**. It is particularly well formed in infants and assists in sucking by increasing the rigidity of the cheek in the absence of teeth. Numerous **buccal glands** lie in the connective tissue beneath the mucosa, and four or five larger mucous **molar glands** lie external to the buccinator around the entry of the parotid duct. The **parotid duct** passes above the buccal pad of fat, pierces the buccinator and its fasciae, and enters the mouth opposite the second upper molar tooth [see Fig. 3.6].

## Gums and teeth

The gums are composed of dense fibrous tissue covered with a smooth, vascular mucous membrane. They are attached to the alveolar margins of the jaws and the neck of the teeth. At the neck of a tooth, the fibrous tissue of the gum is continuous with the **periodontal membrane** which attaches the tooth to its socket.

In the adult, there are eight **permanent teeth** in each half of the jaw. These are the two incisors, one canine, two premolars, and three molars. The complete **primary dentition** consists of five teeth in each half of the jaw. Two incisors, one canine, and two molars. The first of these to erupt are the lower central incisors which erupt at approximately six months of age. The last milk teeth to erupt are the second milk molars at approximately two years of age. The first permanent tooth to erupt is the first molar. It erupts at approximately six years of age.

## Floor of the mouth

The floor of the mouth is covered by mucous membrane. Laterally, this mucous membrane passes from the side of the tongue on to the mandible. Anteriorly, it stretches from one half of the mandible to the other, beneath the free anterior part of the tongue. In the midline, it forms a fold—the **frenulum of the tongue**—between the floor of the mouth and the inferior surface of the tongue. On both sides of the frenulum, the sublingual gland bulges upwards, forming the **sublingual fold** which ends anteriorly in the **sublingual papilla**. The submandibular duct opens on the apex of the papilla. The sublingual ducts open in a series of minute apertures on the top of the sublingual fold [Fig. 16.1].

## Roof of the mouth

The roof of the mouth is formed by the vaulted palate [Figs. 16.2, 16.3]. The anterior two-thirds of the palate is bony—the **hard palate**; the posterior third is made up of soft tissue—the **soft palate**.

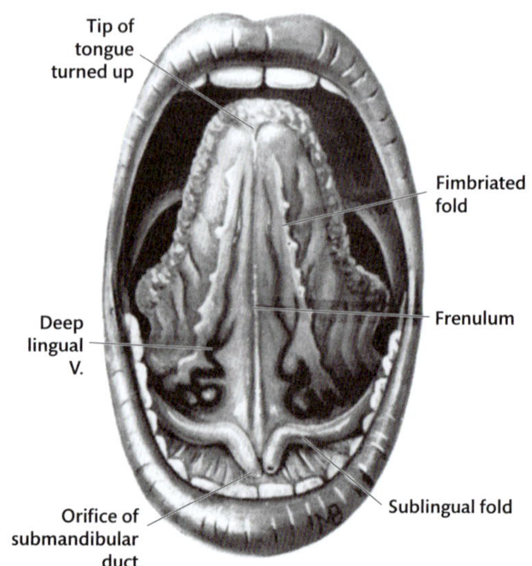


**Fig. 16.1** The inferior surface of the tongue.

The soft palate has a free posterior margin from which hangs down the median **uvula**. A poorly marked median raphe, representing the line of embryological fusion between the two halves of the palate, extends from the incisive fossa to the uvula. The mucous membrane of the anterior part of the hard palate is thrown into 3–4 **transverse palatine folds**. The mucous membrane of the posterior part is comparatively smooth. The **pterygoid hamulus** can be palpated posterior to the lingual surface of the third upper molar tooth.

## Oropharyngeal isthmus

Posteriorly, the oral cavity continues with the oropharynx at the oropharyngeal isthmus bounded by the soft palate, the palatoglossal arches, and the dorsum of the tongue [Fig. 16.2].

The palatoglossal arches are formed by mucous membrane covering the palatoglossus muscle from the soft palate to the posterior part of the side of the tongue [Fig. 16.2].

## The pharynx

The pharynx is a wide muscular tube, about 12 cm long. It extends from the base of the skull above

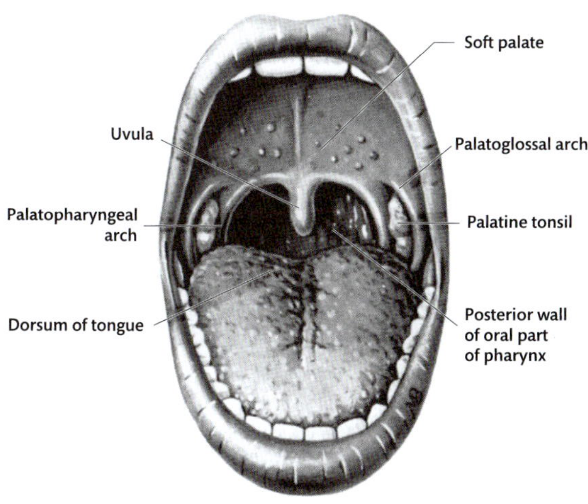


Fig. 16.2 The structures seen through the widely open mouth.

to the level of the body of the sixth cervical vertebra below [Fig. 16.3] where it is continuous with the oesophagus. The pharynx lies posterior to the nasal cavities and septum (**nasopharynx**), the mouth (**oropharynx**), and the larynx (**laryngopharynx**). It conducts air to and from the larynx, and food to the oesophagus. The oral part of the pharynx is common to both functions.

The pharynx is widest at the base of the skull, posterior to the orifices of the auditory tubes. From there, it narrows to the level of the palate (**pharyngeal isthmus**), widens again in the oral and laryngeal parts, and then rapidly narrows to the oesophagus.

The walls of the pharynx above the opening of the larynx are not in contact with each other and allow the passage of air through the mouth or nasal cavities to the larynx. Below the opening of the larynx, the anterior and posterior walls are in contact.

## Position

The pharynx lies anterior to the prevertebral fascia. The retropharyngeal space allows the pharynx to slide freely on the prevertebral fascia during swallowing. Lateral to the pharynx is the neurovascular bundle of the neck (common and internal carotid





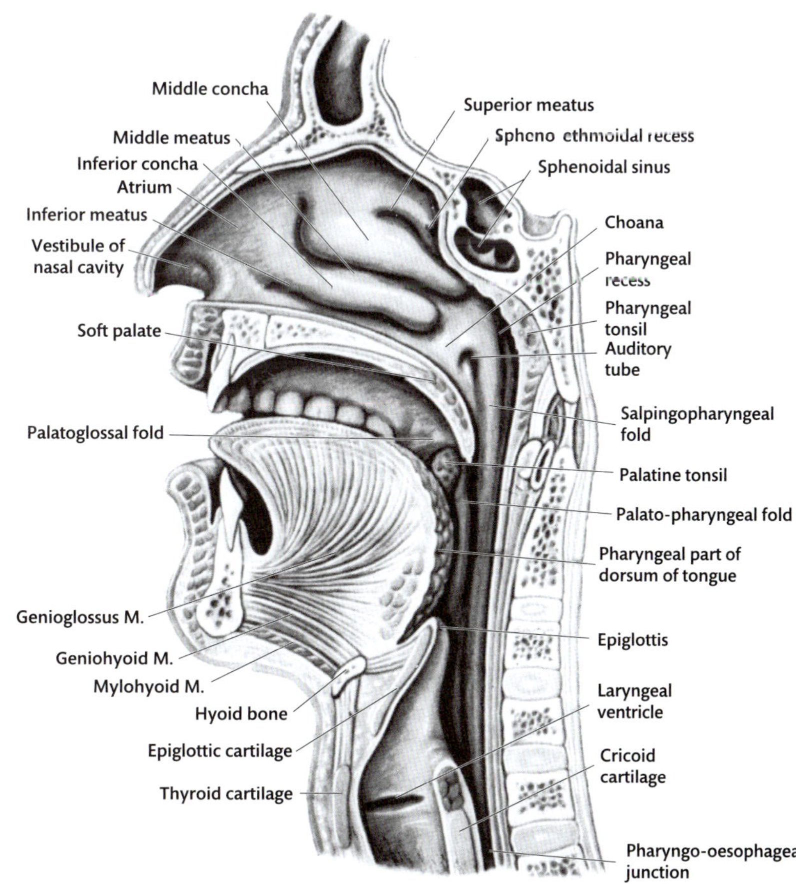


Fig. 16.3 Paramedian section through the nose, mouth, pharynx, and larynx.

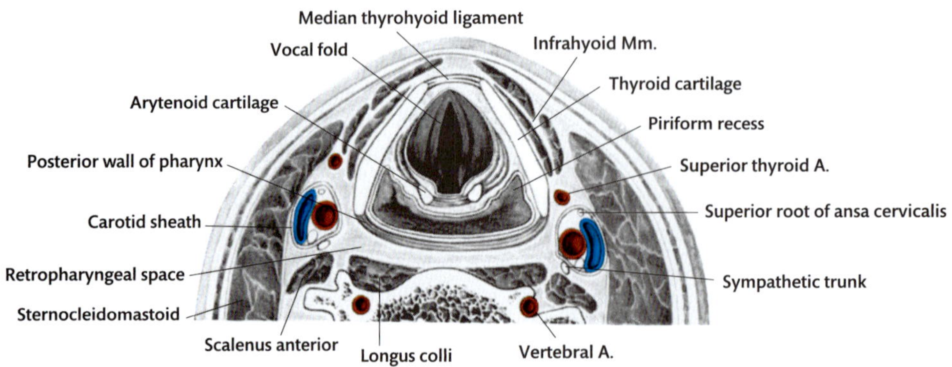


**Fig. 16.4** Transverse section through the anterior part of the neck at the level of the upper part of the thyroid cartilage.

arteries, internal jugular vein, and vagus nerve) in the carotid sheath [Fig. 16.4], and the styloid process of the temporal bone and its muscles. The pharyngeal plexus of nerves ramifies on the pharynx and supplies it with motor and sensory fibres. Anteriorly, the pharynx opens into the nasal cavities, mouth, and larynx. The pharyngeal muscles are attached to structures in the lateral walls of these apertures.

## Pharyngeal wall

The wall of the pharynx consists of five layers. From within out, they are the: (1) mucous membrane; (2) submucosa; (3) pharyngobasilar fascia; (4) pharyngeal muscles; and (5) buccopharyngeal fascia.

The **buccopharyngeal fascia** covers the external surfaces of the buccinator and the pharyngeal muscles. The **pharyngobasilar fascia** lines the internal surface of the pharyngeal muscles and attaches the pharynx to the base of the skull, the auditory tubes, and the lateral margins of the posterior nasal apertures (choanae). It also fills the gap in the pharyngeal wall above the free superior margin of the superior constrictor muscle [Fig. 16.5].

The muscles of the pharynx consist of the three constrictors—the superior, middle, and inferior constrictors—and three longitudinal muscles—the stylopharyngeus, salpingopharyngeus, and palatopharyngeus [Fig. 16.5].

Using the instructions given in Dissection 16.1 (and Fig. 16.6), dissect the muscles of the pharynx.

## Pharyngeal plexus of veins

The pharyngeal plexus of veins lies on the posterior wall of the pharynx and receives blood from the pharynx and soft palate. Two or more veins drain from the plexus to each internal jugular vein. It also communicates with the pterygoid plexus and the cavernous sinuses.

## Constrictor muscles of the pharynx–overview

The three constrictor muscles—the superior, middle, and inferior constrictors—form a curved sheet on the posterior and lateral walls of the pharynx. They overlap each other from below upwards [Fig. 16.5]. They take origin from a series of bones and ligaments on the lateral wall and are inserted posteriorly into a median fibrous **raphe** which descends from the **pharyngeal tubercle** on the base of the skull to the oesophagus [Fig. 16.7]. **Nerve supply**: the pharyngeal plexus of the glossopharyngeal and vagus nerves, with an additional supply to the inferior constrictor from the external and recurrent laryngeal nerves. **Actions**: constriction of the pharynx to move the bolus of food down during swallowing. This is preceded by relaxation of muscles to receive the bolus. (Details of swallowing and action of muscles at each stage are described below.)

Dissection 16.2 provides instructions on dissection of the superior constrictor.

### Superior constrictor

The superior constrictor lies in the wall of the nasal and oral parts of the pharynx. **Origin**: it arises from the lower part of the posterior margin of the medial pterygoid lamina, the pterygoid hamulus, the pterygomandibular raphe, the mandible near the posterior end of the mylohyoid line, and the mucous membrane of the mouth and side of the tongue. The **pterygomandibular raphe** is formed by the interlacing tendinous fibres of the superior constrictor and buccinator muscles. It extends from the pterygoid hamulus to the

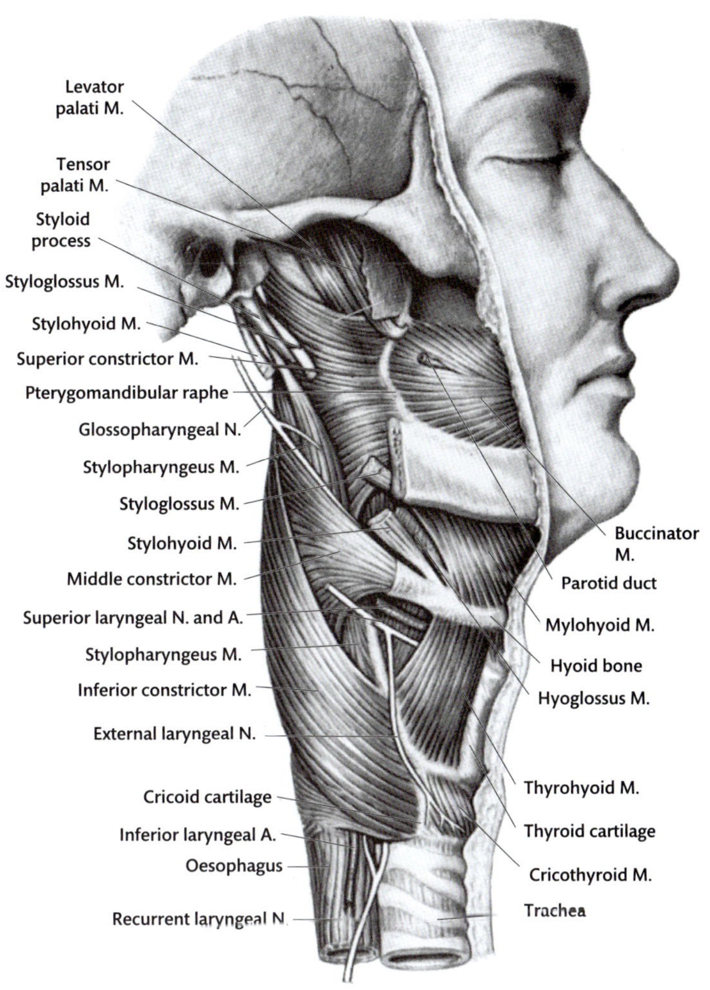


**Fig. 16.5** Lateral view of the constrictors of the pharynx and associated muscles.

mandible near the posterior end of the mylohyoid line. The tendinous fibres run horizontally and are capable of separating and allowing the raphe to stretch when the mouth is opened [Fig. 16.5]. **Insertion**: the superior constrictor curves posteriorly to the median raphe. The upper fibres ascend to the pharyngeal tubercle [see Fig. 2.11]; the lower fibres descend internal to the middle constrictor. The stylopharyngeus muscle and glossopharyngeal nerve enter the pharynx between the superior and middle constrictors [Fig. 16.5].

The free **upper border** of the superior constrictor extends from the medial pterygoid lamina to the pharyngeal tubercle, leaving a gap between it and the skull. This gap is filled by the pharyngobasilar fascia, the tensor and levator palati muscles, and the auditory tube between them [Fig. 16.5]. The **auditory tube** and the **levator muscle** of the palate enter the pharynx above the superior margin of the superior constrictor, together with the ascending palatine artery. The **tensor palati** descends external to the upper part of the superior constrictor.

**Nerve supply**: the pharyngeal plexus of the glossopharyngeal and vagus nerves. **Actions**: acting with the horizontal fibres of the palatopharyngeus, it causes constriction of the pharynx, and separates the nasopharynx from the oropharynx during swallowing.

## Middle constrictor

The middle constrictor is a fan-shaped muscle. **Origin**: it takes origin from the greater and lesser horns of the hyoid bone, and the lower part of the

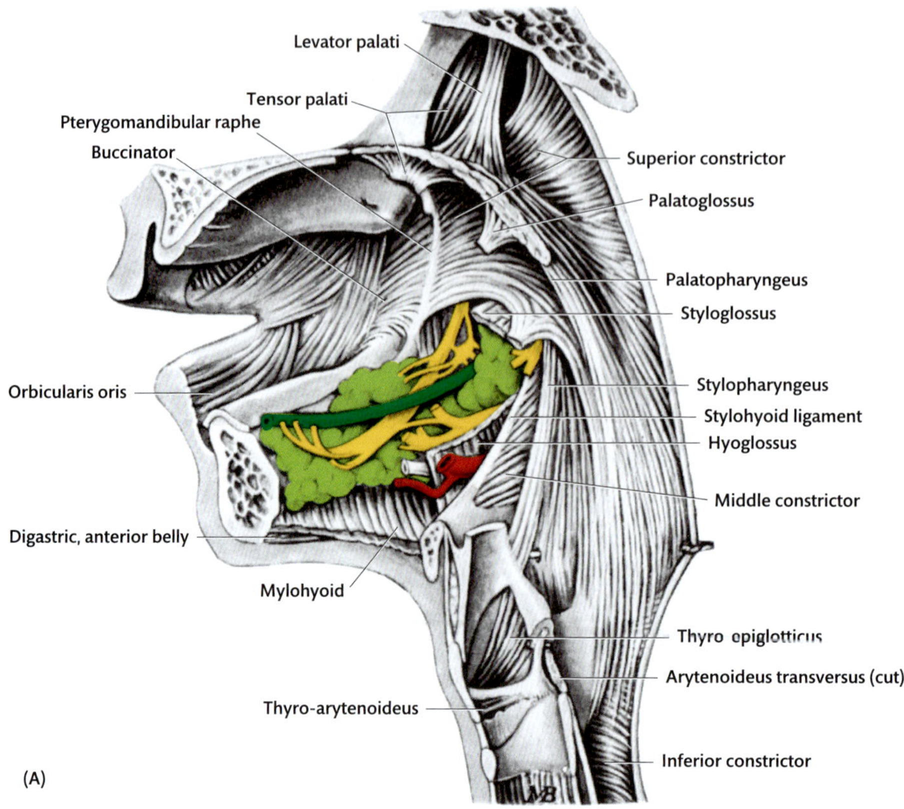


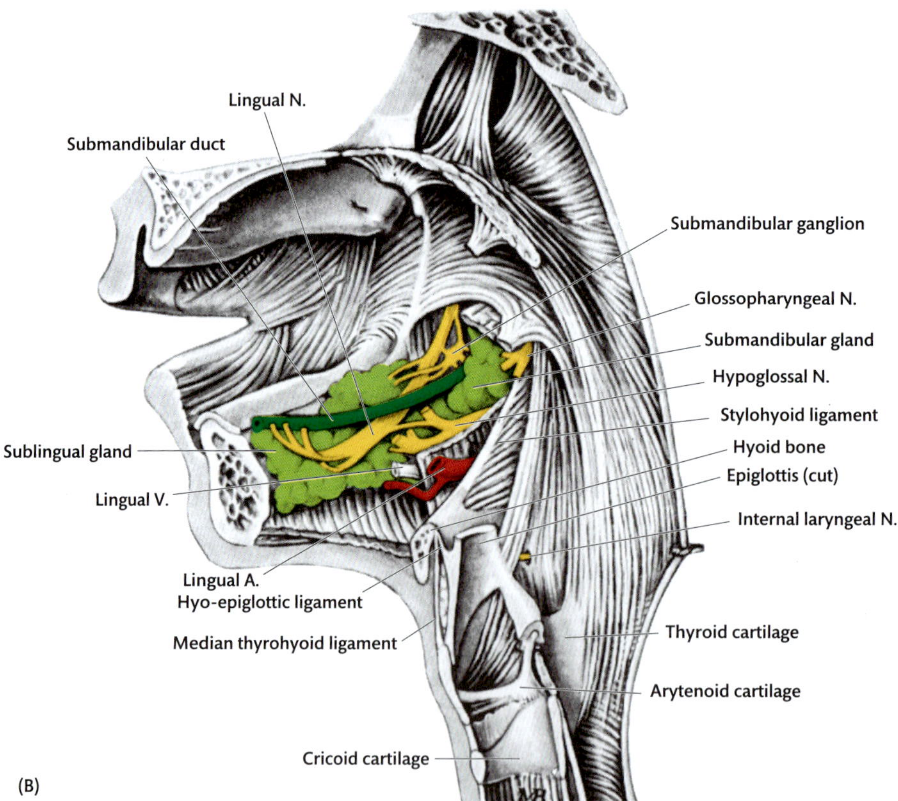


**Fig. 16.6** (A) and (B) Structures lying adjacent to the mucous membrane of the mouth, pharynx, and larynx, seen from the medial side. The tongue has been removed to expose the structures which lie between it and the mylohyoid muscle.

## DISSECTION 16.1 Muscles of the pharynx

### Objectives

**I.** To identify the three constrictors of the pharynx.
**II.** To identify and trace the stylopharyngeus muscle and glossopharyngeal nerve.

### Instructions

1. On the right side, remove the buccopharyngeal fascia from the external surfaces of the pharyngeal muscles [Fig. 16.5].
2. Note the plexus of nerves and veins, and then remove them.
3. On the posterior surface of the pharynx at the level of the angle of the mandible, find the stylopharyngeus muscle entering the pharynx between the superior and middle constrictor muscles [Fig. 16.5].
4. Expose the glossopharyngeal nerve winding spirally round the posterior surface of the stylopharyngeus. Trace the branch to the stylopharyngeus. The nerve will be followed into the posterior part of the tongue later.
5. Find the upper border of the inferior constrictor. Turn this downwards, and expose the lowest fibres of the middle constrictor arching upwards from the hyoid bone.
6. On the left side, examine the interior of the pharynx, and strip off its mucous membrane to expose the pharyngeal muscles from the medial side [Fig. 16.6].



stylohyoid ligament [Figs. 16.5, 16.6]. **Insertion**: from this curved origin, the fibres fan out into the pharyngeal wall and the upper fibres curve up; the middle fibres run horizontally, and the lower fibres curve down. The inferior part of the muscle passes deep to the inferior constrictor posteriorly but is separated from it laterally by a gap. The internal branch of the superior laryngeal nerve and the superior laryngeal artery pass through this gap to pierce the thyrohyoid membrane and enter into the pharynx [Fig. 16.5].

**Nerve supply**: the pharyngeal plexus of the glossopharyngeal and vagus nerves. **Actions**: constriction of the pharynx to move the bolus of food down. Prior to this, the muscles is relaxed to receive the bolus from the oropharynx.

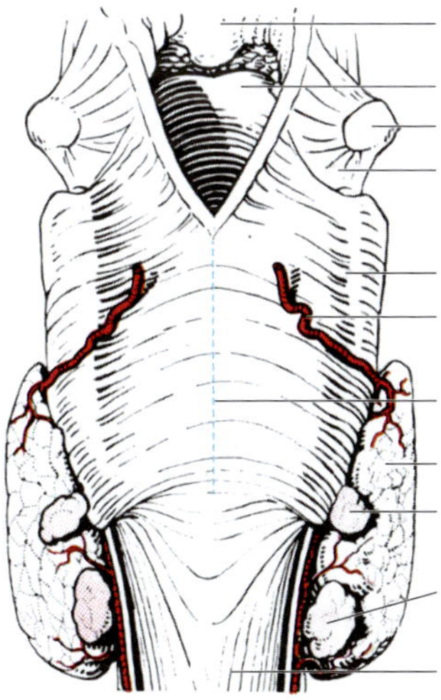

**Fig. 16.7** Posterior surface of the inferior part of the pharynx. The upper part of the posterior wall has been cut to show the interior of the oropharynx.

### Inferior constrictor

**Origin**: the inferior constrictor takes origin from the side of the cricoid cartilage, the fascia covering the cricothyroid, and the oblique line on the thyroid cartilage [Fig. 16.5]. The part of the muscle arising from the thyroid cartilage is the **thyropharyngeus**, and that arising from the fascia over the cricothyroid and the cricoid cartilage is the **cricopharyngeus**. **Insertion**: its fibres sweep posteriorly to the median raphe; the lowest fibres are horizontal, but the upper fibres ascend with increasing obliquity. The highest fibres almost reach the base of the skull, external to the other two constrictors. Inferiorly, the inferior constrictor overlaps the beginning of the oesophagus, the recurrent laryngeal nerve, and the inferior laryngeal artery [Figs. 16.7, 16.5].

## DISSECTION 16.2 Superior constrictor of the pharynx

### Objective

**I.** To expose the superior constrictor of the pharynx.

### Instructions

1. On the right side, detach the medial pterygoid muscle from its origin and turn it down. This exposes the full extent of the superior constrictor.

**Nerve supply**: the pharyngeal plexus of the glossopharyngeal and vagus nerves, with an additional supply to the inferior constrictor from the external and recurrent laryngeal nerves. **Actions**: constriction of the pharynx during swallowing.

➲ The fibres of the cricopharyngeus form two bands. The upper fibres run obliquely backwards and upwards to the median raphe. The lower fibres run transversely to encircle the pharynx. An area of intrinsic weakness exists between the two bands—the **Killian's triangle**. **Hypopharyngeal diverticula**—protrusions of the mucosa through the muscle layers—commonly occur through this part of the pharyngeal wall.

Hypopharyngeal diverticula can also occur above the cricopharyngeus (between the cricopharyngeus and the thyropharyngeus) or below the cricopharyngeus (between the cricopharyngeus and the oesophagus).

## Salpingopharyngeus

**Origin**: this slender muscle arises by one or two slips from the inferior border of the pharyngeal end of the auditory tube. **Insertion**: it descends in the salpingopharyngeal fold to join the palatopharyngeus and is inserted into the posterior border of the thyroid cartilage. **Nerve supply**: the vagus nerve through the pharyngeal plexus **Action**: opens the auditory tube.

## Palatopharyngeus

**Origin**: the palatopharyngeus arises from the superior surface of the soft palate and the posterior margin of the hard palate. The fibres of the palatopharyngeus spread over the internal surface of the constrictors. **Insertion**: the superior margin of the palatopharyngeus passes almost horizontally backwards around the pharyngeal isthmus. Most of the muscle fibres converge on the palatopharyngeal arch and run inferiorly in it, on the internal surfaces of the constrictors of the pharynx. It is inserted into the posterior border of the lamina of the thyroid cartilage and fans out into the posterior pharyngeal wall [Fig. 16.6]. Superiorly, the palatopharyngeus is joined by the salpingopharyngeus, and inferiorly by the stylopharyngeus at the interval between the middle and superior constrictors.

➲ The part which surrounds the pharyngeal isthmus is greatly hypertrophied in persons with cleft palate, in an attempt to separate the oral and nasal parts of the pharynx.

**Nerve supply**: the pharyngeal plexus formed by the glossopharyngeal and vagus nerves. **Actions**: the main mass of the palatopharyngeus depresses the palate onto the posterior part of the dorsum of the tongue and prevents the soft palate from being forced into the nasal part of the pharynx when blowing against resistance through the mouth. The horizontal fibres, with those of the superior constrictor, narrow the pharyngeal isthmus. They also raise a ridge in the pharyngeal wall, against which the soft palate is elevated by the levator palati to separate the oropharynx and nasopharynx.

## Stylopharyngeus

The stylopharyngeus is the longest of the three styloid muscles. **Origin**: it arises from the medial surface of the styloid process close to its root. It runs anteroinferiorly, between the internal and external carotid arteries, and passes obliquely through the pharyngeal wall between the superior and middle constrictor muscles [Fig. 16.5]. **Insertion**: within the pharynx, it blends with the anterior fibres of the palatopharyngeus and is inserted partly with it and partly into the lateral aspect of the epiglottis [Fig. 16.5]. **Nerve supply**: the glossopharyngeal nerve. **Actions**: it helps to raise the larynx and pulls the base of the epiglottis upwards and backwards during swallowing and speaking.

## Interior of the pharynx

The pharynx is lined by a mucous membrane, and the submucosa contains numerous mucous **pharyngeal glands** and nodules of lymph tissue. Aggregations of these **lymph follicles** form the pharyngeal, tubal, palatine, and lingual **tonsils**.

# Nasopharynx

The nasal part of the pharynx, or nasopharynx, lies superior to the soft palate and is continuous inferiorly with the oral part, or oropharynx, through the narrow **pharyngeal isthmus** [Fig. 16.3]. The opening of the nasal cavities into the nasopharynx is known as the **choana**. Each choana is oval in shape, approximately 2.5 cm high and 1.5 cm wide, and extends from the base of the skull to the posterior edge of the hard palate. They are separated from each other by the nasal septum [Fig. 16.3].

The **roof** and **posterior wall** of the nasopharynx form a continuous curved surface. This surface extends over the inferior aspect of the sphenoid, the basilar part of the occipital bone, and the superior part of the longus capitis muscle. The **pharyngeal tonsil** bulges the mucous membrane into the cavity of the pharynx where the roof becomes continuous with the posterior wall [Fig. 16.3]. ➲ This lymph tissue is often enlarged in children—the **adenoids**. It may be large enough to block the nasal part of the pharynx and give a 'nasal' quality to the voice.

The **pharyngeal orifice of the auditory tube** lies on the **lateral wall** of the pharynx, at the level of the inferior concha of the nose [Fig. 16.8]. It is bound superiorly and posteriorly by a firm, rounded **tubal ridge** around which lies the **tubal tonsil**. The slender **salpingopharyngeus muscle** descends from the tubal ridge into

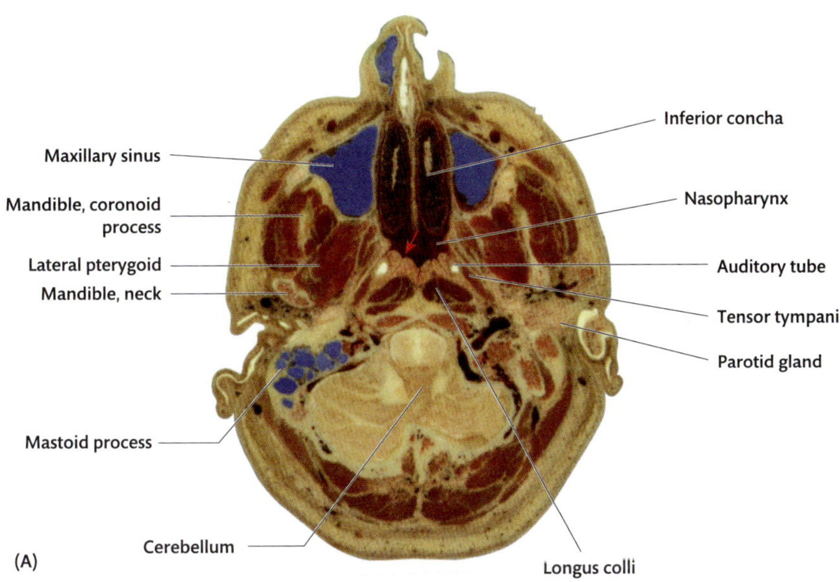


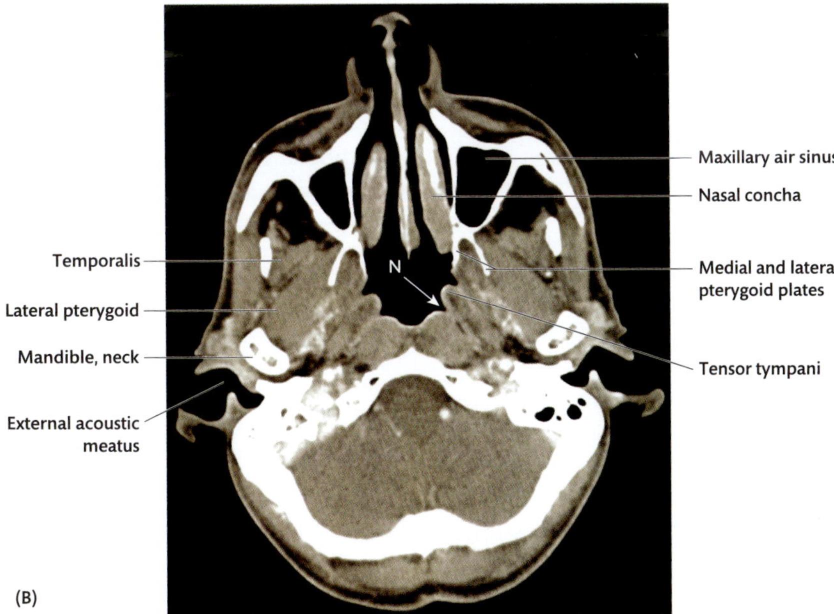


**Fig. 16.8** (A) Transverse section of the head at the level of the nasopharynx. (B) Axial contrast computerized tomography (CT) through the head at the level of the nasopharynx. N = nasopharynx; arrow = opening of auditory tube.

(A) Image courtesy of the Visible Human Project of the US National Library of Medicine.

the lateral wall of the pharynx. It is covered by the salpingopharyngeal fold of mucous membrane. Posterior to the tubal ridge, and the levator palati immediately behind it, is the deep **pharyngeal recess** which extends laterally, above the upper margin of the superior constrictor [Fig. 16.3]. The **pharyngeal isthmus** lies at the lower end of the nasopharynx, posterior to the palate. It is limited laterally by the **palatopharyngeal arches**.

➲ The nasopharynx can be illuminated by light reflected from a mirror introduced through the mouth. A view of the orifices of the auditory tubes, the side walls and roof of the nasopharynx, the choanae, and the posterior ends of the middle and inferior conchae can be obtained.

## Oropharynx

The oral part of the pharynx, or oropharynx, lies posterior to the palatoglossal arch. The posterior one-third of the dorsum of the tongue forms the anterior boundary [Figs. 16.2, 16.3]. Small, scattered collections of lymphocytes in the dorsum of the posterior third of the tongue give the pharyngeal part of the tongue its nodular appearance. These are the **lingual tonsil**. Immediately posterior to the tongue is the **epiglottis**—a curved, leaf-shaped plate of elastic cartilage covered with mucous membrane. The upper part of the epiglottis is posterior to the tongue and is readily visible through the mouth in children. Pull the epiglottis backwards to expose the **median glosso-epiglottic fold**—a median ridge of mucous membrane between the front of the epiglottis and the back of the tongue. On each side of this fold is a depression—the **epiglottic vallecula**. The **lateral glosso-epiglottic folds** are ridges of mucous membrane which form the lateral boundaries of the epiglottic valleculae. They extend from the margins of the epiglottis to the side walls of the pharynx at their junction with the tongue [see Fig. 17.1].

### Palatine tonsils

The palatine tonsils are masses of lymphoid tissue which lie in the mucous membrane on the lateral walls of the oropharynx, between the palatoglossal and palatopharyngeal folds. They are deep to the angle of the mandible, between the back of the tongue and the soft palate. In children, they are larger than the fossae between the arches and bulge into the pharynx. They also extend superiorly into the soft palate and anteriorly lateral to the palatoglossal arch [Fig. 16.3].

The medial surface of the palatine tonsils is covered by mucous membrane which forms about 12 deep **tonsillar crypts**. Superiorly, the tonsil is bounded by a mucosal fold under which lies the **supratonsillar fossa**.

The lateral surface of the palatine tonsils is covered by a thin fibrous **capsule**. The capsule is attached to the pharyngobasilar fascia by loose areolar tissue. The superior constrictor of the pharynx and the facial artery lie further laterally [see Fig. 8.15; Fig. 16.9].

#### Vessels and nerves of the palatine tonsil

The main artery of the palatine tonsils is the **tonsillar branch of the facial artery** [see Fig. 8.15]. It pierces the superior constrictor and enters the inferior part of the lateral surface. One or more inconstant **veins** descend from the soft palate, lateral to the tonsillar capsule. They pierce the superior constrictor near the artery, and either end in the pharyngeal plexus or unite to form a single vessel which drains into the facial vein. ➲ These veins may be a source of troublesome bleeding at tonsillectomy, especially when they unite to form a single larger vein.

Efferent lymph vessels from the palatine tonsils pierce the superior constrictor and pass to nodes on the carotid sheath, including the jugulodigastric at the angle of the mandible and the posterior submandibular nodes. **Nerve supply**: sensory nerves are from the glossopharyngeal and lesser palatine nerves.

➲ Inflammation of the palatine tonsils is called **tonsillitis**. It is usually caused by a viral or bacterial infection and presents with pain in the throat—especially while swallowing—fever, and swelling. It is more common in children.

➲ A complication of tonsillitis is the formation of a **peritonsillar abscess** (collection of pus), also known as **quinsy**. The collection of pus is deep to the tonsils, between it and the lateral pharyngeal wall. It requires treatment with antibiotics. Drainage of the abscess or tonsillectomy may be required.

➲ The surgical procedure done to remove the tonsils is **tonsillectomy**. It is usually done to prevent recurrent or chronic tonsillitis, or to treat a peritonsillar abscess.

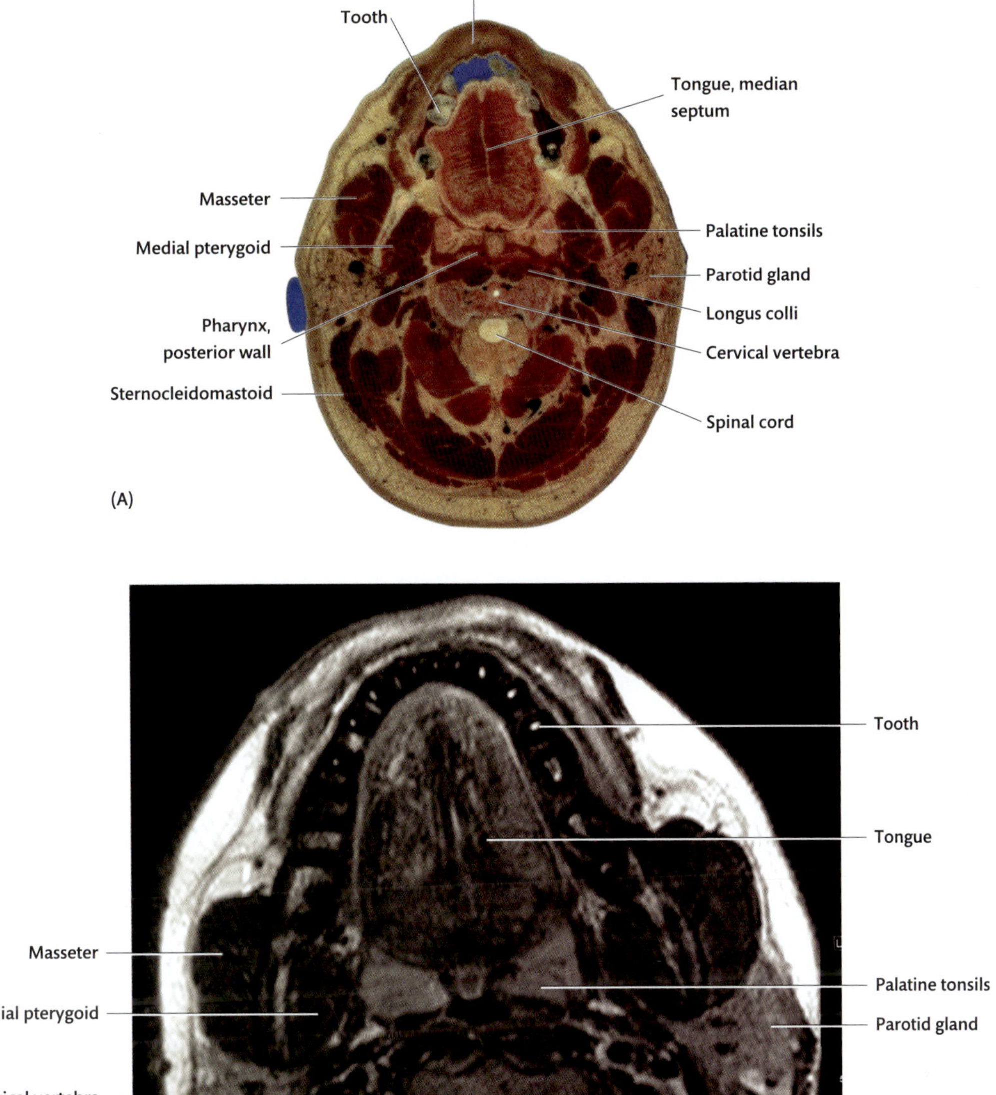


**Fig. 16.9** (A) Transverse section through the oropharynx showing the palatine tonsils. (B) Magnetic resonance image.

(A) Image courtesy of the Visible Human Project of the US National Library of Medicine.



## Lymphoid aggregations in the pharynx

Collections of lymphoid tissue in the pharynx form the pharyngeal and tubal tonsils in the nasopharynx, and the palatine and lingual tonsils in the oropharynx. These masses of lymphoid tissue form an almost complete ring—the **Waldeyer's lymphatic ring**—in the wall of the pharynx into which the nasal and oral cavities open. ➲ This tissue, like similar tissue in the small and large intestines, appears to be concerned with protection against ingested and inspired pathogens and is involved in the production of antibodies to invading organisms. The volume of this lymphoid tissue is normally much greater in children than in adults.

## Soft palate

The soft palate is a flexible, muscular flap which extends posteroinferiorly from the posterior edge of the hard palate. Laterally, it is attached to the lateral walls of the pharynx, and the **uvula** hangs down from the middle of its free posterior border. The lateral edge of the free border is continuous with the palatopharyngeal arch on each side [Fig. 16.2].

The soft palate acts as a flap valve. It can be raised and pulled posteriorly against the posterior pharyngeal wall, to shut off the nasopharynx from the oropharynx. This movement permits such actions as: (1) blowing a balloon or coughing, without air escaping through the nose; and (2) swallowing, without food and fluid regurgitating into the nose.

When the soft palate is pulled inferiorly against the posterior part of the tongue, it cuts off the mouth from the pharynx and permits respiration to continue during sucking or chewing, without danger of food or fluid entering the trachea. The uvula (somewhat like the nodules on the pulmonary and aortic valves [Vol. 2, pp. 70–71]) helps to prevent the soft palate from being forced into the nasopharynx in coughing when the pressure difference between the nasopharynx and the oropharynx is high, or into the mouth in sneezing when the pressure difference between the mouth and the nasopharynx is high. When tensed, the soft palate assists the tongue in directing food and fluids towards the laryngeal part of the pharynx in swallowing.

### Muscles of the soft palate

The soft palate is made up of a fold of mucous membrane enclosing parts of five pairs of muscles—the tensor palati, levator palati, palatoglossus, palatopharyngeus, and musculus uvulae. The musculus uvulae is an intrinsic muscle of the soft palate. Each of the remaining pairs of muscles forms a sling between the muscles of the right and those of the left, at the attachment to the **palatal aponeurosis**. The convex superior surface of the soft palate is continuous with the floor of the nasal cavities. Posteriorly, it abuts on the posterior pharyngeal wall. The **mucous membrane** on the oral surface of the soft palate is thick and has a layer of tightly packed **mucous glands**.

### Tensor palati (tensor veli palatini)

The tensor palati takes **origin** from: (1) the scaphoid fossa at the base of the medial pterygoid lamina; (2) the spine of the sphenoid; (3) the auditory tube; and (4) the margin of the greater wing of the sphenoid. It passes downwards, anterior to the auditory tube, converges on a tendon, hooks around the **pterygoid hamulus** [see Fig. 14.7; Figs. 16.5, 16.6], and spreads out horizontally into the soft palate. **Insertion**: in the soft palate, the tensor palati tendons of the two sides meet in the midline and form the **palatal aponeurosis** [see Fig. 12.6]. Anteriorly, this aponeurosis is attached to the palatine crests on the inferior surface of the hard palate and is thick and rigid. Posteriorly, it is thin. **Nerve supply**: mandibular division of the trigeminal nerve. **Action**: the tensor palati makes the anterior part of the soft palate rigid.

### Musculus uvulae

**Origin**: the musculus uvulae take origin from the posterior nasal spine of the palatine bones and are **inserted** into the mucous membrane of the uvula. They lie on the superior surface of the palatal aponeurosis and run side by side in the midline. **Nerve supply**: the pharyngeal plexus formed by the glossopharyngeal and vagal nerves. **Actions**: the musculus uvulae shorten and tense the uvula.

### Levator palati (levator veli palatini)

**Origin**: the levator palati arises from the medial side of the auditory tube and the adjacent part of the petrous temporal bone. It descends behind the auditory tube, medial to the free upper border of the superior constrictor muscle, and curves medially to join the opposite muscle. **Insertion**: it joins the opposite muscle in the midline. It is partially attached to the superior surface of the palatal aponeurosis. **Nerve supply**: the pharyngeal plexus formed by the glossopharyngeal and vagus nerves. **Action**: the two muscles acting together raise the palate symmetrically [Figs. 16.5, 16.6].

### Palatoglossus

The **palatoglossus** is a small counterpart of the levator palati on the inferior surface of the palate.

**Origin**: it takes origin from the inferior surface of the palatal aponeurosis. **Insertion**: it converges on the palatoglossal arch, and runs through the arch to merge with the muscles of the posterolateral part of the tongue [Figs. 16.3, 16.6]. **Nerve supply**: the pharyngeal plexus formed by the glossopharyngeal and vagus nerves. **Action**: the two muscles acting together draw the soft palate inferiorly onto the posterior part of the dorsum of the tongue.

### Palatopharyngeus

The palatopharyngeus arises from the superior surface of the soft palate, and its fibres spread over the internal surface of the constrictors. It is described above with muscles of the pharynx.

### Vessels and nerves of the soft palate

The **ascending palatine branch of the facial artery** ascends on the lateral pharyngeal wall to the superior border of the superior constrictor, hooks over this border, and descends with the levator palati to the palate. This is the main arterial supply to the soft palate and is supplemented by the lesser palatine branches of the greater palatine artery.

The **lesser palatine** and **glossopharyngeal nerves** supply the mucous membrane. The tensor palati is supplied by the **mandibular nerve** through the otic ganglion. All the other muscles are supplied by the **pharyngeal plexus**—a glossopharyngeal/vagal complex.

## Laryngopharynx

The laryngeal part of the pharynx, or laryngopharynx, lies posterior to the larynx. It decreases in width from above downwards, so that the **oesophageal orifice** is the narrowest part of the pharynx and lies opposite the inferior border of the cricoid cartilage [Fig. 16.3].

The **posterior** and **lateral walls** of the laryngopharynx are formed by the middle and inferior constrictor muscles, with the palatopharyngeus and stylopharyngeus on the inner aspect [Fig. 16.6].

The **anterior wall** is formed superiorly by: (1) the inlet of the larynx; and (2) the piriform recess which extends forwards on each side of the inlet. Inferiorly, the anterior wall is formed by: (3) the mucous membrane on the posterior surfaces of the arytenoid and cricoid cartilages [Fig. 16.10]. The interarytenoid muscles, the posterior crico-arytenoid muscles, and the attachment of the longitudinal muscles of the oesophagus lie in the anterior wall of the laryngopharynx [see Fig. 19.10].



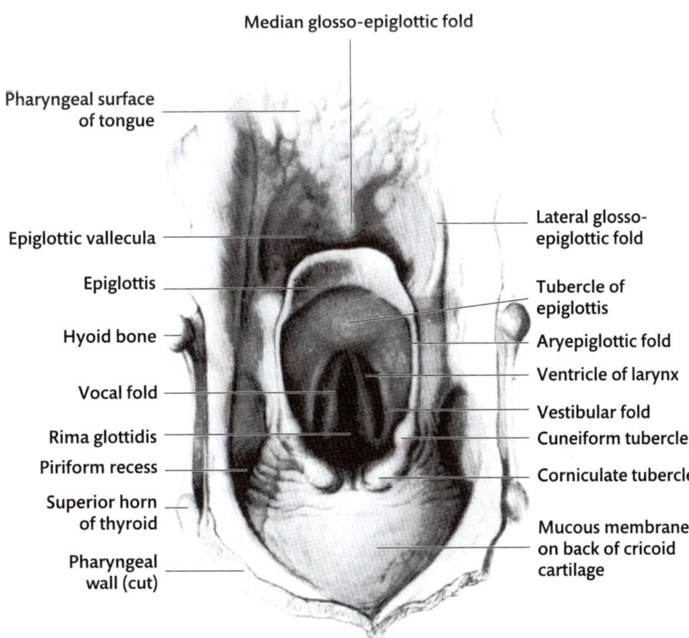


**Fig. 16.10** Anterior wall of the laryngopharynx seen from above. The tongue and epiglottis are pulled forwards.

## Inlet of the larynx

The inlet of the larynx is an almost vertically placed opening on the anterior wall of the laryngopharynx. It is bound anterosuperiorly by the epiglottis, on each side by the aryepiglottic fold of mucous membrane, and inferiorly by the interarytenoid fold of mucous membrane [Fig. 16.9].

Each **aryepiglottic fold** is a thin fold that extends inferiorly from the margin of the epiglottis to the arytenoid cartilage. It contains the thin aryepiglottic muscle. Near the inferior end of the fold are two small pieces of cartilage which form the **corniculate** and **cuneiform tubercles** on the free edge of the fold [Fig. 16.9].

The **arytenoid cartilages** are paired three-sided cartilages placed side by side on the superior border of the lamina of the cricoid cartilage [see Fig. 19.3]. The interarytenoid fold of mucous membrane passes between them and forms the inferior boundary of the inlet. The interarytenoid fold encloses the muscles which pass between the posterior surfaces of the arytenoid cartilages [see Fig. 19.10].

## Piriform recess

The deep piriform recess separates the aryepiglottic fold from the posterior surface of the lamina of the thyroid cartilage and the thyrohyoid membrane. It is lined with mucous membrane and ends as a blind sac inferiorly.

➲ Foreign bodies may lodge in the piriform recess or the sac which extends inferiorly, and pierce the mucous membrane of the recess.

## Stylopharyngeus

The stylopharyngeus muscle lies in the wall of the laryngopharynx. It is described above with the other pharyngeal muscles.

Using the instructions given in Dissection 16.3, dissect the pharynx.

## Swallowing

The walls of the pharynx have been seen from the inner medial aspect and it is possible to visualize the mechanism of swallowing.

In the first phase of swallowing, the mouth is closed, the tip of the tongue is raised against the hard palate, anterior to the bolus of food or fluid, and the bolus is squeezed posteriorly by pressing progressively more posterior parts of the tongue against the palate (intrinsic muscles of the tongue, mylohyoid, and styloglossus). As this movement passes backwards, elevation of the posterior part of the tongue against the tensed anterior part of the soft palate (tensor palati) is achieved by raising the hyoid bone (digastric, stylohyoid). At the same time, the geniohyoid carries the hyoid bone anteriorly, and this increases the anteroposterior diameter of the oropharynx to receive the bolus. The middle and inferior constrictor muscles are simultaneously relaxed. At this stage, the superior constrictor muscle and horizontal fibres of the palatopharyngeus contract to draw the upper part of the posterior pharyngeal wall against the raised posterior part of the soft palate (levator palati). This movement effectively shuts off the nasopharynx from the oropharynx and prevents food or fluid from entering the nasopharynx.

The second phase of swallowing is very rapid. There is considerable elevation of the larynx and the attached inferior part of the pharynx to the raised hyoid bone. (The hyoid bone is raised by the digastric, stylopharyngeus, and palatopharyngeus muscles.) This movement brings the thyroid cartilage within the concavity of the hyoid bone and approximates the arytenoid cartilages to the epiglottis, thus closing the laryngeal orifice. Contraction of the aryepiglottic muscles [see Fig. 19.10] may help to draw the epiglottis down on the arytenoid cartilages. More importantly, elevation of the base of the **epiglottis** through its attachment to the thyroid cartilage, and by contraction of the stylopharyngeus, pushes the apex of the epiglottis against the bulging posterior surface of the tongue and tips it backwards over the closed laryngeal orifice. The bolus of food from the back of the tongue now slips onto the lingual surface of the epiglottis (which now faces superiorly) and is carried down by the contracting middle and inferior constrictor muscles. This is aided by the rapid downward displacement of the larynx and pharynx (brought about by the infrahyoid muscles) which follows immediately and reopens the laryngeal orifice.

The importance of elevation of the hyoid bone and of the digastrics in this movement is shown by the difficulty in swallowing with the mouth open when the digastrics cannot act effectively on the hyoid bone because they are already shortened.

## DISSECTION 16.3 Pharynx

**Objective**

**I.** To identify and trace the muscles and vessels of the pharynx.

**Instructions**

1. Remove the mucous membrane from the palatopharyngeal and palatoglossal arches and from the salpingopharyngeal fold, to expose the muscles within them [Figs. 16.3, 16.6]. (The palatoglossus and salpingopharyngeus are small and often difficult to display.)
2. Remove the mucous membrane, connective tissue, and pharyngobasilar fascia from the wall of the pharynx, anterior and posterior to the opening of the auditory tube.
3. Identify the levator palati, posterior to the auditory tube, and follow it into the palate.
4. The ascending palatine artery may be seen descending beside the levator palati to the palate.
5. Trace the tensor palati inferiorly, lateral to the medial pterygoid lamina [Fig. 16.6], by turning the cartilage of the auditory tube backwards.
6. Identify the superior constrictor, lateral to the levator palati. Expose its superior border, and remove the mucous membrane from the parts of its medial surface which are not covered by the palatal muscles.
7. Dissect out the palatine tonsil.
8. Uncover the anterior part of the superior constrictor muscle. This part is difficult to define, as some of its fibres sweep inferiorly into the tongue, and it is often partly covered by thin sheets of muscle fibres passing inferiorly from the palate, lateral to the tonsil.
9. Follow the palatopharyngeus upwards into the soft palate, stripping off the thick glandular mucous membrane from its inferior surface as far as the hard palate.
10. Identify the pterygoid hamulus with the tendon of the tensor palati spreading medially from its base to form the palatal aponeurosis.
11. Identify the pterygomandibular raphe passing from the pterygoid hamulus to the mandible, and follow the superior constrictor anteriorly to the raphe.
12. Anterior to the pterygomandibular raphe, strip the mucous membrane from the internal surface of the buccinator, and identify its attachments.
13. Identify the opening of the parotid duct.
14. Identify the greater horn of the hyoid bone. Remove the mucous membrane from the medial surface of the middle constrictor, leaving the palatopharyngeus in position on its medial aspect.
15. Follow the **palatopharyngeus** to the posterior border of the lamina of the thyroid cartilage.
16. Anterior to the palatopharyngeus, identify the **stylopharyngeus** entering the pharynx between the middle and superior constrictor muscles. It spreads anteroposteriorly in such a manner that its posterior fibres are inserted with those of the palatopharyngeus, and the anterior fibres pass to the lateral aspect of the epiglottis.
17. Look for the internal laryngeal nerve entering the pharynx through the thyrohyoid membrane below the fibres of the stylopharyngeus [Fig. 16.6].
18. Find the **glossopharyngeal nerve**, anterolateral to the stylopharyngeus, where it enters the pharynx, and trace the nerve to the tongue.
19. Finally remove the mucous membrane from the medial surface of the inferior constrictor, the upper part of the oesophagus, and the piriform recess.
20. In the piriform recess, identify the medial surface of the thyroid cartilage and the thyrohyoid membrane with the superior laryngeal vessels and the internal laryngeal nerve piercing it.

## Auditory tube

Dissection 16.4 provides instructions on dissection of the auditory tube.

The auditory, or pharyngotympanic, tube connects the nasopharynx to the middle ear cavity. The tube is approximately 3.5 cm long. The bony posterolateral 1.5 cm lies between the tympanic and the petrous parts of the temporal bone and opens into the middle ear cavity. The cartilaginous anteromedial part lies in the groove between the petrous part of the temporal bone and the posterior border of the greater wing of the sphenoid.

The superior and medial walls of the pharyngeal opening of the tube are formed by a folded plate of **cartilage**. The inferolateral part of the tube is

## DISSECTION 16.4 Auditory tube

**Objective**

**I.** To study the course of the auditory tube.

**Instructions**

1. Identify the groove for the cartilaginous part, and the bony part of the auditory tube on a dried skull [see Fig. 2.11].
2. Ascertain the direction of the cartilaginous part of the tube by passing a probe into its pharyngeal orifice. At first, it runs superiorly and then posterolaterally between the tensor and the levator palati muscles [see Figs. 12.6, 12.10, 14.7].
3. Note that the levator palati forms a rounded prominence, inferior to the opening of the auditory tube. Remove the mucous membrane from the mouth of the tube, and note that the superior and medial walls are formed by a folded plate of **cartilage**.





completed by dense fibrous tissue joining the edges of the cartilage. The tubal ridge is formed by the base of the cartilage plate. The lumen of the auditory tube is narrowest (**isthmus**) where the cartilaginous and bony parts meet, and widest at the pharyngeal orifice. The tube functions to equalize the pressure in the middle ear with the atmospheric pressure.

Using the instructions given in Dissection 16.5, expose the otic ganglion from the medial side.

## Carotid canal

The carotid canal lies in the petrous part of the temporal bone. It contains the internal carotid artery, the internal carotid plexus of sympathetic nerve fibres, and a plexus of veins. Its position and course can be seen best on a macerated skull.

## Internal carotid artery in carotid canal

The part of the internal carotid artery in the carotid canal is approximately 2cm long. At first, it ascends vertically, then bends anteromedially, and runs horizontally to the apex of the petrous temporal bone [Fig. 16.11]. It enters the foramen lacerum through its posterior wall, turns upwards, and pierces the dura mater in the middle cranial fossa. In the carotid canal, it lies anteromedial to the middle ear, inferior to the

## DISSECTION 16.5 Otic ganglion

**Objective**

**I.** To study the otic ganglion and mandibular nerve.

**Instructions**

1. If the otic ganglion has not yet been seen, free the opening of the auditory tube from the medial pterygoid lamina and turn it posteriorly.
2. Separate the cartilaginous part of the tube from the base of the skull and the tensor palati. This exposes the tensor tympani—a small slip of muscle arising from the petrous temporal bone, superomedial to the tube and passing posterolaterally with it.
3. Detach the tensor palati from the base of the skull, and turn it inferiorly.
4. Remove the layer of fascia which is exposed, and uncover the mandibular nerve with the otic ganglion on its anteromedial aspect.
5. Immediately posterior to the mandibular nerve lies the middle meningeal artery at the foramen spinosum.
6. Identify the branches of the mandibular nerve as far as possible from this aspect, and note the close relation to the pharyngeal wall.
7. Confirm this relation on the base of a macerated skull.

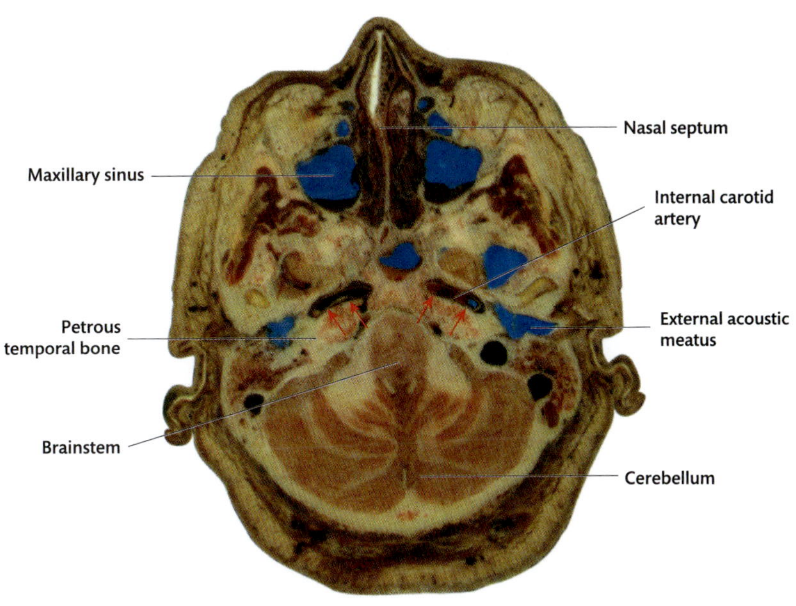


**Fig. 16.11** Transverse section through the petrous temporal bone showing the internal carotid artery in the carotid canal (red arrows).

Image courtesy of the Visible Human Project of the US National Library of Medicine.

cochlea, greater petrosal nerve, and trigeminal ganglion [see Fig. 12.6], and superior to the auditory tube.

## Internal carotid nerve and plexus

The internal carotid nerve is a large branch of the superior cervical ganglion which enters the carotid canal. It forms the internal carotid plexus around the internal carotid artery. Secondary plexuses extend from it around the branches of the artery [see Fig. 12.8]. The internal carotid plexus consists mainly of post-ganglionic sympathetic fibres.

The internal carotid nerve supplies a large area. The deep petrosal branch of the internal carotid plexus joins the pterygopalatine ganglion and, through it, is distributed to the nose, palate, air sinuses, and pharynx. Branches of the internal carotid nerve also join the third, fourth, ophthalmic branch of the fifth, and sixth cranial nerves, and the ophthalmic artery to supply the contents of the orbit, the forehead, and the anterior part of the scalp.

See Clinical Applications 16.1 and 16.2 for the practical implications of the anatomy discussed in this chapter.

**CLINICAL APPLICATION 16.1 Cancer, oral mucosa**

A 58-year-old man presented with a swelling in the right side of the vestibule of his mouth. Clinical examination led to suspicion of cancer of the oral mucosa, and computerized tomography (CT) was done. The images revealed a neoplastic mass of the buccal mucosa [Fig. 16.12].

Study question 1: study the image, and identify the structures marked 1, 2, 3, 4, and 5. (Answer: 1 = vestibule of the mouth in the unaffected side; 2 = masseter; 3 = facial vein; 4 = mandible; 5 = sublingual gland.)

Study question 2: state the sensory nerves, motor nerves, arteries, and lymph nodes likely to be involved. (Answer: sensory nerves = inferior alveolar nerve and its mental branch; motor nerve = facial nerve; arteries = inferior alveolar branch of the maxillary artery, inferior labial branch of the facial artery; lymph nodes = submental and submandibular lymph nodes.)

Cancer of the oral mucosa is very common in India. Chewing tobacco mixed with betel leaves, areca nut (pan masala), and lime shell is one of the main risk factors for this cancer.

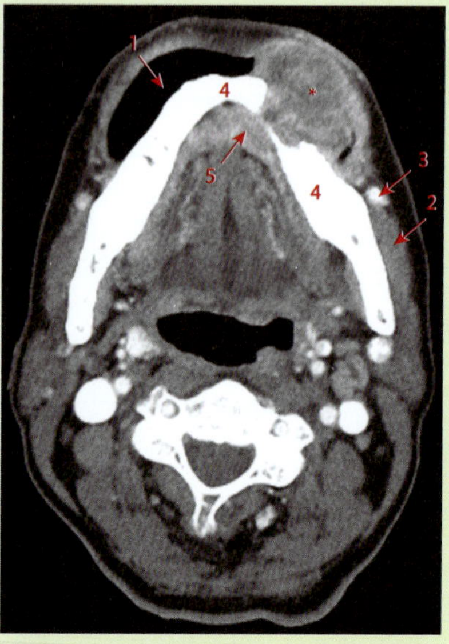


**Fig. 16.12** Computerized tomography scan of the head showing a neoplastic growth in the buccal mucosa (asterisk).

**CLINICAL APPLICATION 16.2 Gag reflex**

Accidently touching the back of the tongue or the mucosa over the palatoglossal arch (e.g. while brushing one's teeth) could stimulate the gag reflex. The gag reflex results in reflex contraction of the pharyngeal muscles, soft palate, and oropharyngeal isthmus. In extreme cases, it is accompanied by retching and vomiting. The afferent limb for the reflex is through the glossopharyngeal nerve. The efferent limb is through the pharyngeal plexus—the vagus and glossopharyngeal nerves.

CHAPTER 17

# The tongue

## Introduction

The tongue is a mobile organ which bulges upwards from the floor of the mouth. Its posterior part forms the anterior wall of the oropharynx [see Figs. 16.2, 16.3]. It is covered by stratified squamous epithelium and consists mainly of skeletal muscle, interspersed with a little fat and numerous glands.

The tongue is separated from the teeth by a deep **alveololingual sulcus**. Posterior to the last molar tooth, this sulcus is filled by the palatoglossal fold. The sulcus partly undermines the lateral margins of the tongue and extends beneath its free anterior third. The smooth mucous membrane in the alveololingual sulcus passes from the root of the tongue across the floor of the mouth to the internal aspect of the mandible and becomes continuous superiorly with that on the gum. Internal to the sulcus, the **root of the tongue** contains the muscles which connect the tongue to the hyoid bone and mandible, and transmits the nerves and vessels which supply it [see Fig. 16.1].

## Dorsum of the tongue

The dorsum of the tongue extends from the tip of the tongue to the anterior surface of the epiglottis. It is arbitrarily divided into an anterior palatine part and a posterior pharyngeal part by a V-shaped sulcus—the **sulcus terminalis**. The apex of the sulcus terminalis points posteriorly and is marked by a pit—the **foramen caecum**. A shallow median groove extends from the tip of the tongue to the foramen caecum [Fig. 17.1].

The thick mucous membrane of the palatine part is rough due to the presence of papillae. In the pharyngeal part, the covering mucosa is smooth, thin, and finely nodular in appearance, due to the presence of the underlying **lymphoid follicles**—the lingual tonsil. Posteriorly, the lingual mucous membrane is continuous with that on the anterior surface of the epiglottis over the median and lateral glosso-epiglottic folds and the valleculae of the epiglottis [Fig. 17.1].



### Lingual papillae

There are three types of lingual papillae—**circumvallate papillae**, **fungiform papillae**, and **filiform papillae**. The largest of these are the 7–12 **circumvallate papillae**, which lie immediately anterior to the sulcus terminalis. Each has the shape of a short cylinder, sunk into the surface of the tongue, with a deep trench surrounding it. The opposing walls of the trench have numerous taste buds.

**Fungiform papillae** are smaller and more numerous than circumvallate papillae. They are seen as bright red spots principally on the tip and margins of the living tongue, but also scattered over the remainder of the dorsum. Each fungiform papilla is attached by a narrow base and expands into a rounded, knob-like free extremity. Most of them carry taste buds.

**Filiform papillae** are numerous minute, pointed projections which cover all of the palatine part of the dorsum and the margins of the tongue. They are in rows parallel to the sulcus terminalis posteriorly, but transverse anteriorly.

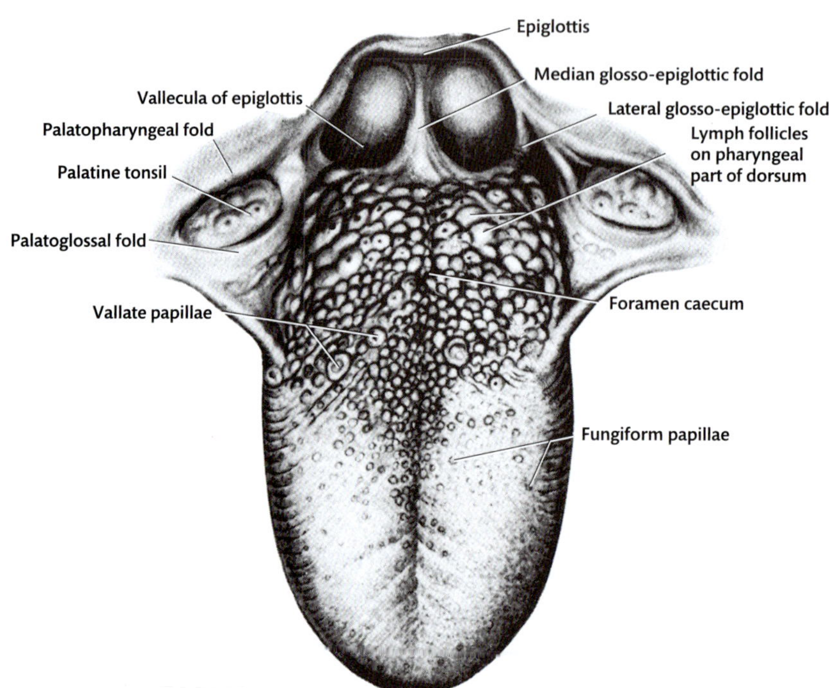


**Fig. 17.1** The dorsum of the tongue, epiglottis, and palatine tonsils.

On the sides of the tongue, anterior to the lingual attachment of the palatoglossal arch, are five short, vertical folds of mucous membrane—the **foliate papillae**.

## Inferior surface of the tongue

The inferior surface and sides of the tongue are covered by a smooth, thin mucous membrane. In the midline, anteriorly the mucosa is raised into a sharp fold which joins the inferior surface of the tongue to the floor of the mouth. This is the **frenulum of the tongue** [see Fig. 16.1]. On the tongue, on each side of the frenulum is the deep lingual vein, which is seen through the mucous membrane in the living subject. Lateral to the deep lingual vein is a fringed **fimbriated fold** of mucous membrane. On each side of the frenulum, on the floor of the mouth, is the **sublingual papilla**, with the opening of the submandibular duct on it. Passing posterolaterally from the sublingual papilla is the rounded **sublingual fold** (which contains the sublingual gland and the submandibular duct) and has the openings of the ducts of the sublingual gland [see Fig. 16.1].

## Muscles of the tongue

The tongue is divided into two halves by a median fibrous septum. The muscles of each half consist of an extrinsic and an intrinsic group. The extrinsic muscles take origin from parts outside the tongue and can move the tongue and change its shape. The intrinsic muscles are solely inside the tongue and can only change its shape.

The extrinsic muscles of the tongue are the genioglossus, hyoglosssus, styloglossus [Chapter 15], and palatoglossus [Chapter 16]. The intrinsic muscles are the superior longitudinal, inferior longitudinal, vertical, and transverse muscles.

Using the instructions given in Dissection 17.1, trace the extrinsic muscles of the tongue.

## Extrinsic muscles of the tongue

The extrinsic muscles of the tongue have been described in Chapters 15 and 16. Review their positions using Fig. 17.2.

**DISSECTION 17.1 Extrinsic muscles of the tongue**

**Objective**

**I.** To identify and trace the extrinsic muscles of the tongue.

**Instructions**

1. On the cut surface of the tongue, identify the genioglossus and geniohyoid. Confirm their attachments and position [see Fig. 16.3].
2. On the right side, separate the buccinator, pterygomandibular raphe, and superior constrictor from their attachments to the mandible, and turn the remainder of the body of the mandible downwards to expose the lateral surface of the tongue. Avoid injury to the lingual nerve and the palatoglossus muscle.
3. Remove the remainder of the mucous membrane from the lateral surface of the tongue, and follow the extrinsic muscles into its substance.

## Movements of the tongue

The posterior part of the tongue is attached to the hyoid bone. Hence the muscles which move the hyoid bone also move this part of the tongue [Chapter 15].

The **hyoglossus** and **genioglossus muscles** enter the tongue from below. The hyoglossus runs vertically along the lateral side of the tongue. The genioglossus is in a paramedian position. Both muscles depress the tongue [see Fig. 13.6; Fig. 17.2]. The genioglossus is fan-shaped when seen in the sagittal section [see Fig. 16.3]. Its posterior fibres pull the tongue forwards and help to protrude it (as does the geniohyoid). Its anterior fibres depress and retract the tip of the tongue.

The **palatoglossus** and **styloglossus** enter the lateral part of the tongue from above. The palatoglossus passes almost transversely and is continuous with the intrinsic transverse fibres. The styloglossus runs anteriorly along the lateral margin [Fig. 17.2].

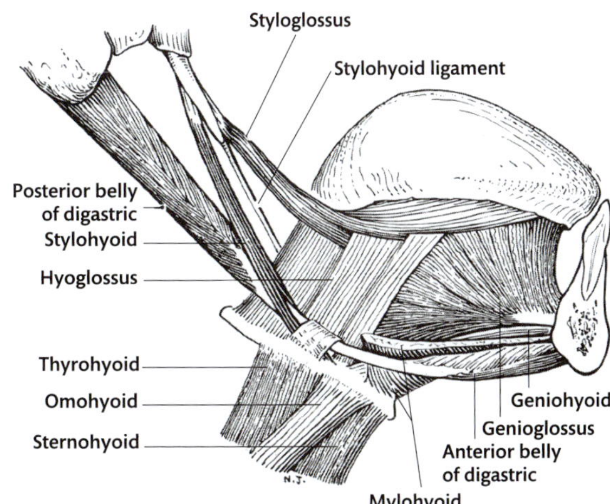


**Fig. 17.2** The extrinsic muscles of the tongue.

Both muscles can elevate the posterior part of the tongue. The styloglossus also retracts the tongue. The palatoglossus draws the palate down onto the tongue, narrows the oropharyngeal isthmus, and helps to isolate the mouth from the pharynx.

The **superior longitudinal muscle** lies close to the dorsum of the tongue. It curls the tip of the tongue upwards and rolls it posteriorly. The **inferior longitudinal muscle** lies in the lower part of the tongue, one on either side of the genioglossus [Fig. 17.3]. It curls the tip of the tongue inferiorly and act with the superior muscle to retract and widen the tongue.

The **transverse muscle fibres** lie inferior to the superior longitudinal muscle and run from the septum to the margins of the tongue between the vertical fibres of the genioglossus, hyoglossus, and intrinsic vertical muscles [see Fig. 16.9]. They narrow the tongue and increase its height.

The **vertical muscle fibres** run inferolaterally from the dorsum. They flatten the dorsum, increase the transverse diameter, and tend to roll up the margins. Acting with the transverse muscles, they increase the length of the tongue and assist with protrusion.

The actions given above represent only a few of the possible movements. Many other complex movements are produced by combinations of these muscles acting together. The tongue is bilaterally symmetrical, and unilateral action of any one muscle or group of muscles will cause the tongue to deviate from the midline.

Table 17.1 provides an overview of the movements of the tongue.

➲ **Hypoglossal nerve palsy**: hypoglossal nerve injury leads to paralysis of the muscles of the tongue (except for the palatoglossus which is sup-

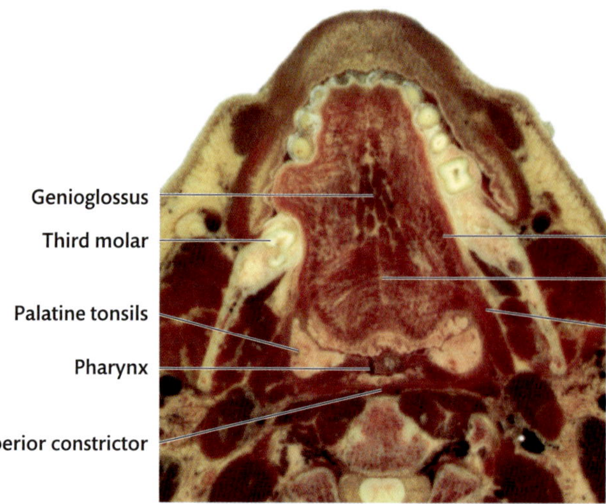


**Fig. 17.3** Horizontal section through the tongue and pharynx.

Image courtesy of the Visible Human Project of the US National Library of Medicine.





**Table 17.1** Movements of the tongue

| Movement | Muscles | Nerve supply |
|---|---|---|
| **Tip** | | |
| Elevation | Superior longitudinal* | Hypoglossal |
| Depression | Inferior longitudinal* and genioglossus | Hypoglossal |
| Retraction | Genioglossus (anterior fibres) and longitudinal muscles* | Hypoglossal |
| Turning to one side | Longitudinal* of that side with protrusors of opposite side | Hypoglossal and C. 1 |
| **Body** | | |
| Widening | Longitudinal* and vertical* | Hypoglossal |
| Heightening | Longitudinal* and transverse* | Hypoglossal |
| Shortening | Longitudinal* | Hypoglossal |
| Elongation | Transverse* and vertical* | Hypoglossal |
| Depression of median part | Genioglossus | Hypoglossal |
| Depression of edges | Hyoglossus | Hypoglossal |
| Depression of all | Lowering of hyoid bone [see Table 8.2] | |
| Elevation | Elevation of hyoid bone [see Table 8.2] | |
| | Styloglossus | Hypoglossal |
| | Mylohyoid | Trigeminal |
| | Palatoglossus | Pharyngeal plexus |
| Protrusion in the midline | Geniohyoid† | Ventral ramus C. 1 |
| | Genioglossus (posterior fibres)† | Hypoglossal |
| | Vertical* | Hypoglossal |
| | (Transverse*) | Hypoglossal |
| Protrusion to one side | Action of above muscles on opposite side ± retractors of same side | |
| Retraction | Longitudinal* | Hypoglossal |
| | Styloglossus | Hypoglossal |

* Intrinsic muscles.

† These muscles help to maintain the patency of the airway when lying supine.

plied by the vagus). The patient's attempt to protrude the tongue results in the tip of the tongue deviating to the paralysed side. The protrusion is brought about by the active muscle, but the tip of the tongue deviates to the paralysed side which is stationary.

## Septum of the tongue

The median fibrous septum of the tongue is best seen in a transverse section. It is strongest posteriorly where it is attached to the hyoid bone and is separated from the mucous membrane of the dorsum by the superior longitudinal muscle [see Figs. 15.2B, 16.9].

## Glands of the tongue

Small serous and mucous glands lie between the muscle fibres deep to the mucous membrane of the pharyngeal surface, tip, and margins. Small serous glands lie near the vallate papillae and open into their trenches. Mucous and serous glands lie on the inferior surface of the tongue near its tip—the **anterior lingual glands**.

## Nerves of the tongue

**Sensory nerves**: the tongue can perceive both **general sensation**—pain, temperature, touch—and **special sensation**—taste. In the anterior two-thirds of the tongue, (1) general sensation is carried by the **lingual nerve**, and (2) taste sensation is carried by the **chorda tympani** branch of the facial nerve. (The chorda tympani runs with the lingual nerve in the mouth [see Fig. 14.6].)

In the posterior one-third of the tongue, (3) the **glossopharyngeal** nerve carries taste and general sensation. The glossopharyngeal nerve also carries sensations from the circumvallate papillae. (4) Small branches of the internal laryngeal branch of





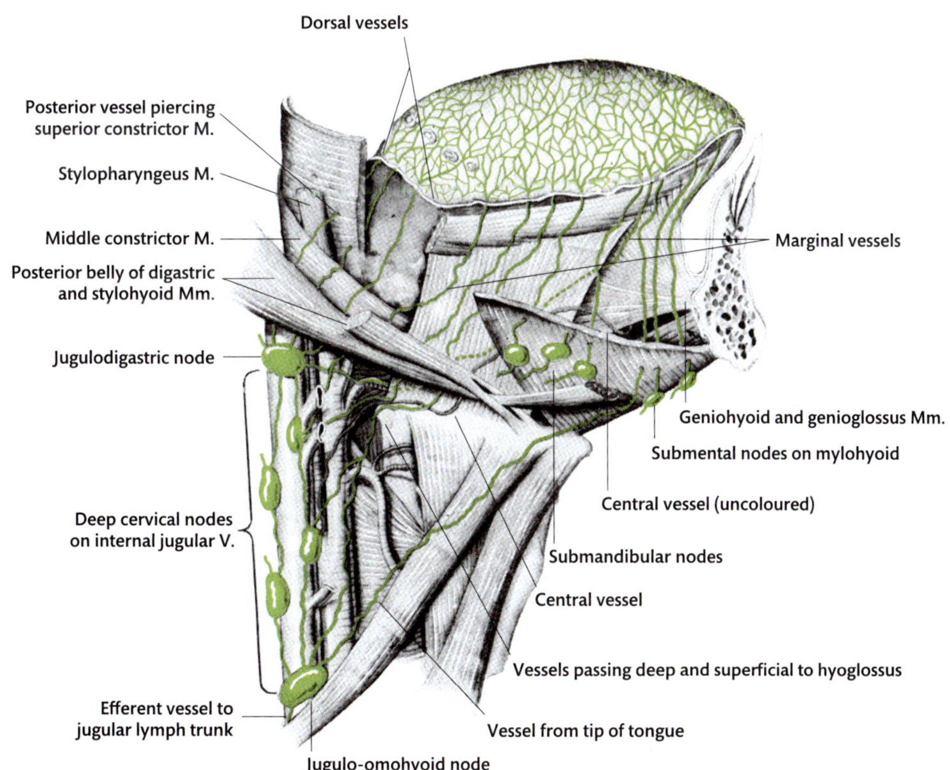


**Fig. 17.4** Lymph vessels and nodes of the tongue.

the superior laryngeal nerve supply a small area of the tongue adjacent to the epiglottis.

**Parasympathetic supply**: the lingual and glossopharyngeal nerves carry parasympathetic secretomotor fibres to the glands in the substance of the tongue.

**Motor supply**: the motor supply to the muscles of the tongue is from the **hypoglossal nerve** which innervates all the intrinsic and extrinsic muscles of the tongue, except the palatoglossus. (The palatoglossus is innervated by the vagus.)

## Vessels of the tongue

The main **arteries** supplying the tongue are branches of the lingual artery. The deep artery of the tongue supplies the anterior part, and the dorsales linguae arteries supply the posterior part. The **deep lingual vein** and other veins drain the tongue. They are described in Chapter 15.

## Lymph vessels of the tongue

These vessels cannot be dissected, but they are important because cancer of the tongue is common and it spreads through lymph vessels.

Lymph vessels from the tongue drain into the **jugulodigastric** and **jugulo-omohyoid** deep cervical lymph nodes. The lymph from the anterior part of the tongue (in front of the circumvallate papilla) drains through two sets of lymph vessels—the marginal and central vessels. Lymph from the posterior part drains through the dorsal lymph vessels. Lymph from the marginal vessels may pass through the **submental nodes** or **submandibular** nodes [Fig. 17.4]. Lymph from the median and paramedian tissue may cross the midline and drain bilaterally.

CHAPTER 18

# The cavity of the nose

## Cavity of the nose

Each nasal cavity is approximately 5 cm in height and 5–7 cm in length. It is narrow transversely, measuring approximately 1.5 cm at the floor and only 1–2 mm at the roof. The width is further reduced by the conchae, which project into the cavity from the lateral wall [Figs. 18.1, 18.2, 18.3].

The oval anterior apertures, or nostrils **(nares)**, open on the inferior surface of the external nose. The posterior apertures, or **choanae**, open into the nasopharynx and face posteroinferiorly [Fig. 18.3]. The **vestibule of the nose** [Fig. 18.1] lies immediately above the nostril. It is lined with skin, from which stout hairs, or vibrissae, project, forming a coarse filter.

## Septum of the nose

The nasal septum lies between the two nasal cavities. It is formed mainly by the perpendicular plate of the ethmoid, vomer, and septal cartilage [Fig. 18.1]. The nasal septum is seldom exactly in the midline but bulges to one or other side. Immediately above the nostril, the septum is slightly concave where it forms the medial wall of the vestibule of the nose. The skin of this part carries a number of stiff hairs, or vibrissae. The remainder of the septum is covered with mucous membrane which is tightly adherent to the underlying periosteum and perichondrium (**mucoperiosteum** and **mucoperichondrium**, respectively). The lower, larger area of the septum is the **respiratory region**. The upper third is the **olfactory region** and its epithelium contains olfactory nerve cells. The respiratory mucous membrane is thick, spongy, and highly vascular. It contains numerous mucous glands and is capable of swelling to a considerable thickness when the vascular spaces in it are filled with blood. It also contains many arteriovenous anastomoses which increase the flow of blood through it to warm the air passing over it. The olfactory mucous membrane is more delicate and is yellowish in the fresh state [Figs. 18.1, 18.2].

Using the instructions given in Dissection 18.1, remove the mucous membrane and expose the components of the nasal septum.



## Roof of the nasal cavity

The roof of the nasal cavity is curved and approximately 7–8 cm long. The anterior and posterior parts are sloping, and the middle part is nearly horizontal. The anterior part is formed by the nasal part of the frontal bone, the nasal bone, and the junction of lateral and septal cartilages. The middle part is formed by the cribriform plate of the ethmoid. The posterior part is formed by the anterior and inferior surfaces of the body of the sphenoid [Fig. 18.3].

## Floor of the nasal cavity

The floor is about 5 cm long and 1–1.5 cm wide. It is formed by the palatine process of the maxilla and the horizontal process of the palatine bone. It is

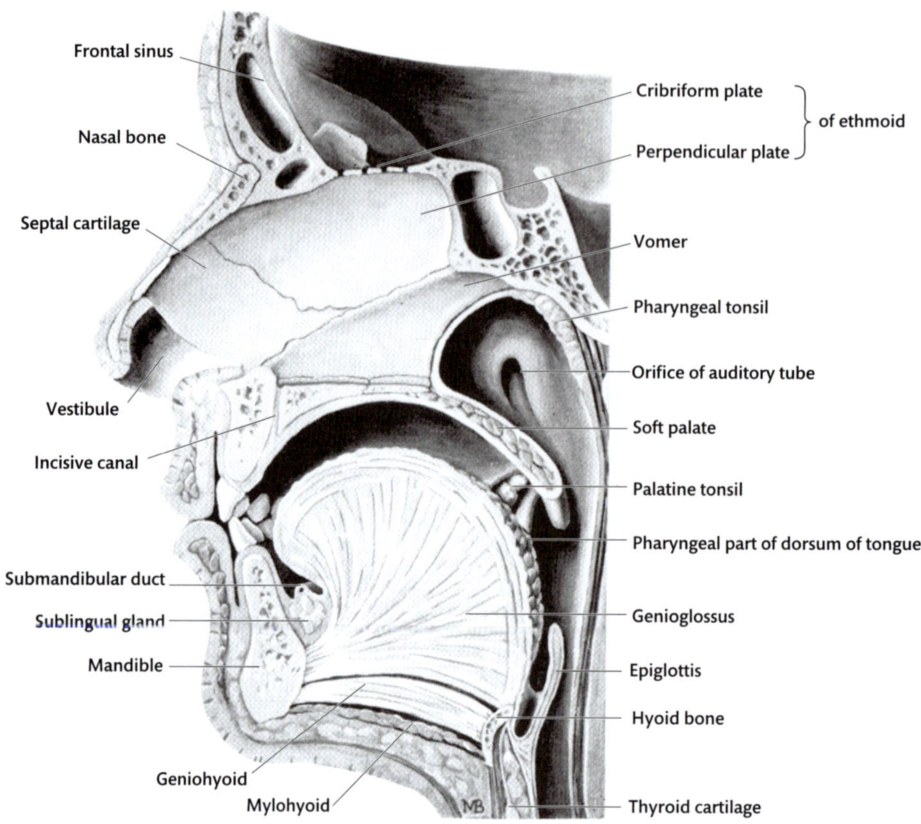


**Fig. 18.1** Sagittal section through the nose, mouth, and pharynx, a little to the left of the median plane.





concave transversely and is slightly higher anteriorly than posteriorly [Figs. 18.2, 18.3].

## Lateral wall

Begin your study of the lateral wall by identifying the bones that form it on a dry skull. The lateral wall of the nasal cavity is irregular due to the presence of three projecting **conchae** or turbinates—the superior, middle, and inferior conchae. The meatuses are the spaces inferior to the conchae—the superior, middle, and inferior meatuses. The space above the superior meatus is the spheno-ethmoidal recess. Adjoining the lateral wall are the air sinuses (air-filled spaces in the bones) which communicate with the nasal cavity. These air sinuses open into

### DISSECTION 18.1 Nasal septum

**Objective**

**I.** To identify the bony and cartilaginous components of the nasal septum.

**Instructions**

1. Strip the mucous membrane off the nasal septum on one side, and expose: (1) the vomer; (2) the perpendicular plate of the ethmoid; (3) the septal cartilage; and (4) small parts of the maxillary, palatine, nasal, and sphenoid bones. The relative positions of these parts are shown in Fig. 18.1.
2. Note that the anterior angle of the septal cartilage is blunt and rounded, and does not reach the point of the nose. The point of the nose is formed by the greater alar cartilages.
3. Remove the septum piecemeal from the mucous membrane, taking care not to damage the structures in that mucous membrane.

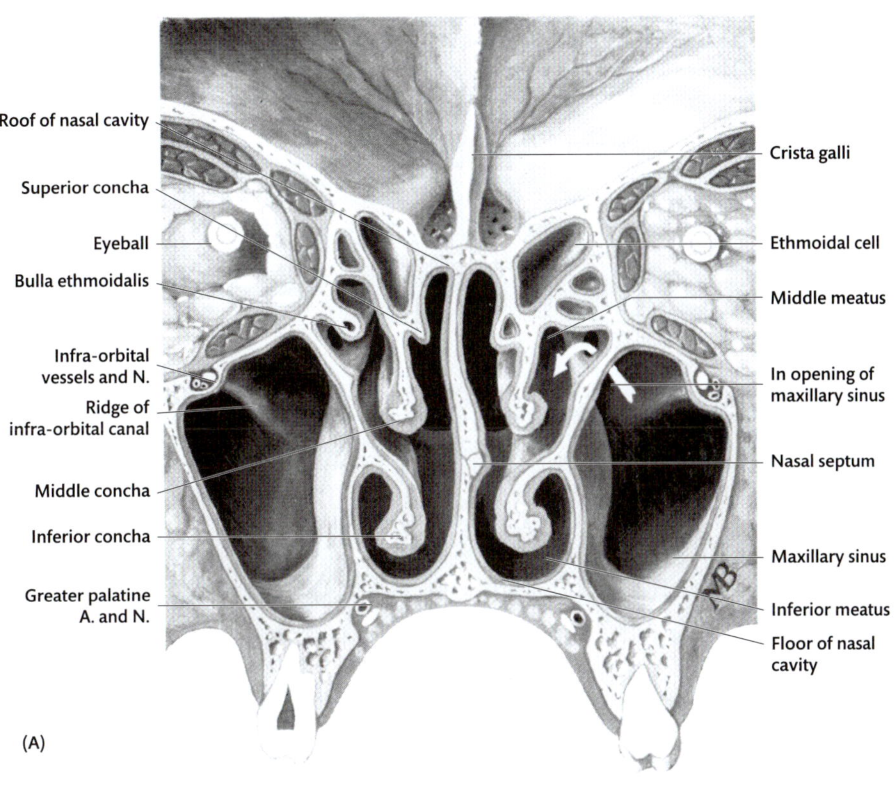


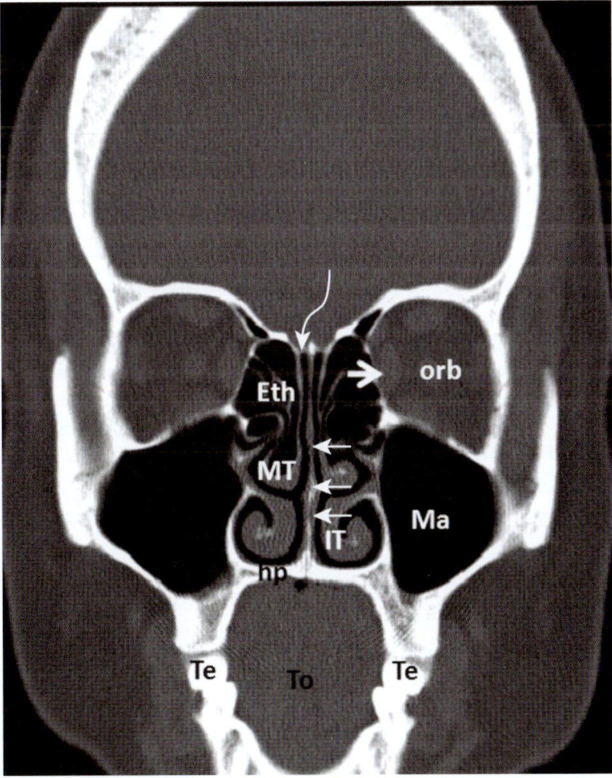


**Fig. 18.2** (A) Coronal section through the nasal cavities, paranasal sinuses, and orbits, seen from behind. (B) Computerized tomography through the nasal cavity. Eth = ethmoid; hp = hard palate; IT = inferior turbinate (concha); Ma = maxillary antrum; MT = middle turbinate (concha); orb = orbit; Te = teeth; To = tongue. Curved arrow = cribriform plate of the ethmoid. Thick arrow = medial wall of the orbit. Thin arrow = nasal septum.

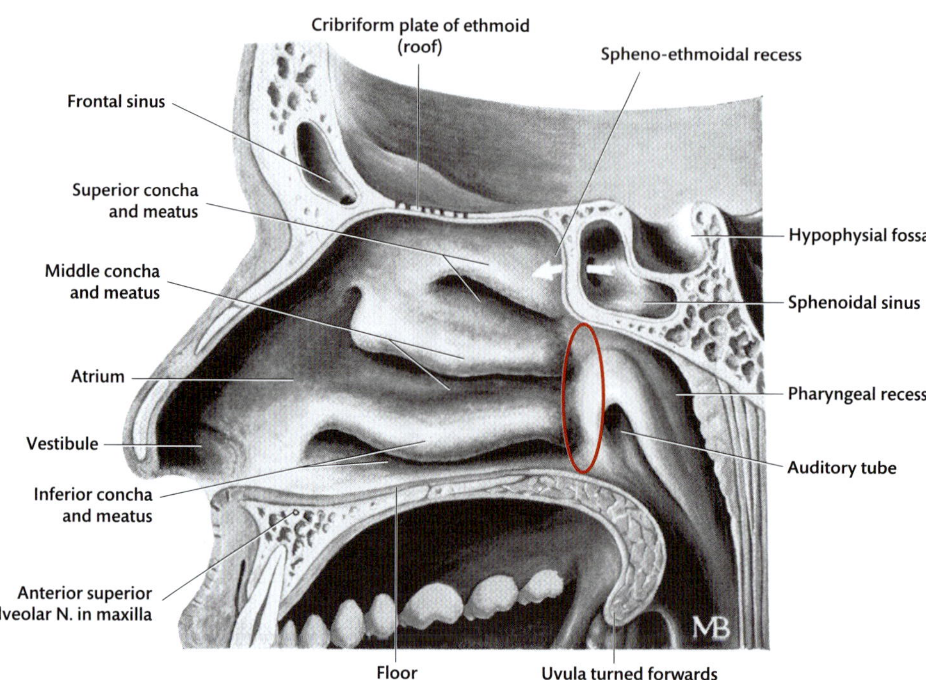


**Fig. 18.3** Sagittal section through the nose and palate to show the lateral wall of the nose.

the nasal cavity through openings in the lateral wall which are better seen when the conchae are removed.

There are three distinct regions in the lateral wall of the nose [Fig. 18.3]:

1. The **vestibule of the nose** lies immediately above the nostril.
2. The **atrium of the middle meatus** is above and slightly behind the vestibule. It lies immediately anterior to the middle meatus. The lateral wall of the atrium is concave, except close to the nasal bone where there is a small elevation—the agger nasi.
3. The **nasal conchae and meatuses** [Figs. 18.2, 18.3]. The **superior concha** lies in the postero-superior part of the nasal cavity and is very short. It is a part of the ethmoid bone. Anteriorly, its free border begins a little inferior to the middle of the cribriform plate, and it passes posteroinferiorly to end immediately anterior to the lower part of the body of the sphenoid. The **middle concha** is much larger than the superior concha and extends from the atrium to the level of the choanae. Like the superior concha, the middle concha is part of the ethmoid bone. The **inferior concha** is slightly longer than the middle concha and lies about midway between the middle concha and the floor of the nose. It is a separate bone and articulates with the maxilla.

The space posterosuperior to the superior concha is the **spheno-ethmoidal recess**. The sphenoidal air sinus opens into it [Fig. 18.3]. The **superior meatus** is a narrow space between the superior and middle conchae. The posterior ethmoidal cells open into it by one or more orifices. These openings can be exposed by forcing the margin of the superior concha upwards [Fig. 18.4].

The **middle meatus** is much longer and deeper than the superior meatus. To expose it, tilt the middle concha forcibly upwards [Fig. 18.4]. The anterosuperior part of the middle meatus has a funnel-shaped opening—the **infundibulum**—which leads to the frontal air sinus. On the lateral wall of the middle meatus is a deep, curved groove which begins at the infundibulum and runs posteroinferiorly. This is the **hiatus semilunaris**. The anterior ethmoidal and maxillary air sinuses open into it. The upper margin of the hiatus semilunaris is formed by a prominent bulge—the **bulla ethmoidalis**—on which is the opening of the middle ethmoidal air cells. The **opening of the maxillary sinus** [see Fig. 10.1; Figs. 18.2, 18.4] lies in the posterior part of the hiatus semilunaris and leads to the upper medial wall of the sinus. ➲ Infective material tends to flow from the frontal into the maxillary sinus because of the relative

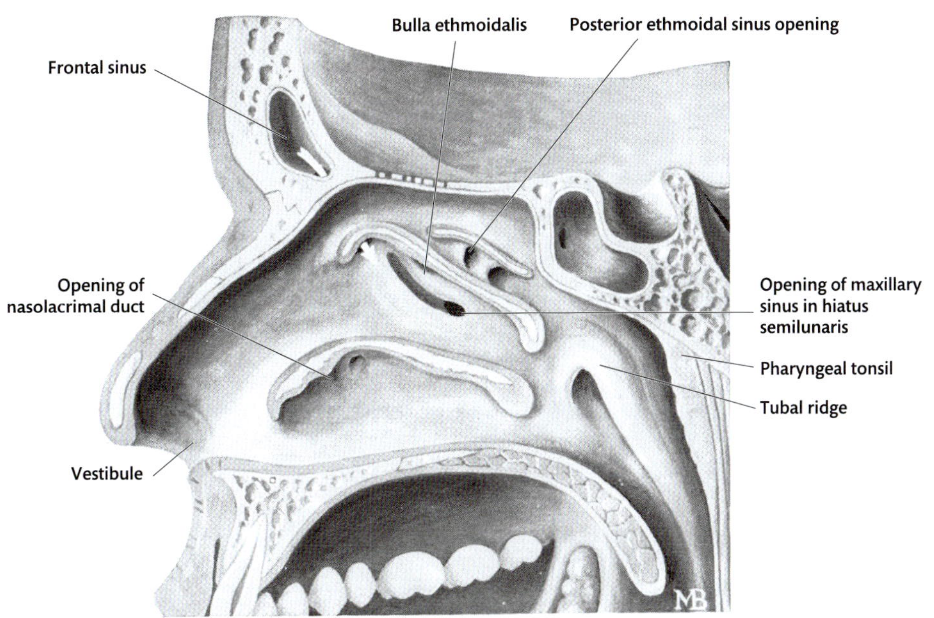


**Fig. 18.4** Sagittal section through the nose and palate. The conchae have been cut away to expose the meatuses and the openings into them.





positions of the two openings on the lateral wall of the nose.

The **inferior meatus** is the horizontal passage between the inferior concha and the floor of the nose. The nasolacrimal duct opens into the anterior part of the inferior meatus, close to the attached border of the inferior concha [Fig. 18.4]. The opening of the nasolacrimal duct may be wide, patent, and circular, or it may be covered by a fold of membrane.

Using the instructions given in Dissection 18.2, dissect out the nasolacrimal duct [Fig. 18.5].

## Mucosa of the lateral wall of the nasal cavity

Apart from the vestibule, the lateral wall is covered with mucous membrane which is tightly adherent to the underlying periosteum and forms a **mucoperiosteum**. This mucoperiosteum is continuous: (1) through the nasolacrimal duct, with the ocular conjunctiva; (2) through the openings of the sinuses with the lining of the air sinuses in the frontal, ethmoid, maxilla, and sphenoid bones; and (3) through the choanae with the mucous membrane of the nasopharynx.

The mucoperiosteum on the lateral wall is divisible into the upper yellowish **olfactory region** in the area of the superior concha, and the remainder which comprises the **respiratory region**. These regions cannot be differentiated by the naked eye. In the respiratory region, the mucoperiosteum is thick and spongy, especially on the free margins and posterior extremities of the middle and inferior conchae, due to the presence of a rich venous plexus

### DISSECTION 18.2 Nasolacrimal duct

**Objective**

I. To expose the nasolacrimal duct.

**Instructions**

1. Remove the anterior part of the inferior concha with scissors, and expose the opening of the nasolacrimal duct. Pass a probe upwards along the duct to confirm its continuity with the lacrimal sac [Fig. 18.5].
2. Break away the thin plate of bone which separates the duct from the nose, and expose the length of the duct. Expose the lacrimal sac by continuing the bone removal upwards to the level of the eye.

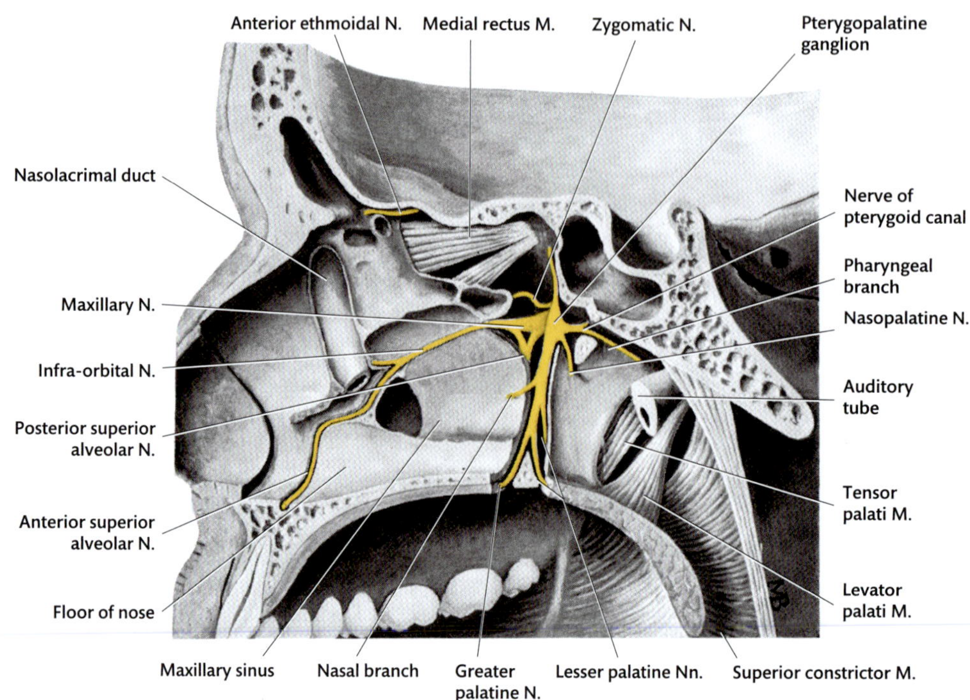


Fig. 18.5 The mucous membrane and a large part of the bone of the lateral wall of the nose have been removed to expose the maxillary sinus. The maxillary, infraorbital, anterior superior alveolar, and palatine nerves have been exposed by removal of the bony wall of their canals. The pterygopalatine fossa and ganglion are also exposed. The ethmoid has been broken into to expose the orbit.





in it. The venous channels and many arteriovenous anastomoses in the mucoperiosteum ensure that the inspired air is warmed and moistened. Dust particles in the inspired air are trapped on the mucus covering the surface and moved posteriorly towards the choanae by the cilia. ➲ The mucoperiosteum on the inferior concha may be swollen by distended venous channels. It may impinge on the nasal septum and effectively reduces the cross-sectional area of the nasal cavity.

## Sensory nerves of the nasal cavity

The mucosa of the nasal cavity has nerves to perceive general sensation and smell. General sensation is carried by the maxillary nerve and the anterior ethmoidal branch of the ophthalmic nerve. Fibres of the maxillary nerve reach the walls of the nasal cavity through branches of the pterygopalatine ganglion and the anterior superior alveolar nerve [Figs. 18.5, 18.6].

### Anterior ethmoidal nerve

The **anterior ethmoidal nerve** arises from the nasociliary nerve in the orbit. It reaches the anterosuperior part of the lateral wall of the nose through the anterior ethmoidal foramen and the cribriform plate of the ethmoid [see Fig. 10.1]. It supplies the anterior part of the lateral wall of the nose. The medial nasal branches of the **anterior ethmoidal nerve** run on the anterosuperior part of the nasal septum as far as the vestibule [Fig. 18.6].

### Branches from the pterygopalatine ganglion

The **nasopalatine nerve** is a long, slender nerve on the deep surface of the mucous membrane of the septum. It arises from the pterygopalatine ganglion and enters the nasal cavity through the sphenopalatine foramen with the sphenopalatine branch of the maxillary artery. It runs medially across the roof of the nasal cavity, and then anteroinferiorly on the septum, in a groove on the surface of the vomer. On reaching the floor of the nasal cavity, it runs through the incisive canal and median incisive foramen with its fellow from the opposite side, and supplies the mucous membrane in the anterior part of the hard palate. The lateral branches of the nasopalatine nerve supply the posterior parts of the lateral wall [Fig. 18.6].

The medial **posterosuperior nasal branches** of the pterygopalatine ganglion, together with

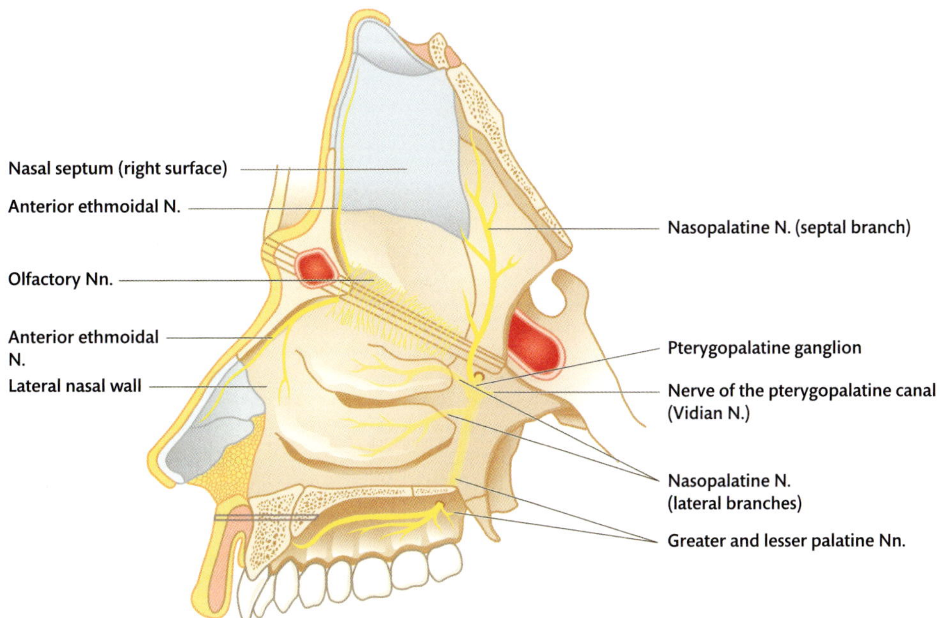


Fig. 18.6 Nerve supply of the nasal septum and lateral wall of the nose.





small branches from the nerve of the pterygoid canal, supply the posterosuperior parts of the septum. They are too small to be dissected easily.

### Olfactory nerves

The **olfactory nerves** are the nerves of smell. They are the central processes of the olfactory cells in the epithelium of the olfactory area. These fine, non-myelinated nerve fibres run in shallow grooves and small canals in the bone, deep to the mucous membrane. They unite to form 12–20 olfactory nerves which pass through the cribriform plate of the ethmoid and pierce the meninges to enter the olfactory bulb [Fig. 18.6].

## Autonomic nerves to nasal mucosa

The maxillary nerve also carries post-ganglionic sympathetic fibres from the carotid plexus (via the deep petrosal nerve) and post-ganglionic parasympathetic nerve fibres from the pterygopalatine ganglion to the glands in the lateral wall.

## Arteries supplying the nasal mucosa

The nasal mucosa is supplied by: (1) the sphenopalatine artery, a branch of the maxillary artery; (2) ethmoidal branches of the ophthalmic artery; and (3) branches of the superior labial arteries [Fig. 18.7].

➲ Epistaxis is the medical term for nosebleeds. It commonly occurs from rupture of small blood vessels in the anterior part of the nose where four or five small arteries form an arterial anastomosis—Keisselbach's area or Little's area.

Dissection 18.3 provides instructions on dissecting the nerves and vessels of the nasal cavity.

## Important relations of the lateral wall of the nose

The **pterygopalatine ganglion** and its branches, a short segment of the **maxillary nerve**, and the terminal part of the **maxillary artery** lie adjacent to the lateral wall of the nose [Fig. 18.5]. The pterygopalatine ganglion lies in the pterygopalatine fossa, lateral to the sphenopalatine foramen and the perpendicular plate of the palatine bone.

The greater and lesser palatine branches of the pterygopalatine ganglion will be dissected, following the instructions provided in Dissection 18.4.

## Greater palatine nerve

The greater palatine nerve is the largest branch of the pterygopalatine ganglion [Fig. 18.5]. It descends vertically through the greater palatine

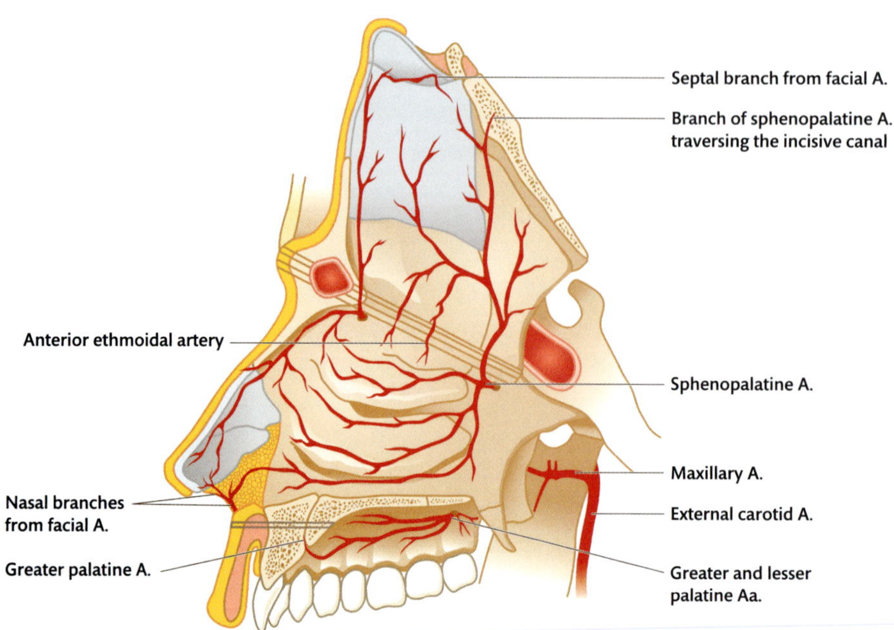


**Fig. 18.7** Arterial supply of the nasal septum and lateral wall of the nose.

canal and foramen with the **descending palatine branch** of the maxillary artery and enters the inferior surface of the hard palate at its posterolateral corner. It runs forwards in a groove on the inferior surface of the bony palate, close to its lateral margin. At the incisive fossa, it communicates with the terminal branches of the nasopalatine nerve. It supplies the gum and the mucous membrane of the hard palate, including the palatine mucous glands which indent the inferior surface of the bone.

The greater palatine nerve gives: (1) two **posterior nasal** branches through the perpendicular plate of the palatine bone to the mucous membrane

## DISSECTION 18.3 Vessels and nerves of the nasal cavity

### Objective

**I.** To expose the vessels and nerves of the nasal cavity.

### Instructions

1. Trace the **nasopalatine nerve** from the nasal septum across the roof of the nasal cavity to the sphenopalatine foramen in the lateral wall.
2. By careful dissection, attempt to display one or more of the nasal branches of the pterygopalatine ganglion and the sphenopalatine artery running with the nasopalatine nerve.
3. Carefully reflect the mucous membrane on the medial pterygoid lamina anteriorly.
4. Attempt to find the **posterior nasal branches of the pterygopalatine ganglion**. These are minute twigs which pass through the sphenopalatine foramen and supply the mucous membrane on the posterior part of the septum, the superior and middle conchae, some ethmoidal cells, and the lateral wall of the nasal part of the pharynx [Fig. 18.6].
5. Two **nasal branches of the greater palatine nerve** pierce the perpendicular plate of the palatine bone. They supply the mucous membrane on the posterior parts of the conchae and meatuses.
6. The **anterior ethmoidal nerve** [Fig. 18.6] descends in a groove on the deep surface of the nasal bone. Its branches supply the anterosuperior parts of the septum, roof, and lateral wall of the nose.
7. The **sphenopalatine branch of the maxillary artery** is the main arterial supply to the mucous membrane. It enters the nasal cavity through the sphenopalatine foramen and is distributed with the various nerves [Fig. 18.7].
8. The anterior and posterior **ethmoidal arteries** also supply the anterosuperior region, the anterior reaching as far inferiorly as the anterior end of the inferior concha.

### DISSECTION 18.4 Greater and lesser palatine nerves

**Objective**

**I.** To expose the greater and lesser palatine nerves.

**Instructions**

1. The mucoperiosteum has already been stripped from the perpendicular plate of the palatine bone. Find the greater palatine nerve which is seen shining through this very thin plate of bone, as it descends on the lateral side of the bone to reach the palate. It runs with the **descending palatine branch** of the maxillary artery.
2. Break through the perpendicular plate of the palatine bone, and expose part of the greater palatine nerve. Then open up the whole length of the canal by levering off the remainder of the lamina lying medial to the nerve. Superiorly, the **greater palatine nerve** joins the pterygopalatine ganglion at the level of the sphenopalatine foramen.
3. Inferiorly, where the canal reaches the hard palate, cut out a narrow, transverse strip of the hard palate to open into the palatine foramen, through which the greater palatine nerve reaches the hard palate.
4. Remove the fibrous sheath covering the greater palatine nerve, and expose the **lesser palatine nerves** which run with it in the upper part of their course. Inferiorly, the lesser palatine nerves pass through separate bony canals.
5. Turn to the inferior surface of the palate, and follow the greater palatine nerve and artery in it.

of the nose; and (2) the **lesser palatine nerves** which descend through the lesser palatine canals. The more medial of the lesser palatine nerve emerges immediately posterior to the palatine crest and enters the soft palate to supply its mucous membrane and glands. The more lateral nerve, when present, supplies the mucous membrane of the soft palate near the palatine tonsil.

Using the instructions given in Dissection 18.5, dissect the pterygopalatine ganglion and maxillary nerve.

## Pterygopalatine ganglion

The pterygopalatine ganglion is one of the four parasympathetic ganglia of the head. It is small and triangular in shape and lies in the superior part of the pterygopalatine fossa near the sphenopalatine foramen. It is surrounded by the terminal branches of the maxillary artery [see Fig. 14.3; Fig. 18.5].

### DISSECTION 18.5 Pterygopalatine ganglion and maxillary nerve

**Objectives**

**I.** To remove the lateral wall of the nasal cavity. **II.** To expose the ethmoidal air cells. **III.** To expose the maxillary nerve and its branches. **IV.** To identify the pterygopalatine ganglion.

**Instructions**

1. Remove the three nasal conchae.
2. Beginning just posterior to the infundibulum, strip away the thin medial wall of the ethmoidal air cells, noting their continuity with the nasal mucous membrane through the apertures already described.
3. Remove the mucous membrane lining the individual cells and the bony walls between them, and expose the medial surface of the orbital lamina of the ethmoid.
4. Break away the medial wall of the maxillary sinus between the nasolacrimal duct and the greater palatine canal, and examine the interior of the maxillary sinus [see Fig. 14.3].
5. Expose the maxillary nerve in the pterygopalatine fossa by removing the intervening bone through the maxillary sinus. This also exposes the anterior surface of the pterygopalatine ganglion and the terminal parts of the maxillary artery.
6. Chip away the sphenoid medial to the ganglion, taking care to preserve the pharyngeal branch of the ganglion and the nerve of the pterygoid canal which enters the posterior surface of the ganglion.
7. Follow the infraorbital nerve anteriorly by chipping away the floor of the infraorbital groove and canal.
8. Find the **anterior superior alveolar branch** of the infraorbital nerve, and trace it forwards. Attempt to find its branches to the upper teeth, gums, and mucous membrane of the maxillary sinus.

## Roots of the pterygopalatine ganglion

The pterygopalatine ganglion is suspended from the inferior aspect of the maxillary nerve by two stout **ganglionic roots**, which are nerves entering the ganglia. The sensory trigeminal fibres in these roots pass directly through the ganglion into its branches.

Sympathetic and parasympathetic nerve fibres enter the ganglion in the **nerve of the pterygoid canal**. This nerve is formed by the union of the greater petrosal nerve and deep petrosal nerve. The greater petrosal branch of the facial nerve carries preganglionic parasympathetic fibres to the ganglion. The deep petrosal nerve is a branch of the internal carotid plexus and carries post-ganglionic sympathetic fibres to the ganglion [see Fig. 12.8]. The preganglionic parasympathetic fibres synapse in the ganglion.

## Branches of the pterygopalatine ganglion

Branches of the pterygopalatine ganglion contain post-ganglionic parasympathetic, post-ganglionic sympathetic, and sensory nerves. They supply the lacrimal gland and glands in the nose, palate, and pharynx. The named branches are: (1) the palatine branches—the **greater** and **lesser palatine nerves**; (2) the **orbital branches**—2–3 thin filaments which enter the orbit through the inferior orbital fissure to supply the orbital periosteum (sensory) and the lacrimal gland (secretory); (3) the **nasopalatine** and **posterior nasal branches** passing through the sphenopalatine foramen to the mucous membrane of the nose; and (4) the **pharyngeal branch** which passes posteriorly through the palatovaginal canal to the mucous membrane of the sphenoidal air sinus and the roof of the pharynx.

# Termination of the maxillary artery

The third part of the maxillary artery enters the pterygopalatine fossa through the pterygomaxillary fissure [see Fig. 14.2]. It breaks up into branches which accompany the nerves arising in the pterygopalatine fossa (infraorbital, posterior superior alveolar, greater palatine, nasopalatine, pharyngeal, and nerve of the pterygoid canal) and have the same names.

# Paranasal air sinuses

Review the general features of the paranasal air sinuses and the details of the frontal air sinus described in Chapter 7.

## Ethmoidal air sinus

The **ethmoidal sinus** lies between the upper part of the nasal cavity and the orbit. It consists of anterior, middle, and posterior **ethmoidal air cells**. Superiorly lies the anterior cranial fossa, and inferiorly is the **maxillary air sinus** which lies below the orbit [Fig. 18.2]. The posterior ethmoidal cells open into the superior meatus of the nose through one or more orifices. The anterior ethmoidal cells open into the hiatus semilunaris in the middle meatus, and the middle ethmoidal air cells open on the bulla ethmoidalis [Fig. 18.4].

## Maxillary air sinus

The maxillary air sinus is the largest of the paranasal air sinuses. It occupies the whole of the body of the maxilla and has the shape of an irregular three-sided pyramid. The **apex** is directed laterally and extends into the zygomatic process of the maxilla. The **base** is the lower part of the lateral wall of the nose. The surfaces of the sinus are the **orbital**, **anterior**, and **infratemporal surfaces** and they lie against the corresponding surfaces of the body of the maxilla. The sinus lies inferior to the orbit, lateral to the nasal cavity and superior to the molar and premolar teeth. The lowest part of this sinus is opposite the second premolar and first molar tooth, and is approximately 1 cm below the level of the floor of the nose [see Figs. 10.1, 12.11, 16.8, 16.11; Figs. 18.2, 18.5].

The infraorbital groove and canal run forwards in the bone of the roof of the sinus. The canal bends inferiorly towards the infraorbital foramen and produces a marked ridge in the angle between the orbital and anterior surfaces of the sinus. The posterior superior alveolar nerve and vessels run in the lower part of the infratemporal and anterior walls of the sinus. The anterior superior alveolar nerve and vessels are in the orbital and anterior surfaces [see Fig. 14.3; Fig. 18.5]. The **mucous membrane** of the sinus is supplied by branches of these nerves and by branches of the greater palatine nerve. ➲ In some situations, the bone which separates the nerves from the mucous membrane of the sinus may be absent, and this, combined with the fact that the alveolar nerves supply both the teeth and the mucous lining of the sinus, may be responsible for the sensation of toothache which frequently accompanies inflammation in the sinus.

**Opening of the maxillary sinus**: the maxillary air sinus opens into the middle meatus of the nasal cavity through an aperture in the superior part of its base [see Fig. 10.1; Fig. 18.2].

## Sphenoidal air sinus

Using the instructions given in Dissection 18.6, dissect the sphenoidal air sinus.

The paired sphenoidal air sinuses occupy a variable extent of the body of the sphenoid bone. They may extend into the wings and pterygoid processes, and even into the basilar part of the occipital bone. Each opens with a small, round hole into the spheno-ethmoidal recess [see Fig. 7.12; Fig. 18.3].

Each sinus lies posterior to the nasal cavity and superior to the nasopharynx. Posteriorly, a thick layer of bone usually separates it from the cranial cavity, the basilar artery, and the pons. Above the sphenoidal sinus lie the pituitary gland, intercavernous sinuses, and the cavernous sinuses further laterally [see Figs. 2.7B, 7.12, 7.13A; Fig. 18.3].

**DISSECTION 18.6 Sphenoidal air sinus**

**Objective**

**I.** To study the sphenoidal air sinus.

**Instructions**

1. Examine these sinuses on the two halves of the bisected skull [Fig. 18.3]. As the septum between them is not median, it may be necessary to break down the septum to open the sinus which is not exposed by the cut through the skull.
2. Find the nasal openings in the anterior walls of the sphenoid sinuses.

## Sinusitis

➲ Infections commonly spread from the nasal cavity into the paranasal air sinuses. Inflammation and swelling of the mucous lining of the paranasal sinuses are known as **sinusitis**.

➲ The opening of the maxillary sinus into the nasal cavity is situated high on the medial wall. It is also small and easily blocked by swelling of the mucosa. These factors lead to an accumulation of secretions within the sinus, associated with pain and heaviness of the head. The proximity of the floor of the sinus to the upper molars [Fig. 18.2A] and the common sensory nerves to both often make it difficult to locate the primary pathology.

➲ Fluid in the maxillary sinus may drain at night when the patient lies on one side. (The position of the ostia is such that the right sinus will drain when the patient lies on the left, and vice versa.) In contrast, the frontal air sinus drains best when the head is erect and is often painful and heavy early in the morning.

➲ The relation of the ostia of the frontal sinus to that of the maxillary sinus in the middle meatus is such that infection from the frontal sinus often tracks into the maxillary sinus.

➲ **Squamous cell carcinomas** can occur in the maxillary sinus. They present with frequent headaches, nasal obstruction, pain over the maxilla, and epistaxis (nosebleeds).

See Clinical Application 18.1 for the practical implications of the anatomy discussed in this chapter.

## CLINICAL APPLICATION 18.1 Pollen allergy

An 8-year-old girl returned from a school outing, looking tired and feverish. By the evening, she complained of a headache, itching of her nose and eyes, and a sore throat. She also started coughing and had watering of her eyes and a running nose. She told her parents that it all started when she was playing in a field and had begun with a bout of repeated sneezing. The family physician examined her and treated her for pollen allergy.

Study question 1: which part of the nervous system supplies the glands in the nasal cavity? (Answer: the parasympathetic system.)

Study question 2: what nerves are responsible for secretions of the glands in the nasal cavity? Trace the entire secretomotor pathway. (Answer: preganglionic parasympathetic fibres run in the facial nerve. They leave the facial nerve in the greater petrosal nerve, run in the nerve of the pterygoid canal, reach the pterygopalatine ganglion, and synapse with cells in the ganglion. Post-ganglionic fibres from the ganglion reach the walls of the nasal cavity through branches of the maxillary nerve and medial posterior superior nasal branches of the ganglion.) The lacrimal glands are supplied by parasympathetic nerves from the pterygopalatine ganglion, which run through the zygomatic and lacrimal nerves.

Pollen allergy also causes conjunctivitis and sinusitis, which could account for the itching of the eyes and headache in this patient.

# CHAPTER 19
# The larynx

## Introduction to the larynx

The larynx is the upper expanded part of the airway which is modified for sound production. Its walls are supported by a number of cartilages [Figs. 19.1, 19.2, 19.3, 19.4, 19.5, 19.6]: (1) the unpaired leaf-shaped epiglottis behind the tongue; (2) the V-shaped thyroid cartilage consisting of two laminae set at an angle to each other; (3) the ring-like cricoid cartilage in the midline below the thyroid cartilage; (4) the paired arytenoid cartilages on the superior margin of the cricoid; and (5, 6) in addition, two small paired nodules of cartilage—the corniculate and cuneiform cartilages—are seen on the inlet of the larynx. Familiarize yourself with the location and inter-relations of these cartilages using the figures. Also review the position of the epiglottis in relation to the tongue, and the thyroid and cricoid cartilages in the front of the neck.



The lower part of the larynx is vertical and parallel to the laryngeal part of the pharynx which lies posterior to it. The upper part (within the concavity of the thyroid cartilage) curves [see Fig. 16.3]

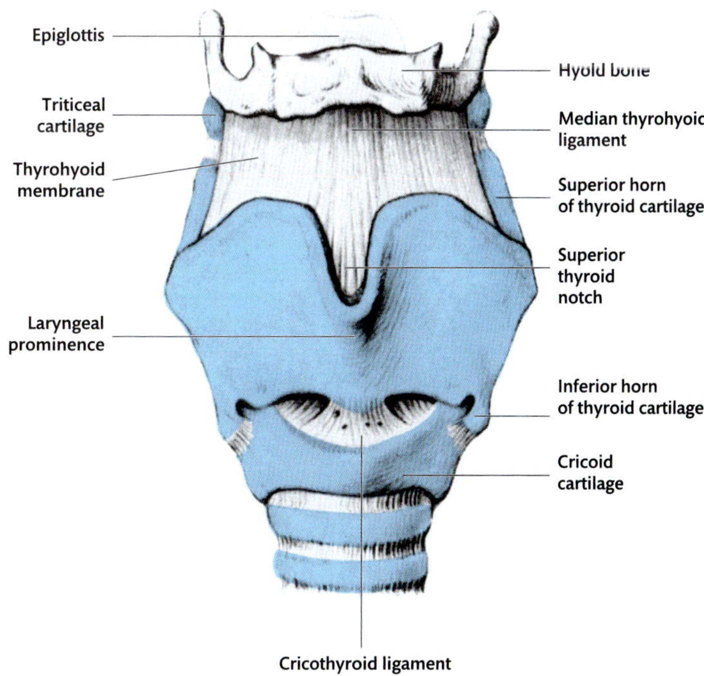


**Fig. 19.1** Anterior aspect of the cartilages (blue) and ligaments of the larynx.

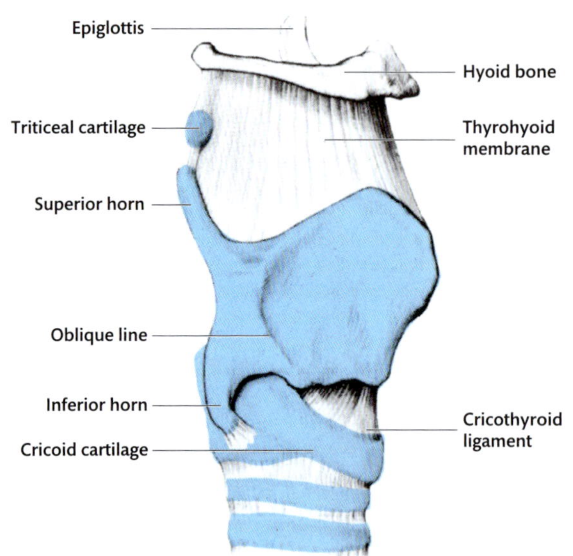


**Fig. 19.2** Lateral view of the cartilages (blue) and ligaments of the larynx.



back to open into the pharynx through a vertical orifice—the **inlet of the larynx**. On either side of the inlet, part of the pharyngeal cavity projects forwards as the **piriform recess** [see Fig. 16.10].

## Cartilages, ligaments, and joints of the larynx

### Thyroid cartilage

The thyroid cartilage is the largest of the laryngeal cartilages and consists of two laminae or plates of hyaline cartilage. In the midline anteriorly, the inferior parts of the two laminae are fused together. The superior parts of the laminae are separated from each other by the deep **superior thyroid notch** [Fig. 19.1] and project anteriorly to form the **laryngeal prominence**. The laryngeal prominence is more acute in the male as the angle at which the laminae meet is smaller.

The thyroid laminae diverge posteriorly and end in the posterior margins, which are lateral to the **piriform recesses** of the pharynx. Each posterior margin extends superiorly and inferiorly as slender horns (**cornua**) of the thyroid cartilage [Figs. 19.2, 19.3]. The **superior horns** are attached to the corresponding greater horns of the hyoid bone by the thyrohyoid ligaments. The **inferior horns** articulate with the cricoid cartilage at the cricothyroid joint.

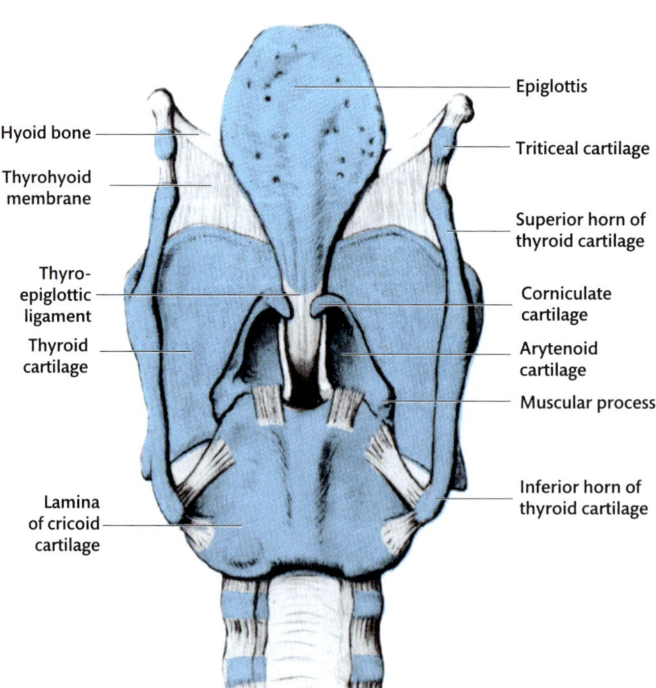


**Fig. 19.3** Posterior aspect of the cartilages (blue) and ligaments of the larynx.

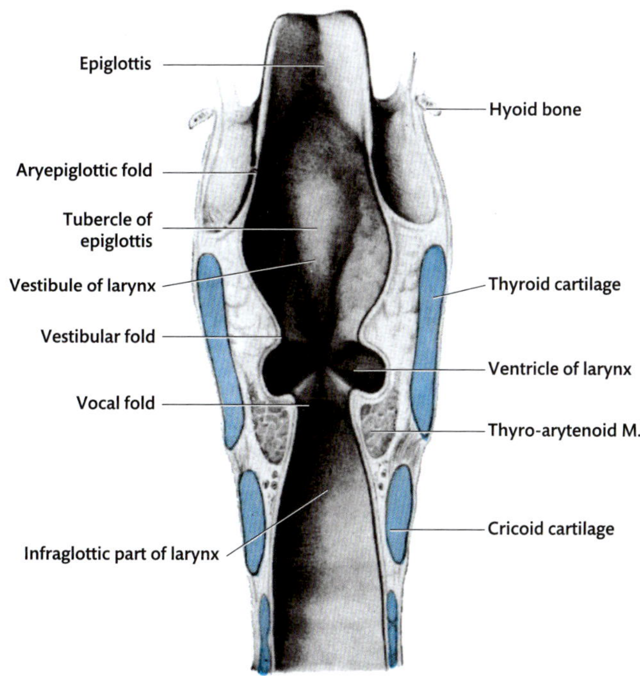


**Fig. 19.4** Coronal section through the larynx to show its parts. Cartilage = blue.

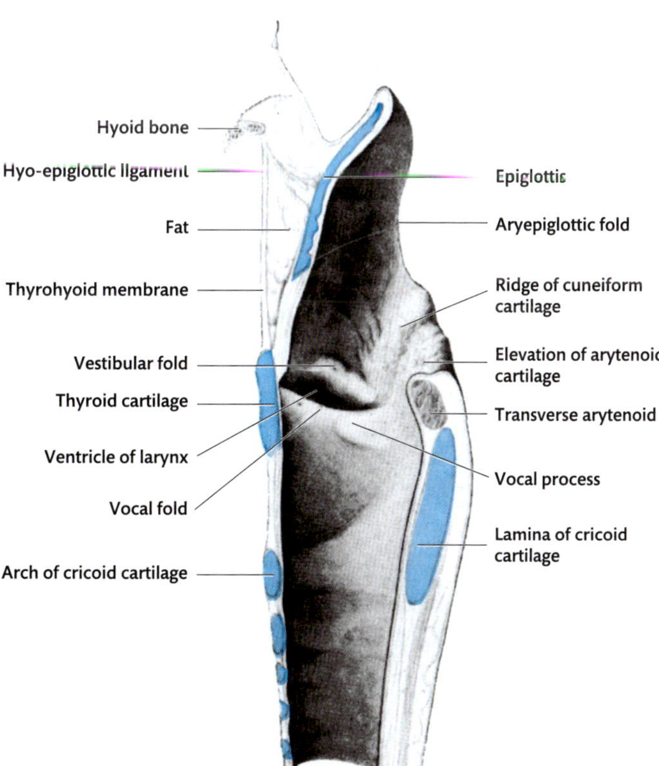


**Fig. 19.5** Median section through the larynx to show the lateral wall of its right half. Cartilage = blue.

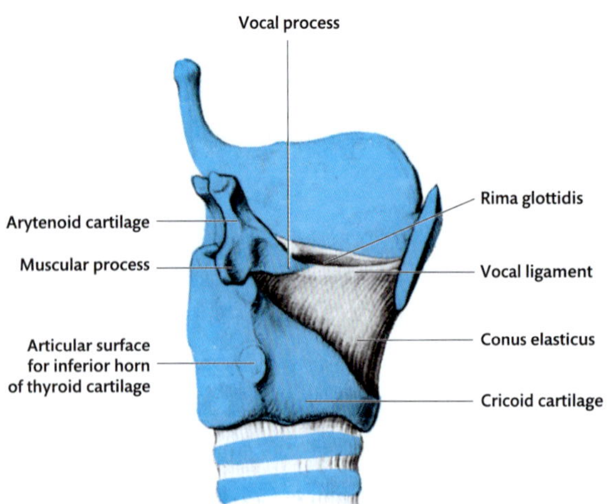


**Fig. 19.6** Dissection to show the conus elasticus and vocal ligament. The right lamina of the thyroid cartilage has been removed. Cartilage = blue.

The lateral surfaces of the thyroid cartilage are relatively flat, except for a raised, oblique line on each lamina [Fig. 19.2]. The inferior constrictor of the pharynx, the pre-tracheal fascia, and the sternothyroid and thyrohyoid muscles are attached to the oblique line.

## Thyrohyoid membrane and ligaments

The thyrohyoid membrane ascends from the superior border of the thyroid cartilage, passes deep to the concavity of the hyoid bone, and is attached to the upper margin of the hyoid bone. Anteriorly, the membrane is thickened to form the **median thyrohyoid ligament**. This ligament is separated from the posterior surface of the body of the hyoid bone by a bursa, which lessens the friction between the ligament and the hyoid when the thyroid cartilage is drawn up behind the hyoid bone in swallowing. The lateral thyrohyoid ligaments are thickened posterior margins of the thyrohyoid membrane. Each contains a small cartilaginous nodule—the **triticeal cartilage** [Figs. 19.1, 19.2, 19.3]. The thyrohyoid ligament is pierced by the internal laryngeal branch of the superior laryngeal nerve and the superior laryngeal vessels.

Using the instructions given in Dissection 19.1, study the thyrohyoid membrane.

## Cricoid cartilage

The cricoid cartilage is shaped like a signet ring. The horizontal inferior margin is at the level of the sixth cervical vertebra. The narrow **arch of the cricoid**

### DISSECTION 19.1 Thyrohyoid membrane

**Objective**

**I.** To expose the thyrohyoid membrane and study its attachments.

**Instructions**

1. Cut through the thyrohyoid muscle to expose the thyrohyoid membrane and the vessels and nerve piercing it.
2. Define the attachments of the membrane.

lies anteriorly [Fig. 19.1]. Traced laterally from the arch, the upper margin of the cricoid cartilage [Fig. 19.6] slopes upwards, deep to the thyroid cartilage, to form the **lamina of the cricoid cartilage** [Fig. 19.3]. The cricothyroid membrane extends upwards from the upper margin of the cricoid cartilage to the thyroid cartilage. It is thickened in the midline anteriorly to form the **cricothyroid ligament**. The cricoid is attached to the trachea by the membranous, elastic **cricotracheal ligament** [Fig. 19.1].

## Arytenoid cartilages

Each of the paired arytenoid cartilages is shaped like a three-sided pyramid [Fig. 19.3]. The base rests on the superior surface of the cricoid lamina and forms a synovial joint with it [Figs. 19.3, 19.6].

Each arytenoid cartilage has a **muscular process** which projects laterally and gives attachment to the crico-arytenoid muscles, and a **vocal process** which projects anteriorly and gives attachment to the vocal ligament [Fig. 19.6]. The apex of the arytenoid cartilage extends upwards, curves posteromedially, and has the corniculate cartilage resting on it. The transverse arytenoid muscle is attached to the posterior surface of each arytenoid cartilage [see Fig. 19.10]. The thyro-arytenoid and vocalis muscles are attached to the anterolateral surfaces [Fig. 19.4; see also Fig. 19.11].

Clean and define the cricothyroid muscle and cricothyroid membrane by following the instructions provided in Dissection 19.2.

## Cricothyroid joint

The inferior horns of the thyroid cartilage articulate with the lamina of the cricoid cartilage by a synovial joint—the cricothyroid joint [Fig. 19.3]. The two cricothyroid joints allow the cricoid cartilage to rock around a horizontal axis passing through them.

**DISSECTION 19.2 Cricothyroid muscle and cricothyroid membrane**

**Objectives**

**I.** To expose the cricothyroid muscle. **II.** To expose the cricothyroid membrane. **III.** To identify the cricothyroid joint.

**Instructions**

1. Turn the sternothyroid muscle upwards, and define its attachment to the thyroid cartilage.
2. Identify the attachments of the inferior constrictor to the thyroid and cricoid cartilages and to the fascia covering the cricothyroid muscle.
3. Expose the cricothyroid muscle by removing the fascia over it and reflecting the divided parts of the inferior constrictor [see Fig. 16.5].
4. Trace the inferior horn of the thyroid cartilage to its articulation with the cricoid cartilage.
5. Expose the cricothyroid ligament at the anterior border of the cricothyroid muscle.
6. Note that the cricothyroid membrane passes deep to the cricothyroid muscle.

This movement swings the superior margin of the cricoid lamina and the attached arytenoid cartilages either towards or away from the anterior part of the thyroid, and slackens or tightens the elastic vocal ligament which is attached to it [Fig. 19.6].

➲ **Cricothyrotomy** is an emergency procedure done to establish an airway by making a surgical incision through the cricothyroid membrane.

## Epiglottis

The epiglottis is a thin, leaf-shaped cartilage. It forms the upper part of the anterior wall of the larynx, and the superior margin of the inlet of the larynx [Fig. 19.3]. It is posterior to the base of the tongue, hyoid bone, and median thyrohyoid ligament. The epiglottis tapers inferiorly and is attached to the posterior surface of the thyroid cartilage in the midline by the strong **thyro-epiglottic ligament**. It is convex anteriorly in its superior part, and convex posteriorly in the lower part. The lower part bulges into the larynx as the **epiglottic tubercle** [Fig. 19.4]. Numerous mucous and serous glands lie on the surface of the epiglottis.

## Ligaments of the epiglottis

The thyro-epiglottic ligament has been described earlier. In addition, the anterior surface of the epiglottis is also attached to the upper surface of the hyoid bone by the loose, fibro-elastic **hyo-epiglottic ligament** [Fig. 19.5]. This is separated from the thyro-epiglottic and median thyrohyoid ligaments by fat, which is displaced when the thyroid cartilage is drawn up inside the hyoid bone. The epiglottis is also attached to the tongue by the median and lateral **glosso-epiglottic folds** of mucous membrane [see Figs. 16.10, 17.1] and to the arytenoid cartilages by the **aryepiglottic folds** [see Fig. 16.10].

Dissection 19.3 provides instructions on dissection of the ligaments of the epiglottis.

## Crico-arytenoid joints

The crico-arytenoid joints are synovial joints between the base of the arytenoid cartilage and the lamina of the cricoid cartilage. At these joints, the arytenoid cartilages: (1) slide transversely on the lamina of the cricoid to come closer together or move apart from each other; and (2) rotate around a vertical axis [Figs. 19.7, 19.8], so as to approximate or separate the vocal processes (and hence the vocal ligaments). The arytenoid cartilages are prevented from slipping anteriorly on the cricoid lamina by the strong posterior capsule of the joint [Fig. 19.3].

**DISSECTION 19.3 Epiglottis and the ligaments**

**Objectives**

**I.** To study the epiglottis. **II.** To identify the thyro-epiglottic and hyo-epiglottic ligaments.

**Instructions**

1. On the sectioned surface of the larynx, identify the epiglottis and the thyro-epiglottic and hyo-epiglottic ligaments.
2. Note the relationship of these ligaments to the thyroid cartilage, the hyoid bone, and the thyrohyoid ligament.

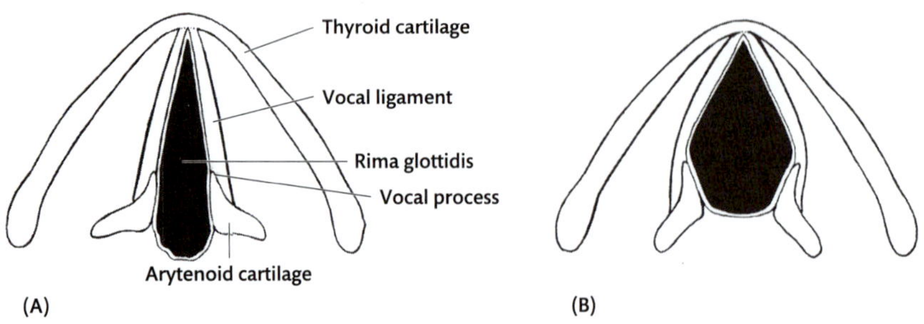


**Fig. 19.7** Diagrams to show movements of the arytenoid cartilages. (A) Position during quiet breathing—the rima glottidis is partially open. (B) Position during forced respiration—the rima glottidis is wide open.





## Structure of laryngeal cartilages

The thyroid, cricoid, and basal parts of the arytenoid cartilages are composed of hyaline cartilage and tend to ossify, even in early adult life. In old age, they may be completely ossified. The apex and vocal process of the arytenoid cartilage and the other cartilages are made up of elastic fibrocartilage and do not ossify.

## Exterior of the larynx

The inlet of the larynx is an almost vertically placed opening. It is bound anterosuperiorly by the epiglottis, on each side by the aryepiglottic fold of mucous membrane, and inferiorly by the interarytenoid fold of mucous membrane. The vertical posterior wall of the larynx below the inlet is made up of the lamina of the cricoid cartilage, surmounted by the two arytenoid cartilages, covered by mucous membrane [see Fig. 16.10]. The anterior wall of the larynx is made up of: (1) the epiglottis which curves upwards and backwards from its attachment to the internal surface of the thyroid cartilage; (2) the thyroid cartilage; and (3) the arch of the cricoid cartilage [Fig. 19.1]. The lateral wall of the upper part is formed by the **aryepiglottic fold**. Each fold has two small nodules of cartilage—the **corniculate** and **cuneiform cartilages**—embedded in its margin near the arytenoid cartilage [see Fig. 16.10].

## Interior of the larynx

The interior of the larynx is divided into superior and inferior parts by anteroposterior folds projecting from the lateral walls—the **vocal folds**. Above each vocal fold is a subsidiary **vestibular fold** which is separated from the vocal fold by a narrow, horizontal groove—the **ventricle of the larynx** [Fig. 19.4]. The two pairs of folds narrow the middle part of the laryngeal cavity. The part of the laryngeal cavity above the vestibular folds is the **vestibule of the larynx**. The part below is the **infraglottic part of the larynx**.

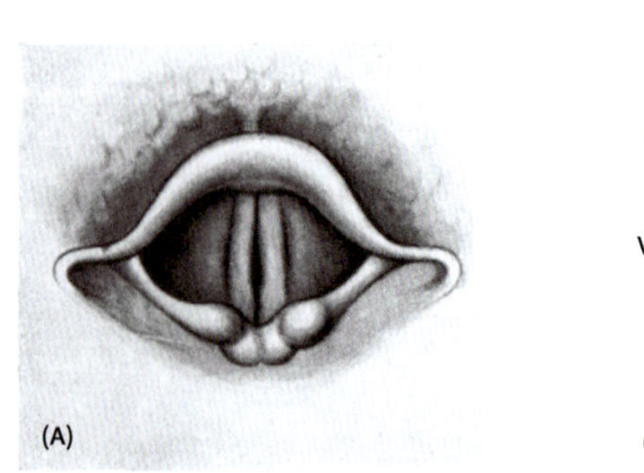


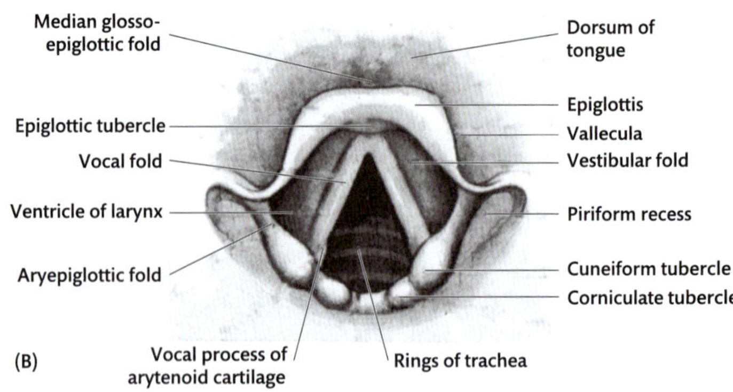


**Fig. 19.8** Laryngoscopic view of the cavity of the larynx. (A) During phonation. The rima glottidis is closed by approximation of the vocal folds. (B) During moderate respiration. The rima glottidis is widely open.

## Vestibule of the larynx

The superior part, or vestibule, of the larynx extends from the inlet of the larynx to the vestibular folds. It has a long **anterosuperior wall** consisting of the mucous membrane covering the epiglottis and thyro-epiglottic ligament, and a short **posterior wall** formed by the mucous membrane covering the apex of the arytenoid and corniculate cartilages. The lateral walls are the aryepiglottic folds which slope inwards towards the vestibular folds and separate the vestibule of the larynx from the piriform recess of the pharynx [Figs. 19.4, 19.5].

➲ Inflammation of the mucosa of the larynx results in **laryngitis**. It is often caused by viral infections and presents as a sore throat, cough, and difficulty in swallowing.

## Vestibular folds and rima vestibuli

Vestibular folds are soft, flaccid folds of mucous membrane which extend from the thyroid to the arytenoid cartilages. They contain: (1) numerous mucous glands; (2) a thin band of fibro-elastic tissue; and (3) a few muscle fibres. They lie further apart than the vocal folds and play little or no part in sound production [Fig. 19.5]. The space between the two vestibular folds is the **rima vestibuli**.

## Ventricle and saccule of the larynx

The ventricle of the larynx is the narrow groove between the vestibular and vocal folds [Figs. 19.4, 19.5]. The saccule of the larynx is a narrow, blind diverticulum which passes posterosuperiorly between the vestibular fold and the thyroid cartilage. It may reach up to the upper border of the thyroid cartilage.

Dissection 19.4 provides instructions on dissection of the ventricle and saccule of the larynx.

## Vocal folds

Each vocal fold is wedge-shaped in the coronal section [Fig. 19.4]. The apex projects medially into the laryngeal cavity. The base lies against the lamina of the thyroid cartilage. The superior surface is nearly horizontal and forms the inferior wall of the ventricle. The inferior surface slopes inferolaterally to the superior border of the cricoid cartilage. Each fold contains the: (1) conus elasticus; (2) vocal ligament; (3) muscle fibres; and (4) covering mucous membrane.

### DISSECTION 19.4 Ventricle and saccule of the larynx

**Objective**

**I.** To explore the ventricle and saccule of the larynx.

**Instructions**

1. Pass a blunt seeker along the roof of the ventricle into the saccule of the larynx.
2. Cut the vestibular fold away from the upper part of the arytenoid cartilage, and strip it carefully forwards from the wall of the larynx. Avoid injury to the underlying muscle—the thyro-epiglotticus.
3. Separate the vestibular fold from the thyroid cartilage, and open the saccule.

## Conus elasticus and vocal ligament

The **conus elasticus** is a thin layer of fibro-elastic tissue on the inferomedial surface of each vocal fold, immediately deep to the mucous membrane. It is an elastic membrane which is attached inferiorly to the arch of the cricoid cartilage. It slopes superomedially to end in a free margin which stretches from the back of the thyroid cartilage (close to the midline) to the vocal process of the corresponding arytenoid cartilage [Fig. 19.6]. The free edge of each membrane is a thickened elastic band known as the **vocal ligament**. The membranes on the right and left sides together form the conus elasticus. Anteriorly, the conus elasticus is continuous with the cricothyroid ligament. The mucous membrane covering the vocal ligament is tightly bound to it.

The muscle fibres in the vocal fold lie between the conus elasticus and the lamina of the thyroid cartilage. They arise from the thyroid cartilage and vocal ligament anteriorly. Most of them pass horizontally backwards to the arytenoid cartilage (**thyro-arytenoideus**). The most medial fibres arise from the vocal ligament and form the **vocalis muscle**. The most lateral fibres sweep superiorly to the epiglottis—the **thyro-epiglotticus** [see Fig. 19.11].

Using the instructions given in Dissection 19.5, expose the vocal fold and conus elasticus.

## Rima glottidis

The rima glottidis is a midline fissure between the free margins of the vocal folds and the vocal

**DISSECTION 19.5 Vocal fold and conus elasticus**

**Objective**

**I.** To expose the vocal fold and conus elasticus.

**Instructions**

1. Strip the mucous membrane from the inferior surface of the vocal fold, and expose the conus elasticus and vocal ligament.
2. Strip the mucous membrane from the superior surface of the vocal fold, thus exposing the upper surface of the thyro-arytenoid muscle and its continuity with the thyro-epiglotticus. The thyro-epiglotticus was exposed when the vestibular fold was removed.

processes of the arytenoid cartilages. The anterior part of the rima lies between the two vocal folds, and the posterior part between the two arytenoid cartilages [Figs. 19.7, 19.8]. It is the narrowest part of the laryngeal cavity and lies behind the thyroid cartilage.

## Movement of the vocal cords

The shape of the rima glottidis is continually changing [Fig. 19.8] due to movements of the arytenoid cartilages on the cricoid and of the cricoid relative to the thyroid cartilage. These movements are essential for breathing and sound production. **Abduction of the vocal cords**: separation of the vocal cords to allow air to enter and leave the lungs is abduction. The posterior part of the rima is progressively widened when: (1) the arytenoid cartilages are displaced laterally on the cricoid; and (2) the arytenoids are rotated such that their vocal processes turn laterally [Figs. 19.7B, 19.8B]. When the lamina of the cricoid is tilted forwards with the vocal cords abducted, the vocal ligaments are slackened and the opening can be widened further to allow the free passage of air in forced respiration.

**Adduction of the vocal cords**: the rima glottidis is narrowed or closed when the arytenoid cartilages are: (1) drawn together; and (2) rotated so that their vocal processes come into apposition [Figs. 19.7A, 19.8A]. The additional tightening of the vocal ligaments by tilting of the cricoid lamina backwards effectively prevents the passage of air. This tightly closed position is taken up prior to the explosive discharge of air in coughing and sneezing. During these actions, the intrathoracic pressure is raised by contraction of the expiratory muscles, following which the tension in the vocal folds is released suddenly.

When the rima glottidis is closed, attempts to draw air into the thorax push the sloping vocal folds more firmly together and prevent inspiration, a situation which arises in laryngeal spasm.

Delicate variations in the following factors are responsible for changes in the pitch and volume of the voice: (1) the tension and length of the vocal cords; (2) the width of the rima glottidis; and (3) the intensity of expiratory effort. The lower pitch of the male voice is due to the greater length of the vocal folds in them (approximately 2.5 cm), as compared with those in the female (approximately 1.7 cm).

Table 19.1 provides an overview of the movements of the vocal cords.

## Infraglottic part of the larynx

The **infraglottic part of the larynx** extends from the vocal folds to the level of the arch of the cricoid cartilage where it becomes continuous with the trachea.

**Table 19.1** Movements of the vocal cords

| Movement | Muscles involved | Nerve supply |
|---|---|---|
| Abduction | Posterior crico-arytenoid | Recurrent laryngeal |
| Adduction | Lateral crico-arytenoid | Recurrent laryngeal |
| | Oblique and transverse arytenoid | Recurrent laryngeal |
| Tightening | Cricothyroid | External laryngeal |
| | Vocalis | Recurrent laryngeal |
| Slackening | Thyro-arytenoid | Recurrent laryngeal |
| | Vocalis | Recurrent laryngeal |

# Muscles of the larynx

The muscles of the larynx include the cricothyroid, posterior crico-arytenoid, transverse and oblique interarytenoids, lateral crico-arytenoid, thyro-arytenoid, vocalis, aryepiglottic, and thyro-epiglottic muscles. The muscles of the larynx act to alter the length and tension of the vocal folds, and change the size of the rima glottidis or the size of the inlet of the larynx.

## Cricothyroid

The **cricothyroid** is seen on the external surface of the larynx anteriorly. **Origin**: it takes origin from the anterolateral part of the cricoid cartilage. **Insertion**: the fibres pass posterosuperiorly to the inferior horn, inferior margin, and lower part of the deep surface of the lamina of the thyroid cartilage [Fig. 19.9]. **Nerve supply**: external branch of the superior laryngeal nerve. **Action**: it rotates the cricoid at the cricothyroid joints such that the arch is drawn posterosuperiorly and the lamina is tilted posteriorly. This movement causes stretching and tightening of the vocal ligaments and raises the pitch of the voice.

Using the instructions given in Dissection 19.6, identify the muscles of the larynx [Fig. 19.10].

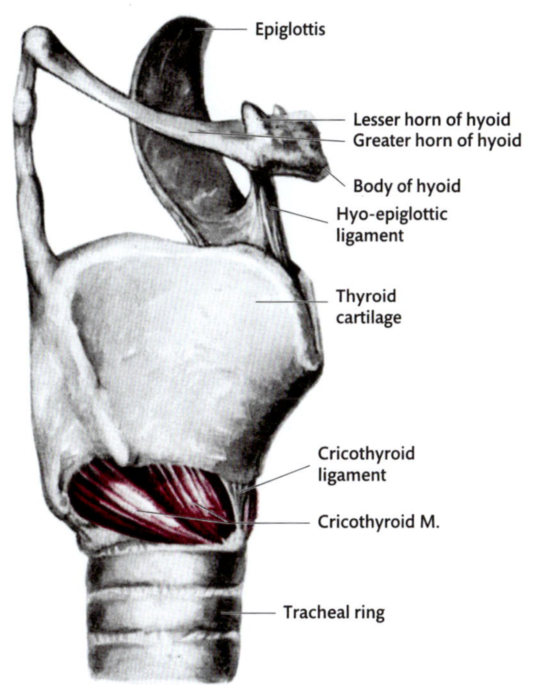


**Fig. 19.9** The right cricothyroid muscle.

## Posterior crico-arytenoid

**Origin**: the posterior crico-arytenoid arises from the posterior surface of the lamina of the cricoid cartilage. **Insertion**: it runs laterally and converges on the laterally directed muscular process of the arytenoid cartilage [Fig. 19.10]. **Nerve supply**: recurrent laryngeal branch of the vagus. (All intrinsic muscles of the larynx, except the cricothyroid, are supplied by the recurrent laryngeal nerve.) **Action**: the upper, more horizontal fibres rotate the arytenoid, so that its vocal process is directed laterally and the rima glottidis is opened. The lower, more vertical fibres pull the arytenoid laterally, further increasing the size of the rima. It is the sole abductor of the vocal folds.

### DISSECTION 19.6 Muscles of the larynx

#### Objectives

**I.** To identify and study the posterior crico-arytenoid, thyro-arytenoid, and oblique arytenoid muscles. **II.** To identify and trace the recurrent laryngeal nerve.

#### Instructions

1. Identify the recurrent laryngeal nerve entering the larynx, deep to the inferior constrictor muscle.
2. Strip the mucous membrane from the posterior surface of the arytenoid and cricoid cartilages. Note the attachment of the longitudinal oesophageal muscle fibres to the median part of the cricoid lamina.
3. Identify the posterior crico-arytenoid, transverse arytenoid, and oblique arytenoid muscles [Fig. 19.10]. The transverse arytenoid and oblique arytenoid have been divided in the midline, but the oblique arytenoid can be followed into continuity with the aryepiglottic muscle by stripping the mucous membrane from the margin of the aryepiglottic fold.

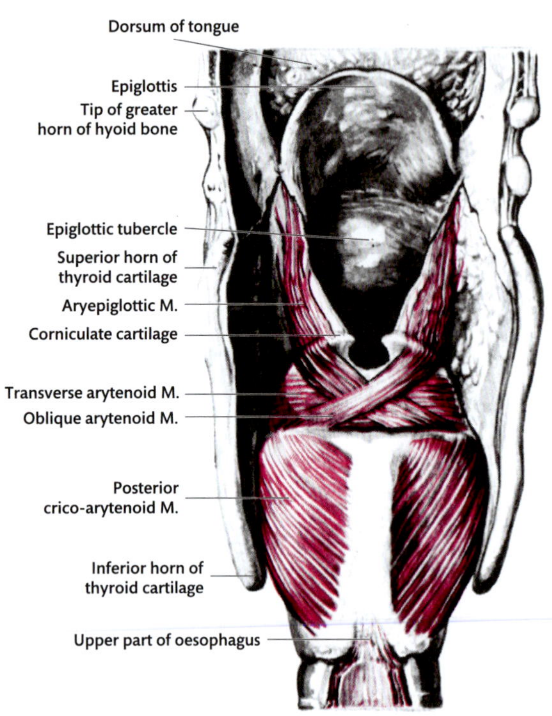


**Fig. 19.10** Muscles on the posterior surface of the larynx.

## Transverse and oblique arytenoids, and aryepiglottic muscles

**Origin** and **insertion**: the **transverse** and **oblique arytenoids (interarytenoids)** extend between the two arytenoid cartilages and draw them together. The aryepiglottic muscle are fibres of the oblique arytenoid which extend into the aryepiglottic fold and attach to the epiglottis. **Nerve supply**: recurrent laryngeal branch of the vagus. **Action**: the interarytenoids close the rima glottidis. The continuity of the oblique arytenoid and aryepiglottic muscles ensures that the arytenoid cartilages are drawn together, closing the rima, while the epiglottis is pulled down over the laryngeal inlet, during passage of food or fluid into the pharynx [Fig. 19.10].

Using the instructions given in Dissection 19.7, study the cricothyroid joint [Fig. 19.11].

## Lateral crico-arytenoid muscle

**Origin**: the lateral crico-arytenoid muscle takes origin from the superior border of the posterior part of the arch of the cricoid cartilage. **Insertion**: it is inserted into the muscular process of the arytenoid cartilage [Figs. 19.11, 19.12]. **Nerve supply**: recurrent laryngeal branch of the vagus. **Action**: it pulls the muscular process anteriorly, rotating the arytenoid so that its vocal process swings medially and closes the rima glottidis—adduction.

## Thyro-arytenoid, thyro-epiglottic, and vocalis

**Origin**: the **thyro-arytenoid** takes origin from the posterior surface of the thyroid cartilage, close to the midline. **Insertion**: it is inserted into the anterolateral surface of the arytenoid cartilage. The upper lateral fibres sweep superiorly to the epiglottis, forming the **thyro-epiglottic** muscle.

**Origin**: the **vocalis** is constituted by some of the deeper fibres of the thyro-arytenoid which arise from the vocal ligament. **Insertion**: these fibres pass to the vocal process of the arytenoid cartilage [Figs. 19.11, 19.12]. **Action**: the thyro-arytenoid pulls the arytenoid anteriorly and slackens the vocal ligament. The vocalis tends to tighten the anterior part of the ligament, while simultaneously slackening the posterior part—a position taken up by the vocal cords in whispering. The thyro-epiglottic and aryepiglottic muscles play a minor role in closing the laryngeal inlet.

### DISSECTION 19.7 Cricothyroid joint

**Objectives**

**I.** To open the cricothyroid joint. **II.** To examine the thyro-arytenoid and lateral crico-arytenoid muscles.

**Instructions**

1. On one side, remove the cricothyroid muscle, the lower part of the lamina, and the inferior horn of the thyroid cartilage, thus opening the cricothyroid joint. Take care not to cut the recurrent laryngeal nerve (the inferior laryngeal nerve) which is deep to the posterior part of the thyroid cartilage.
2. Examine the thyro-arytenoid muscle in the vocal fold which is now exposed [Fig. 19.11], with the lateral crico-arytenoid muscle inferior to it.

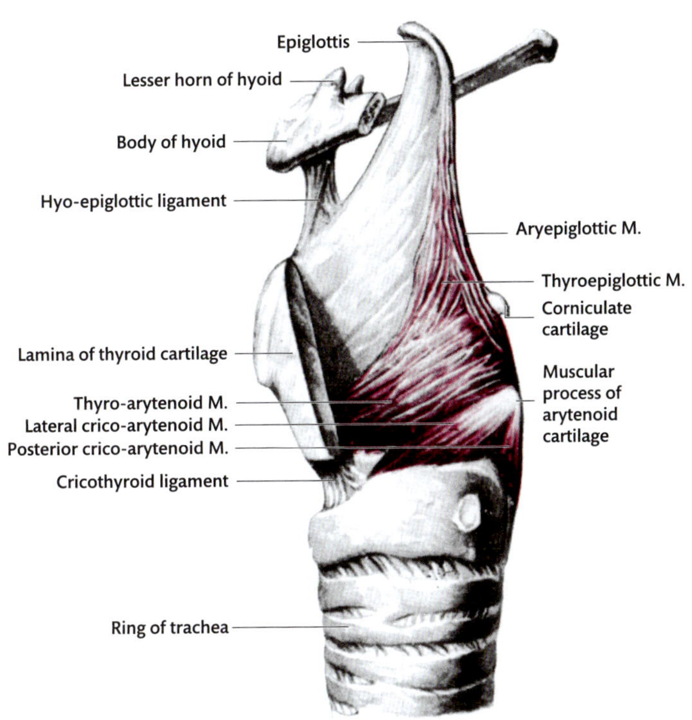


**Fig. 19.11** Muscles in the lateral wall of the larynx.





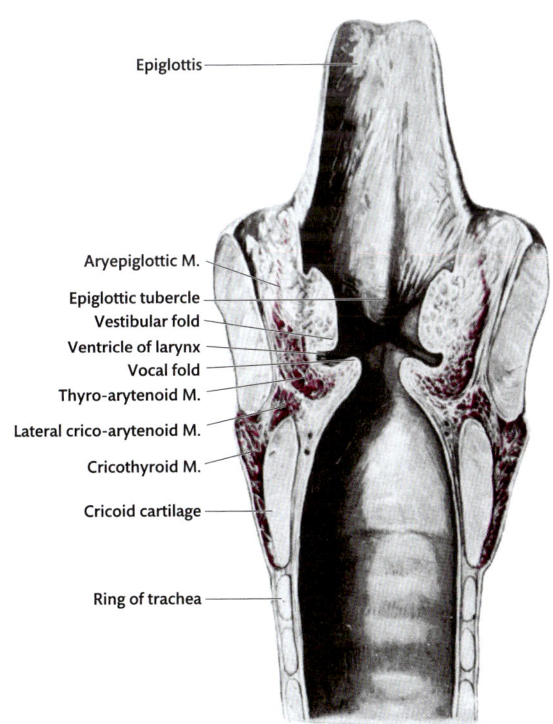


**Fig. 19.12** Coronal section of the larynx to show the position of the muscles.

## Extrinsic muscles

The extrinsic muscles of the larynx raise and lower the larynx during swallowing. The **thyrohyoid**, acting from a fixed hyoid bone and assisted by the **stylopharyngeus** and **palatopharyngeus**, raises the larynx inside the hyoid bone. The elevated epiglottis is tipped backwards by the bulging posterior surface of the tongue (assisted by the aryepiglottic and thyro-epiglottic muscles). It comes into contact with the elevated arytenoid cartilages, closes the laryngeal orifice, and allows the tip of the epiglottis to direct the bolus away from the larynx. The **sternothyroid** returns the larynx to its original position and opens the laryngeal orifice.

# Nerves and vessels of the larynx

## Superior laryngeal nerve

The **superior laryngeal** branch of the vagus supplies the larynx through its branches—the internal and external laryngeal nerves [see Fig. 16.5]. The **internal laryngeal nerve** pierces the thyrohyoid membrane with the superior laryngeal artery and supplies the lateral wall of the piriform recess, through a number of small branches. Some branches pass in the aryepiglottic fold to the base of the tongue and epiglottis. Others descend to supply the mucous membrane on the internal surface of the larynx, as far as the vocal folds, and the mucous membrane covering the posterior surfaces of the arytenoid and cricoid cartilages. One branch descends deep to the thyroid cartilage to join a branch from the recurrent laryngeal nerve. The superior laryngeal nerve contains sensory and autonomic fibres. The **external laryngeal nerve** supplies the cricothyroid muscle.

## Inferior laryngeal nerve

The inferior laryngeal nerve is a continuation of the recurrent laryngeal branch of the vagus. It ascends in the groove between the trachea and the oesophagus, and enters the larynx by passing posterior to the cricothyroid joint and the lower border of the inferior constrictor [see Fig. 16.5]. It gives motor branches to all the intrinsic muscles of the larynx, except the cricothyroid, and sensory branches to the mucous membrane below the rima glottidis. It communicates with the internal laryngeal branch of the superior laryngeal nerve and is accompanied by the inferior laryngeal branch of the inferior thyroid artery.

➲ Injury to the **recurrent laryngeal nerve** on one side leads to hoarseness of voice, due to paralysis of the vocal cord on that side. The paralysed vocal cord cannot adduct to close the rima. Some degree of compensatory movement of the vocal cord on the other side will occur with time.

➲ In bilateral paralysis of the cords, the voice is almost totally lost. In such cases, abduction of the cords is also lost (paralysis of the posterior crico-arytenoids), and the patient will not be able to take a deep breath. Attempt to do so will result in stridor—a loud, high-pitched sound—and a sense of anxiety.

➲ Injury to the **superior laryngeal nerve** will result in loss of sensation in the vestibule. Accidental aspiration of food particles during swallowing will not be detected, and the aspirate will enter the larynx. In addition, paralysis of the cricothyroid muscle will make it hard to raise the pitch of the voice.

## Vessels of the larynx

The larynx is supplied by the **superior laryngeal branch** of the superior thyroid artery, and the **inferior laryngeal branch** of the inferior thyroid artery. It is drained by the corresponding veins.

Figs. 19.13A and 19.13B show the vocal cords, cartilages, and relations of the larynx in a cross-sectional view.

See Clinical Application 19.1 for the practical implications of the anatomy discussed in this chapter.

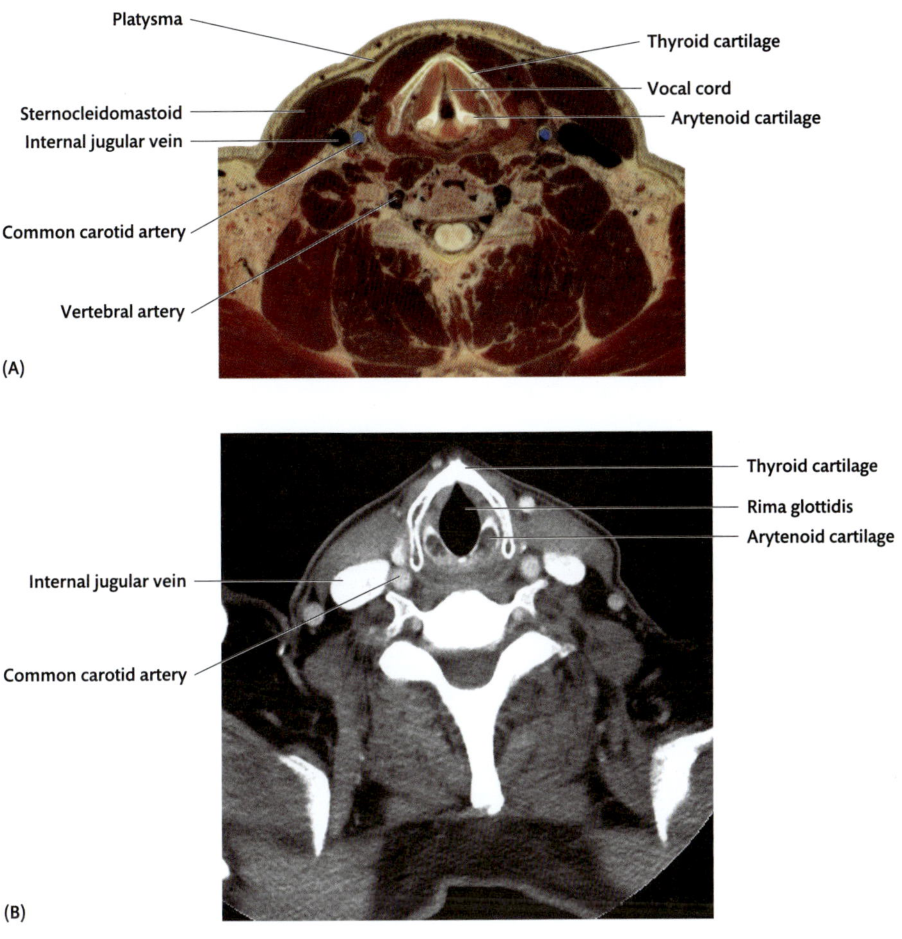


**Fig. 19.13** (A) Horizontal section through the neck at the level of the vocal cords. (B) Contrast-enhanced axial computerized tomography (CT) section at the level of the vocal cords.

(A) Image courtesy of the Visible Human Project of the US National Library of Medicine.



### CLINICAL APPLICATION 19.1 Laryngoscopy

The larynx can be visualized in the living by a procedure known as laryngoscopy. In direct laryngoscopy, an instrument—the laryngoscope—is inserted into the mouth, past the tongue and epiglottis, towards the inlet of the larynx. The laryngoscope allows the doctor to visualize the vestibule of the larynx, the vestibular fold, and the vocal folds. When the rima glottidis is open, the infraglottic part of the larynx can also be seen through the laryngoscope [Fig. 19.8].

In indirect laryngoscopy, a small handheld mirror is held at the back of the throat and a light is shone into the patient's mouth. The mirror is angulated, so as to get a reflection of the larynx in the mirror. The piriform recess of the pharynx can also be examined in this way.

# CHAPTER 20

# The contents of the vertebral canal

## Introduction

The vertebral canal lies behind the vertebral bodies and intervertebral discs, and in front of the spines and laminae of the vertebrae [Fig. 20.1]. The main content of the vertebral canal is the spinal cord, the meninges surrounding the spinal cord, the blood vessels supplying the cord, and the spinal nerves. The external features of the spinal cord and its coverings and blood supply are described in this chapter. The internal features are described later in the section on the brain and spinal cord.

Using the instructions given in Dissection 20.1, remove the vertebral spines and laminae to open into the vertebral canal.



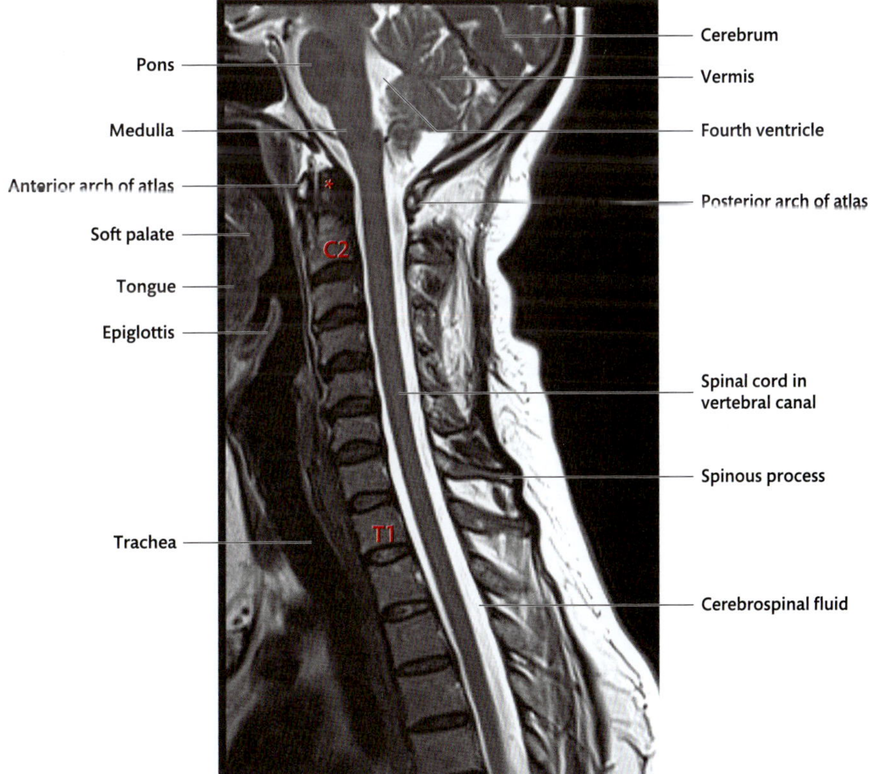


**Fig. 20.1** T2-weighted sagittal magnetic resonance imaging (MRI) of the cervical spine in the midline, showing the cervical and upper thoracic vertebrae (C. 2–T. 4). The spinal cord is seen within the vertebral canal, surrounded by the hyperintense (bright) cerebrospinal fluid.

**DISSECTION 20.1 Opening of the vertebral canal**

**Objectives**

**I.** The lower lumbar and sacral parts of the vertebral canal may have been opened already. In this session, you will: (1) open the remainder of the vertebral canal to see the entire length of the spinal cord; and (2) see the course of the spinal nerves within the vertebral canal.

**Instructions**

1. Remove all the remaining muscles of the back to expose the laminae and spines of the vertebrae and the dorsum of the sacrum.
2. Follow the dorsal rami of the spinal nerves towards the intervertebral foramina, noting their course relative to the vertebrae and especially the articular processes.
3. Remove the posterior wall of the vertebral canal by sawing through the lateral parts of the laminae and dividing the ligamentum flava in a coronal plane. Do not saw completely through the laminae, but complete the division with a chisel or bone forceps to avoid cutting the spinal cord and its coverings (meninges). (It is often possible to cut the cervical laminae entirely with bone forceps by starting at the upper end where the right half of the skull has been removed.)
4. When a length of spines, laminae, and ligamentum flava has been removed, test the elasticity of these ligaments by stretching the specimen.
5. Note the extensive venous plexus which surrounds the spinal dura mater. It is very obvious when filled with blood.

## Epidural space

The epidural space lies between the periosteum of the vertebral canal and the spinal dura mater. The space is filled with loose areolar tissue, semi-liquid fat, a network of veins—the internal vertebral venous plexus—and the small arteries which supply the structures in the vertebral canal [Fig. 20.2]. The veins correspond to the dural venous sinuses in the cranium and are continuous with them through the foramen magnum.

### Spinal arteries in the epidural space

Small spinal arteries arise from arteries in the cervical, thoracic, lumbar, and sacral regions from the

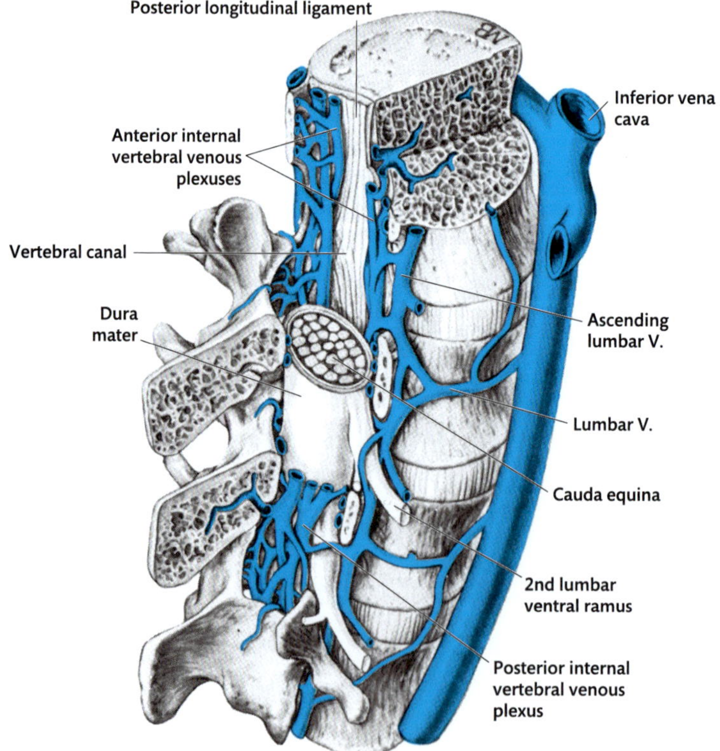


Fig. 20.2 Dissection of the upper four lumbar vertebrae to show the internal vertebral venous plexuses and their communications with the inferior vena cava.

ascending cervical, vertebral [see Fig. 8.8], posterior intercostal [see Fig. 5.14 in Vol. 2], lumbar [see Fig. 15.1 in Vol. 2], and lateral sacral arteries. They enter the vertebral canal through the intervertebral foramina and join the anterior and posterior spinal arteries [p. 260] to supply the spinal cord, its nerve roots and meninges, and the surrounding bone and ligaments.

## Internal vertebral venous plexus

The **internal vertebral venous plexus** extends throughout the length of the vertebral canal and may be divided into four subordinate longitudinal channels—two anterior and two posterior venous channels [Fig. 20.2].

The posterior plexuses lie on the deep surfaces of the laminae and ligamentum flava. The anterior plexuses are on the posterior aspect of the vertebral bodies near the edges of the posterior longitudinal ligament. The four plexuses are united to each other by dense transverse plexuses opposite the laminae and receive the veins from the bones and contents of the vertebral canal. The **basivertebral veins** from the back of each vertebral body are especially large [see Fig. 1.9 in Vol. 2. The internal vertebral venous plexus communicates through the intervertebral foramina with the body wall veins—the vertebral, posterior intercostal, lumbar, and lateral sacral veins. The plexus contains no valves and is capable of considerable distension. It may drain into, or receive blood from, any of the body wall veins, transmitting blood from areas of high venous pressure to areas of lower venous pressure. For example, the internal vertebral venous plexus may transmit blood from tributaries of the inferior vena cava (lateral sacral and lumbar veins) to tributaries of the superior vena cava (posterior intercostal and vertebral veins) when there is a pressure difference between the two. ➲ Because of its multiple communications, the internal vertebral venous plexus is implicated in the spread of some pelvic tumours (e.g. spread of cancer of the prostate to the vertebral bodies, and even to the skull).

## Meninges of the spinal cord

The spinal cord is covered by the same three layers of meninges as the brain—the pia mater, arachnoid mater, and dura mater. The meninges extend from the foramen magnum down the vertebral canal as three separate tubular sheaths around the spinal cord. The sheaths terminate at different levels, as described below.

Using the instructions given in Dissection 20.2 (and Fig. 20.3), identify the spinal meninges and the spinal nerve roots.

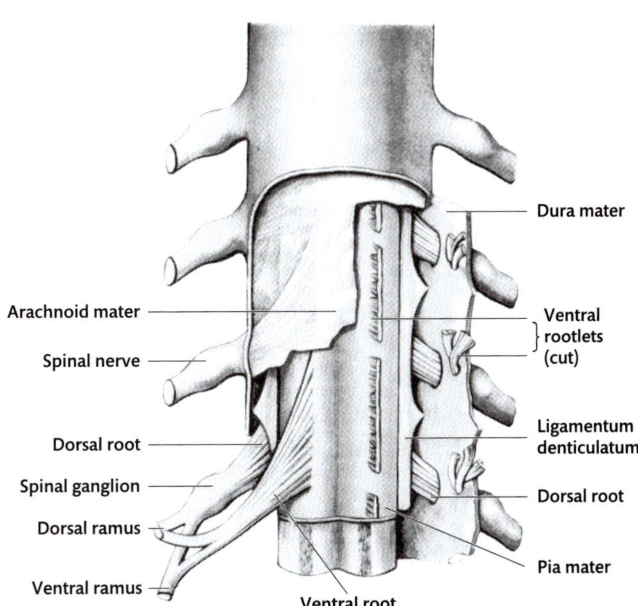


Fig. 20.3 Meninges of the spinal cord and mode of origin of spinal nerves. The contribution of each root to both rami is shown diagrammatically in the lowest spinal nerve on the left.

**DISSECTION 20.2 Spinal meninges and spinal nerve roots**

**Objectives**

**I.** To study the spinal meninges in the vertebral canal. **II.** To identify and trace the dorsal and ventral nerve roots.

**Instructions**

1. Remove the veins and fat from the external surface of the **dura mater**.
2. Follow one of the prolongations of the dura over a spinal nerve into an intervertebral foramen by cutting away the articular processes.
3. Make a small incision in the dura mater in the midline. This allows the **arachnoid** to fall away from it. Introduce the blade of scissors into the incision, and split the dura mater longitudinally, taking care not to damage the underlying transparent arachnoid.
4. If the arachnoid is not damaged, the subarachnoid space should be inflated by injecting water or air beneath the arachnoid.
5. Split the arachnoid longitudinally, and pull its edges apart. Note the trabeculae attaching it to the pia mater on the surface of the spinal cord.
6. Below the first lumbar vertebra, note a collection of the lower lumbar and sacral spinal nerve roots. This is the **cauda equina** [Fig. 20.2]. The cauda equina descends in the subarachnoid space, and individual nerve roots of the cauda exit the vertebral canal at each vertebral level.
7. Gently pull the spinal cord to one side to expose the projection of the pia mater from its lateral aspect—the **denticulate ligament**. The denticulate ligament sends pointed, teeth-like extensions through the arachnoid to the dura between the points of emergence of the spinal nerves [Fig. 20.3]. These extensions are more easily seen if the dorsal rootlets of one or two spinal nerves are cut away from the spinal cord and reflected laterally.
8. Fold the cut edges of the dura mater and arachnoid laterally to expose the emergence of one or more spinal nerves through them. Note that each spinal nerve makes two separate openings in the dura and arachnoid—one for the dorsal root, and one for the ventral root.
9. Follow the dorsal root to the spinal cord, and note how the rootlets enter it.
10. Follow one or more ventral roots in a similar manner, dividing one or more teeth of the denticulate ligament so that the spinal cord may be rotated to expose the exit of the rootlets which make up the ventral root.

## Spinal dura mater

The tough fibrous sleeve of the dura extends from the margin of the foramen magnum to the second sacral vertebra. It is closely applied to the underlying arachnoid mater throughout its length. At the foramen magnum, it is fused with the meningeal layer of the cranial dura. At the second sacral vertebra, the spinal dura mater and arachnoid close onto the filum terminale [Fig. 20.4]. (The filum terminale is an extension of the pia mater beyond the caudal end of the spinal cord. It is attached inferiorly to the coccyx.) The dura is separated from the walls of the vertebral canal by the epidural space, except at certain locations. It is attached: (1) to the posterior longitudinal ligament on the bodies of the second and third cervical vertebrae; and (2) to the intervertebral foramina by the extensions around the roots of the spinal nerves. These attachments hold the dural sheath close to the vertebral bodies, so that the spinal cord is as close to the axis of movement between the vertebrae as possible, and is not greatly affected by these movements [Fig. 20.3].

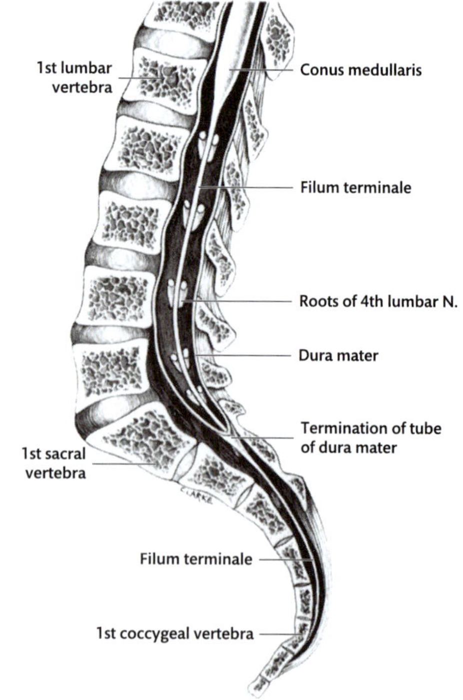


**Fig. 20.4** Sagittal section through the lower part of the vertebral canal.

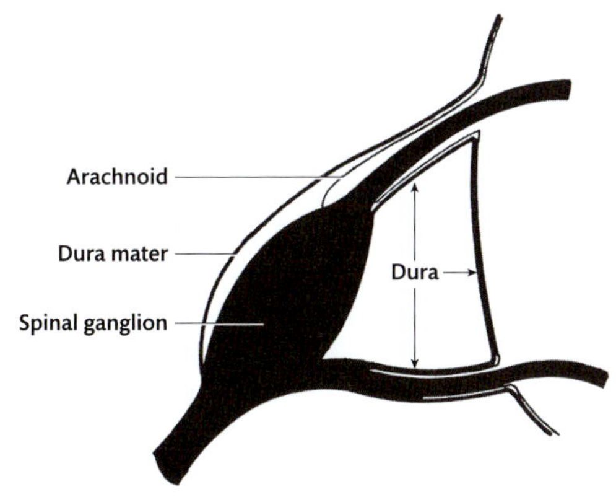


Fig. 20.5 Diagram to represent the meningeal relation of a spinal nerve.

The dura mater forms a separate sheath for each dorsal and ventral root. The adjacent surfaces of these sheaths fuse at the medial surface of the spinal ganglion [Figs. 20.3, 20.5]. But the dura on the posterior surface of the dorsal root remains as a separate layer until it fuses with the distal part of the ganglion and becomes continuous with the **epineurium** of the nerve [Fig. 20.5].

## Spinal arachnoid

The thin, transparent arachnoid membrane lines the dural sac throughout its length, but is separated from it by the potential subdural space. The dura and arachnoid mater fuse with each other: (1) at the intervertebral foramen around the spinal nerves; (2) on the filum terminale at S. 2 level; and (3) where the teeth of the denticulate ligament pass through the arachnoid to the dura mater. The arachnoid mater extends along each spinal nerve root and usually fuses with the medial part of the spinal ganglion [Fig. 20.5].

## Subarachnoid space

Deep to the arachnoid lies a relatively wide **subarachnoid space** containing **cerebrospinal fluid**. Only a few strands of connective tissue pass from the deep surface of the arachnoid to the pia mater around the spinal cord, and these are mainly on the posterior aspect of the cord. The space is also crossed by the denticulate ligament.

## Spinal pia mater

The pia mater around the spinal cord is a firm vascular membrane closely adherent to the spinal cord. At the lower end of the spinal cord, it continues over the filum terminale. The pia ensheathes each rootlet of the spinal nerve, as it crosses the subarachnoid space and becomes continuous with the **perineurium** of the spinal nerves. The pia mater also extends into the nervous tissue for a short distance over each vessel entering the spinal cord and carries a short sleeve of subarachnoid space around the vessel—the **perivascular space**. The pia extends into the anterior median fissure of the spinal cord and is thickened at the mouth of the fissure to form a median longitudinal, glistening band—the **linea splendens**.

## Denticulate ligament

The denticulate ligament is a thin ridge of pia mater on each side of the spinal cord, midway between the attachments of the ventral and dorsal nerve roots. This ligament extends from the foramen magnum to the first lumbar vertebra (the lower limit of the spinal cord). It is made up of 21 pointed projections of pia mater which extend laterally from the surface of the spinal cord. The projections cross the subarachnoid space, pierce the arachnoid mater, and get attached to the dura mater in the interval between two adjacent spinal nerves. The first projection is at the foramen magnum; the last is between the twelfth thoracic and first lumbar nerves. The two ligaments (right and left) together suspend the spinal cord in the subarachnoid space from these points of attachments and allow some movement of the dura mater without corresponding movement of the spinal cord [Fig. 20.3].

## Filum terminale

The filum terminale is a thin filament which extends from the narrowed end of the spinal cord (**conus medullaris**) to the coccyx. It lies among the descending roots of the lumbar and sacral nerves (the cauda equina) but is readily differentiated from them by its silvery appearance and attachments [Fig. 20.4]. The part of the filum terminale within the dural sac is called the **filum terminale internum**, and the part outside the dural sac is called the **filum terminale externum**.

The filum terminale is composed chiefly of the pia mater surrounding a continuation of the central canal, and some neural elements which can be traced in it for nearly half of its length. At the level of the second sacral vertebra, the spinal arachnoid and dura mater fuse with the filum (and the subdural and subarachnoid spaces end). The filum continues through the sacral canal and fuses with the periosteum on the back of the coccyx or the last piece of the sacrum [Fig. 20.4].

## The spinal cord

The spinal cord begins at the foramen magnum as the inferior continuation of the medulla oblongata of the brain. In the adult, it ends opposite the intervertebral disc between the first and second lumbar vertebrae, and approximately one vertebra lower in the newborn. From its termination, the spinal cord rapidly tapers to a point, forming the **conus medullaris**.

The average length of the spinal cord is 45 cm. It is nearly cylindrical in shape. The diameter increases in regions which give rise to the large nerves of the limbs, because of the increased number of nerve cells within the spinal cord at these regions. These enlargements occur in the cervical and lumbar regions and are known as the cervical and lumbar swellings. The **cervical swelling** extends from the fourth cervical vertebra to the first thoracic vertebra (it has a maximum transverse diameter of 14 mm at the sixth cervical vertebra). The **lumbar swelling** extends from the tenth to twelfth thoracic vertebrae (it has a maximum transverse diameter of 12 mm at the twelfth thoracic vertebra).

## Spinal nerves

Thirty-one pairs of spinal nerves are attached to the spinal cord: eight cervical, 12 thoracic, five lumbar, five sacral, and one coccygeal nerve [Figs. 20.2, 20.3]. The first seven cervical nerves leave the vertebral canal above the corresponding vertebrae; the eighth emerges between the seventh cervical and first thoracic vertebrae; and the remaining nerves emerge below the corresponding vertebrae.

### Spinal nerve roots

Each spinal nerve is formed by the union of the dorsal and ventral roots. The roots are made up of a series of dorsal and ventral rootlets [Fig. 20.3]. The **dorsal root** is larger than the ventral root (except in the first cervical nerve which frequently has no dorsal root) and has an oval swelling—the **spinal ganglion**—on it where it joins the ventral root. The dorsal root is composed of afferent (sensory) nerve fibres which are processes of the cells in the spinal ganglion. The ventral rootlets arise from cells in the spinal cord and unite to form the **ventral root**. It consists of efferent (motor) nerve fibres. The dorsal and ventral roots unite beyond the spinal ganglion to form the **spinal nerve**, which contains both sensory and motor fibres [see Fig. 6.7].

**Attachment to spinal cord**: the rootlets of the dorsal roots enter the spinal cord on the dorsolateral aspect, on a slight furrow—the **posterolateral sulcus**. The rootlets of the ventral roots emerge from the ventrolateral aspect of the spinal cord over a broader strip [Figs. 20.3, 20.5]. The part of the spinal cord to which any one pair of nerves is attached is called a **spinal segment**. There are 31 spinal segments in the spinal cord.

**Size of root**: the size of a root is directly proportional to the amount of tissue it supplies. The roots of nerves contributing to the limb plexuses are large, especially those which innervate the lower limb. The roots of the thoracic and upper cervical segments are small, except the first thoracic nerve which innervates part of the upper limb.

**Length of root**: the roots of the spinal nerve vary in length because the spinal cord is shorter than the vertebral canal (due to differential growth between the two during intrauterine life). By birth, the lower end of the spinal cord has moved from its original position in the coccyx to the third lumbar vertebra; and by adulthood, it has ascended to the lower border of the first lumbar vertebra. Despite the shortening of the spinal cord, the spinal nerves continue to exit the vertebral canal at the intervertebral foramen below the numerically corresponding vertebra. As the upper part of the spinal cord is relatively fixed during development, the upper spinal roots are short (approximately 1.5–2 cm) and horizontal. The nerve roots of the lower spinal nerves run obliquely downwards and laterally to the intervertebral foramen and are progressively elongated (approximately 27 cm in S. 5). The **cauda equina** is made up of dorsal and ventral roots of the lumbar, sacral, and coccygeal nerves. These nerves descend as a leash around the filum terminale in the subarachnoid space, inferior to the termination of the spinal cord [Figs. 20.2, 20.6].

#### Radiculopathy

➲ **Radiculopathy** is sensory or motor disturbance caused by pathology of a nerve root. The

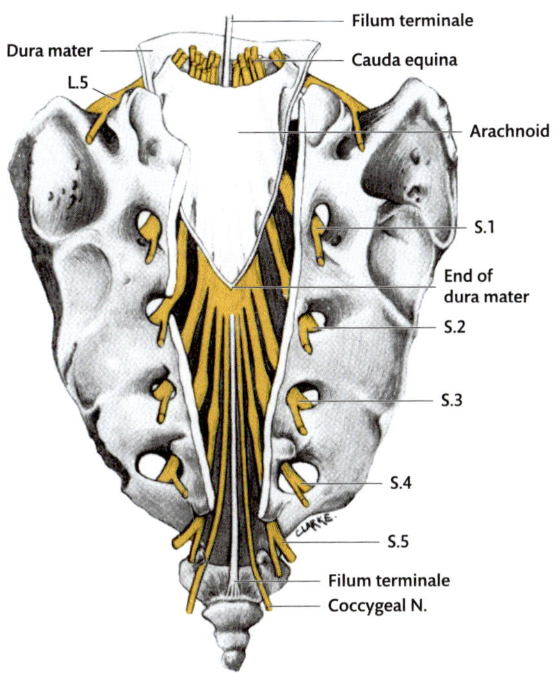


Fig. 20.6 Posterior view of the meninges and spinal nerves in the sacral canal.

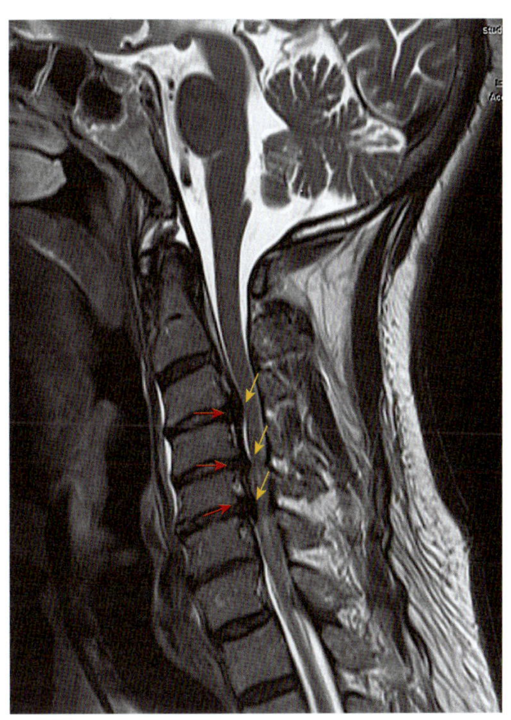

Fig. 20.7 T2-weighted sagittal magnetic resonance imaging (MRI) of the cervical spine, showing intervertebral disc prolapse between C. 3/C. 4, C. 4/C. 5, and C. 5/C. 6 (red arrows) and compression of the dural sac (yellow arrows).

most common cause of radiculopathy is intervertebral disc herniation. Fig. 20.7 shows herniation of the intervertebral discs between C. 3/C. 4, C. 4/C. 5, and C. 5/C. 6. [See also Fig. 1.7 in Vol. 2 for disc herniation between L. 4/L. 5 and L. 5/S. 1.]

Other causes of radiculopathy are presence of osteophytes, spinal stenosis, and trauma.

## Vertebral levels of spinal segments

Shortening of the spinal cord results in individual spinal segments lying at a higher level than the corresponding vertebra, as shown in Table 20.1.

➲ In patients with spinal cord injury following a vertebral fracture, the level of the spinal injury can be predicted from the level of vertebral injury using information given in Table 20.1. For example, a fracture of T. 9 vertebra is likely to affect T. 12 segment of the spinal cord (T. 9 spinal segment will be unaffected).

### Significance of high termination of the spinal cord

➲ The high termination of the spinal cord and the presence of only a leash of roots in the subarachnoid space inferior to it have a number of clinical significance. (1) Injuries to the vertebral column below the second lumbar vertebra can damage only spinal nerve roots (and not the spinal cord itself), though the roots of many nerves may be damaged by an injury at one level. (2) Samples of cerebrospinal fluid can be obtained for diagnostic purposes from the subarachnoid space below L. 1 level without fear of injuring the spinal cord. This procedure is a lumbar puncture and is done by introducing a hollow needle into the subarachnoid space between the laminae of the lower lumbar vertebrae.

### Exit of spinal nerves

Most of the spinal nerves emerge through an intervertebral foramen [see Fig. 1.5 in Vol. 2]. The first cervical nerve emerges between the posterior arch of the atlas and the occiput, and the second between the posterior arch of the atlas and the vertebral arch of the axis. The fifth sacral and coccygeal

Table 20.1 Vertebral levels of spinal segments

| Vertebral levels (spines) | Spinal segments |
|---|---|
| Foramen magnum–sixth cervical | Cervical 1-8 |
| Sixth cervical–fourth thoracic | Thoracic 1-6 |
| Fourth thoracic–ninth thoracic | Thoracic 7-12 |
| Tenth thoracic–first lumbar | Lumbar and sacral |

nerves emerge through the lower end of the sacral canal. The other sacral nerves additionally have a separate sacral foramen (ventral and dorsal sacral foraminae) for the ventral and dorsal rami.

## Meningeal branch of the spinal nerve

A slender meningeal branch arises at each level from the spinal nerve and the sympathetic trunk. It runs back into the vertebral canal through the intervertebral foramen. It is sensory to the walls and contents of the vertebral canal and its blood vessels [see Fig. 6.7].

## Spinal ganglia

The **spinal ganglion** is also known as the **dorsal root ganglion** or **sensory ganglion**. It is made up of a collection of nerve cell bodies on the dorsal root [Figs. 20.3, 20.5]. It lies in the intervertebral foramina, except for the sacral and coccygeal ganglia which lie in the sacral canal [Fig. 20.6]. The first two cervical ganglia lie above and below the atlas, behind the articular facets. Each ganglion contains pseudounipolar neurons which have the peripheral process in the peripheral nerve, and the central process in the dorsal root. There are no synapses in the ganglia.

Using the instructions given in Dissection 20.3, study the spinal cord.

# Arteries of the spinal cord

The spinal cord is supplied by a single median **anterior spinal artery** and paired **posterior spinal arteries**. Throughout its length, many thin-walled arteries reach the anterior and posterior spinal arteries on the roots of the spinal nerves. These arteries arise from the vertebral arteries, ascending cervical arteries (in the cervical region), posterior intercostal arteries (in the thoracic region), lumbar arteries (in the lumbar region), and lateral sacral arteries (in the sacral region). They are smaller and more numerous on the dorsal roots.

## Anterior spinal artery

**The anterior spinal artery** is formed on the anterior surface of the medulla oblongata of the brain by the union of two roots, one from each vertebral artery [see Fig. 26.2]. It descends on the anterior surface of the spinal cord, through the length of the spinal cord, dorsal to the linea splendens. It receives 3–10 spinal arteries from the vessels on the ventral roots. The largest of these supplies the lumbar swelling and usually enters from the left, frequently on the tenth thoracic ventral root—the **artery of Adamkiewicz**.

The anterior spinal artery gives rise to many small perforating vessels which enter the spinal cord at the anteromedian fissure. They branch to supply the central parts of the spinal cord, including most of the grey matter (nerve cell bodies) and the deeper parts of the surrounding white matter (nerve fibres). Small vessels also pass backwards on the surface of the spinal cord to anastomose with the **posterior spinal arteries** which course

### DISSECTION 20.3 Spinal cord

#### Objectives

**I.** To remove the spinal cord and its meninges. **II.** To identify and trace the spinal accessory nerve. **III.** To identify and trace the branches of the anterior spinal artery.

#### Instructions

1. Cut across the spinal nerves in the intervertebral foramina, leaving as long a piece attached to the dura as possible.
2. Pull on the dura, and divide its attachments to the posterior longitudinal ligament.
3. Remove the spinal cord and meninges in one piece.
4. Split the dura mater along the middle anteriorly to expose the arachnoid and pia mater, and the ligamenta denticulata.
5. Find the rootlets of the **spinal part of the accessory nerve**, posterior to the denticulate ligament in the upper cervical region. Follow them to the nerve, and trace the nerve cranially in front of the dorsal roots [see Fig. 7.8].
6. Remove the linea splendens from the ventral surface of the anterior median fissure, and expose the anterior spinal artery.
7. Follow the artery cranially and caudally, and try to expose the arteries joining it on the ventral roots.
8. With a hand lens, examine the small branches of the artery on the surface of the spinal cord, and the perforating branches passing into the anterior median sulcus when the artery is lifted gently away from the spinal cord.

longitudinally beside the entry point of the dorsal rootlets.

### Posterior spinal arteries

The **posterior spinal arteries** arise as branches of the posterior inferior cerebellar or vertebral arteries on the medulla oblongata [see Fig. 26.2]. They run down along the entry points of the dorsal rootlets. They are fed by numerous small arteries on the dorsal roots and are much smaller than the anterior spinal artery. The posterior spinal arteries send branches onto the posterior surface of the spinal cord to complete an irregular, circular anastomosis, from which branches pass radially into the white matter.

All the arteries which enter the spinal cord are end-arteries. This pattern of surface anastomosis with perforating end-arteries is present throughout the central nervous system.

## Veins of the spinal cord

The veins of the spinal cord, though small, numerous, and tortuous, are larger than the arteries. They anastomose freely on the surface of the spinal cord and form six more or less perfectly longitudinal channels—one anteromedian, one posteromedian, two close to the attachment of the dorsal rootlets, and two close to the attachment of the ventral rootlets. They are continuous above with the veins of the medulla oblongata and drain laterally along the spinal nerve roots to the internal vertebral venous plexus.

The internal structure of the spinal cord is described in Chapter 27 in the section on the brain and spinal cord.

See Clinical Application 20.1 for the practical implications of the anatomy discussed in this chapter.





**CLINICAL APPLICATION 20.1 Cauda equina syndrome**

A 45-year-old man was lifting a heavy load when he coughed and immediately experienced sharp pain in both gluteal regions. Over the next few days, he continued to have pain and developed loss of sensation over his buttock and genitalia. He also developed constipation and urinary retention.

On examination, his motor function was normal. He had decreased sensation (touch, pain, and temperature) over the buttock, genitalia, anal region, and back of the upper thigh (saddle anaesthesia). Sensation in all other areas was normal. Superficial abdominal reflexes and the cremasteric reflex were normal.

Study question 1: what spinal segments receive sensation from the skin of the gluteal region, perineum, and back of the upper thigh? [Refer to Fig. 24.2 in Vol. 1] (Answer: S. 2 to S. 5/Co.)

Study question 2: what can you deduce about spinal cord function from the finding that the abdominal and cremasteric reflexes are intact? [Refer to Clinical Application 10.2 in Vol. 2] (Answer: spinal segments T. 7–L. 2 are normal.)

Spinal computerized tomography/myelography done on the patient revealed a L. 5–S. 1 central disc prolapse compressing the nerves of the cauda equina. (Herniation of the disc posteriorly into the vertebral canal is a central disc herniation. Rootlets of lower segments are located more medially in the cauda equina and are more likely to be affected by a central disc herniation. A posterolateral disc prolapse affects upper segment rootlets, as they lie closer to the intervertebral foramen.) The mass was removed surgically, and the dural sac decompressed, and the patient made a good recovery.

CHAPTER 21
# The joints of the neck

## Cervical joints

Each cervical vertebra articulates with the adjacent vertebrae by joints between the bodies and the articular processes. The first cervical vertebra (atlas) articulates with the skull at the atlanto-occipital joint. The joints between the atlas and the skull allow nodding movements of the skull on the vertebral column (as in flexing and extending the head). The joints between the first and second cervical vertebrae are designed to allow rotation of the head from side to side (as in turning the face to the right and left). The occipital bone and the axis are firmly bound to each other by strong ligaments, so that the atlas is held between them like a washer.

The joints between the second to fifth cervical vertebrae are similar to those in the other parts of the vertebral column and allow flexion, extension, lateral flexion, and some rotation. Begin the study of this region by reviewing the cervical joints exposed earlier and exposing the remaining joints.

Dissection 21.1 provides instructions on reviewing the atlanto-occipital joint and dissecting the remaining cervical joints [Fig. 21.1].

### Typical cervical joints

The joints between the lower six cervical vertebrae are typical cervical joints [Fig. 21.2]. **Joints between the vertebral bodies**: the bodies of these vertebrae are firmly bound to each other by a flexible intervertebral disc and small, paired synovial joints at the lateral margin. The intervertebral discs are strengthened anteriorly and posteriorly by the anterior and posterior longitudinal ligaments, which are attached principally to the discs and the adjacent parts of the bodies [see Fig. 21.4]. The discs do not cover the entire surface of the vertebral bodies but are replaced laterally by small synovial joints where the margins of one vertebra overlap the vertebral body above [Fig. 21.2].



**Joints between the vertebral arches**: the vertebral arches are united by the synovial joints between the superior and inferior articular processes and by a number of ligaments [Fig. 21.2]. The cervical articular facets lie in an oblique coronal plane which passes anterosuperiorly, and the facets on the two sides are parallel to each other [see Fig. 2.19]. The capsules of these joints are lax and permit a considerable range of movement. **Movements**: the typical cervical joints allow flexion, extension, and lateral flexion. Rotation is minimal at the typical cervical joints.

### Intervertebral ligaments

The joints between the lower six cervical vertebrae are strengthened by the intervertebral ligaments—ligamentum flavum [Fig. 21.3], anterior longitudinal ligament, posterior longitudinal ligament [Fig. 21.4], and interspinous and supraspinous ligaments [Vol. 2, p. 7].

The interspinous ligaments are weak in the cervical region. They pass between adjacent spines and are directly continuous with the supraspinous ligaments and the ligamentum nuchae [see Fig. 6.6]. The **anterior longitudinal ligament** [Vol. 2, p. 7] narrows superiorly to be attached to the anterior tubercle of the atlas.

Following the instructions in Dissection 21.2, expose the membrana tectoria, and cruciate and atlanto-axial ligaments.

**DISSECTION 21.1 Cervical joints**

**Objectives**

**I.** To review the joints already opened. **II.** To expose the remaining cervical joints.

**Instructions**

Instructions

1. The joints of the neck have already been partly dissected when the right half of the head was removed. The right atlanto-occipital joint has been opened, and the right alar ligament and the longitudinal fibres of the cruciate ligament have been cut [Fig. 21.1].
2. Expose the ligaments uniting the cervical vertebrae by removing the remnants of muscle from the cervical articular processes and from the laminae and spines which have been removed in one piece.

## Ligaments connecting the axis, atlas, and occiput

A number of important ligaments connect the axis, atlas, and occiput, and stabilize and strengthen the atlanto-axial and atlanto-occipital joints.

### Membrana tectoria

The membrana tectoria is a broad ligamentous sheet. It is the superior continuation of the posterior longitudinal ligament. It passes from the posterior surface of the body of the axis to the cranial surface of the occipital bone [Figs. 21.2, 21.4]. It holds the axis to the skull and covers the posterior surface of the dens and its ligaments, and the anterior margin of the foramen magnum.

### Ligamentum flavum and posterior atlanto-occipital membrane

Between the atlas and the axis, the ligamentum flavum is thin. Between the posterior arch of the atlas and the occipital bone, the ligamentum flavum forms the **posterior atlanto-occipital membrane** [Fig. 21.4]. It passes from the part of the posterior arch of the atlas to the margin of the foramen magnum and the atlanto-occipital joints [see Fig. 6.4]. The lateral edges arch over the vertebral artery to the posterior surface of the lateral mass of the atlas. These edges may be ossified.

### Anterior atlanto-occipital membrane

The anterior atlanto-occipital membrane passes from the superior margin of the anterior arch of the

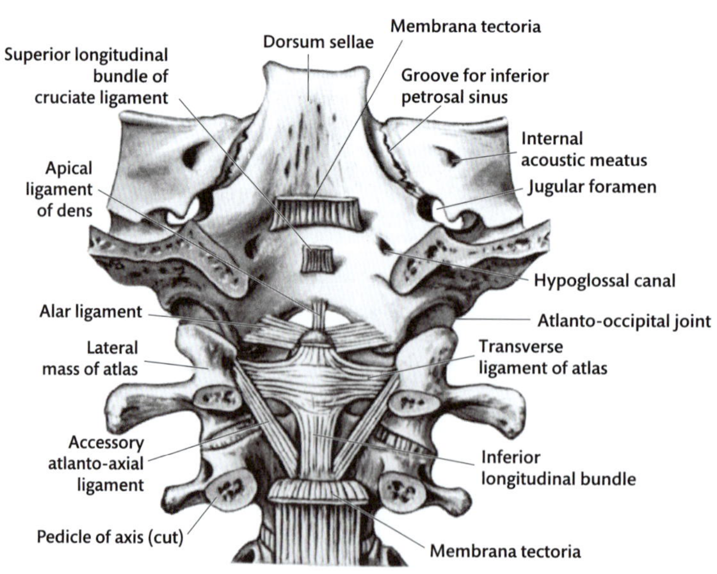


**Fig. 21.1** Diagram showing the main ligaments that connect the occipital bone, atlas, and axis.

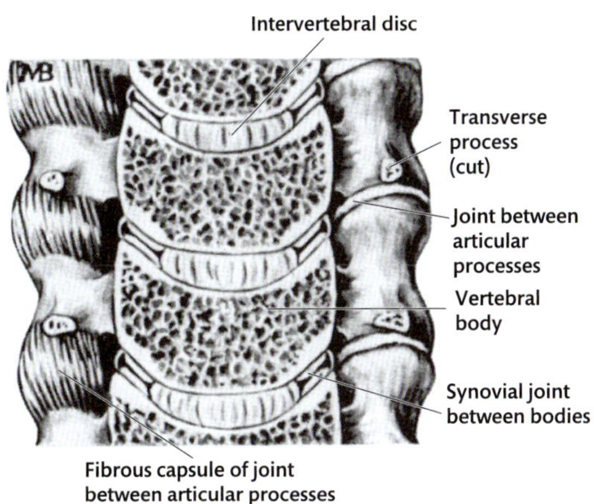


**Fig. 21.2** Coronal section through the joints between the bodies of the cervical vertebrae.

atlas to the base of the skull, anterior to the foramen magnum [Fig. 21.4].

## Accessory atlanto-axial ligaments

The **accessory atlanto-axial ligaments** [Fig. 21.1] pass from the posterior surface of the body of the axis to the corresponding lateral mass of the atlas. These strong ligaments help to limit rotation of the atlas on the axis.

## Transverse ligament of the atlas

The **transverse ligament of the atlas** stretches between two tubercles on the medial side of the lateral masses of the atlas [see Fig. 2.20]. It extends across the posterior surface of the dens and holds it firmly against the posterior surface of the anterior arch of the atlas. There is a synovial joint between the dens and the ligament, and another between the dens and the anterior arch of the atlas [Fig. 21.4].

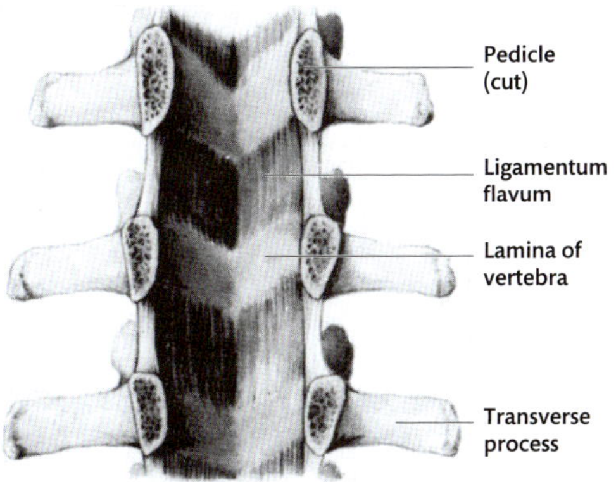


**Fig. 21.3** Ligamentum flavum seen from the front after removal of the bodies of the vertebrae in the lumbar region.

**DISSECTION 21.2 Ligaments connecting the axis, atlas, and occiput**

**Objective**

**I.** To expose the membrana tectoria, and cruciate and atlanto-axial ligaments.

**Instructions**

1. Remove any remaining parts of the posterior arch of the atlas and the laminae of the axis, to expose the parts of the membrana tectoria [Figs. 21.2, 21.4] not damaged during removal of the right half of the head.
2. Cut through the membrana tectoria, and reflect it to expose the undamaged parts of the cruciate ligament and the accessory atlanto-axial ligaments.

## Cruciate ligament

The cruciate ligament is formed by the transverse ligament of the atlas and the superior and inferior longitudinal bands. The **superior longitudinal band** passes from the transverse ligament to the cranial surface of the occipital bone. The **inferior longitudinal band** passes from the transverse ligament to the body of the axis [Figs. 21.1, 21.4].

Using the instructions given in Dissection 21.3, expose the apical and alar ligaments of the dens.

## Apical ligament of the dens

The apical ligament of the dens is a weak, cord like ligament which stretches from the apex of the dens to the cranial surface of the occipital bone, immediately above the margin of the foramen magnum. It lies anterior to the superior band of the cruciate ligament but does not play a significant part in strengthening the joints [Fig. 21.1]. (It develops around a part of the notochord.)

## Alar ligaments

The **alar ligaments** are very powerful ligaments which arise from the sloping sides of the top of the dens. They pass laterally and slightly upwards to the medial sides of the occipital condyles. They hold the skull to the axis and tighten when the atlas, carrying the skull, rotates round the dens. The alar ligaments are attached to the skull on the axis of the nodding movements which the skull makes on the atlas, and do not hinder these movements [Fig. 21.1].

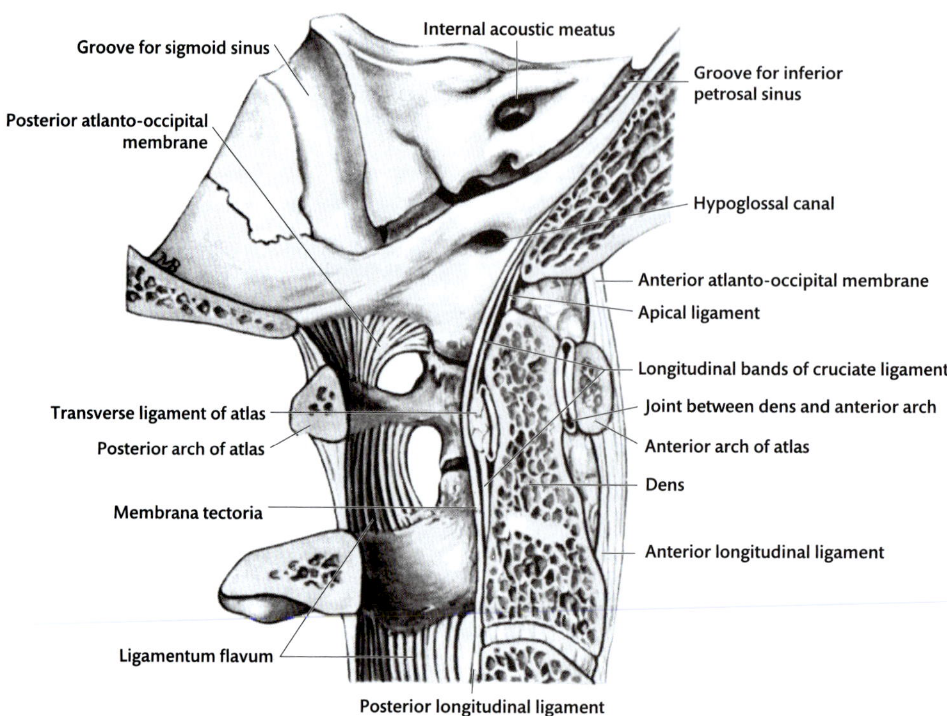


**Fig. 21.4** Median section through the foramen magnum and first two cervical vertebrae.

## Atlanto-occipital joints

The **atlanto-occipital joints** are synovial joints between the atlas and the occiput. The occipital condyles are kidney-shaped and lie on the antero-lateral aspects of the foramen magnum. The articular surfaces are directed laterally and downwards [see Fig. 2.10]. They fit into the superior articular facets of the atlas which are also kidney-shaped. **Movements**: the atlanto-occipital joints allow flexion, extension, and slight side-to-side rocking of the head, but no rotation. These movements are brought about by a complex play of interactions of muscles surrounding the joints [see Figs. 6.4, 9.1]. Flexion is brought about by the longus capitis and rectus capitis anterior; extension by the rectus capitis posterior major, rectus capitis posterior minor, and obliquus capitis superior; and lateral flexion by the action of the rectus capitis lateralis, trapezius, splenius capitis, semispinalis capitis, and sternocleidomastoid. **Ligaments**: the stability of these joints depends on the alar ligaments, the membrana tectoria, and the longitudinal bands of the cruciate ligament, all of which bind the skull to the axis.

## Atlanto-axial joints

The **atlanto-axial joints** are synovial joints between the atlas and the axis. The **median**

### DISSECTION 21.3 Ligaments of the dens—apical and alar ligaments

**Objective**

**I.** To expose the apical and alar ligaments of the dens.

**Instructions**

1. If the division of the skull was to the right of the midline, the apical ligament of the dens [Figs. 21.1, 21.4] should still be present with the left half. It may be exposed by removing the superior band of the cruciate ligament.
2. Identify the divided right alar ligament, and expose the left alar ligament passing from the side of the apex of the dens to the occipital condyle.

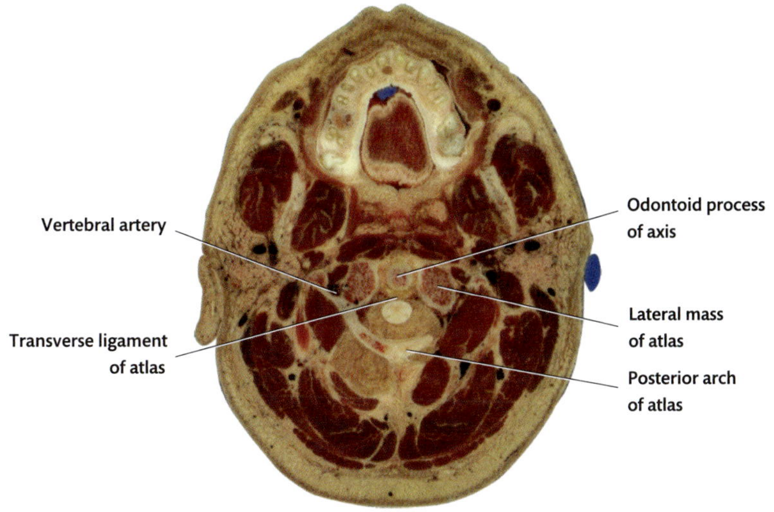


**Fig. 21.5** Horizontal section through the dens showing the median atlanto-axial joint.
Image courtesy of the Visible Human Project of the US National Library of Medicine.





**atlanto-axial joint** lies in the midline where the dens of the axis articulates with the anterior arch and the transverse ligament of the atlas [Fig. 21.5].

The **lateral atlanto-axial joints** are formed between the large, nearly circular, slightly curved facets on the inferior surface of the lateral mass of the atlas and the superior articular facet of the axis. These facets slope downwards and laterally [Fig. 21.1]. The lateral atlanto-axial joints are stabilized by the ligaments which bind the axis and the skull together.

**Movements**: the atlanto-axial joints allow rotation of the atlas and the skull around the dens of the axis. Rotation is brought about by the suboccipital muscles, mainly the ipsilateral obliquus capitis inferior and rectus capitis posterior major. Flexion, extension, and lateral flexion also occur between the atlas and the axis. **Ligaments**: the alar ligaments are important ligaments that hold the skull to the axis and tighten when the atlas, carrying the skull, rotates round the dens. They are the main factor in limiting rotation at the atlanto-axial joints. The transverse ligament of the axis plays an important role in holding the dens apposed to the anterior arch of the atlas. The apical ligament of the dens and the cruciate ligament strengthen the joint.

See Clinical Application 21.1 for the practical implications of the anatomy discussed in this chapter.

**CLINICAL APPLICATION 21.1 Fracture of the dens versus rupture of the transverse ligament of the atlas**

Fracture of the dens commonly occurs at its base where the dens is united to the body. In an isolated fracture of the dens, the transverse ligament of the atlas is intact. It holds the fractured dens against the anterior arch of the atlas and prevents the fractured segment from impinging on the spinal cord. The most common complication in a fracture of the dens is avascular necrosis of the fractured segment.

Rupture of the transverse ligament of the atlas is a result of pathological softening of the ligament. It results in the dens being free to move posteriorly and impinge on the spinal cord. Spinal cord compression between the posterior arch of the atlas and the dens could result in quadriplegia (paralysis of all four limbs).

CHAPTER 22

# Surface marking of the head and neck

## Introduction

Having studied the important structures in the head and neck, it is essential to gain the knowledge and skills to mark their position on the surface of the body. Clinical examination of a patient includes inspection, palpation, and auscultation of the neck, and a sound knowledge of the surface anatomy of the carotid arteries, jugular veins, and thyroid and parotid glands is fundamental to doing a proper examination. This chapter deals with the surface marking of clinically important head and neck structures. Before you start, review the surface anatomy of face, front and side of the neck [Figs. 22.1, 22.2], and back of the head described in Chapters 3, 4, and 5.

## Thyroid gland

The thyroid gland is made up of two lobes on either side of the midline, and the midline isthmus.

### Isthmus of the thyroid gland

- Mark the isthmus of the thyroid gland by two transverse parallel lines, 2 cm apart, below the first tracheal ring (lines 1 and 2). Note: the first tracheal ring is felt below the arch of the cricoid cartilage [Fig. 22.3].

### Lobes of the thyroid gland

To mark the lobes of the thyroid gland on the surface of the body:



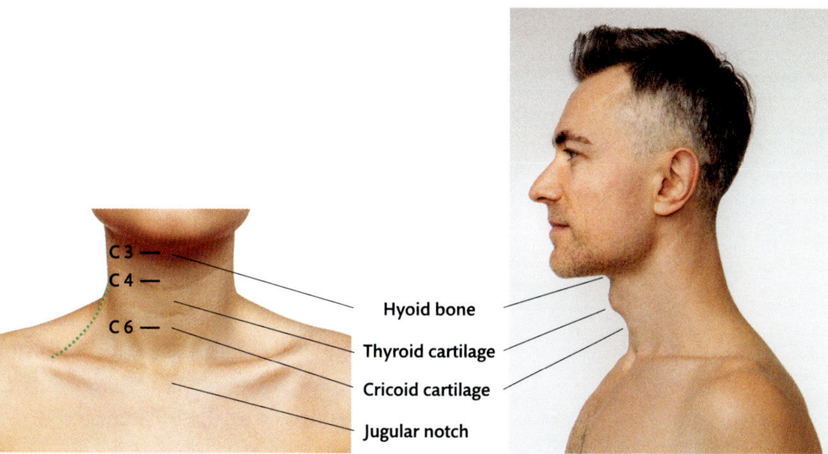


Fig. 22.1 Midline skeletal structures of the neck, seen from the front and from the side. The hyoid bone lies at the level of the third cervical vertebra—C3; the upper border of the thyroid cartilage lies at the level of C4, and the cricoid cartilage lies at the level of C6. The anterior border of the right trapezius is shown by a dotted green line.

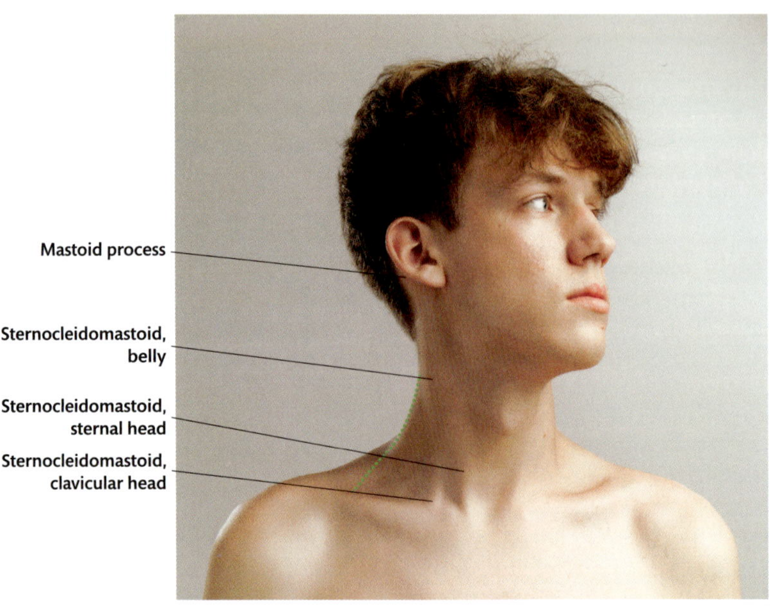


**Fig. 22.2** Side of the neck to show the extent of the sternocleidomastoid. The anterior border of the right trapezius is shown by a dotted green line.





- Mark two points on the middle of the thyroid laminae to represent the superior extent of the right and left lobes (3 and 3′).
- Mark two points at the level of the clavicle, the same distance from the midline, as points 3 and 3′ to represent the inferior extent of the right and left lobes (4 and 4′).

Draw a line joining the right end of line 1 to point 3, point 4, and the right end of line 2, to mark the right lobe of the thyroid gland. Similarly, draw a line joining the left end of line 1 to point 3′, point 4′ and the left end of line 2, to mark the left lobe of the thyroid gland [Fig. 22.3]. The upper end of the lobe should be drawn pointed, and the lower end should be drawn flat.

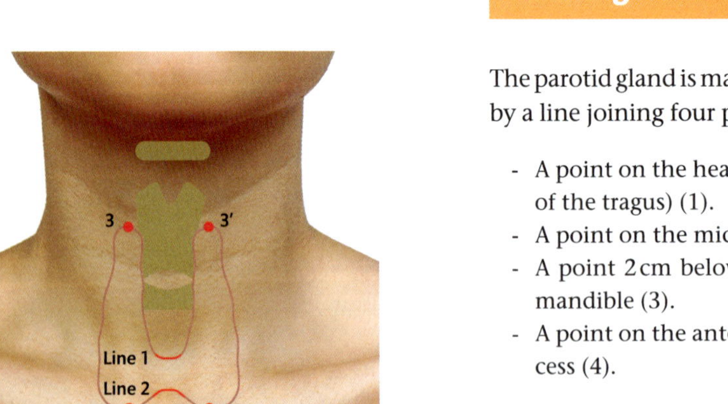


**Fig. 22.3** Surface marking of the thyroid gland.



## Parotid gland

The parotid gland is marked on the surface of the body by a line joining four points shown in Fig. 22.4A.

- A point on the head of the mandible (just in front of the tragus) (1).
- A point on the midpoint of the masseter (2).
- A point 2cm below and behind the angle of the mandible (3).
- A point on the anterior border of the mastoid process (4).

Join points 1, 2, and 3 to represent the anterior border of the parotid gland. Join points 3 and 4 to represent the posterior border of the parotid gland. Join points 1 and 4 by a curved line with a convexity directed downwards to represent the superior border of the parotid gland (which curves below the external acoustic meatus) [Fig. 22.4A].

## Parotid duct

To mark the parotid duct on the surface of the body, first draw a line joining two points shown in Fig. 22.4A:

- A point on the tragus (5).
- A point at the angle of the mouth (6).

The middle one-third of this line marks the position of the parotid duct [Fig. 22.4A].

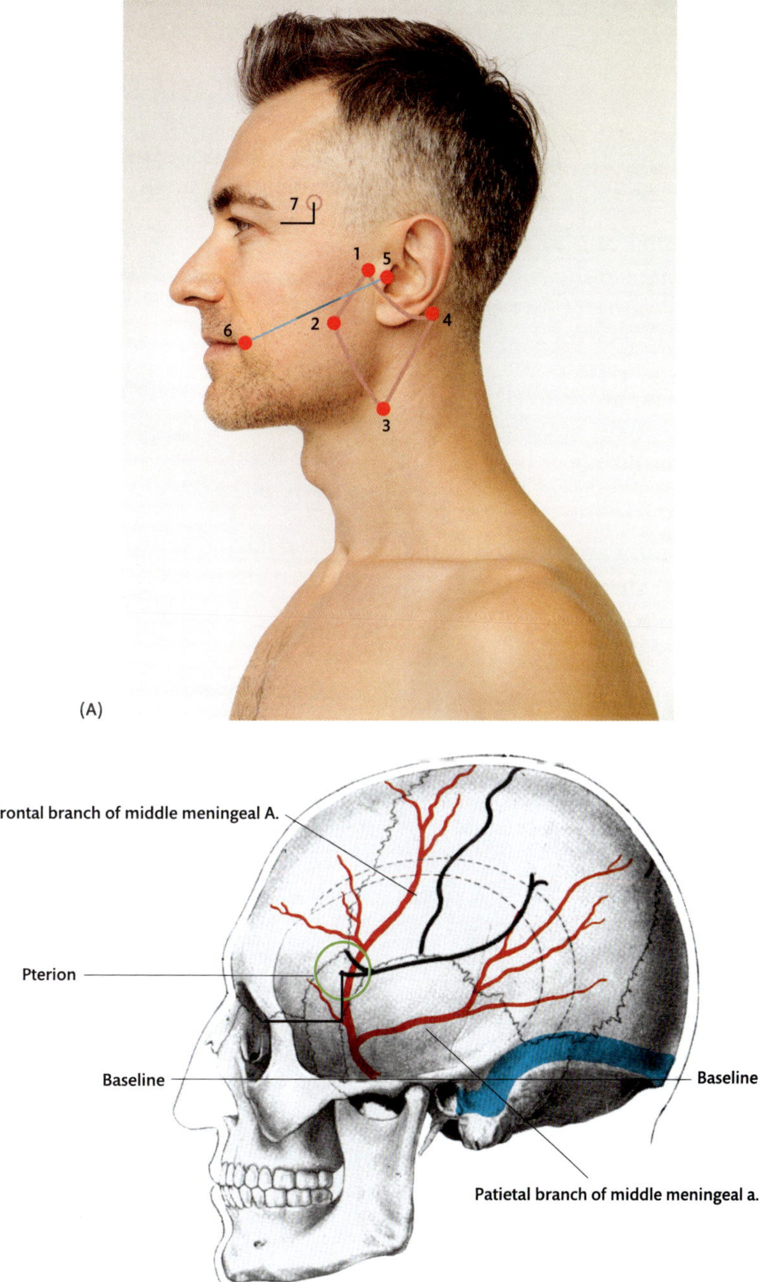


**Fig. 22.4** (A) Surface marking of the parotid gland, parotid duct, and pterion. (B) Lateral side of the skull showing the pterion in relation to the frontozygomatic suture and branches of the middle meningeal artery.

## Pterion

The pterion is marked by a circle 1 cm in diameter [Fig. 22.4A]. The centre of the pterion is marked by a point 2.5 cm posterior, and 1.5 cm superior, to the frontozygomatic suture (7). Fig. 22.4B shows the position of the pterion and the anterior branch of the middle meningeal artery on the lateral side of the skull.

## Common carotid artery

The position of the common carotid artery in the neck is marked on the surface of the body by a vertical line joining the following points shown in Fig. 22.5:

- A point on the sternoclavicular joint (1).
- A point on the anterior border of the sternocleidomastoid at the level of the upper border of the thyroid cartilage (2).

The pulsation of the carotid artery can be felt at the anterior border of the sternocleidomastoid at the level of the cricoid cartilage.

## Internal jugular vein

The position of the internal jugular vein is marked on the surface of the body by a vertical line joining the following points shown in Fig. 22.5:

- A point on the sternoclavicular joint (1).
- A point on the neck behind the lobule of the ear (3).

The terminal part of the internal jugular vein lies between the sternal and clavicular heads of the sternocleidomastoid. This landmark is used for placing a cannula in the vein.

## Subclavian vein

The subclavian vein lies deep to the medial part of the clavicle. Its position is marked on the surface of the body by a line joining the following points shown in Fig. 22.5:

- A point on the sternoclavicular joint (1).
- A point on the clavicle at the junction of the medial and middle thirds (4).

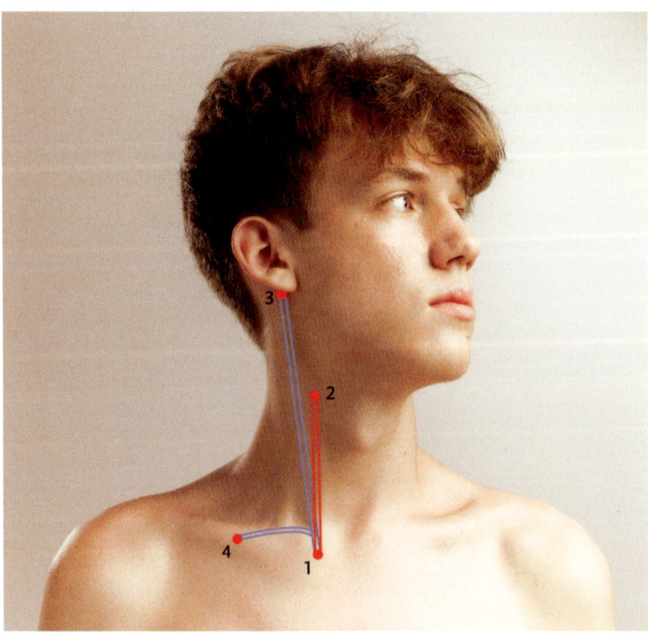


**Fig. 22.5** Surface marking of the common carotid artery, internal jugular vein, and subclavian vein.

## External jugular vein

The external jugular vein is marked on the surface of the body by a line joining the following points shown in Fig. 22.6:

- A point immediately behind the below the angle of the mandible (1).
- The midpoint of the clavicle (2).

## Facial artery in face

The facial artery is marked on the side of the face by a wavy line joining the following points shown in Fig. 22.6:

- A point on the lower margin of the body of the mandible at the anteroinferior angle of the masseter (3).
- A point 1 cm lateral to the angle of the mouth (4).
- A point at the medial angle of the eye (5).

The pulsations of the facial artery can be felt at the lower border of the mandible at the anteroinferior angle of the masseter.

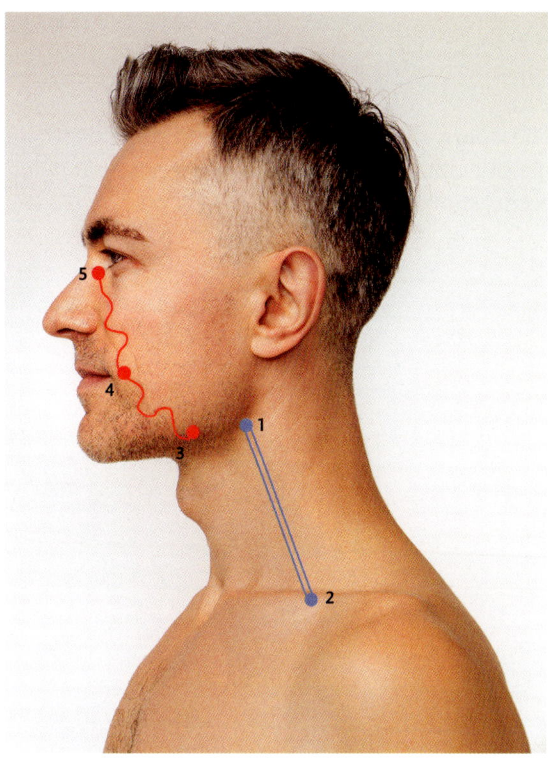


**Fig. 22.6** Surface marking of the external jugular vein and facial artery.







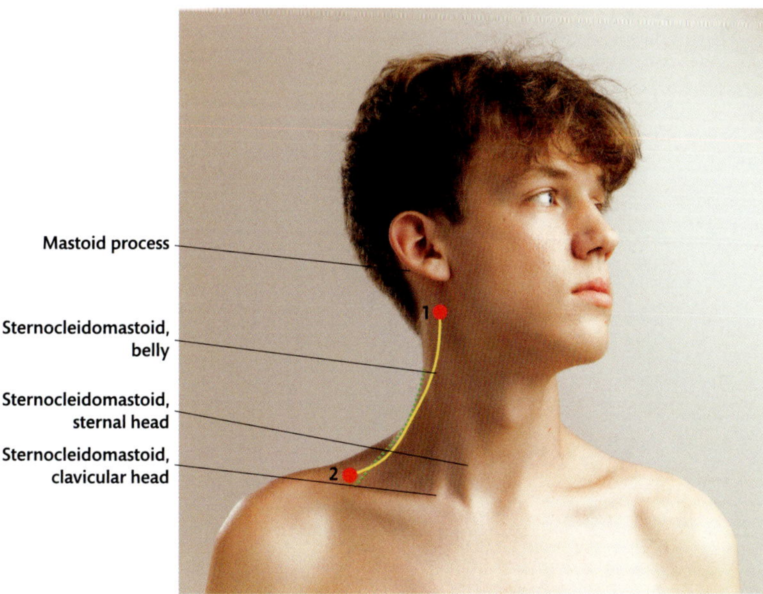


**Fig. 22.7** Surface marking of the accessory nerve.

## Accessory nerve

The course of the accessory nerve is marked on the side of the neck by a line joining the following points shown in Fig. 22.7:

- A point on the anterior border of the sternocleidomastoid, 4 cm below the mastoid process (1).
- A point on the anterior border of the trapezius, 2 cm above the clavicle (2).

CHAPTER 23

# MCQs on head and neck

Each of the following questions have four options. Please choose the most correct answer.

1. **The sensory innervation to the lower part of the medial surface of the auricle is by the**

   A. Facial nerve
   B. Auriculotemporal nerve
   C. Greater auricular nerve
   D. Lesser occipital nerve



2. **The three cutaneous nerves that pierce the deep fascia at the middle of the posterior border of the sternocleidomastoid include all the following, EXCEPT the**

   A. Supraclavicular nerve
   B. Lesser occipital nerve
   C. Great auricular nerve
   D. Transverse nerve of the neck

3. **The nerve that accompanies the submental artery is the**

   A. Cervical branch of the facial nerve
   B. Mylohoid nerve
   C. Transverse cervical nerve
   D. Great auricular nerve

4. **All of the following statements are true concerning the middle meningeal artery, EXCEPT**

   A. It enters the cranial cavity through the foramen ovale
   B. It has no role in supplying the pia and arachnoid mater
   C. It grooves the inner table of the skull
   D. Rupture of it results in extradural haematoma

5. **The straight sinus is formed by the union of the**

   A. Superior sagittal sinus and inferior sagittal sinus
   B. Superior sagittal sinus and transverse sinus
   C. Superior sagittal sinus and great cerebral vein
   D. Inferior sagittal sinus and great cerebral vein

**6. The emissary vein that traverses through the foramen ovale connects the cavernous sinus with the**

A. Superior ophthalmic vein
B. Inferior ophthalmic vein
C. Pterygoid plexus of veins
D. Pharyngeal plexus of veins

**7. The following are branches of the hypoglossal nerve, EXCEPT the**

A. Superior root of the ansa cervicalis
B. Nerve to the geniohyoid
C. Nerve to the genioglossus
D. Nerve to the palatoglossus

**8. In Horner's syndrome, ptosis is due to paralysis of the**

A. Orbital part of the orbicularis oculi
B. Palpebral part of the orbicularis oculi
C. Striated part of the levator palpebrae superioris
D. Smooth muscle component of the levator palpebrae superioris

**9. The otic ganglion receives preganglionic fibres from the**

A. Oculomotor nerve
B. Facial nerve
C. Glossopharyngeal nerve
D. Vagus nerve

**10. The muscle that retracts the mandible is the**

A. Masseter
B. Temporalis
C. Medial pterygoid
D. Lateral pterygoid

**11. The nerve that pierces the sphenomandibular ligament is the**

A. Auriculotemporal nerve
B. Lingual nerve
C. Chorda tympani
D. Mylohyoid nerve

**12. The muscle that hooks round the pterygoid hamulus is the**

A. Medial pterygoid
B. Lateral pterygoid
C. Tensor palati
D. Levator palati

**13. The sinuses that open into the hiatus semilunaris are the**

A. Frontal and anterior ethmoidal
B. Anterior and middle ethmoidal
C. Anterior ethmoidal and maxillary
D. Middle and posterior ethmoidal

**14. The muscle that is responsible for raising the pitch of the voice is the**

A. Cricothyroid
B. Posterior crico-arytenoid
C. Lateral crico-arytenoid
D. Vocalis

**15. Which one of the following is the remnant of the notochord?**

A. Alar ligament
B. Apical ligament
C. Cruciate ligament
D. Transverse ligament of the atlas

Please see Chapter 35 for the answers.

Find additional MCQs online by searching for *Cunningham's Manual of Practical Anatomy Volume 3 Head, Neck and Brain, 17th edition* at https://academic.oup.com/ and go to the endmatter to find the free online appendix at the end of the book.

## PART 2

# The brain and spinal cord

# CHAPTER 24
# Introduction to the brain and spinal cord



## Introduction

The nervous system consists of two main parts—the central nervous system (CNS) made up of the brain and spinal cord, and the peripheral nervous system (PNS) made up of the spinal nerves, cranial nerves, and peripheral part of the autonomic nervous system. The brain and spinal cord are discussed in this section.

## Structure of the nervous tissue

Begin the study of the CNS by reviewing the parts of the neuron, types of nerve fibres, types of glial cells, and other general features of the nervous system [Vol. 1, pp. 24–7].

### Grey matter and white matter

The brain and spinal cord are largely made up of nerve cells. The nerve cell bodies are grouped together and make up the **grey matter**. A collection of nerve cell bodies within the CNS, often having shared functions and connections, are referred to as **nuclei**. Axons of nerve cells are grouped together to form the **white matter**. Groups of axons coming from the same origin, or going to the same destination, often run together in definite pathways and are called **tracts** or **fasciculi**. Dendrites and nerve synapses are usually confined to the grey matter.

In the spinal cord and most of the brainstem, the grey matter lies internally and is covered by a layer of white matter, which consists of longitudinally running axons. In the cerebellum and cerebrum, there is an additional layer of nerve cells on the external surface. This covering of grey matter, or **cortex**, greatly increases the number of nerve cells and the complexity of their interactions.

Functionally, the CNS is concerned with the receipt and integration of sensory information (sensory system), production of movement (motor system), memory, emotions, and many other complex higher functions. These complex activities are achieved by passage of impulses through the interconnected networks of cells in the CNS. Each cellular unit is linked into the system by cell junctions, or **synapses**, where nerve cells come together and neuronal impulse from one cell is transferred to another. Passage of impulses can be facilitated or inhibited at the synapse.

It is not possible to give a detailed account of this complex system in this book. But a knowledge of the arrangement of the parts of the CNS and of the major tracts by which they are interconnected is provided. The external features, meninges, and gross structure of the spinal cord have been discussed in Chapter 20. The internal features of the spinal cord are described in Chapter 27.

## The brain

The **brain** lies within the cranial cavity. It is surrounded by the **meninges**—dura mater, arachnoid mater, and pia mater. The meninges are continuous with their spinal counterparts at the foramen magnum. As you saw when you removed the brain, the cranial dura mater remains fused with the skull, the arachnoid is separated from the dura by the subdural space, and the pia and arachnoid mater come away with the brain [Chapter 7].

The main **blood vessels** of the brain and spinal cord and their principal branches lie in the subarachnoid space between the arachnoid and pia mater. The smaller vessels ramify on the pia mater before sinking into the substance of the brain.

Before examining the arachnoid, pia mater, and blood vessels which lie between them, you must have some knowledge of the main parts of the brain. With the help of Figs. 24.1 and 24.2, identify the major parts of the brain. Having a brain from which the meninges and blood vessels have been removed will be helpful. If such a specimen is not available, study the brain which was removed in Chapter 7, but avoid damage to the meninges during this preliminary examination. Confirm the relations of the parts of the brain to the skull by using a dry skull.

### Parts of the brain

The brain is made up of the cerebrum, cerebellum, diencephalon, midbrain, pons, and medulla oblongata [Figs. 24.1, 24.2]. The midbrain, pons, and medulla together constitute the brainstem.

### External features of the cerebrum

The **cerebrum** is the largest part of the brain. It is composed of the two **cerebral hemispheres** which are partially separated from each other by the falx cerebri in the midline. The hemispheres cover the other parts of the brain superiorly, so that these parts can only be seen on the inferior surface [Fig. 24.2]. The surface area of each hemisphere is increased by extensive folding and the presence of a number of grooves known as **sulci**, between which are blunt ridges known as **gyri**.

Each hemisphere has three surfaces: (1) the convex **superolateral surface** [Fig. 24.1]; (2) the medial surface, partly in contact with the falx cerebri; and (3) the **inferior surface** [Fig. 24.2]. The superolateral surface is convex. It ends anteriorly at the frontal pole and posteriorly at the occipital pole. The temporal pole is the most anterior part of the temporal lobe [Fig. 24.1]. The medial surface is not seen on the external aspect of the brain. The inferior surface consists of **orbital** and **tentorial** parts. The orbital part lies in the anterior cranial fossa, on the roof of the orbit, and the nasal cavity [see Fig. 2.14]. It is separated from the tentorial part of the inferior surface by a deep horizontal fissure known as the stem of the lateral sulcus, into which the lesser wing of the sphenoid fits. Posteriorly, the tentorial part rests on the tentorium cerebelli and ends in the occipital pole [see Fig. 7.7]. The occipital pole fits into the fossa on the occipital bone in

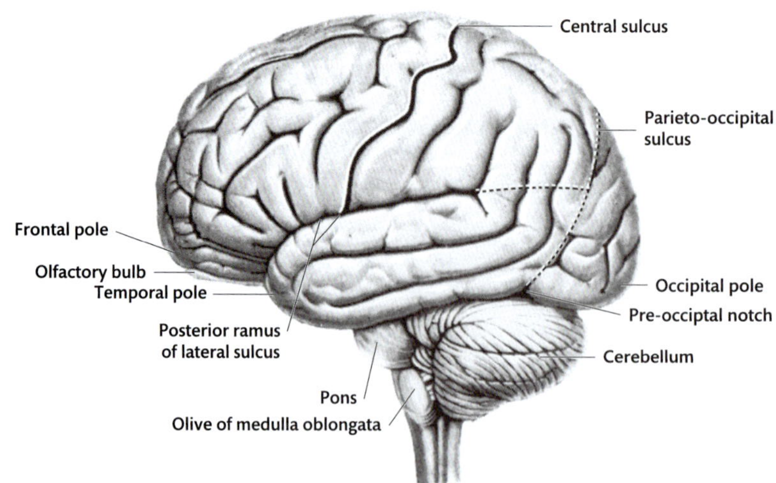


Fig. 24.1 Lateral surface of the brain to show the main sulci and gyri. The division of the superolateral surface into lobes by the central sulcus and two arbitrary lines is shown.

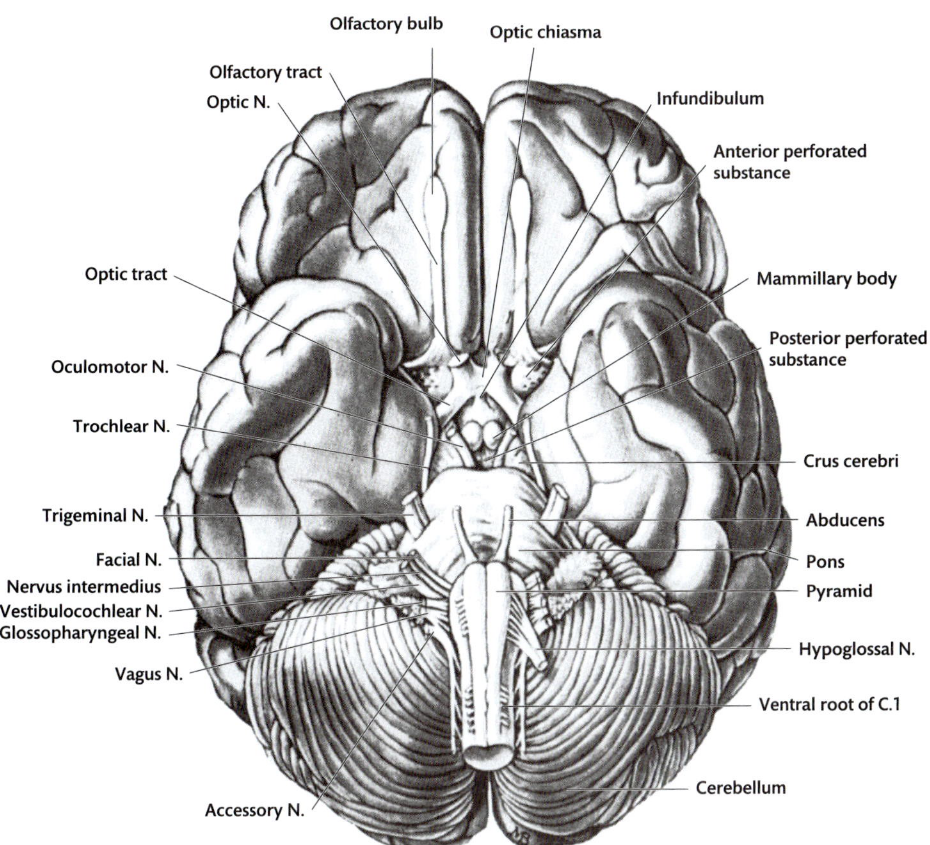


**Fig. 24.2** The base of the brain and the cranial nerves.



the area between the grooves for the superior sagittal and transverse sinuses [see Fig 7.9]. Anteriorly, the tentorial surface lies on the floor of the middle cranial fossa and extends forwards below the lesser wing of the sphenoid into the anterior extremity of the fossa.

## External features of the diencephalon

The **diencephalon** consists of the **epithalamus** and **thalamus** superiorly, and the **hypothalamus** and **subthalamus** inferiorly. It is almost entirely hidden from view by the cerebral hemispheres. The inferior surface of the hypothalamus is visible on the inferior surface of the brain between the optic chiasma anteriorly, the optic tracts anterolaterally, and the crus cerebri posterolaterally [Fig. 24.2]. This quadrangular space is the **interpeduncular fossa**. It lies superior to the sella turcica of the sphenoid bone.

## External features of the cerebellum

The **cerebellum** is the second largest part of the brain. It lies in the posterior cranial fossa, inferior to the tentorium cerebelli, and overlaps the posterior surfaces of the midbrain, pons, and medulla oblongata [Fig. 24.2]. A large number of closely set transverse **fissures** run across the surface of the cerebellum. The cerebellum consists of two cerebellar hemispheres and a median portion—the **vermis** [Figs. 24.1, 24.2]. On the inferior surface, the vermis is deeply placed between the cerebellar hemispheres in a median groove called the **vallecula cerebelli**. The vallecula is partly filled by the falx cerebelli.

## External features of the midbrain

The **midbrain** is part of the brainstem. It is the narrow segment which passes through the tentorial notch and joins the diencephalon above to the pons below. The anterior surface of the midbrain can be seen in continuity with the base of brain. It consists of the **crus cerebri** which are two broad bundles of nerve fibres, descending from the cerebral hemispheres and entering the pons inferiorly [Figs. 24.2, 24.3]. The posterior part of the interpeduncular fossa lies between them [p. 285]. The

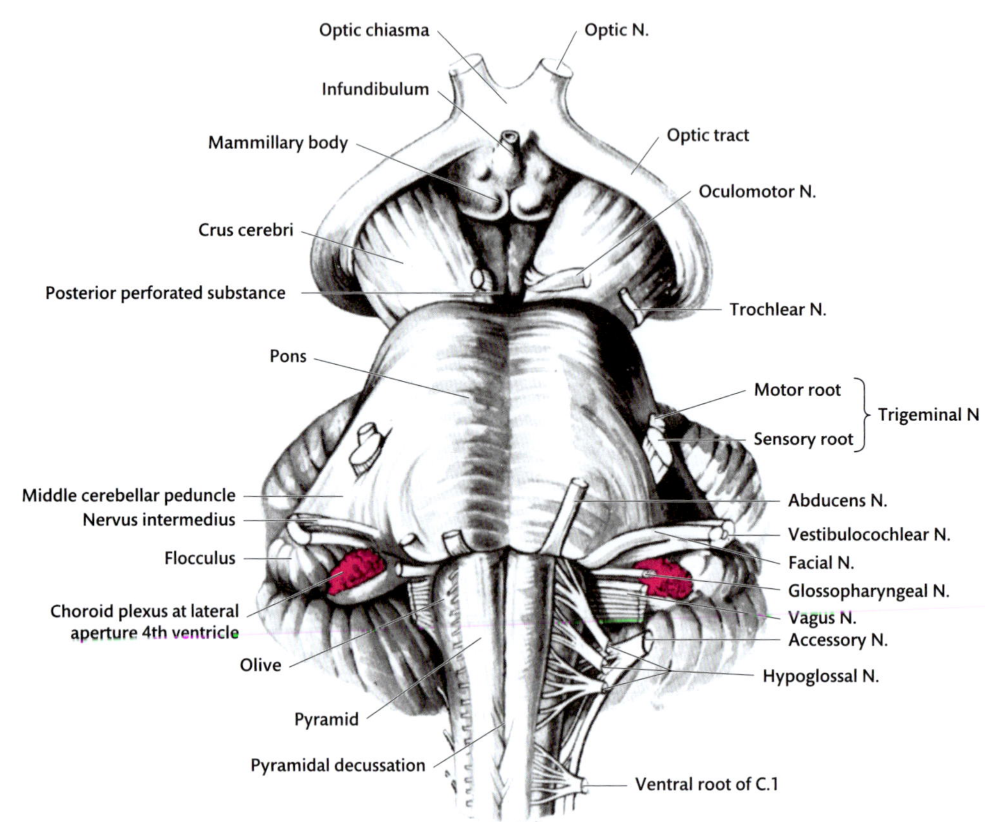


**Fig. 24.3** Anterior surface of the brainstem.

oculomotor—the third cranial nerve—emerges from the anterior surface of the midbrain, medial to the crus cerebri [Fig. 24.2]. The posterior surface of the midbrain is hidden from view in the whole brain. It is known as the **tectum** and consists of four small swellings—the **colliculi**. They are the paired **superior** and **inferior colliculi**. The tectum is deeply buried between the cerebellum and the cerebral hemispheres and will be seen later [Fig. 24.4].

## External features of the pons

The **pons** is the part of the brainstem between the midbrain and the medulla. Seen from the ventral aspect, it is a broad band of transversely running fibres. On each side, it narrows to form the rounded **middle cerebellar peduncle**, which extends posteriorly into the cerebellum. The thick **trigeminal nerve**—the fifth cranial nerve—marks the junction of the pons and middle cerebellar peduncle [Figs. 24.2, 24.3, 24.5]. The dorsal aspect of the pons is not seen on the external surface. It forms the upper part of the floor of the fourth ventricle [Fig. 24.4].

## Medulla oblongata

The **medulla oblongata** is the conical, white structure which extends inferiorly from the pons and joins the spinal cord at the foramen magnum. A **median fissure** divides the ventral surface of the medulla into right and left halves. The **pyramid** is a longitudinal ridge on each side of the fissure. Posterolateral to the pyramid is an oval swelling—the **olive** [Figs. 24.3, 24.5]. The dorsal surface of the medulla is hidden from view. The upper part forms the floor of the fourth ventricle. The lower part is in direct continuation with the dorsal aspect of the spinal cord [Fig. 24.4].

The sixth, seventh, and eighth cranial nerves are attached to the junction of the pons and medulla. The sixth cranial nerve is attached ventrally (in line with the groove between the pyramid and the olive), and the seventh and eighth laterally. The ninth, tenth, and eleventh cranial nerves are attached to the lateral surface of the medulla, posterior to the olive, in a series of linear rootlets. The twelfth cranial nerve is attached as a series of

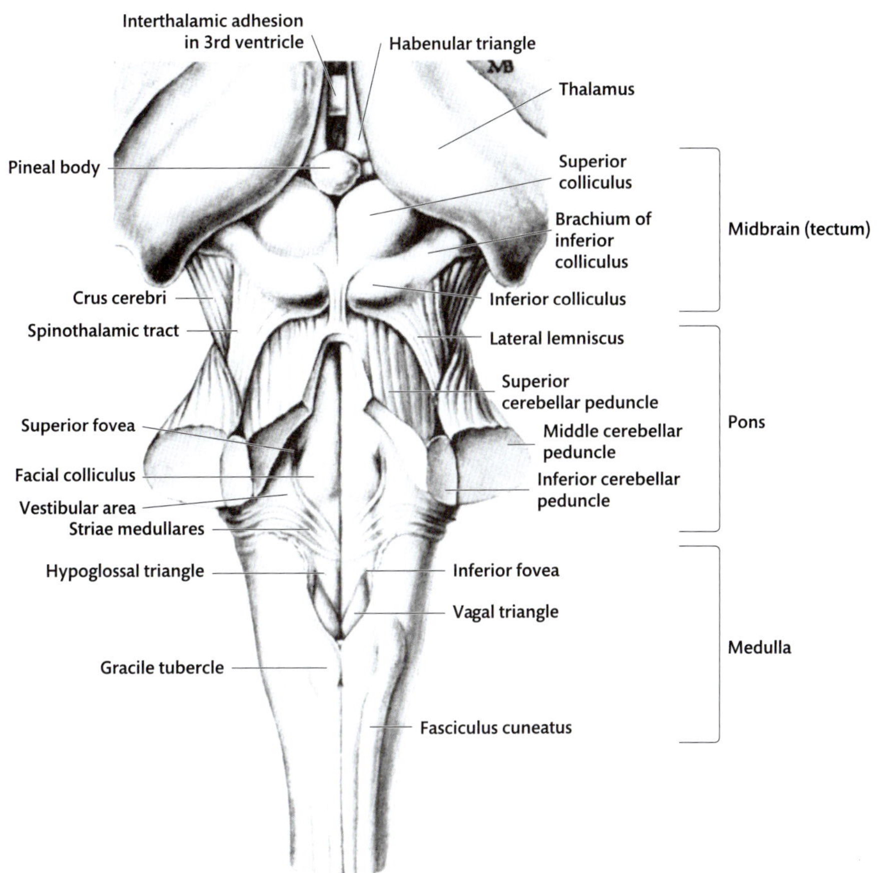


**Fig. 24.4** Posterior view of the brainstem.





rootlets in the groove between the pyramid and the olive.

Use the instructions given in Dissection 24.1 to identify the parts and salient features of the brain.

# Base of the brain

Having identified the parts of the brain and salient surface projections, it is useful to study in further detail the base of the brain.

## Interpeduncular fossa

The interpeduncular fossa is a rhomboid-shaped space on the base of the brain, bounded by the pons posteriorly, the crus cerebri (or cerebral peduncles) posterolaterally, the optic tracts anterolaterally, and the optic chiasma anteriorly [Fig. 24.3]. The crus cerebri project down from the cerebral hemispheres and converge into the pons. They are crossed laterally by the optic tracts.

## Structures in the interpeduncular fossa

The following structures are seen in the interpeduncular fossa: (1) the **oculomotor nerves**, which emerge immediately dorsomedial to the corresponding crura; (2) the **posterior perforated substance**, a layer of grey matter in the angle between the crus cerebri—it is pierced by branches of the posterior cerebral arteries; (3) the **mammillary bodies**, a pair of small, white, spherical bodies which protrude, side by side, from the ventral surface of the hypothalamus, immediately anterior to the posterior perforated substance; and (4) the **tuber cinereum**, a slightly raised area of grey matter between the mammillary bodies and the optic chiasma. The **infundibulum**, a narrow stalk which connects the hypothalamus to the hypophysis (pituitary gland), rises from the tuber cinereum. (The infundibulum was cut when the brain was removed.)

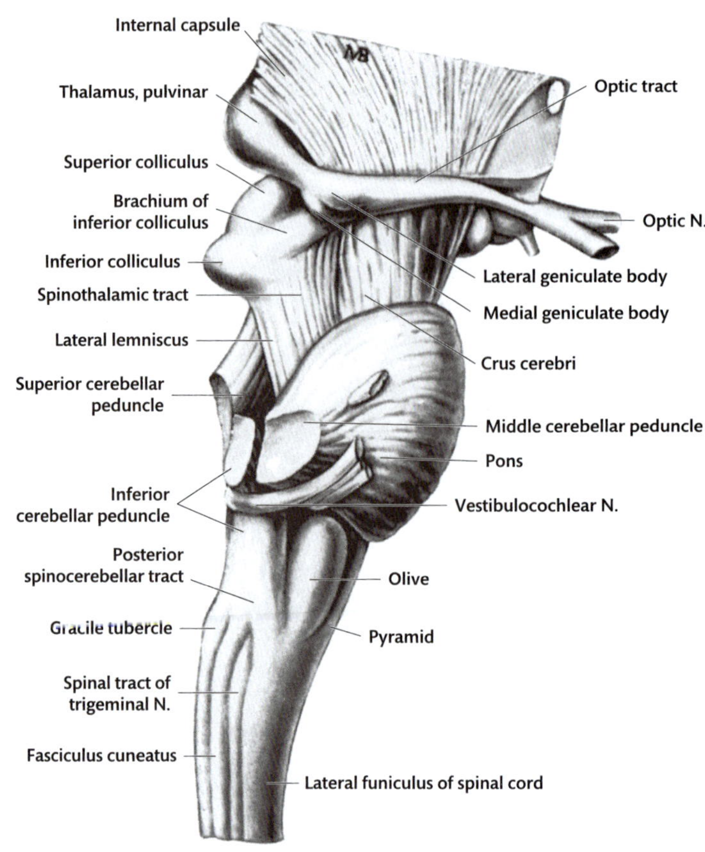


Fig. 24.5 Lateral view of the brainstem.

## Anterior perforated substance

The **anterior perforated substance** is a small area of grey matter. It is bound anteriorly by the diverging striae of the olfactory tract, medially by the optic chiasma and tract, and posteriorly by the uncus—a part of the cortex of the temporal lobe [Fig. 24.6].

## Optic chiasma

The optic chiasma lies across the midline between the anterior perforated substance of either side. It

### DISSECTION 24.1 Parts of the brain

**Objective**

**I.** To identify the cerebrum, cerebellum, midbrain, pons, and medulla oblongata on the exterior of the brain.

**Instructions**

1. Identify the superolateral surface of the cerebral hemisphere, and the frontal, occipital, and temporal poles.
2. Identify the inferior surface of the cerebral hemisphere and the temporal pole. The posterior part is hidden from view by the cerebellum. Raise the cerebellum gently to visualize this part.
3. Identify the two cerebellar hemispheres and the vermis.
4. Identify the midbrain, pons, and medulla oblongata [Fig. 24.3].
5. Identify the crus cerebri of the midbrain and the oculomotor nerve.
6. Trace the ventral aspect of the pons laterally, and identify the middle cerebellar peduncle and the cut end of the trigeminal nerve.
7. On the ventral aspect of the medulla, identify the median fissure, pyramid, and olive.
8. Identify the cut ends of the sixth to twelfth cranial nerves.

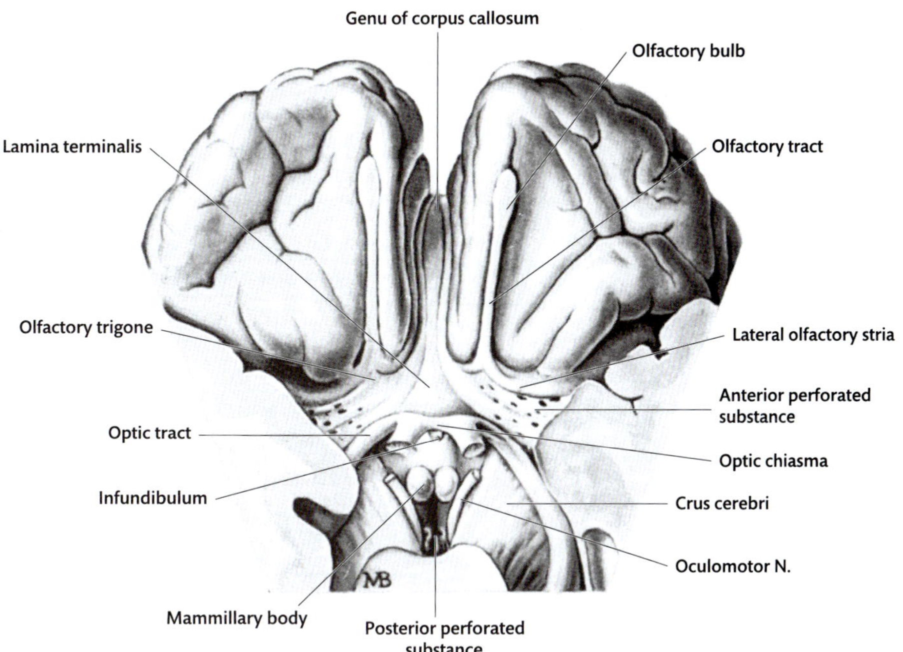


**Fig. 24.6** Orbital surfaces of the hemispheres and the interpeduncular fossa. The frontal lobes have been separated slightly to show the genu of the corpus callosum, and the optic chiasma has been turned inferiorly to uncover the lamina terminalis.





receives the optic nerves anteriorly and gives rise to the optic tracts posteriorly. It is made up of crossing fibres from the nasal half of each retina [Figs. 24.2, 24.6].

## Optic tracts

Each optic tract begins at the posterolateral corner of the optic chiasma. It passes posterolaterally between the anterior perforated substance and the tuber cinereum. It then lies superior to the medial aspect of the temporal lobe on the lateral aspect of the crus cerebri [Figs. 24.2, 24.6].

## Lamina terminalis

The lamina terminalis is a thin, grey membrane which extends superiorly from the optic chiasma and forms the anterior wall of the third ventricle. It can be seen by bending the optic chiasma gently downwards. Confirm the continuity of the lamina terminalis with the anterior perforated substance on both sides [Fig. 24.6].

## Superficial attachments of the cranial nerves

Twelve pairs of cranial nerves are attached to the brain. They are the: (1) olfactory; (2) optic; (3) oculomotor; (4) trochlear; (5) trigeminal; (6) abducens; (7) facial; (8) vestibulocochlear; (9) glossopharyngeal; (10) vagus; (11) accessory; and (12) hypoglossal.

Each cranial nerve enters or leaves the brain at its superficial attachment. Nerve fibres in the motor nerves arise within the brain and leave at the superficial attachment. Nerve fibres in the sensory nerves enter the brain at the superficial attachment and terminate on nuclei within the brain. The first pair of cranial nerves (olfactory nerve) is attached to the cerebrum, the second (optic nerve) to the diencephalon, the third and fourth (oculomotor and trochlear nerves) to the midbrain, the fifth (trigeminal nerve) to the pons, the sixth to eighth (abducens, facial, and vestibulocochlear nerves) to the junction of the pons and medulla, and the ninth to twelfth (glossopharyngeal, vagus, spinal accessory, and hypoglossal nerves) to the medulla oblongata. The eleventh (spinal accessory nerve) is attached to the cervical spinal cord as well. The cranial nerves may be attached to the ventral, lateral, or dorsal surface of the brain. The nerves with ventral and lateral attachments are seen on the base of the brain.

### Cranial nerves with ventral attachments

#### Olfactory nerves

Approximately 20 **olfactory nerves** on each side pass through the cribriform plate of the ethmoid to the olfactory bulb. They are unusual in that they arise from the olfactory cells in the nasal mucous membrane and consist of bundles of minute, non-myelinated nerve fibres [Fig. 24.2].

### Optic nerve

The **optic nerve** is a thick, cylindrical nerve. It is composed of myelinated nerve fibres which arise in the retina. The optic nerve ends by joining the anterolateral angle of the optic chiasma [Fig. 24.2].

### Oculomotor nerve

The **oculomotor nerve** arises as a compact bundle of rootlets at the medial aspect of the cerebral peduncle in the posterior part of the interpeduncular fossa [Fig. 24.3].

### Abducens nerve

The **abducens nerve** emerges at the inferior border of the pons, immediately lateral to the pyramid [Fig. 24.3].

### Hypoglossal nerve

The **hypoglossal nerve** is formed by the union of rootlets which arise from the anterior aspect of the medulla oblongata in the groove between the pyramid and the olive [Fig. 24.3]. They are directly in line with the ventral rootlets of the first cervical nerve.

## Cranial nerves with lateral attachments

### Trigeminal nerve

The **trigeminal nerve**, the largest of the cranial nerves, is attached to the junction of the pons and the middle cerebellar peduncle. It consists of two roots: a larger posterolateral **sensory root** consisting of loosely packed nerve bundles; and a smaller anterosuperior **motor root** which is compact and closely applied to the sensory root [Fig. 24.3].

### Facial and vestibulocochlear nerves

The **facial** and **vestibulocochlear nerves**, with the small **nervus intermedius** between them, emerge on the inferior border of the pons, posterior to the olive, and in the same vertical line as the other laterally attached cranial nerves [Fig. 24.3].

The facial nerve is motor. The nervus intermedius [Fig. 24.3] carries sensory and parasympathetic fibres associated with the facial nerve. It lies between the facial and vestibulocochlear nerves. The vestibulocochlear nerve is sensory. It splits at the medulla oblongata into a cochlear part passing posterior to the inferior cerebellar peduncle [Fig. 24.5] and a vestibular part passing anterior to it.

### Glossopharyngeal, vagus, and accessory nerves

The **glossopharyngeal**, **vagus**, and **accessory nerves** arise as a series of rootlets from a groove posterior to the olive in the medulla oblongata, and from the lateral aspect of the spinal cord as far inferiorly as the fifth cervical spinal segment. The rootlets which form the glossopharyngeal nerves can only be differentiated from the others because they pierce the dura mater separately at the jugular foramen. A part of the accessory nerve may still be attached to the brain in the specimen. If a portion of the spinal cord is present, the spinal and cranial roots may be seen [Figs. 24.2, 24.3].

## Cranial nerve with dorsal attachment

### Trochlear nerve

The thin **trochlear nerve** is the only cranial nerve with a dorsal attachment. It decussates within the midbrain and emerges from the dorsal surface, lateral to the median plane. The proximal part will be seen later when the anterior lobe of the cerebellum is removed. A part of it may be seen here winding around the lateral aspect of the crus cerebri towards the interpeduncular fossa, immediately superior to the pons [Fig. 24.2].

Use the instructions given in Dissection 24.2 to identify the 12 pairs of cranial nerves.

**DISSECTION 24.2 Surface attachment of cranial nerves**

**Objective**

**I.** To identify the surface attachment of the cranial nerves.

**Instructions**

1. Identify the surface attachments of the cranial nerves.
2. Remove the small blood vessels and pia mater from the medulla oblongata, leaving the nerve roots in position as far as possible.

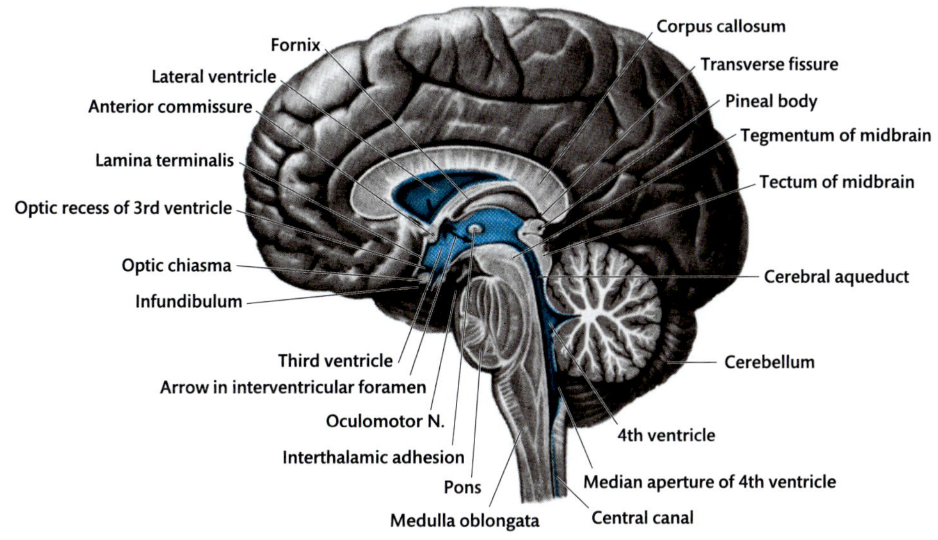


**Fig. 24.7** Medial surface of the right half of a bisected brain to show the ventricles. The arrow passes through the interventricular foramen from the lateral to the third ventricle. (The septum pellucidum has been removed to expose the lateral ventricle.) Ependymal lining of ventricles = blue.

## The ventricular system

The **ventricular system** is a hollow, fluid-filled system derived from the cavities of the primitive brain vesicles. It is lined by ependyma. Each cerebral hemisphere has a **lateral ventricle** which communicates with the single midline third ventricle through the interventricular foramen, or **foramen of Monro** [Fig. 24.7]. The **third ventricle** is a narrow slit-like cavity of the diencephalon. Posteriorly, it continues with the **cerebral aqueduct** of the midbrain, which in turn communicates with the fourth ventricle. The **fourth ventricle** is a wide tent-shaped cavity between the pons and medulla and the cerebellum [see Figs. 32.1, 32.2]. Inferiorly, the cavity of the fourth ventricle is continuous with the central canal in the inferior part of the medulla and the spinal cord.

The ventricles are filled with cerebrospinal fluid (CSF) and contain the choroid plexus which produces it. The roof of the fourth ventricle has one median and two lateral apertures. Through these apertures, CSF leaves the ventricle and enters the subarachnoid space around the brain and spinal cord [see Fig. 25.1].

## Development of the brain and spinal cord

The brain and spinal cord develop from the neural tube. The cavity of the neural tube persists as the ventricular system in the brain and as the central canal of the spinal cord. The parts of the brain developed from each of the primitive brain vesicles (forebrain, midbrain, and hindbrain vesicles) and the cavity enclosed within them are listed in Table 24.1.

**Table 24.1** Developmental origin and ventricular system in parts of the brain

| During development | In the adult | Ventricular system |
|---|---|---|
| Forebrain | Cerebrum | Lateral ventricle |
| | Diencephalon | Third ventricle |
| Midbrain | Midbrain | Cerebral aqueduct |
| Hindbrain | Medulla oblongata<br>Pons<br>Cerebellum | Fourth ventricle |

CHAPTER 25

# The meninges of the brain

## Introduction

The brain is surrounded by the same three membranes which surround the spinal cord—the dura mater, arachnoid mater, and pia mater [see Fig. 7.1]. The meninges of the brain and spinal cord are continuous with each other at the foramen magnum.

## Dura mater

The cranial dura mater, including the two layers and the folds, has been seen and described during the dissection of the cranial cavity [Chapter 7], but its parts should be reviewed in relation to the brain.

## Arachnoid mater

The arachnoid mater is an exceedingly thin, almost transparent membrane which lines the internal surface of the dura mater and, for the most part, has exactly the same shape as the dural sac. The arachnoid is separated from the dura mater by a capillary space—the **subdural space**—which contains a film of fluid. This arrangement allows movement between the dura mater and the brain (enclosed in the arachnoid and pia mater), except where the arachnoid and dura are fused. Fusion of the arachnoid and dura occurs where both meninges are pierced by structures entering or leaving the brain (e.g. nerves and blood vessels), where the arachnoid granulations pierce the dura mater, and where the ligamentum denticulatum is attached to the spinal dura mater [Chapter 20].

## Subarachnoid space



The subarachnoid space, between the arachnoid and pia mater, is filled with **cerebrospinal fluid** (CSF). The fluid acts as a mobile buffer to distribute and equalize pressures within the skull [Fig. 25.1].

The subarachnoid space is traversed by filaments, or **trabeculae**, from the arachnoid to the pia mater which are numerous on the surfaces of the cerebral hemispheres. The dense trabeculae form a kind of fluid-filled sponge which helps to protect the surface of the brain from damage against the skull or the dural folds, when it moves within the dura mater. The trabeculae also bind the pia and arachnoid tightly together in these situations. Elsewhere, and especially where the pia mater is widely separated from the arachnoid, the mesh is less dense and the CSF can flow more freely. The larger arteries and veins of the brain lie in the subarachnoid space and send branches into the substance of the brain. A sleeve of pia mater and subarachnoid space, called the **perivascular space**, surround each branch for a short distance within the brain substance.

### Subarachnoid cisterns

In certain situations, the subarachnoid space is wide and the brain closely covered by the pia mater lies some distance from the arachnoid lining the dura mater. In these situations, the subarachnoid space

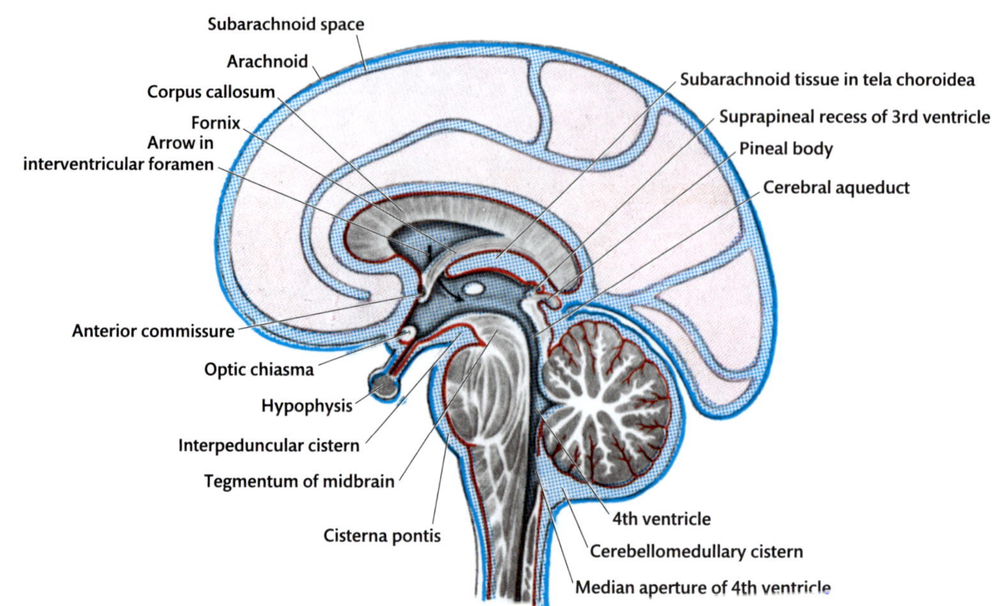


**Fig. 25.1** Diagram of a median section of the brain to show membranes and cisterns. Red = pia mater; blue stipple = subarachnoid space and ventricles; blue = arachnoid; pink = surface view of shallow subarachnoid space. The lines of blue stipple running over the pink area indicate the places where the subarachnoid space is deeper around the branches of the anterior and posterior cerebral arteries.

is large and is known as **subarachnoid cisterns**. Like the subarachnoid space everywhere else, the subarachnoid cisterns are filled with CSF. Cisterns are principally found around the brainstem and cerebellum, on the base of the brain, around the free margin of the tentorium cerebelli, and in association with the major blood vessels [Fig. 25.1].

The **cerebellomedullary cistern** lies in the angle between the cerebellum, medulla oblongata, and occipital bone. It is continuous inferiorly with the posterior part of the spinal subarachnoid space [Fig. 25.1]. ➲ The cerebellomedullary cistern is accessible through a needle introduced through the posterior atlanto-occipital membrane, between the posterior arch of the atlas and the posterior margin of the foramen magnum. This procedure is called a **cisternal puncture.**

The **cisterna pontis** lies anterior to the pons and medulla oblongata [Fig. 25.1]. It contains the vertebral and basilar arteries. It is continuous: (1) posteriorly around the medulla oblongata with the cerebellomedullary cistern; (2) inferiorly with the spinal subarachnoid space; and (3) superiorly with the interpeduncular cistern.

The **interpeduncular cistern** fills the interpeduncular fossa [Fig. 25.1]. At the superior border of the pons, the arachnoid turns anteriorly above the sella turcica and is stretched between the temporal lobes of the hemispheres. Here it forms the floor of the interpeduncular cistern. This cistern contains the arterial circle—the circle of Willis [Fig. 25.2].

## Arachnoid villi and granulations

Arachnoid villi are minute protrusions of the arachnoid mater into the dural venous sinuses through apertures in the dura mater. (They are similar to, but smaller and more numerous than, the arachnoid granulations shown in Fig. 25.3.) They are particularly common in the superior sagittal sinus and its lateral lacunae. The arachnoid villi contain subarachnoid tissue, CSF, and a number of thin tubules which pass through the middle of each villus. The tubules and spaces between the arachnoid trabeculae are continuous with the subarachnoid space at the base of the villus. The tubules open into the venous sinus at the apex of the villus. When the pressure of the CSF exceeds that in the venous sinus, the spaces fill with fluid, the villi bulge into the sinus, and the central tubules become patent and allow CSF to flow into the venous sinus. If the venous pressure exceeds that of the subarachnoid space, the villi collapse, effectively closing the

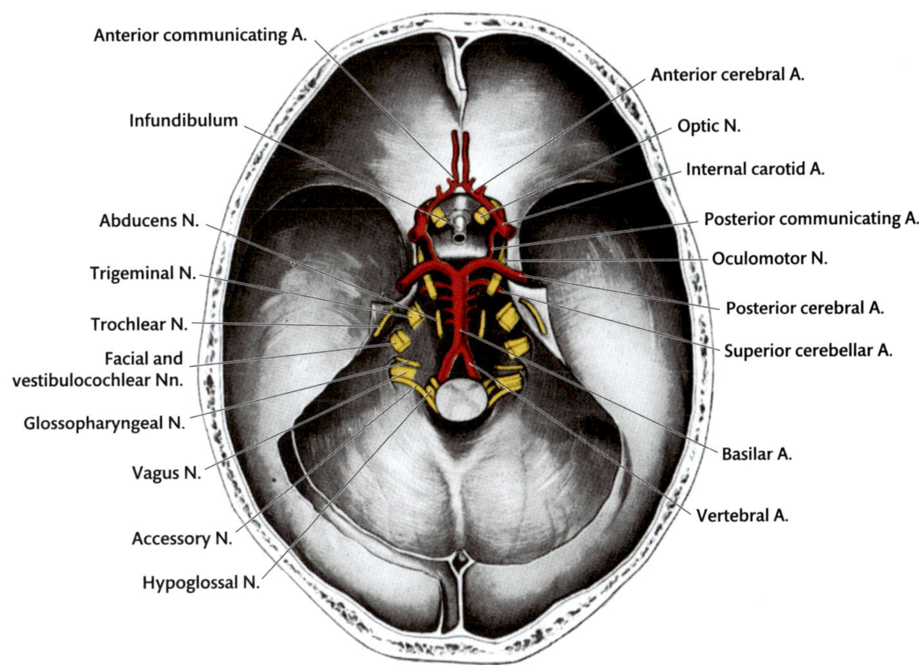


**Fig. 25.2** Floor of the cranial cavity after removal of the brain. The arteries at the base of the brain are intact.





central tubules and preventing the reflux of blood into the subarachnoid space. In effect, the arachnoid villi are one-way valves for the passage of CSF into the venous system. With increasing age, the size of the villi increases till they form arachnoid granulations which often indent the overlying bone of the skull.

## Communications of the subarachnoid space

The subarachnoid space communicates with: (1) the cavity of the dural venous sinus through the arachnoid villi; and (2) the ventricles of the brain through three small openings in the roof of the fourth ventricle.

Using the instructions given in Dissection 25.1 (and Fig. 25.2), explore the extent and contents of the subarachnoid space.

## Pia mater

The pia mater is adherent to the surface of the brain and follows the irregularities of its surface closely.

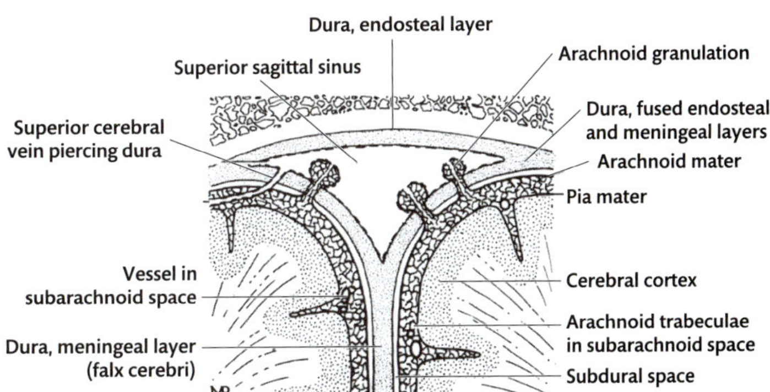


**Fig. 25.3** Diagrammatic transverse section through the superior sagittal sinus and surrounding structures. Note the arrangement of the arachnoid granulations.

**DISSECTION 25.1 Subarachnoid space—major arteries**

**Objectives**

**I.** To study the extent of the subarachnoid space. **II.** To identify and trace the vertebral and basilar arteries.

**Instructions**

1. If the arachnoid is complete, divide it along the anterior aspect of the medulla oblongata and pons to expose the vertebral and basilar arteries and their branches [Fig. 25.2].
2. Note the arachnoid trabeculae.
3. Cut posteriorly through the arachnoid into the cerebellomedullary cistern, and identify the posterior inferior cerebellar branch of the vertebral artery. This branch winds posteriorly on the medulla oblongata, on its way to the cerebellum.
4. Extend the median incision in the arachnoid into the interpeduncular fossa which lodges the **interpeduncular cistern**. Note the blood vessels in the cistern and the fact that its floor is perforated posteriorly by the oculomotor nerves and anteriorly by the internal carotid arteries and the infundibulum (stalk of the pituitary).

The blood vessels of the brain lie in the subarachnoid space on the surface of the pia mater. They break up into branches on the pia mater and anastomose there, before passing into the substance of the brain as end-arteries. If a small piece of the pia mater is stripped from the surface of the brain, a number of minute blood vessels are seen entering the brain substance from its deep surface.

## Choroid plexus and tela choroidea

In specific locations of the developing brain—the transverse and choroid fissure—the pia mater covering the surface of the brain invaginates into the ventricles. The invaginating pia mater is vascularized by a tuft of choroidal vessels and is known as the **tela choroidea**. The choroid plexus is formed by: (1) the invaginating vascularized pia mater; and (2) the ependymal covering. The location, extent, structure, and function of the choroid plexus is described in Chapter 32.

Using the instructions given in Dissection 25.2, identify the protrusions of the choroid plexus of the fourth ventricle into the subarachnoid space.

See Clinical Application 25.1 for the practical implications of the anatomy discussed in this chapter.

**DISSECTION 25.2 Subarachnoid space—choroid plexus**

**Objective**

**I.** To identify the choroid plexus in the median and lateral apertures of the fourth ventricle.

**Instructions**

1. Identify the apertures in the roof of the fourth ventricle by the tuft of finely granular material (**choroid plexus**) which protrudes through each. The **median aperture** can be seen in the depths of the cerebellomedullary cistern by gently depressing the medulla away from the cerebellum [Fig. 25.1]. The **lateral apertures** face anteriorly and lie immediately posterior to the glossopharyngeal nerve. Pick up the tuft of choroid plexus protruding through the lateral aperture, and pull it gently towards the cerebellum—the aperture will be seen immediately anterior to the choroid plexus at the end of a sleeve-like extension of the thin roof of the fourth ventricle [see Figs. 24.3, 29.4].

## CLINICAL APPLICATION 25.1 Subarachnoid haemorrhage

A 54-year-old man complained of sudden onset of severe headache accompanied by vomiting. Soon after, he became unconscious and had a generalized seizure. Clinical examination revealed moderately elevated blood pressure, papilloedema, and focal neurological deficits. Imaging studies showed a bleed in the subarachnoid space—a subarachnoid haemorrhage (SAH).

Study question 1: what are the contents of the subarachnoid space? (Answer: the subarachnoid space contains CSF and the major blood vessels of the brain.)

Study question 2: what are the causes of an SAH? (Answer: the usual causes of an SAH include rupture of an aneurysm [see Clinical Application 26.1], localized dilatation of a vessel, arteriovenous malformation [see Clinical Application 26.2], or head trauma.)

Study question 3: what is the cause for the headache and vomiting? (Answer: headache and vomiting are typical signs of raised intracranial pressure. In this patient, raised intracranial pressure is due to collection of blood in the subarachnoid space. This pressure is transferred around the optic nerve, and also explains the papilloedema.)

Study question 4: how is this condition managed? (Answer: blood pressure is controlled by antihypertensive medication. Bleeding is controlled by applying surgical clips or an endovascular coil.)

## CHAPTER 26

# The blood vessels of the brain

## Introduction

The intracranial vessels (with the exception of the dural venous sinuses—Chapter 7) have much thinner walls than extracranial vessels of comparable size, as they are enclosed in, and supported by, the surrounding cranium. The walls of most of the veins are so thin that they are impossible to see, unless filled with blood.

## Veins of the cerebral hemispheres

Most of the cerebral veins lie on the surface of the hemisphere in the subarachnoid space.

### Veins of the superolateral surface

The **superior cerebral veins** [Fig. 26.1] converge on the superior sagittal sinus, the anterior and posterior veins entering the sinus obliquely from in front and behind. They all pass inferior to the lateral lacunae of the sinus. They drain into the superior sagittal sinus by piercing the arachnoid, crossing the subdural space and piercing the dura [see Fig. 25.3]. The small segments of the cerebral veins in the subdural space are referred to as 'bridging veins' as they bridge the subdural space. ➲ The bridging veins may rupture in a head injury and lead to a **subdural haemorrhage** and haematoma. Most of the **inferior cerebral veins** converge on the superficial middle cerebral vein, but those of the occipital lobe run inferiorly into the transverse sinus [Fig. 26.1A].

The **superficial middle cerebral vein** runs anteriorly between the lips of the posterior ramus of the lateral sulcus [see Fig. 24.1] and curves medially into the stem of the lateral sulcus. It ends in the cavernous sinus. Its cut end will be found piercing the arachnoid near the medial end of the stem of the lateral sulcus. Posteriorly, the superficial middle cerebral vein is frequently connected to the superior sagittal sinus by a wide **superior anastomotic vein**, and to the transverse sinus by the **inferior anastomotic vein** [Fig. 26.1A]. ➲ These anastomotic veins may become important if the cavernous sinus is blocked. The superficial veins also connect with veins in the interior and on the base of the hemisphere by small veins which pierce the hemisphere.



### Veins of the inferior surface of the hemisphere

The veins on the inferior surface drain in a number of different directions: (1) anteriorly to the anterior and superficial middle cerebral veins; (2) posteriorly to the basal vein; and (3) directly to the superior petrosal, straight, and transverse sinuses.

### Veins of the medial surface of the hemisphere

These veins will be seen later when the hemispheres are separated, but parts of this system can be seen now, so a brief description is given.

The main vein on the medial aspect of the hemisphere is the **great cerebral vein**. It is formed by the union of the two **internal cerebral veins**, inferior to the splenium of the corpus callosum, and ends by uniting with the inferior sagittal sinus to form the straight sinus [see Fig. 7.2; Fig. 26.1B]. (The internal cerebral veins are formed by the union of the thalamostriate vein and the veins draining the choroid plexus of the lateral ventricle at the interventricular foramen [see Fig. 32.7].) If

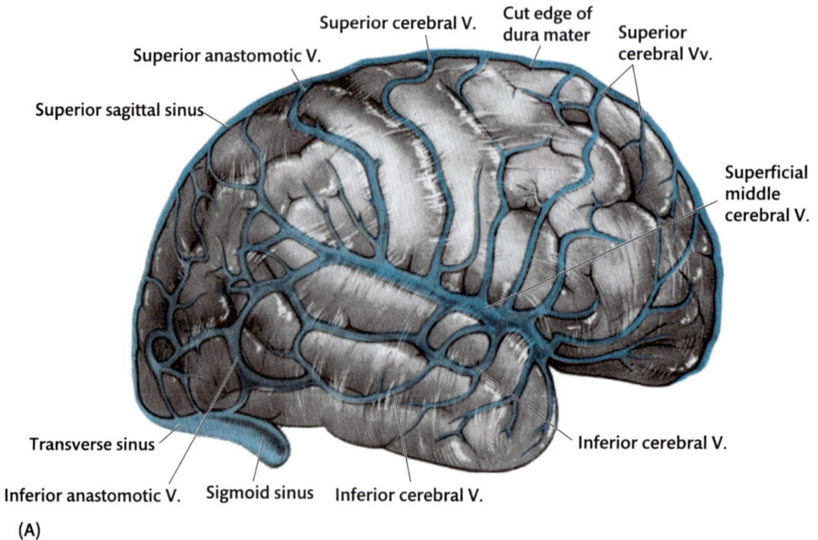


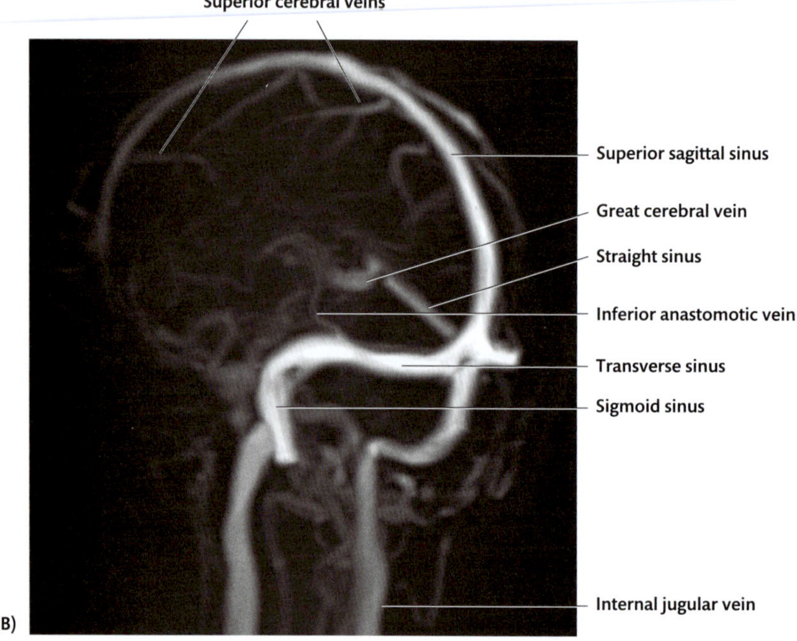


Fig. 26.1 (A) Veins of the superolateral surface of the hemisphere, seen through the arachnoid mater. (B) Magnetic resonance venogram of the brain.

the occipital lobes of the hemispheres are gently separated, the cut end of the great cerebral vein will be seen close to the splenium. The great cerebral vein is joined by a number of symmetrical tributaries from the midbrain and cerebellum, and by the basal veins which curve around the sides of the midbrain to reach it from the inferior surface of the brain.

Each **basal vein** is formed deep in the medial part of the stem of the lateral sulcus by the union of: (1) the **anterior cerebral vein**, which runs with the corresponding artery and enters it from in front; (2) the **deep middle cerebral vein** which lies in the depths of the lateral sulcus on the insula; and (3) the **striate vein** or veins which descend through the substance of the brain and emerge through the anterior perforated substance [see Fig. 24.2].

Using the instructions given in Dissection 26.1, expose the vessels in the lateral sulcus.

> **DISSECTION 26.1 Exposure of arteries and veins in the lateral sulcus**
>
> **Objectives**
>
> **I.** To expose the middle cerebral artery and superficial middle cerebral vein in the stem of the lateral sulcus. **II.** To identify the striate veins and basal veins.
>
> **Instructions**
>
> 1. Divide the arachnoid mater over the stem of the lateral sulcus, and depress the temporal pole to expose the beginning of the middle cerebral artery, the deep middle cerebral vein, the striate veins, and the origin of the basal vein.
> 2. If the basal vein is filled with blood, it will be seen passing posteriorly close to the optic tract. Trace it as far as possible towards the great cerebral vein.

## Veins of the cerebellum and brainstem

The veins of the brainstem and cerebellum drain posteriorly to the basal veins, great cerebral veins, and adjacent dural venous sinuses. The veins of the medulla oblongata communicate with those of the spinal cord.

## Arteries of the brain

Two **internal carotid arteries** and two **vertebral arteries** supply the brain. The vertebral arteries enter the skull through the foramen magnum [see Fig. 25.2]. Each internal carotid artery runs through the skull in the carotid canal and the superior part of the foramen lacerum. It then takes a sinuous course through the cavernous sinus and pierces the dural roof of the sinus. It ends immediately lateral to the optic chiasma, inferior to the anterior perforated substance, by dividing into its terminal branches—the anterior and middle cerebral arteries [see Figs. 7.12, 25.2].

### Vertebral arteries

Each **vertebral artery** enters the subarachnoid space in the upper part of the vertebral canal by piercing the lateral aspect of the spinal dura and arachnoid mater. It ascends anterosuperiorly through the foramen magnum, curves around the ventrolateral aspect of the medulla oblongata, and unites with the vertebral artery of the other side to form the **basilar artery** at the lower border of the pons. The two vertebral arteries are often of very different calibre [see Fig. 25.2].

### Intracranial branches of the vertebral artery

1. The **posterior spinal artery** is the first intracranial branch. It passes inferiorly on the spinal cord among the dorsal rootlets of the spinal nerves. It commonly arises from the posterior inferior cerebellar artery.
2. The **posterior inferior cerebellar artery** is the largest branch [Fig. 26.2]. It arises from the vertebral artery, soon after it pierces the meninges, and pursues a tortuous course posteriorly on the side of the medulla oblongata, among the rootlets of the hypoglossal, vagus, and glossopharyngeal nerves. It supplies branches to the lateral part of the medulla oblongata, occasionally as far cranially as the inferior border of the pons. It reaches the posterior surface of the medulla oblongata, between the roof of the fourth ventricle and the cerebellum, and supplies the choroid plexus of the fourth ventricle and the inferior surface of the cerebellum. It varies inversely in size with the anterior inferior cerebellar artery but is usually much larger.
3. The **anterior spinal artery** [Fig. 26.2] is formed by the union of a branch from each of the verte-

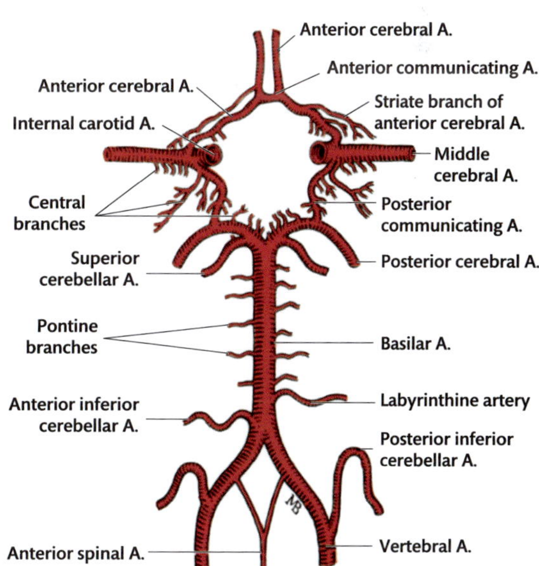


**Fig. 26.2** Diagram of the arteries on the base of the brain.

bral arteries on the ventral surface of the medulla oblongata, close to the pons. It supplies the median part of the medulla oblongata and continues inferiorly throughout the length of the spinal cord.

## Basilar artery

The **basilar artery** is formed at the inferior border of the pons by the union of the two vertebral arteries. It ends at the superior border of the pons by dividing into the two posterior cerebral arteries. It lies in the median groove of the pons in the cisterna pontis, on the basilar part of the occipital bone and the dorsum sellae of the sphenoid [Fig. 26.2].

### Branches of the basilar artery

1. The **anterior inferior cerebellar artery** arises at the lower border of the pons and runs laterally, superficial to the sixth, seventh, and eighth cranial nerves. It then loops over the flocculus [see Fig. 24.3] and supplies the anteroinferior part of the cerebellar surface.
2. The **artery of the labyrinth** arises close to, or from, the anterior inferior cerebellar artery [Fig. 26.2]. It accompanies the vestibulocochlear nerve to the internal ear and also supplies the adjacent part of the facial nerve.
3. Numerous slender **pontine branches** pierce the pons, some close to the midline, others further laterally [Fig. 26.2].
4. The large **superior cerebellar artery** arises close to the superior border of the pons. It winds posteriorly along the superior border of the pons and the middle cerebellar peduncle, supplying them and the adjacent part of the midbrain. It also sends many branches to the superior surface of the cerebellum, inferior to the tentorium cerebelli.
5. The two large **posterior cerebral arteries** are the terminal branches of the basilar artery. They diverge at the superior border of the pons. On the anterior surface of the midbrain, each posterior cerebral artery receives a slender **posterior communicating** branch from the corresponding internal carotid artery [Fig. 26.3].

The posterior cerebral and superior cerebellar arteries run parallel to each other and lie on, and supply, the superior and inferior parts of the midbrain, respectively. The posterior cerebral artery lies above the third and fourth cranial nerves, which

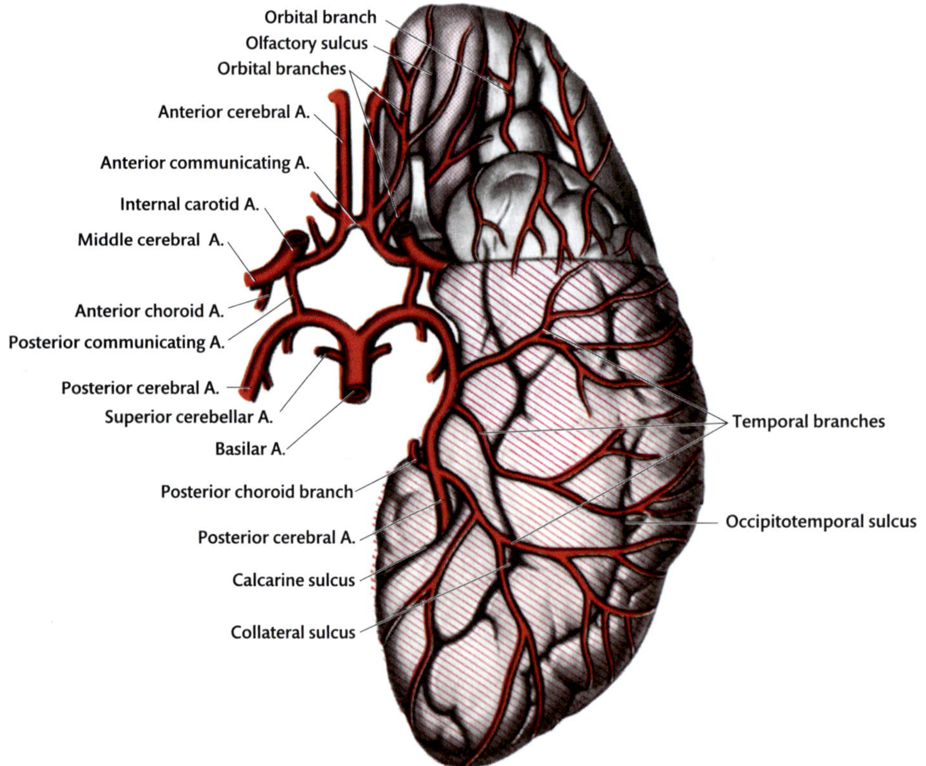


**Fig. 26.3** Arteries of the inferior surface of the left hemisphere. The areas supplied by the three cerebral arteries are indicated by: red stipple = anterior cerebral artery; red cross-hatching = posterior cerebral artery; and no colour = middle cerebral artery.

arise from the midbrain, and the superior cerebellar artery lies below these nerves [see Fig. 25.2].

## Posterior cerebral artery

Each posterior cerebral artery arises as a terminal branch of the basilar artery.

### Branches of the posterior cerebral arteries

1. Small **posteromedial central branches** pierce the ventral surface of the midbrain in the interpeduncular fossa. (The passage of these branches creates the **posterior perforated substance**—the perforated tissue in the floor of the interpeduncular fossa.) Similar branches pierce the lateral surface of the midbrain and caudal diencephalon [Fig. 26.2].
2. **Posterior choroid branches** arise on the lateral surface of the midbrain and pass forwards to supply the greater part of the choroid plexus of the lateral and third ventricles [Fig. 26.3].
3. **Cortical branches** supply mainly the inferior surface of the cerebral cortex through the temporal branches and occipital branches [Figs. 26.3, 26.4].

## Internal carotid arteries

The cut end of each internal carotid artery can be seen immediately lateral to the optic chiasma. The artery passes into a shallow pit, immediately inferior to the anterior perforated substance [see Figs. 24.2, 25.2].

### Branches of the internal carotid artery

1. The **posterior communicating artery** passes posteriorly across the crus cerebri to join the posterior cerebral artery [Fig. 26.2]. It is usually a thin vessel, but it may be large on one or both sides and form the major source of blood in the posterior cerebral artery. The posterior communicating artery gives minute branches to the crus, optic tract, hypophysis, and hypothalamus.

➲ When the posterior communicating artery's contribution to the posterior cerebral artery is significant, occlusion of the internal carotid artery may lead to damage in the territory of the posterior cerebral artery as well.

2. The **anterior choroid artery** arises superior to the posterior communicating artery and passes posterolaterally, close to the optic tract [Fig. 26.3]. It gives branches into the crus cerebri and turns laterally [see Fig. 32.5] to enter the choroid plexus of the inferior horn of the lateral ventricle.
3. **Ophthalmic artery**.
4. **Middle cerebral arteries**.
5. **Anterior cerebral arteries** [Figs. 26.2, 26.3].

### Anterior cerebral artery

Only a small part of this artery can be seen at this stage. (The remainder will be seen when the medial aspect of the hemisphere is exposed.) This initial part of the anterior cerebral artery runs horizontally in an anteromedial direction [Fig. 26.3] to the longitudinal fissure. Here it is joined to the anterior cerebral artery by the short **anterior communicating artery** anterosuperior to the optic chiasma [Figs. 26.2, 26.3]. The anterior cerebral artery then bends sharply upwards into the median longitudinal fissure and runs on the medial surface of the cerebral hemisphere [Fig. 26.4].

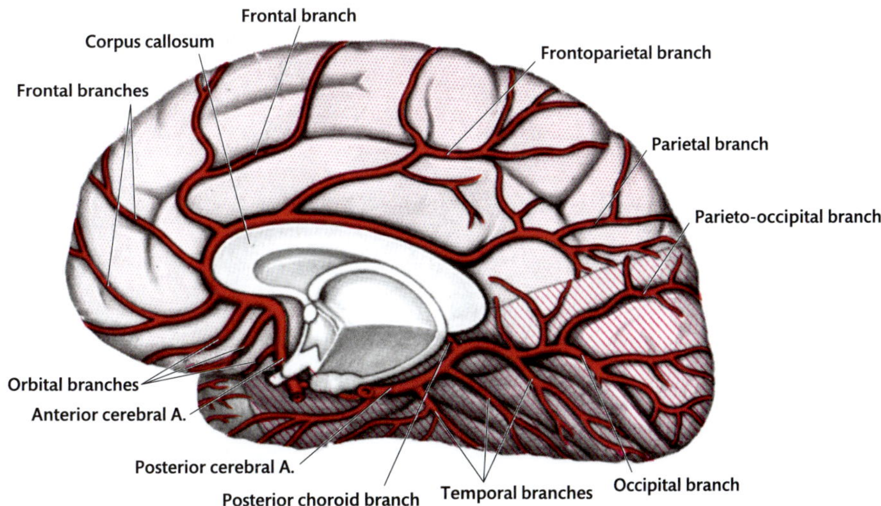


Fig. 26.4 The arteries of the medial and tentorial surfaces of the right hemisphere. Area supplied by the: anterior cerebral artery = red stipple; posterior cerebral artery = red cross-hatching; and middle cerebral artery = no colour.

Branches of the anterior cerebral artery

1. Several thin **central** branches pierce the brain, anterior to the optic chiasma, and enter the anterior hypothalamus.
2. Branches pass to the optic chiasma and the optic nerve.
3. One or more larger recurrent branches arise close to the anterior communicating artery and run to the medial part of the anterior perforated substance. Here they send **medial striate** (**anteromedial central**) branches into the brain substance [Fig. 26.2].
4. Several **cortical branches**—frontal, frontoparietal, parietal, and parieto-occipital—are given to the cerebral cortex [Figs. 26.3, 26.4].

## Middle cerebral artery

The middle cerebral artery continues in line with the internal carotid artery [Fig. 26.2]. ➲ As such, particulate matter in the internal carotid artery enters the middle cerebral artery more frequently than the anterior cerebral. The middle cerebral artery runs laterally in the stem of the lateral sulcus and breaks up into a number of branches on the **insula**—a submerged part of the parietal lobe not seen on the surface. These branches emerge through the lateral sulcus and supply most of the superolateral surface of the cerebral hemisphere.

Branches of the middle cerebral artery

1. Branches to the **insular cortex**.
2. **Cortical branches** to the superolateral surface through the frontal, parietal, parietotemporal, and temporal branches [Fig. 26.5]; to the inferior surface through the orbital and tentorial branches [Figs. 26.3, 26.4]; and to the medial surface through branches to the temporal pole.
3. The **central branches** of the middle cerebral artery are the numerous small **lateral striate** (**anterolateral central**) **arteries** [Fig. 26.2]. They pass superiorly through the anterior perforated substance to the deep nuclei of the hemisphere.

## Cortical and central branches of the cerebral arteries

Two types of branches arise from the three cerebral arteries: the cortical and central branches. The **central branches** are numerous and slender, and tend to arise in groups which immediately pierce the surface of the brain to supply the deeper parts. The largest collections of central branches pass through the anterior and posterior perforated substances [Fig. 26.2]. They do not anastomose to any significant extent within the brain substance. The **cortical branches** ramify over the surface of the cortex and anastomose freely on the pia mater. They give rise to numerous small branches which enter the cortex at right angles and, like the central branches, do not anastomose in it [Figs. 26.3, 26.4, 26.5].

➲ It follows that blockage of an artery on the pia mater may produce little, if any, damage to the brain, but damage to branches entering the substance of the brain leads to the destruction of brain tissue.

➲ The arteries of the brain are supplied with **sympathetic nerves** which reach them from the carotid and vertebral plexuses. They are extremely sensitive to injury and react by passing into prolonged spasm.

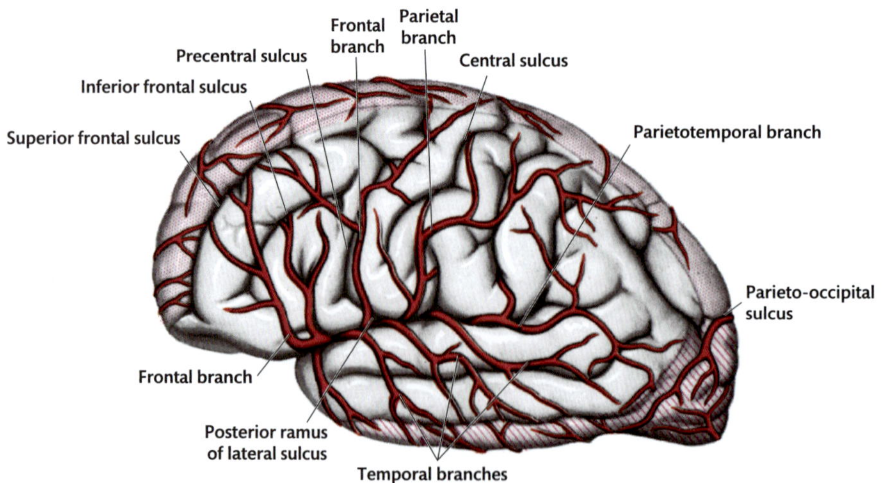


**Fig. 26.5** Arteries of the superolateral surface of the left cerebral hemisphere. The areas supplied by the three arteries are indicated by: red stipple = anterior cerebral artery; no colour = middle cerebral artery; and red cross-hatching = posterior cerebral artery.

## Carotid angiogram

A **carotid angiogram** is a medical imaging procedure done to visualize the internal carotid artery. It helps to diagnose blockages or narrowing of the artery. A thin, flexible tube is inserted into the femoral artery and guided to the internal carotid artery, using real-time X-rays. When the tip of the catheter is in place, a contrast dye is injected into the artery and X-ray images are taken. In digital subtraction angiography, X-rays are taken before and after the dye is injected. A computer digitally subtracts the image taken before the dye from the image taken after the dye is injected, leaving only the contrast-filled blood vessels visible. Fig. 26.6A shows a digital subtraction angiogram of the left internal carotid artery. The internal carotid artery, anterior and middle cerebral arteries, and branches of the anterior and middle cerebral arteries are seen.

## Vertebral angiogram

A **vertebral** or **spinal angiogram** is a medical imaging procedure done to visualize the vertebral artery. As in the case of the carotid angiogram, a thin, flexible tube is inserted into the femoral artery and guided to the vertebral artery. When the tip of the catheter is in place, a contrast dye is injected into the artery and X-ray images are taken. Fig. 26.6B shows a digital subtraction angiogram of the left vertebral artery. The second, third, and fourth parts of the vertebral artery, the posterior inferior cerebellar artery, superior cerebellar artery, posterior cerebral artery, and branches of the posterior cerebral artery are visualized.



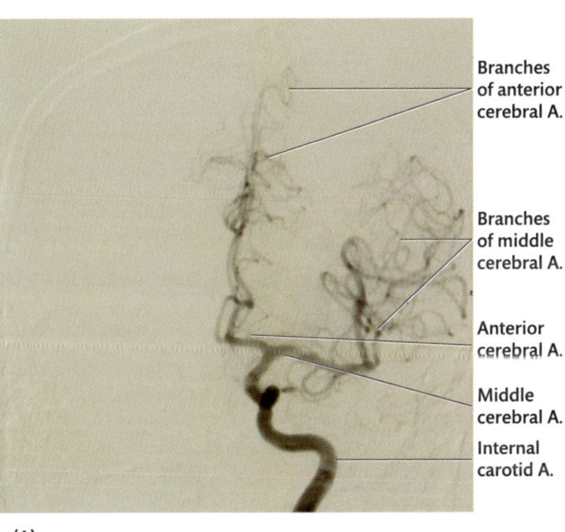


(A)



(B)



(C)

**Fig. 26.6** (A) Digital subtraction angiogram of the left internal carotid artery. (B) Digital subtraction angiogram of the left vertebral artery. (C) Magnetic resonance angiogram of the circle of Willis.

Fig. 26.6C is a magnetic resonance angiogram of the arterial circle.

## Arterial circle of Willis

The arterial circle—**circle of Willis**—is a communicating channel of arteries made up of the posterior cerebral, posterior communicating, anterior cerebral, and anterior communicating arteries. It extends from the superior border of the pons at the posterior end to the longitudinal fissure at the anterior end, and lies principally in the interpeduncular fossa. It forms a means of communication between branches of the two internal carotid arteries and the basilar artery.

See Clinical Applications 26.1 and 26.2 for the practical implications of the anatomy discussed in this chapter.

### CLINICAL APPLICATION 26.1 Aneurysm

An aneurysm of the cavernous part of the right internal carotid artery was noted in a 42-year-old woman who was investigated for double vision [Fig. 26.7]. An aneurysm is a balloon-like swelling in the arterial wall. As it grows, an aneurysm causes pressure symptoms on surrounding structures. A ruptured aneurysm leads to rapid subarachnoid haemorrhage, with high mortality.

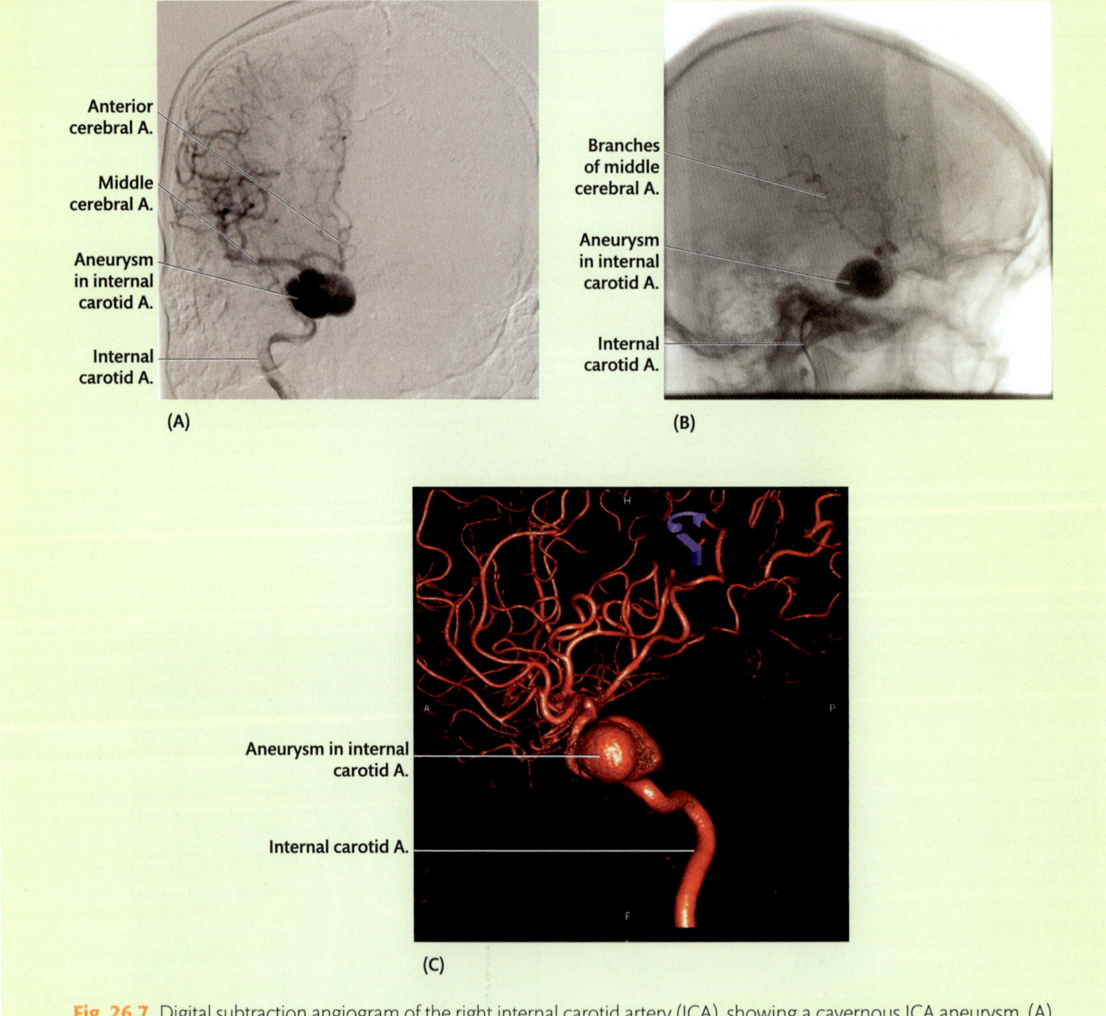


**Fig. 26.7** Digital subtraction angiogram of the right internal carotid artery (ICA), showing a cavernous ICA aneurysm. (A) Anteroposterior view. (B) Lateral view. (C) Three-dimensional imaging.

## CLINICAL APPLICATION 26.2 Arteriovenous malformations

An arteriovenous malformation (AVM) is a tangled mass of abnormal and poorly formed blood vessels—both arteries and veins. It has a high rate of spontaneous rupture and bleeding. AVMs can occur anywhere in the body, but brain AVMs are of special concern because rupture of them causes subarachnoid haemorrhage [see Clinical Application 25.1]. Fig. 26.8 shows an AVM in the middle cerebral artery.

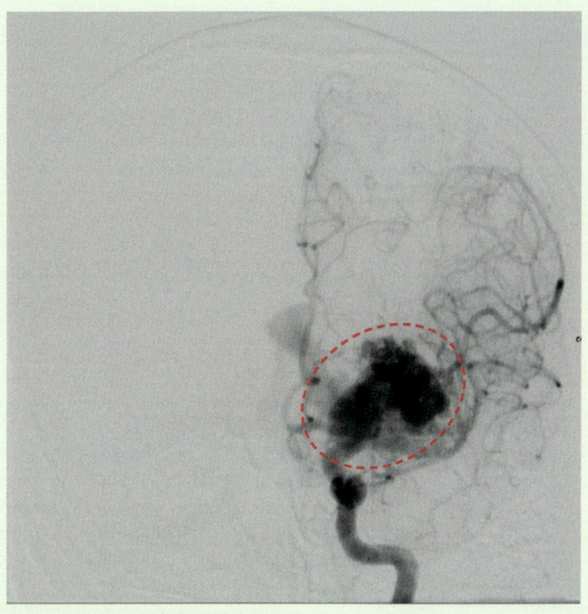

(A)

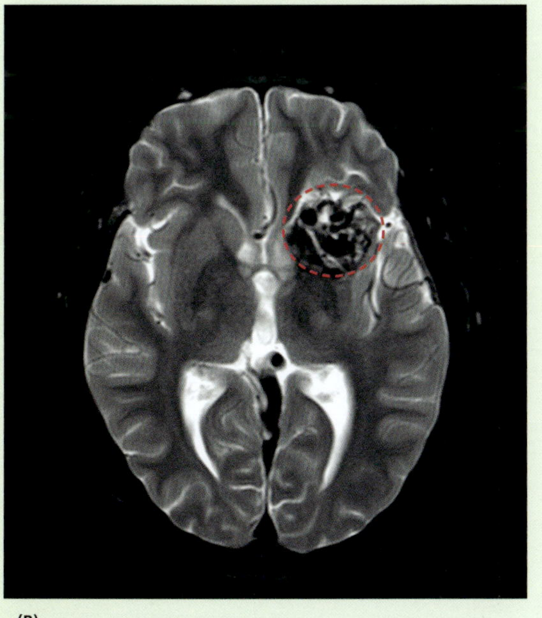

(B)

(C)

**Fig. 26.8** Arteriovenous malformation in the middle cerebral artery = red circle. (A) Digital subtraction angiogram of the right internal carotid artery. (B) T2-weighted axial magnetic resonance imaging (MRI). (C) T2-weighted coronal MRI.

# CHAPTER 27
# The spinal cord

The spinal cord extends from just below the foramen magnum to the intervertebral disc between L. 1 and L. 2. The gross features, coverings, and blood supply of the spinal cord have been described in Chapter 20. The internal arrangement of the grey and white matter of the spinal cord and its connections are described in this chapter.

## General arrangement of white and grey matter

The internal arrangement of neural elements in the spinal cord are best studied on transverse section. In transverse section, the spinal cord is seen to consist of an H-shaped core of **grey matter**, consisting principally of nerve cell bodies, and an external layer of **white matter**—nerve fibres. (Neuroglia, the cellular connective tissue of the central nervous system, is seen in both the grey and white matter.) The horizontal bar of the H in the grey matter is the **grey commissure**, and it surrounds the central canal. Ventral to the grey commissure, nerve fibres cross the midline, forming the **white commissure**. The two commissures are the only neural continuity between the two halves of the spinal cord, which is otherwise separated into right and left halves [Fig. 27.1].

The **anteromedian fissure** on the spinal cord extends from the midline anteriorly inwards to the white commissure. The **posteromedian septum** extends inwards from the posteromedian sulcus to the grey commissure [Fig. 27.1].

The **central canal** is a narrow tube which runs longitudinally in the grey commissure. It is lined by ependyma and is continuous superiorly with the fourth ventricle of the brain. It ends at the filum terminale. The canal contains cerebrospinal fluid.

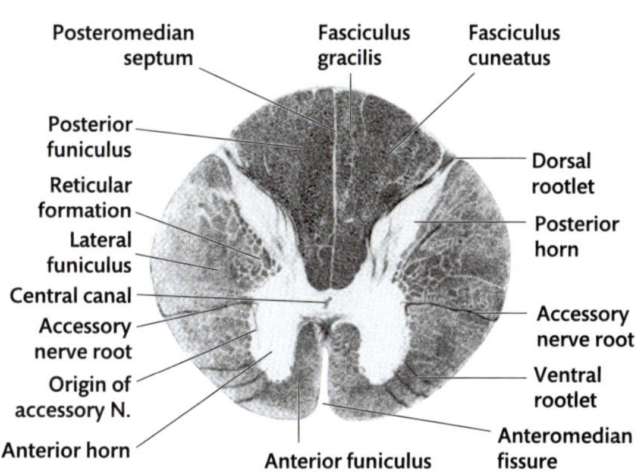


**Fig. 27.1** Transverse section through the upper part of the cervical spinal cord.

The anterior and posterior limbs of the H-shaped grey matter are the **anterior** and **posterior horns**. Since the horns extend throughout the length of the spinal cord, they are also known as **anterior** and **posterior grey columns**. The majority of cells in the posterior horn are associated with the sensory system. The cells in the anterior or ventral horn give rise to motor nerves. The amount of grey matter at any level is proportional to the amount of tissue supplied by the spinal nerves arising there. As a result, the horns are large in the cervical and lumbar swellings (and are mainly responsible for them) [Fig. 27.2].

The **white matter** of the spinal cord is composed of longitudinally running nerve fibres placed superficial to the grey matter. On each side, the white matter is divided into **posterior**, **lateral**, and **anterior columns**, or **funiculi**, by the dorsal and ventral roots [Fig. 27.1].

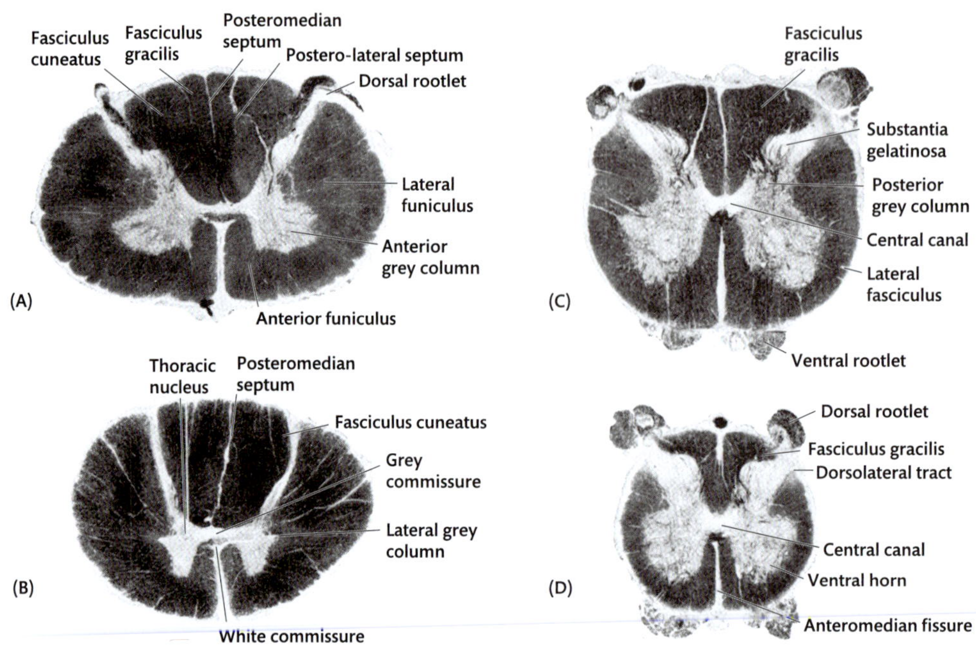


**Fig. 27.2** Transverse sections through the cervical (A), thoracic (B), lumbar (C), and sacral (D) regions of the spinal cord.





The **dorsal roots** on each side enter the **posterolateral sulcus** near the tip of the posterior horn. The **ventral roots** arise mainly from large **motor cells** in the anterior horn.

## Grey matter of the spinal cord

Fig. 27.3 summarizes the main terminations of the afferent nerves entering the spinal cord, and the origin of the efferent nerves leaving the spinal cord.

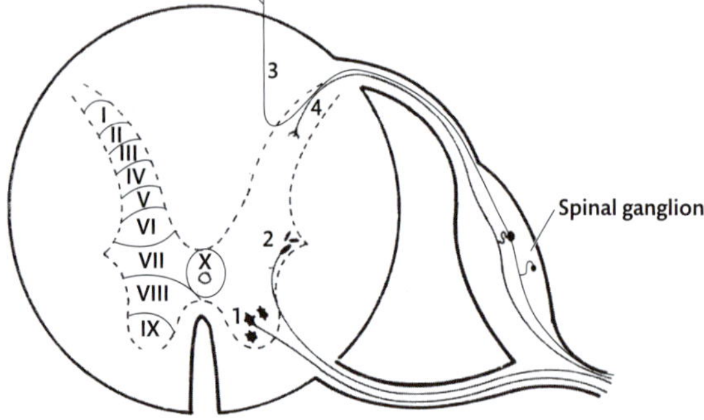


**Fig. 27.3** Thoracic spinal segment. On the right is shown the main terminations of the afferent (sensory) nerves entering the spinal cord and the origin of the efferent (motor) nerves leaving the spinal cord. 1 = somatic efferent fibre; 2 = visceral efferent fibre; 3 = afferent fibres entering the posterior column; 4 = afferent fibres ending in the posterior horn. On the left side is shown the position of laminae I–X of Rexed.

The grey matter of the spinal cord is arbitrarily divided into ten laminae known as Rexed laminae [Fig. 27.3]. Within the grey matter are a series of discontinuous cell groups which correspond approximately to one or more of these laminae. Laminae I–IV are in the dorsal horn and are the main sites of termination of the sensory fibres entering through the dorsal root. Throughout the spinal cord, the tips of the posterior horns, adjacent to the entry of the posterior roots, are composed of a translucent substance—the **substantia gelatinosa** [Fig. 27.2]. The substantia gelatinosa corresponds to laminae II and III. Lamina I lies superficial to the substantia gelatinosa, and laminae V and VI lie at the base of the dorsal horn. The **thoracic nucleus** (also known as Clarke's column) lies in the thoracic and upper lumbar segments at the medial side of the base of the posterior grey column [Fig. 27.2B]. The **lateral grey column**, or **lateral horn**, is a small extension on the lateral aspect of the grey matter, seen in spinal segments between the first thoracic and second or third lumbar segments [Fig. 27.2B]. It contains the nerve cells—the **intermediolateral neurons**—which give rise to the preganglionic fibres of the sympathetic system. Neurons in the **anterior** or **ventral horn** innervate skeletal muscles. These cells may be grouped into *medial, central*, and *lateral columns* within the anterior horn. In the lower cervical and lumbosacral regions, the cells in the lateral group innervate the limb musculature, and the cells in the medial group innervate the axial musculature. The anterior horn is small in the thoracic and upper cervical regions [Fig. 27.1].

## Functional columns of the spinal cord

From the above description of nerve cells in the grey matter, it is seen that cells performing the same function lie in the same position at every level of the spinal cord. For example, all cells in the anterior horn will supply skeletal muscle, and cells in the lateral horn will supply smooth muscle and glands. Based on this arrangement, four **functional columns** are described in the spinal cord: the **general somatic efferent** supplying motor nerves to skeletal muscles; the **general visceral efferent** supplying motor nerves to smooth muscles; the **general visceral afferent**, located in the dorsal horn cells in the thoracic and upper lumbar regions and receiving sensory input from the viscera; and the **general somatic afferent**, located in the dorsal horn of all segments and receiving sensory input from the skin [Fig. 27.2].

# White matter of the spinal cord

The **white matter** of the spinal cord is composed of longitudinally running nerve fibres placed superficial to the grey matter and divided into **posterior**, **lateral**, and **anterior columns** [Fig. 27.1]. The deepest fibres are short and pass from one segment of the spinal cord to another (**fasciculi proprii**) [Fig. 27.4]. The superficial fibres are long.

Fibres with similar origin and termination are grouped together in the white matter to form **tracts**, or **fasciculi**. Tracts which carry motor impulses from the brain to the spinal cord are the **descending tracts**. Tracts which carry sensory impulses from the spinal cord to the brain form the **ascending tracts** [Fig. 27.4]. In each segment of the spinal cord, sensory fibres are added to the ascending tracts, and motor fibres leave the descending tracts to end in the grey matter. As a result, both ascending and descending tracts increase in size superiorly, and the volume of white matter increases from below upwards. Note this change in the four sections of the spinal cord depicted in Fig. 27.2.

## Descending tracts

The descending tracts originate from the brain and carry motor impulses to the anterior horn cells in the spinal cord. Most of these are crossed tracts (i.e. the fibres cross the midline and terminate on the anterior horn cells of the opposite side). The most important of these—the **lateral corticospinal tract**—originates in the cerebral cortex. The other descending tracts are the **rubrospinal**

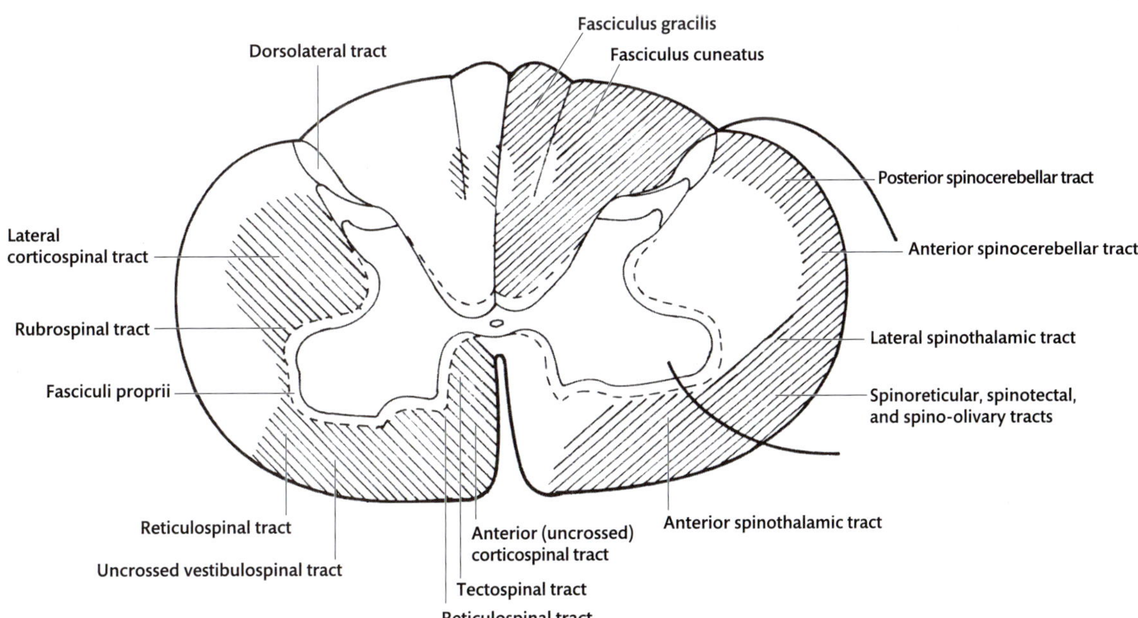


**Fig. 27.4** The main ascending (right) and descending (left) pathways in the white matter of the spinal cord.

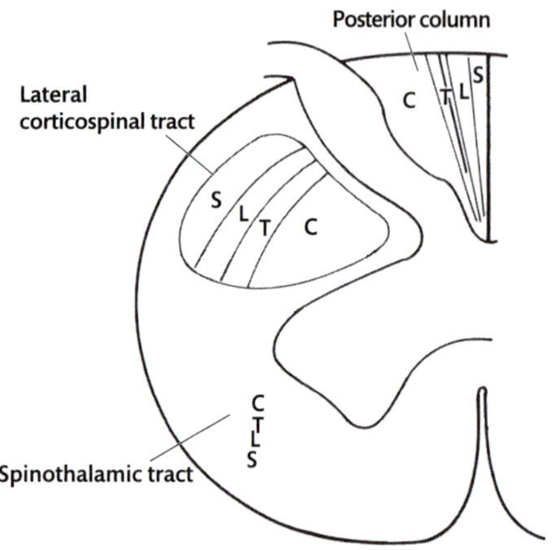


**Fig. 27.5** Diagrammatic transverse section through half of the cervical spinal cord to show the relative positions of the cervical (C), thoracic (T), lumbar (L), and sacral (S) fibres in the posterior column, spinothalamic tract, and lateral corticospinal tract.

(from the red nucleus in the midbrain), **reticulospinal** (from the reticular formation of the brainstem), **vestibulospinal** (from the vestibular nuclei in the medulla), and **tectospinal** (from the tectum of the midbrain) tracts. Note the position of these tracts in Figs. 27.4 and 27.5. The cervical fibres of the lateral corticospinal tract are located most medially, and are the first ones to leave the tract to end on the anterior horn cells. The thoracic, lumbar, and sacral fibres lie sequentially in more lateral positions and reach the anterior horn cells at a lower level [Fig. 27.5]. The exact origin of the descending fibres and the location in different parts of the brainstem will be dealt with in the corresponding sections.

## Ascending tracts

The **dorsal roots** on each side enter the **posterolateral sulcus** near the tip of the posterior horn. Each nerve fibre of the root either enters the posterior column and ascends in it or enters the posterior horn. The ascending tracts carry sensory impulses from the periphery to various parts of the brain. They are the **dorsal column**, consisting of the **fasciculus gracilis** and **cuneatus** [Figs. 27.2, 27.3, 27.4], **anterior** and **posterior spinocerebellar tracts**, and **anterolateral spinothalamic tracts** [Fig. 27.4]. Sensory information reaches the spinal cord through cells in the spinal or dorsal root ganglion. In the dorsal root, the thicker fibres lie medially and carry sensations of crude touch, pressure, and proprioception. Thinner fibres lie laterally and carry sensations of fine touch, pain, and temperature. The cells of the spinal ganglia are **first-order neurons** [Fig. 27.3]. They end by synapsing with other neurons—**second-order neurons**—in the spinal cord or brainstem.

### Posterior column

The **posterior white columns**, or **dorsal columns**, lie between the dorsal roots of the two sides [Fig. 27.2]. In the upper half of the spinal cord, each posterior column is subdivided by a **posterolateral septum** into a slender medial **fasciculus gracilis** (which carries such fibres from the lower half of the body) and a broader lateral **fasciculus cuneatus** which carries fibres from the upper half of the body [Figs. 27.2, 27.4]. The position of this septum is marked on the surface by the **postero-intermediate sulcus**.

Both fasciculi consist of fibres which enter the spinal cord in the dorsal roots and are predominantly concerned with crude touch, vibration, and proprioception. They ascend to the medulla oblongata [Fig. 27.3]. New fibres are added at each level and cause the width of the posterior column to increase as it ascends. The fibres entering through the highest roots, i.e. from the cervical region, lie most laterally [Fig. 27.5]. Both groups of fibres give off collaterals to the grey matter throughout their length and ascend without interruption to the **nucleus gracilis** and **nucleus cuneatus** in the medulla.

### Spinothalamic tract

The finer fibres in the dorsal roots (principally concerned with fine touch, pain, and temperature) enter laterally, divide, and ascend or descend for a short distance. Together, they form the **dorsolateral tract** overlying the lateral part of the substantia gelatinosa [Fig. 27.3]. These fibres end by synapsing on cells in the posterior horn. Second-order neurons arise from cells in the posterior horn, cross the midline in the anterior white commissure, and ascend to the thalamus in the **spinothalamic tract** [Figs. 27.5, 27.6]. (For further details on the course and termination of the spinothalamic tracts, see Chapters 28 and 30.)

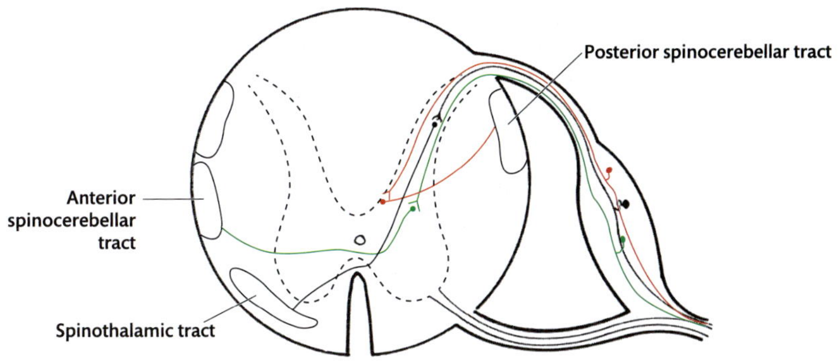


**Fig. 27.6** Diagrammatic representation of the origin of the spinothalamic (black), posterior spinocerebellar (red), and ventral spinocerebellar (green) tracts.

## Spinocerebellar tracts

There are two pathways connecting the spinal cord to the cerebellum—the anterior and posterior spinocerebellar tracts. (The origin of these tracts is shown in Fig. 27.6.) The **posterior spinocerebellar tract** arises from the cells of the thoracic nucleus (lamina VII of the first thoracic to the second lumbar segments). They transmit information from the inferior half of the same side of the body to the cerebellum. This tract ascends in the most posterolateral part of the lateral column of the same side [Figs. 27.4, 27.6].

Fibres of the **anterior** or **ventral spinocerebellar tract** arise from laminae V–VII of the lumbosacral spinal cord [Fig. 27.4]. They cross the midline and ascend in the anterior spinocerebellar tract [Figs. 27.4, 27.6]. They carry information from the lower limb. (For further details on the course and termination of the spinocerebellar tracts, see Chapters 28 and 29.)

## Syringomyelia

**Syringomyelia** is a medical condition that results from the formation of fluid-filled cysts (syrinx) within the spinal cord (myelia) and dilatation of the central canal. These cysts are often found in the cervical region. Syringomyelia may be *congenital* and often associated with Chiari malformations, or *acquired* as a result of spinal cord injuries or tumours.

The syrinx can get big enough to damage nerve fibres and disrupt the tracts. It initially compresses the spinothalamic tract fibres as they cross in the anterior white commissure. This results in bilateral loss of pain and temperature sensation in a 'cape-like' distribution affecting the arms and shoulders. As the syrinx expands laterally, it can damage the corticospinal tracts, and lead to spasticity, weakness, or paralysis.

See Clinical Applications 27.1 and 27.2 for the practical implications of the anatomy discussed in this chapter.



### CLINICAL APPLICATION 27.1 Upper motor neuron and lower motor neuron lesions

The descending motor pathway consists of an upper motor neuron from the motor cortex to the spinal grey matter, and a lower motor neuron located in the anterior horn cell. The clinical presentations of lesions affecting the upper motor neurons and lower motor neurons are different.

*Signs of upper motor neuron lesions:*

1. Hypertonia and exaggerated deep tendon reflexes due to loss of the normal cortical inhibition of the stretch reflex.
2. Absent superficial reflex due to lack of required cortical control.
3. Positive Babinski sign—or upgoing plantar reflex—due to loss of cortical inhibition of primitive reflexes.

*Signs of lower motor neuron lesions:*

1. Hypotonia and diminished deep tendon reflexes due to damage to the lower motor neurons (efferent limb of reflex).
2. Muscle atrophy resulting from loss of trophic factors normally secreted by the alpha motor neurons.
3. Muscle fasciculations in response to spontaneous action potentials produced by damaged alpha motor neurons.

These clinical findings help to differentiate upper and lower motor neuron lesions, and enable the anatomical localization of a lesion in a patient with paralysis.

**CLINICAL APPLICATION 27.2 Hemisection of the spinal cord (Brown-Séquard syndrome)**

A man involved in a car accident sustained an injury to the right half of his spinal cord. On examination, he was found to have:

1. Paralysis of the entire right lower limb.
2. Increased muscle tone and exaggerated deep tendon reflexes in the right lower limb, and an upgoing plantar reflex on the right side.
3. Loss of vibration, joint sense, and two-point discrimination on the right side of the body below the level of the umbilicus.
4. Loss of pain and temperature on the left half of the body below the level of the umbilicus.
5. A band of hyperaesthesia and occasional muscle fasciculations on the right side at the level of the umbilicus.

Study questions 1–5: explain the anatomical basis for each of the clinical features seen in this patient.

(Answer 1: paralysis of the right lower limb indicates damage to the corticospinal tract of the right side. The spinal segments involved in motor supply to the lower limb are L. 2 to S. 1. The fact that all movement of the right lower limb is lost means that the corticospinal tract injury is above the level of L. 2. Note: crossing of the corticospinal fibres occurs above the level of the lesion (in the medulla), which explains why the paralysis is on the same side as the lesion.)

(Answer 2: increased muscle tone, exaggerated deep tendon reflexes, and an upgoing plantar reflex on the right lower limb are features of an upper motor neuron lesion and are consistent with damage to the corticospinal tract.)

(Answer 3: loss of vibration, joint sense, and two-point discrimination on the right side of the body below the level of the umbilicus is due to damage to the posterior column fibres of that side. Fibres carrying these impulses ascend ipsilaterally in the spinal cord. Hence, loss of these sensations is on the same side as the lesion.)

(Answer 4: loss of pain and temperature from the left half of the body below the level of the umbilicus is due to damage of the spinothalamic tract on the right side. The origin of these fibres is on the left side [Fig. 27.6], and the second-order neurons cross the midline to ascend on the right. The sensory loss up to the level of the umbilicus localizes the lesion to the T. 10 dermatome.)

(Answer 5: the band of hyperaesthesia at the T. 10 dermatome and muscle fasciculations at this level are most likely due to involvement of the nerve roots and anterior horn cells at the T. 10 level—a lower motor neuron injury. This further indicates that the spinal cord injury occurred at the T. 10 level.)

The combination of neurological lesions discussed above constitutes the Brown-Séquard syndrome. You should know that cases of spinal cord hemisection rarely present this typically.

# CHAPTER 28
# The brainstem



## Introduction

The brainstem consists of the medulla oblongata, pons, and midbrain. Some of the external features of the brainstem have been described and identified in Chapter 24. Review these features using Figs. 28.1, 28.2, and 28.3.

## External features of the medulla oblongata

The **medulla oblongata** is a conical part of the brainstem which extends from the pons to the spinal cord. It joins the spinal cord approximately at the level of the foramen magnum. (The junction of the medulla and spinal cord is just above the attachment of the first spinal nerve.) It is approximately 2.5 cm long and was once known as the bulb, a term which is still used occasionally.

The anterior surface of the medulla oblongata lies against the basilar part of the occipital bone. The posterior surface is lodged in a groove on the anterior surface of the cerebellum—the vallecula cerebelli. A narrow central canal is present in the inferior half of the medulla. This is the upward continuation of the central canal in the spinal cord. The central canal opens into the fourth ventricle on the posterior surface of the superior half of the medulla oblongata.

### Ventral surface of the medulla

Review the description of the ventral surface of the medulla given in Chapter 24. The medulla oblongata has an **anterior median fissure** which is continuous with that of the spinal cord. The **pyramids** are bundles of corticospinal nerve fibres which originate from cells in the cerebral cortex. In the lower medulla, bundles of fibres from the pyramids cross the midline through the **decussation of the pyramids** [Fig. 28.1]. The **olive** is an oval elevation which lies posterolateral to the pyramid and is separated from it by the rootlets of the hypoglossal nerve [Figs. 28.1, 28.2]. The hypoglossal nerve is attached between the pyramid and the olive. The ninth, tenth, and eleventh cranial nerves are attached to the lateral surface of the medulla, posterior to the olive. The sixth, seventh, and eighth cranial nerves are attached at the upper border of the medulla.

### Lateral surface of the medulla

The **inferior cerebellar peduncle** lies posterolateral to the olive [Figs. 28.1, 28.2]. It is a thick bundle of fibres on the posterolateral margin of the medulla oblongata. It begins near the middle of the medulla oblongata and passes upwards and slightly laterally to the inferior border of the pons. It then curves posteriorly into the cerebellum, medial to the middle cerebellar peduncle. The inferior cerebellar peduncle is covered by a narrow ridge of grey matter—the **dorsal** and **ventral cochlear** nuclei. The inferior cerebellar peduncle forms a route of communication between the medulla oblongata

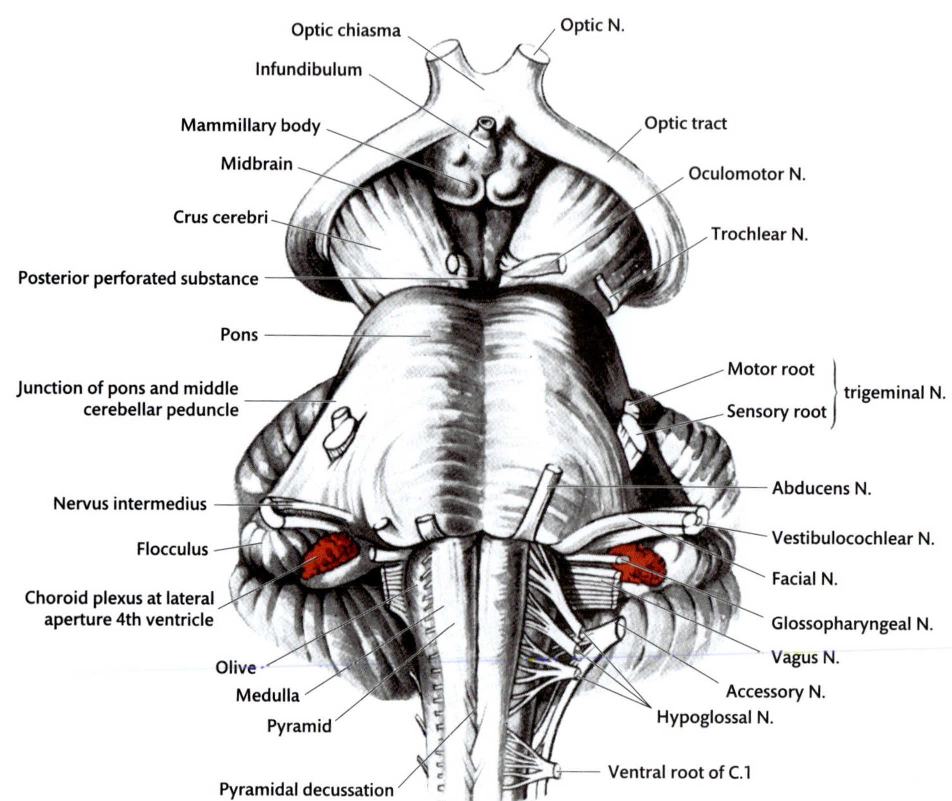


**Fig. 28.1** Anterior surface of the brainstem.

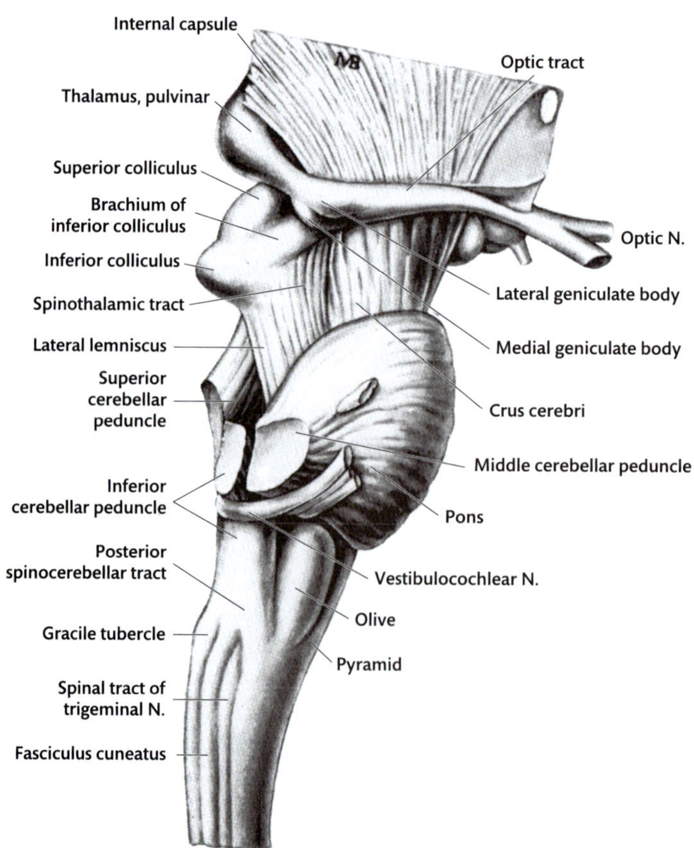


**Fig. 28.2** Lateral view of the brainstem.

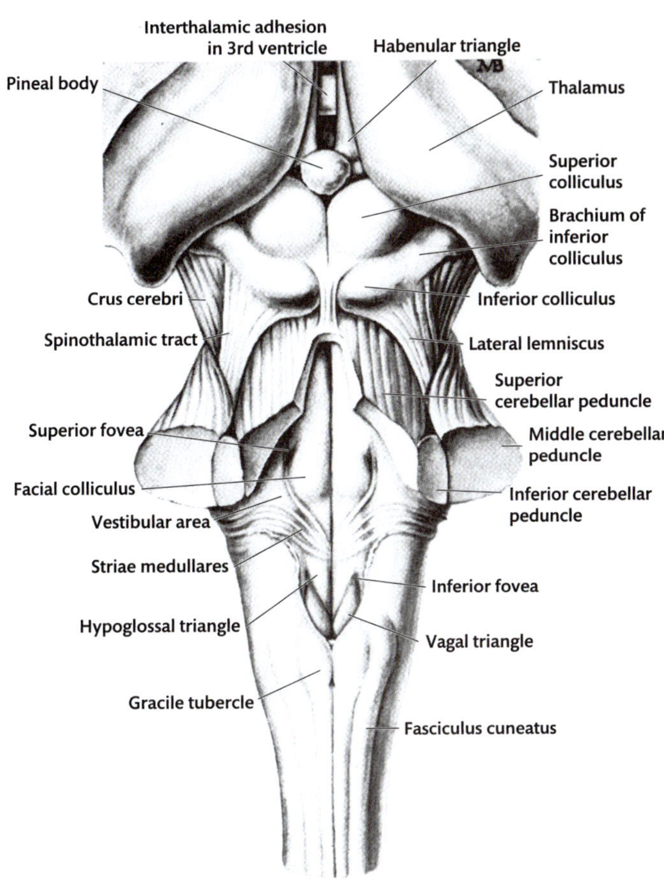


Fig. 28.3 Posterior view of the brainstem.

and spinal cord and the cerebellum. The **spinal tract of the trigeminal** nerve is seen as a poorly defined longitudinal ridge, immediately posterior to the inferior cerebellar peduncle.

## Posterior surface of the medulla

The posterior surface of the medulla is divided into superior and inferior parts. The inferior part of the posterior surface of the medulla oblongata shows the following features. The **posterior median sulcus** of the spinal cord extends upwards to the inferior angle of the fourth ventricle [Fig. 28.3]. The **fasciculi gracilis** and **fasciculi cuneatus** lie on the posterior surface of the inferior half of the medulla oblongata. The fasciculi gracilis lie one on either side of the posterior median sulcus and end superiorly in the **gracile tubercle**. The fasciculus cuneatus lies immediately lateral to each fasciculus gracilis and ends at a slightly higher level in a poorly defined eminence—the **cuneate tubercle** [see Fig. 27.4; Fig. 28.3].

The upper part of the posterior surface of the medulla forms the lower part of the floor of the fourth ventricle. The floor of the fourth ventricle is diamond-shaped and is formed by the posterior surfaces of the pons and the upper half of the medulla oblongata. It is divided into right and left halves by a **median sulcus**, with a ridge on each side called the **medial eminence**. About the middle of the floor, fine bundles of fibres are seen running laterally towards the inferior cerebellar peduncle. These are the **medullary striae**, and they divide the floor of the ventricle into pontine and medullary parts.

In each half of the medullary part, there is a V-shaped depression (the **inferior fovea**) which divides the floor into three triangular areas. The medial area, part of the medial eminence, overlies the superior part of the hypoglossal nucleus and is known as the **hypoglossal triangle**. The intermediate part overlies the dorsal nucleus of the vagoglossopharyngeal complex and is known as the **vagal triangle**. The lateral part is the inferior part of the **vestibular area**—a poorly defined swelling in the lateral part of the floor of the ventricle formed by the **vestibular nuclei** [Fig. 28.3].

## External features of the pons

### Ventral surface of the pons

The ventral aspect of the pons forms a prominent bulge on the inferior aspect of the brain, between the medulla and the midbrain. It lies in the posterior cranial fossa, just behind the clivus, and has the basilar artery on it. The **ventral part of the pons** is made up of a bulky ridge composed of transversely running fibre bundles [Fig. 28.1]. These fibres converge laterally to form the **middle cerebellar peduncle** which enters the cerebellum [Figs. 28.1, 28.2]. The trigeminal nerve is attached to the pons at its junction with the middle cerebellar peduncle. The **crus cerebri** enter the ventral part of the pons at its superior margin, and the **pyramids** leave it at the inferior margin. Anteriorly, the ventral part of the pons is grooved by the **basilar sulcus** (which lodges the basilar artery) [Fig. 28.1].

### Posterior surface of the pons

The posterior aspect of the pons forms the upper part of the floor of the fourth ventricle. A slight swelling in the medial eminence at the inferior part of the pons is the **facial colliculus**. This is produced by the abducens nucleus, with the facial nerve looping round it. Lateral to the facial colliculus, a slight groove represents the remains of the sulcus limitans of the developing neural tube and is slightly accentuated at the level of the facial colliculus to form the **superior fovea**. Above the superior fovea is the **locus coeruleus**, a small, dark-coloured area lateral to the medial eminence. The colour is due to the presence of pigmented cells beneath the ependyma.

## External features of the midbrain

The midbrain is the short, thick part of the brainstem which connects the hindbrain in the posterior cranial fossa with the cerebrum superior to the tentorium cerebelli. It passes through the tentorial notch. It is about 1.5 cm long and slightly more in width. The narrow tubular part of the ventricular system in the midbrain is the **cerebral aqueduct** [see Fig. 25.1]). It connects the third ventricle to the fourth ventricle.

### Ventral surface of the midbrain

The anterior surface of the midbrain can be seen in continuity with the base of the brain. It consists of the **crus cerebri** which descend from the cerebral hemispheres, and enters the pons inferiorly [Fig. 28.1]. The posterior part of the interpeduncular fossa lies between the crus cerebri.

### Posterior surface of the midbrain

The posterior surface of the midbrain shows four small swellings—the colliculi. They are the paired **superior** and **inferior colliculi** [Fig. 28.3]. This surface is overlapped by the anterior lobe of the cerebellum, pineal body, and splenium of the corpus callosum. The **trochlear nerves** emerge from the dorsal surface of the midbrain, immediately inferior to the inferior colliculi. The **pineal body** lies between, and just above, the two superior colliculi [Fig. 28.3].

### Lateral surface of the midbrain

The superior cerebellar peduncles enter the substance of the midbrain, anterior to the inferior colliculi. Each peduncle is crossed obliquely by a ridge of white matter (the **lateral lemniscus** [Fig. 28.2]) which emerges from the superior border of the pons, posterior to the crus cerebri, and passes posterosuperiorly into the inferior colliculus.

A similar ridge (**brachium of the inferior colliculus** [Fig. 28.2]) passes anterosuperiorly from the inferior colliculus to the **medial geniculate body**—a part of the thalamus.

## Internal features of the brainstem

The brainstem contains both grey and white matter. The **grey matter** of the brainstem includes the cranial nerve nuclei, and other nuclear masses like the inferior olivary nucleus in the medulla and the red nucleus in the midbrain. The **white matter** of the brainstem includes the ascending and descending tracts of the spinal cord [Chapter 27] and other tracts formed in the brainstem. The **reticular formation** consists of numerous neurons arranged in ill-defined groups and connected by fine bundles of nerve fibres. It extends from the midbrain to the medulla.

### Cranial nerve nuclei–functional columns

Cranial nerve nuclei of 10 of the 12 cranial nerves lie in the brainstem. The motor nuclei give rise to efferent or motor fibres which leave the brain. The sensory nuclei receive the afferent (sensory) fibres of the cranial nerves. The nuclei subserving similar functions lie in longitudinal groups or columns which are referred to as **functional columns**.

The general arrangement of the cranial nerve nuclei is similar to the arrangement of nuclei in the spinal cord. The motor nuclei are placed ventrally and the sensory nuclei are placed dorsally. In the upper part of the medulla and pons, where the central canal is replaced by the fourth ventricle, the sensory nuclei lie lateral to the motor nuclei. Fig. 28.4 shows the comparative positions of the different groups of nuclei in the spinal cord and upper medulla.

### Position of functional columns

The motor nuclei lie in three columns based on function. From medial to lateral, they are: (1) **somatic efferent**—to skeletal muscles of myotomic origin; (2) **special visceral efferent**—to skeletal muscles of branchiomeric origin; and (3) **general visceral efferent**—to smooth muscles and glands (parasympathetic) [Fig. 28.5].

The sensory nuclei lie in four functional columns. Medial to lateral, they are: (1) **general visceral afferent**, receiving general sensation from the viscera; (2) **special visceral afferent**, receiving taste sensation; (3) **general somatic afferent**, receiving general sensation from the head and neck; and (4) **special somatic afferent**, receiving impulses from the vestibulocochlear system [Fig. 28.5].

➲ The internal features of the brainstem are best studied in thin transverse sections. These sections are stained to differentiate between the white matter and grey matter. Conventionally, the lowest section is at the junction of the spinal cord and medulla, and the highest at the level of the superior colliculus in the midbrain. These sections show the location of the major white matter bundles and the nuclear masses at each level of the brainstem. Knowledge of the structures that lie at each level helps clinicians localize lesions of the brainstem.

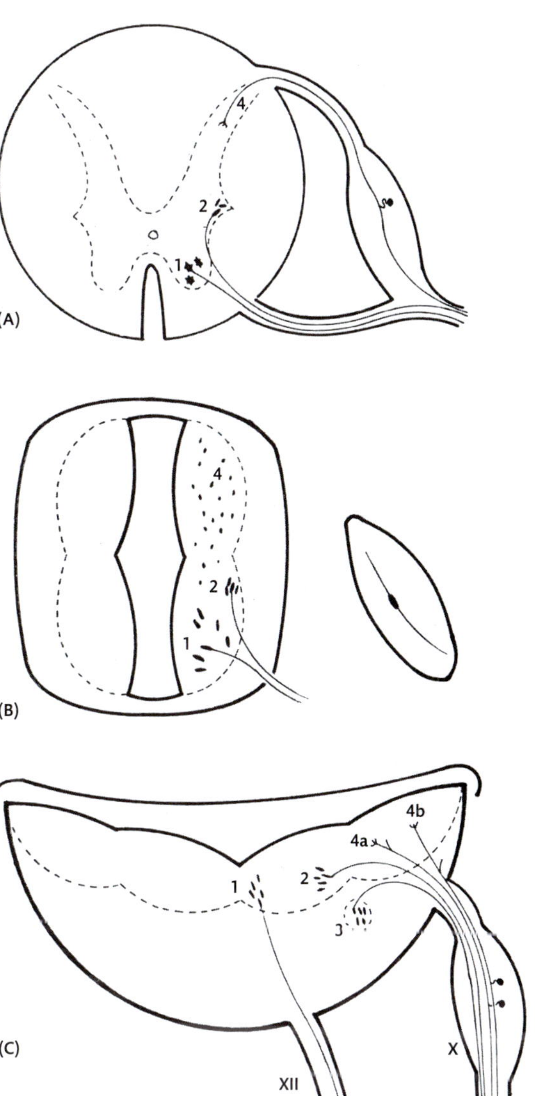


**Fig. 28.4** Diagram to illustrate the difference in development between the spinal cord and the medulla. (B) is the basic structure, from which both (A) the thoracic spinal cord and (C) the medulla oblongata arise. Basal lamina: 1 = motor nerves to striated muscles of somite origin (general somatic efferent—or just somatic efferent); 2 = preganglionic autonomic cells (general visceral efferent); 3 = motor nerves to striated muscles of branchial origin. Alar lamina: 4 = sensory terminations: 4a = special visceral afferent (tractus solitarius); 4b = general somatic afferent (trigeminal system).

## Internal features of the medulla

The internal features of the medulla are shown in Figs. 28.6. 28.7. 28.8, and 28.9. Figs. 28.6 and 28.7 are through the closed section of the medulla and show the central canal. Fig. 28.6 is a section taken through the motor decussation, and Fig. 28.7 is through the sensory decussation. Figs. 28.8 and 28.9 are through the upper part of the medulla bordering the fourth ventricle.

### White matter of the medulla

The following tracts run through the medulla and should be identified at each level.

### Corticospinal tract

Corticospinal fibres originate in the cerebral cortex and descend through the cerebral hemispheres, the crura cerebri, and the pons to form the pyramids in the medulla oblongata. Each lateral corticospinal

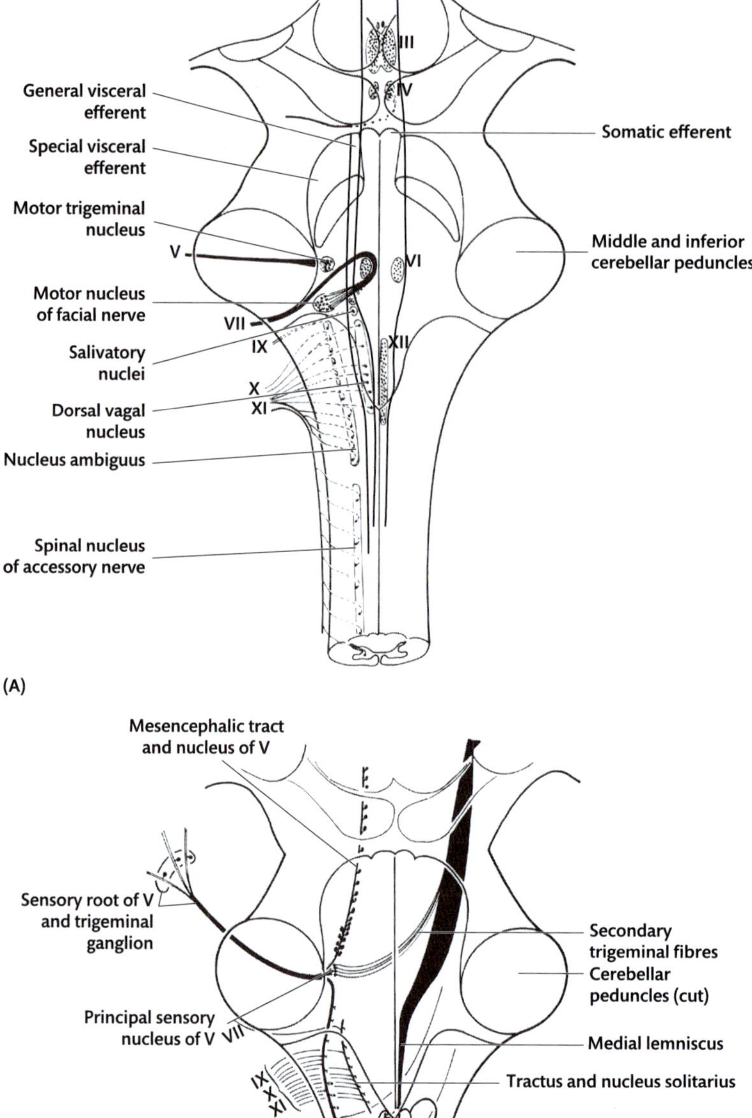


**Fig. 28.5** (A) Posterior view of the brainstem and spinal cord, showing the positions of the motor nuclei. (B) Posterior view of the brainstem and spinal cord, showing the positions of the sensory nuclei. (The nuclei of cranial nerve VIII are not shown.)

tract extends throughout the length of the spinal cord. The corticospinal fibre tracts are commonly called the **pyramidal tracts**.

In the upper part of the medulla, the corticospinal fibres lie on the ventral aspect and account for the pyramid seen on the external surface [Fig. 28.1]. Note the position of the pyramid, starting from the upper medulla and tracing it down in Figs. 28.9, 28.8, and 28.7 to the level of the sensory decussation. In the lower medulla, most of the fibres cross the midline in the **motor decussation** to form the **lateral corticospinal tract** on the opposite side [Figs. 28.6, 28.10]. Review the position of the lateral corticospinal tract in the deeper parts of the lateral column of the spinal cord [see Figs. 27.4, 27.5]. The corticospinal fibres which do not cross in the medulla descend either in the anterior column, as the **anterior corticospinal tract**, or in the lateral column anterior to the lateral corticospinal tract [Fig. 28.10].

## Dorsal column–medial lemniscus pathway

The fasciculus gracilis and cuneatus, nucleus gracilis and cuneatus, internal arcuate fibres, and medial lemniscus are parts of the pathway that carry crude touch and proprioception to the thalamus. Identify the fasciculus gracilis in Fig. 28.6, the nucleus gracilis and cuneatus, internal arcuate fibres, and medial lemniscus in Fig. 28.7, and the medial lemniscus in Figs. 28.8 and 28.9.

Review the formation and position of the fasciculus gracilis and cuneatus in the spinal cord [Chapter 27; see Figs. 27.4, 27.5]. These fasciculi lie on the posterior surface of the inferior half of the medulla oblongata and extend up to the **gracile** and **cuneate tubercles** [Fig. 28.3].

The fibres of the fasciculus gracilis and cuneatus end by synapsing in the **nucleus gracilis** and **nucleus cuneatus** which lie deep to the tubercles of the same name. Second-order neurons arise from the cells of the nucleus gracilis and cuneatus,





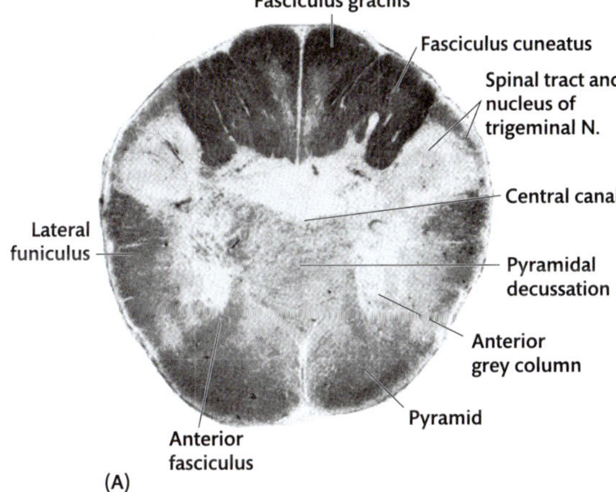


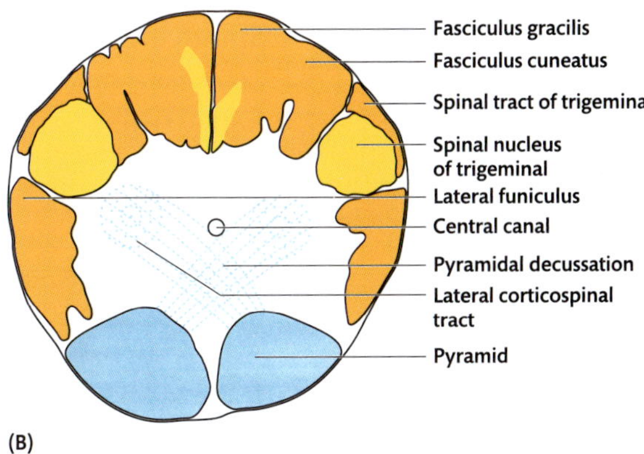


**Fig. 28.6** Transverse section through the lowest part of the medulla oblongata. (A) Histology section. Grey matter = white; white matter = grey to black, depending on the density of the myelinated fibres. (B) Structures of interest in (A) are highlighted.

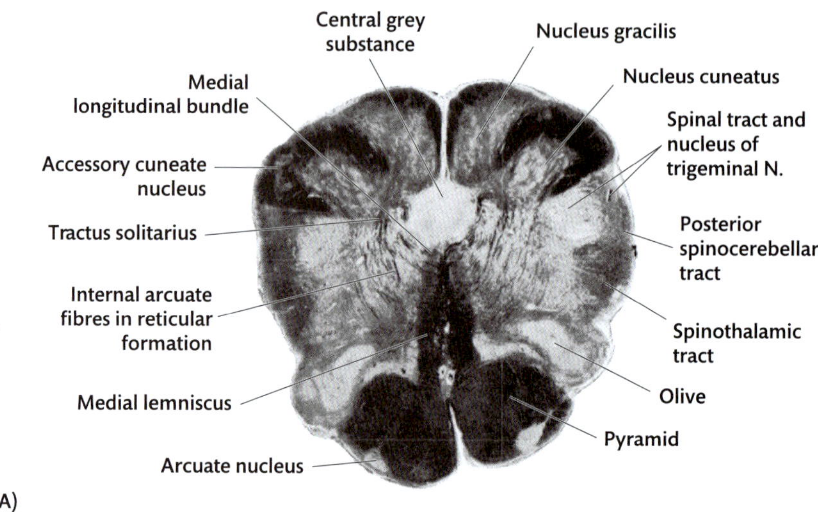


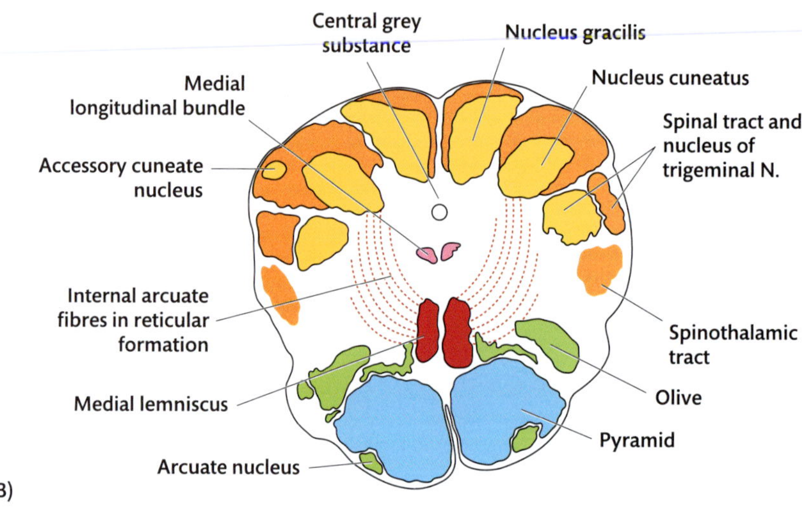


**Fig. 28.7** Transverse section of the medulla through the nuclei cuneatus and gracilis. (A) Histology section. Grey matter = white; white matter = grey to black. (B) Structures of interest in (A) are highlighted.

run ventrally, and cross the midline anterior to the central canal as the **internal arcuate fibres**. They form the great **sensory decussation** [Fig. 28.7]. After crossing the midline, the fibres form the **medial lemniscus** and ascend [see Fig. 31.29] to the thalamus. In the upper medulla, the medial lemnisci are in the form of flat bands, adjacent to the midline and dorsal to the pyramid [Fig. 28.8].

## Spinothalamic tract

The **spinothalamic tract** consists of fibres that arise in the spinal cord from cells in the grey matter [see Figs. 27.4, 27.6]. These fibres retain the lateral position in the medulla. Note the position of the spinothalamic tracts in the medulla at ascending levels [Figs. 28.7, 28.8]. They pass posterior to the inferior olivary nucleus [Fig. 28.8], and give fibres to the reticular formation—the **spinoreticular tract**.

## Spinocerebellar tracts

The origin of the fibres in the **posterior spinocerebellar tract** and their position in the spinal cord are described in Chapter 27. They ascend in the posterolateral part of the lateral column of the spinal cord and enter the medulla oblongata close to the spinal tract of the trigeminal nerve [Fig. 28.7]. At the mid-olivary level, the tract passes posteriorly and enters the inferior cerebellar peduncle [Figs. 28.2, 28.8].

The **anterior spinocerebellar tract** passes through the medulla oblongata and pons, anterior to the spinal tract of the trigeminal nerve, and turns posteriorly into the cerebellum over the superior

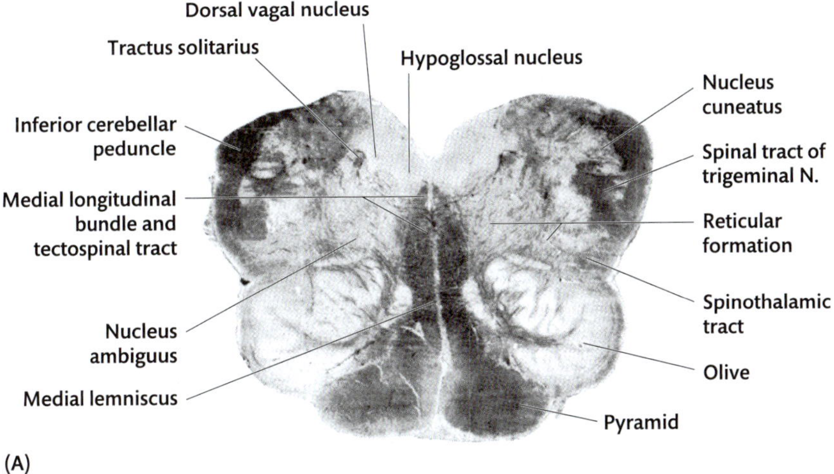


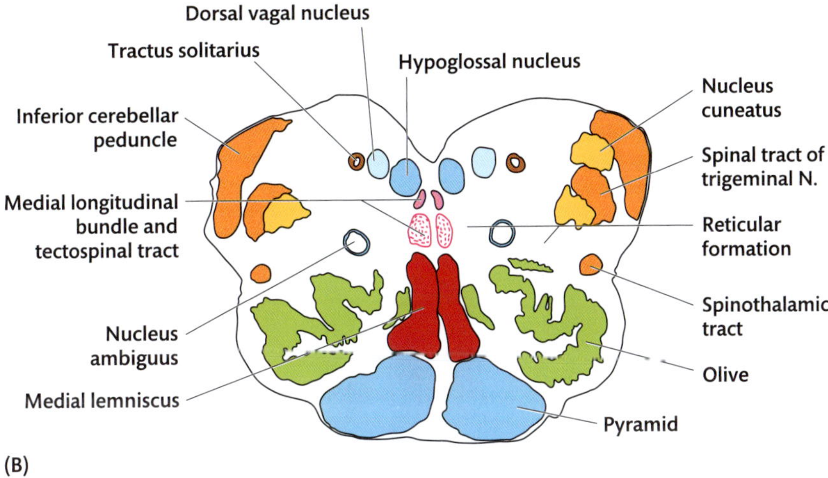


**Fig. 28.8** Transverse section through the upper half of the medulla oblongata. (A) Histology section. Grey matter = white; white matter = grey to black. (B) Structures of interest in (A) are highlighted.

cerebellar peduncle [Fig. 28.2], above the level of entry of the trigeminal nerve.

### Spinal tract of trigeminal nerve

The spinal tract of the trigeminal nerve has fibres which arise from the trigeminal ganglion and descend to the spinal nucleus of the trigeminal. They are seen at all levels in the medulla with the nucleus of the spinal tract [Figs. 28.6, 28.7, 28.8, 28.9].

## Grey matter of the medulla

The named grey matter masses in the medulla include the nuclei of the lower cranial nerves, the nucleus gracilis and cuneatus, and the inferior olivary, accessory olivary, and arcuate nuclei.

### Cranial nerve nuclei in the medulla

The cranial nerve nuclei in the medulla are the: (1) spinal nucleus of the trigeminal (cranial nerve—CN V); (2) nucleus of the tractus solitarius (CN VII, IX, X); (3) nucleus ambiguus (CN IX, X, XI); (4) hypoglossal nucleus (CN XII); (5) dorsal motor nucleus of the vagus (CN X); and (6) cochlear nuclei, and inferior and part of the medial and lateral vestibular nuclei (CN VIII).

#### Spinal nucleus of the trigeminal

The **spinal nucleus of the trigeminal**, also known as the **nucleus of the spinal tract of the trigeminal**, is located in the medulla. (The other trigeminal nuclei are located in the pons and midbrain.) Sensory fibres from the area supplied by the trigeminal nerve enter the brainstem at the pons. Some of these fibres descend in the spinal tract of the trigeminal to end in the nucleus of the spinal tract of the trigeminal. The tract and spinal nucleus extend from the level of the lower pons to the upper part of the spinal cord, and are seen throughout the length of the medulla oblongata. The spinal

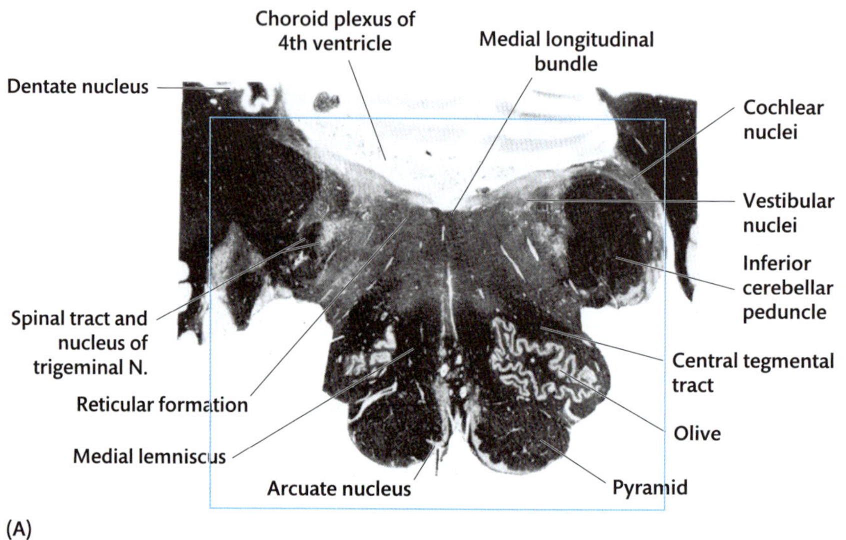


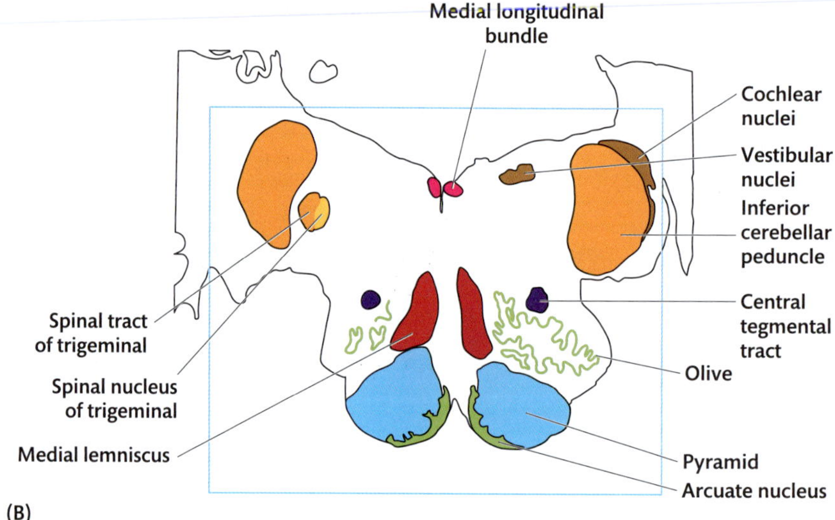


**Fig. 28.9** Transverse section through the uppermost part of the medulla oblongata (enclosed in box). (A) Histology section. Grey matter = white; white matter = grey to black. (B) Structures of interest in (A) are highlighted.

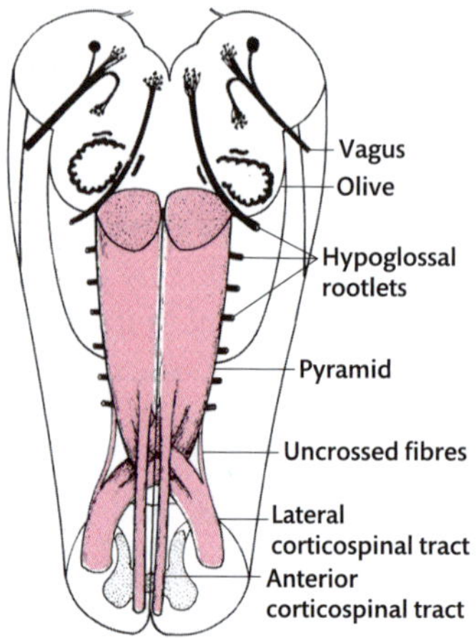


**Fig. 28.10** Diagram of the medulla oblongata and spinal cord to show the decussation of the pyramids (corticospinal tracts).

nucleus lies medial to the tract [Figs. 28.5B, 28.6, 28.7, 28.8, 28.9].

The spinal nucleus and tract of trigeminal are principally concerned with sensations of pain and temperature from the face. They are also concerned general sensation from the territory supplied by the facial, glossopharyngeal, and vagus nerves.

### Nucleus of the tractus solitarius

The **nucleus of the tractus solitarius** lies in the upper part of the medulla [Fig. 28.8]. It receives general sensation from the viscera (GVA), and taste sensation from the tongue, epiglottis, and soft palate (SVA). These sensations are carried by branches of the facial, glossopharyngeal, and vagus nerves which form the **tractus solitarius** in the medulla and end in the nucleus solitarius. Identify the position of the nucleus and tract in Figs. 28.7 and 28.8.

### Cochlear and vestibular nuclei

Sensory fibres from the cochlear nerve end in the **cochlear nuclei** which overlie the superior part of the inferior cerebellar peduncle in the medulla oblongata. The vestibular fibres pass anterior to the same peduncle and spread out into the **vestibular nuclei** in the floor of the fourth ventricle. These nuclei underlie the **vestibular area** [Fig. 28.3] which is partly in the medulla and partly in the pons [Fig. 28.9].

### Dorsal motor nucleus of the vagus and inferior salivatory nucleus

The **dorsal nucleus of the vagus** contains the preganglionic parasympathetic neurons which give rise to the parasympathetic fibres in the vagus (GVE). It lies in the upper part of the medulla [Figs. 28.5A, 28.8]. At the upper end of this nucleus is the **inferior salivatory nucleus** which gives rise to the preganglionic parasympathetic fibres of the glossopharyngeal nerve. The inferior salivatory nucleus lies in the upper medulla.

### Nucleus ambiguus

The **nucleus ambiguus** lies in the upper part of the medulla [Fig. 28.8]. It gives rise to somatic efferent nerve fibres to muscles of branchiomeric origin (SVE). They run in the glossopharyngeal, vagus, and accessory nerves [Fig. 28.5A].

### Hypoglossal nucleus

The hypoglossal nerve arises from a single paramedian **hypoglossal nucleus** in the upper part of the medulla [Figs. 28.5A, 28.8]. It supplies the tongue muscles (GSE or simply SE).

## Summary of cranial nerves CN IX, X, XI, and XII

The **glossopharyngeal nerve** (CN IX):

1. Supplies the stylopharyngeus (SVE) through fibres which rise in the nucleus ambiguus.
2. Supplies preganglionic parasympathetic fibres to the parotid gland through fibres which arise in the inferior salivatory nucleus (GVE).
3. Carries general sensation from the posterior third of the tongue, pharynx, and external ear to the spinal nucleus of the trigeminal (GSA).
4. Carries sensation from the baroreceptors and chemoreceptors of the carotid body and sinus to the nucleus solitarius (GVA).
5. Carries taste sensation from the posterior third of the tongue to the nucleus solitarius (SVA).

The **vagus nerve** (CN X):

1. Supplies the pharyngeal and laryngeal muscles (SVE) through fibres which arise in the nucleus ambiguus.
2. Supplies preganglionic parasympathetic fibres to the heart, lungs, and much of the gastrointestinal tract through fibres which arise in the dorsal motor nucleus of the vagus (GVE).
3. Carries general sensation from the pharynx and external ear to the spinal nucleus of the trigeminal (GSA).
4. Carries taste sensation from the posterior-most part of the tongue to the nucleus solitarius (SVA).

The **accessory nerve** (CN XI):

1. Supplies the pharyngeal and laryngeal muscles (SVE) through fibres which arise in the nucleus ambiguus—cranial part.
2. Supplies the sternocleidomastoid and trapezius (SVE) through fibres which arise in the cervical spinal cord—spinal part.

The **hypoglossal nerve** (CN XII):

1. Supplies muscles of the tongue (SE) through fibres which arise in the hypoglossal nucleus.

## Other nuclei in the medulla

### Inferior olivary nucleus

The **inferior olivary nucleus** lies posterolateral to the pyramid [Figs. 28.8, 28.9]. It has the shape of a crumpled bag of grey matter, with its open mouth facing medially. Its efferent fibres emerge from the mouth and pass to the opposite half of the cerebellum through the inferior cerebellar peduncle [Fig. 28.8].

### Arcuate nucleus

The **arcuate nucleus** lies anterior to the pyramid [Fig. 28.7]. This nucleus and the fibres which arise from it represent an inferior extension of the pontine nuclei and the pontocerebellar fibres. The **anterior external arcuate fibres** and **striae medullares** arise from the arcuate nucleus. The anterior external arcuate fibres pass laterally to the cerebellum in the inferior cerebellar peduncle. Other fibres from the arcuate nucleus [Fig. 28.9] pass posteriorly through the midline of the medulla oblongata and run across the floor of the fourth ventricle to the cerebellum as the striae medullares [Fig. 28.3].

### Accessory cuneate nucleus

The **accessory cuneate nucleus** lies on the lateral aspect of the main cuneate nucleus [Fig. 28.7]. It gives rise to the **posterior external arcuate fibres** which pass superiorly into the inferior cerebellar peduncle. The accessory cuneate nucleus receives collaterals (branches) from the fibres in the fasciculus cuneatus and transmits information carried by the fasciculus cuneatus from the upper half of the body on the same side [Fig. 28.8].

## Neurological lesions in medulla

➲ Having studied the blood supply of the brainstem and the location of important nuclei and white matter in the medulla, it is possible to explain the neurological deficits seen in ischaemic diseases.

## Lateral medullary syndrome

➲ The **lateral medullary syndrome**, or **Wallenberg syndrome (WS)**, is a neurological disorder that is due to damage to the lateral portion of the medulla oblongata (i.e. the lateral medullary syndrome). WS is typically due to ischaemia from a **vertebral artery** or **posterior inferior cerebellar artery** infarction. Primary aetiologies include atherosclerosis, hypertension, and other vascular risk factors. In cases of lateral medullary syndrome, the clinical picture is based on the extent to which the related nuclei and pathways are damaged.

A patient with right-sided infarction would present with the following signs and symptoms:

1. Gait and limb ataxia on the right side due to interruption of the right posterior spinocerebellar tracts in the inferior cerebellar peduncle.
2. Vertigo, nausea, and nystagmus due to ischaemia of the vestibular nuclei.
3. Loss of pain and temperature sensation on the right side of the face due to damage to the left spinal nucleus and tract of the trigeminal nerve.
4. Loss of pain and temperature sensation on the left side of the body due damage to the left spinothalamic tract. The fibres in the left spinothalamic tract carry sensation from the right side of the body [see Fig. 27.6].
5. Hoarseness of voice and difficulty in swallowing are due to damage to the right nucleus ambiguus and right dorsal motor nucleus of the vagus which innervate muscles of the palate, pharynx, and larynx. The gag reflex is also lost on the right side, as the glossopharyngeal nerve forms the efferent limb of the reflex.
6. Ptosis, miosis, and anhidrosis of the head and neck on the right side due to disruption of the fibres descending from the diencephalon to the thoracolumbar sympathetic outflow.

Note the proximity of the damaged structures in the upper part of the medulla [Fig. 28.11].

## Medial medullary syndrome

➲ The **medial medullary syndrome** is a neurological disorder that is due to damage to the midline and medial portion of the medulla oblongata. It is typically due to ischaemia from a **spinal artery** infarction due to atherosclerosis, hypertension, or other vascular risk factors. In cases of medial medullary syndrome, the clinical picture is based on the extent to which the related nuclei and pathways are

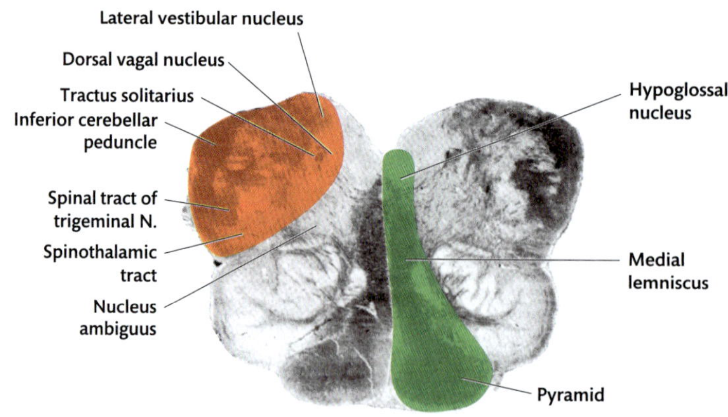


**Fig. 28.11** Diagram to show the structures affected in lateral medullary syndrome (left) and medial medullary syndrome (right).

damaged. A patient with left-sided infarction would present with the following signs and symptoms:

1. Loss of proprioception and vibration on the right side of the body due to interruption of the fibres in the medial lemniscus. The fibres in the left medial lemniscus carry sensation from the right side of the body [Fig. 28.7].
2. Hemiparesis of the right side due to damage of corticospinal fibres in the pyramid.
3. Paralysis of the left side of the tongue due to damage to the hypoglossal nucleus.
4. Vertigo, nausea, and vomiting due to ischaemia of the medial vestibular nuclei.

Note the proximity of the damaged structures in the upper part of the medulla [Fig. 28.11].

## Internal gross features of the pons

The interior of the pons is arbitrarily divided into a ventral and dorsal part which can be appreciated with the naked eye. The bulky ridge seen on the ventral aspect of the external surface of the pons lies in the **ventral part of the pons**. The **dorsal part of the pons**, also known as the **tegmentum**, separates the ventral part from the floor of the fourth ventricle [Fig. 28.12; see Fig. 29.1]. The tegmentum is continuous superiorly with the tegmentum of the midbrain, and inferiorly with the medulla oblongata. The ventral part of the pons contains transverse and longitudinally running fibre bundles. Finer details of the grey and white matter of the pons are appreciated in stained histological sections and are shown in Figs. 28.12, 28.13, and 28.14. Fig. 28.12 is through the lower pons, and Fig. 28.13 is through the upper pons. Fig. 28.14 is a section taken close to the junction of the pons and midbrain.

### White matter of the pons

The ascending and descending tracts seen in the spinal cord and medulla are seen continuing in the pons. In addition, there are fibre bundles such as the pontocerebellar fibres and trapezoid body which are specific to the pons.





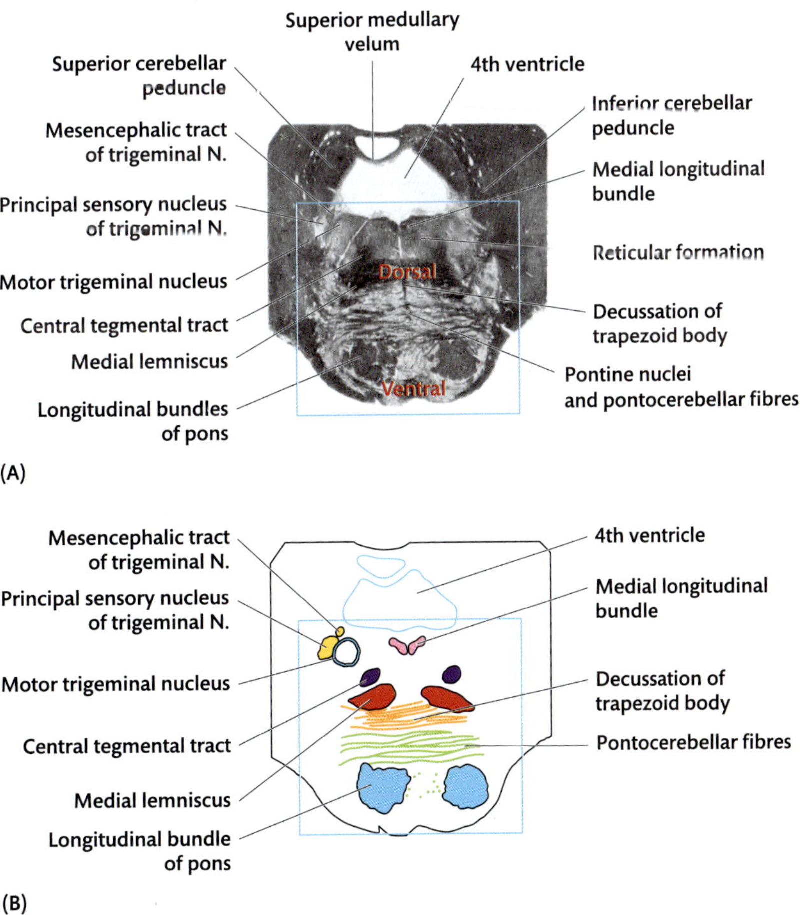


Fig. 28.12 Transverse section through the middle of the pons (enclosed in box). (A) Histology section. Grey matter = white; white matter = grey to black. (B) Structures of interest in (A) are highlighted.

## Corticospinal, corticopontine, and corticonuclear tracts

The **corticospinal**, **corticonuclear**, and **corticopontine fibres** arise in the cerebral cortex and run longitudinally in the ventral part of the pons. The corticospinal fibres to the spinal cord and their position in the upper medulla (pyramid), their decussation in the lower medulla, and the position in the spinal cord have been described. In the pons, these fibres run longitudinally in the ventral part of the pons and are continuous with the crura cerebri of the midbrain and the pyramids of the medulla [Figs. 28.12, 28.13, 28.14]. The **corticopontine fibres** run with the corticospinal tract in the midbrain and end in the pontine nuclei located in the ventral part of the pons. **Corticonuclear fibres** end on the motor nuclei of the cranial nerves situated in the pons and the medulla.

## Medial lemniscus and spinothalamic tract

The **medial lemniscus** and **spinothalamic tract** enter the pons from the medulla and pass into the dorsal part of the pons. Trace these fibres sequentially through Figs. 28.6, 28.7, 28.8, 28.9, 28.12, and 28.13 to get an idea of the course of these fibres [see also Fig. 31.29]. Note that the medial lemniscus which was oriented anteroposteriorly in the medulla is now placed transversely.

## Pontocerebellar fibres

The **pontocerebellar fibres** arise from the **pontine nuclei** scattered in the ventral part of pons, cross the midline, and converge laterally to form the **middle cerebellar peduncle** [Figs. 28.12, 28.13, 28.14].

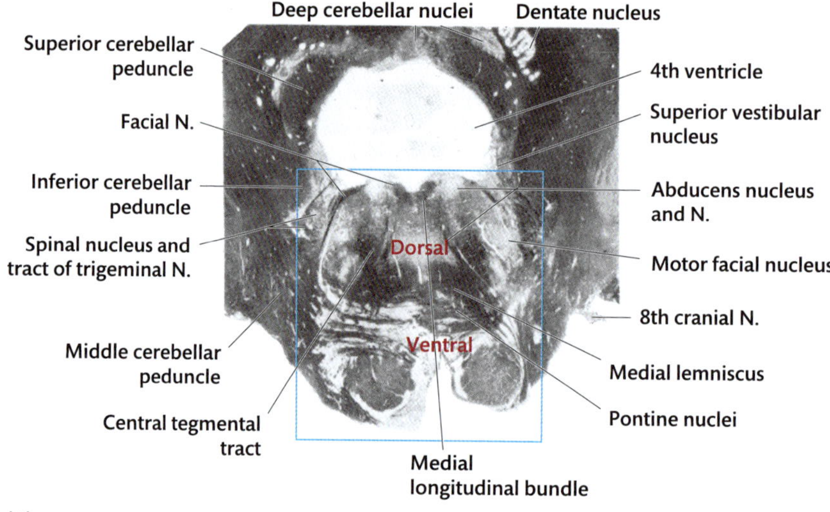


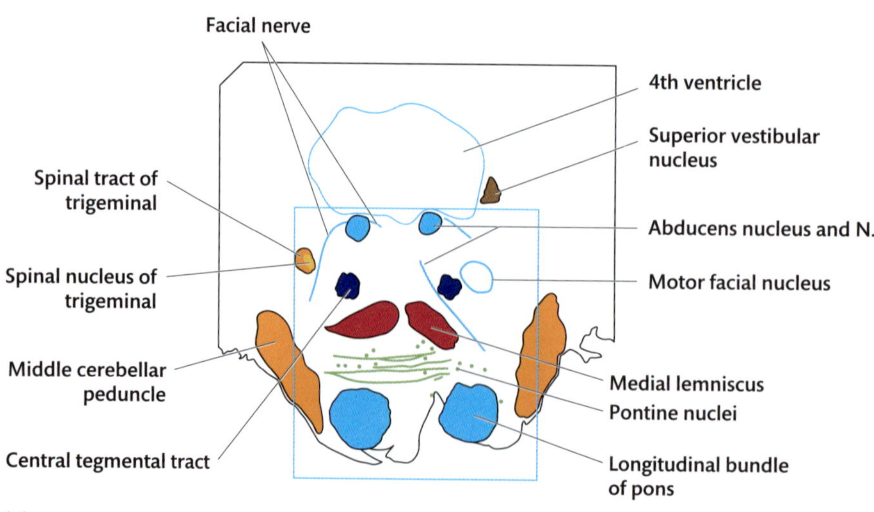


**Fig. 28.13** Transverse section through the inferior part of the pons (enclosed in box). (A) Histology section. Grey matter = white; white matter = grey to black. (B) Structures of interest in (A) are highlighted.

## Trapezoid body

The **trapezoid body** runs transversely just posterior to the ventral part of the pons [Figs. 28.13, 28.12, 28.14]. It consists of auditory fibres which arise in the cochlear nucleus and cross the midline to the opposite side. At the lateral ends of the trapezoid body, these fibres collect to form the **lateral lemniscus** which ascends to the inferior colliculus in the midbrain.

Note: the inferior cerebellar peduncle does not enter the pons but passes dorsally into the cerebellum at the upper border of the medulla [Fig. 28.9].

# Grey matter of the pons

The nuclear masses in the pons includes the nuclei of cranial nerves V, VI, VII, and VIII and the pontine nuclei.

## Cranial nerve nuclei in the pons

The cranial nerve nuclei in the pons are the: (1) motor nucleus of the trigeminal (CN V); (2) main sensory nucleus of the trigeminal nerve (CN V); (3) abducens nucleus (CN VI); (4) facial nucleus (CN VII); (5) superior salivatory nucleus (CN VII); and (6) vestibular and cochlear (CN VIII).

### Motor nucleus of the trigeminal

All four nuclei of the trigeminal nerve—motor, main or chief sensory, mesencephalic, and nucleus of the spinal tract—lie in the pons, but two only partially. The **motor nucleus** lies medially at the level of the upper pons. It gives rise to the nerves which innervate the muscles of mastication and other muscles derived from the first pharyngeal arch [Figs. 28.5, 28.12].

### Main sensory nucleus of the trigeminal

The **main sensory nucleus of the trigeminal nerve** lies lateral to the motor nucleus in the upper pons. It receives fibres carrying sensations of fine touch and pressure from the trigeminal area.

### Spinal nucleus of the trigeminal

The **spinal nucleus of the trigeminal** extends inferiorly from the point of entry of the trigeminal nerve, in the lateral margin of the dorsal part of the inferior pons [Fig. 28.13]. Its continuation in the medulla has been described.

### Mesencephalic nucleus of the trigeminal

The **mesencephalic tract and nucleus of the trigeminal** pass dorsally, between the motor and

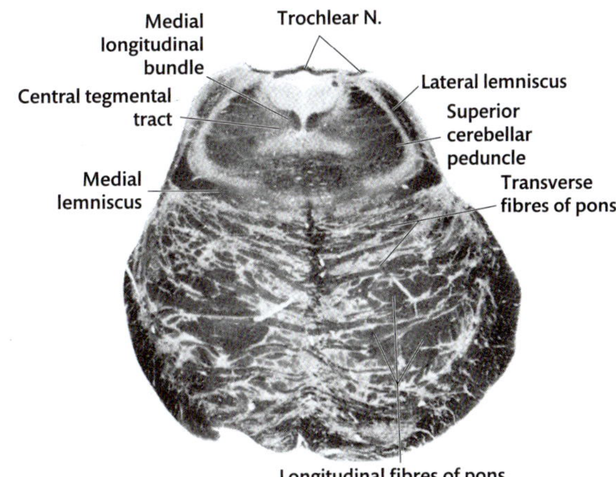


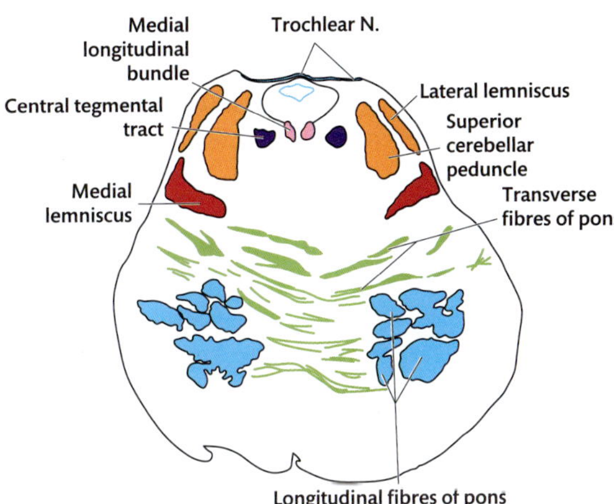


**Fig. 28.14** Transverse section through the upper part of the pons. (A) Histology section. Grey matter = white; white matter = grey to black. (B) Structures of interest in (A) are highlighted.

main sensory nuclei, to the midbrain [Figs. 28.5B, 28.12]. This tract contains proprioceptive fibres from the muscles of mastication and the temporomandibular joint and the cell bodies of the primary sensory neurons. It is unique because cell bodies of primary sensory neurons are usually found in peripheral ganglia.

### Abducens nucleus

This small nucleus lies on the floor of the fourth ventricle, in the lower pons, close to the midline [Figs. 28.5, 28.13]. It raises the **facial colliculus** on the floor of the ventricle where the facial nerve curves around this nucleus [Figs. 28.3, 28.5A, 28.13]. The abducens nerve can be seen running anterolaterally from the nucleus.

### Facial nucleus

The **motor nucleus of the facial nerve** lies immediately anteromedial to the spinal nucleus of the trigeminal nerve in the lower part of the pons [Fig. 28.13]. It supplies the muscles of facial expression and other muscles derived from the second pharyngeal arch. The facial nerve passes posteromedially from the nucleus, curves around the medial and posterior aspects of the abducens nucleus, forming the **genu of the facial nerve**, and passes anterolaterally to emerge at the inferior border of the pons [Fig. 28.5A].

### Superior salivatory nucleus

The preganglionic parasympathetic fibres of the facial nerve arise from the **superior salivatory nucleus**, which lies in the lower part of the pons, superior to the inferior salivatory nucleus [Fig. 28.5A]. Fibres from this nucleus join the facial nerve as it runs through the pons.

### Vestibular nuclei

The vestibular fibres of the vestibulocochlear nerve pass anterior to the inferior cerebellar peduncle and fan out into the **superior**, **lateral**, **medial**, and **inferior vestibular nuclei** in the floor of the fourth ventricle [Figs. 28.3, 28.13]. These nuclei underlie the **vestibular area** which is partly in the medulla and partly in the pons [Fig. 28.9].

### Cochlear nuclei

Sensory fibres from the cochlear divisions of the vestibulocochlear nerve have already been seen passing into the **cochlear nuclei** which overlie the superior part of the inferior cerebellar peduncle in the medulla oblongata [Fig. 28.9].

## Summary of cranial nerves CN V, VI, VII, and VIII

The **trigeminal nerve** (CN V):

1. Supplies the muscles of mastication (SVE) through fibres which arise in the motor nucleus of the trigeminal.
2. Carries general sensation from the face, nasal and oral cavities, and meninges to the main sensory and spinal nucleus of the trigeminal (GSA).
3. Carries proprioception from the muscles of mastication and the temporomandibular joint to the mesencephalic nucleus of the trigeminal (GSA).

The **abducens nerve** (CN VI):

1. Supplies the lateral rectus (GSE) through fibres which arise in the abducens nucleus.

The **facial nerve** (CN VII):

1. Supplies the muscles of facial expression (SVE) through fibres which arise in the motor nucleus of the facial nerve.
2. Supplies preganglionic parasympathetic fibres to the submandibular, sublingual, lacrimal, nasal, and oral mucosal glands through fibres which arise in the superior salivatory nucleus (GVE).
3. Carries taste sensation from the anterior two-thirds of the tongue to the nucleus solitarius (SVA).
4. Carries general sensation from a small area on the external ear to the spinal nucleus of the trigeminal (GSA).

The **vestibulocochlear nerve** (CN VIII):

1. Carries vestibular and cochlear stimuli to the vestibular and cochlear nuclei (SSA).

## Other nuclei in the pons

### Pontine nuclei

The **pontine nuclei** are large clusters of neurons in the ventral part of the pons [Figs. 28.13, 28.12]. They receive impulses from the cortex through the corticopontine tract, and project to the opposite cerebellum as pontocerebellar fibres. The fibres arising from the pontine nuclei cross the midline as pontocerebellar fibres. At the lateral aspect of the pons, they converge to form the **middle cerebellar peduncle** [Figs. 28.1, 28.2].

# Internal features of the midbrain

The gross internal features of the midbrain can be appreciated by a naked-eye examination of the cut surface. The interior of the midbrain is arbitrarily divided into a ventral and dorsal part separated by the cerebral aqueduct. The dorsal part, or **tectum**, lies posterior to the cerebral aqueduct, and the ventral part—the **cerebral peduncle**—lies anterior. Each cerebral peduncle consists of: (1) the crus cerebri anteriorly; (2) the tegmentum posteriorly; and (3) a layer of pigmented cells—**the substantia nigra**—between the two [Figs. 28.15]. The **round red nucleus** is seen in the tegmentum.

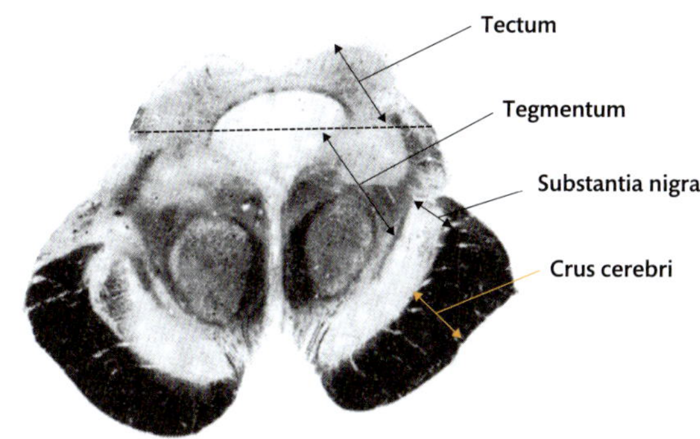


**Fig. 28.15** Transverse section through the midbrain to show the subdivisions—tectum, tegmentum, substantia nigra, and crus cerebri.

The tectum consists of the two superior and two inferior colliculi.

Finer details of the grey and white matter of the midbrain are appreciated in stained histological sections and are shown in Fig. 28.16, a section through the inferior colliculi, in [Fig. 28.17], a section through the superior colliculi, in [Fig. 28.18], a section at the junction of the midbrain and diencephalon.

## Crus cerebri

The **corticospinal, corticonuclear**, and **corticopontine fibres** lie in the crus cerebri. They arise in the cerebral cortex and converge radially on the crus [Fig. 28.19]. Corticopontine fibres from the frontal cortex (frontopontine fibres) lie in the medial part of the crus, and corticopontine fibres from the other parts of the cortex (parietopontine, temporopontine, and occipitopontine) lie in the lateral part. The corticospinal and corticonuclear fibres which arise in the posterior part of the frontal lobe (i.e. near the middle of the hemisphere) lie in the intermediate part of the crus. Of these, the corticonuclear fibres are the most medial, and the corticospinal fibres to the lower limb are the most lateral.

## Substantia nigra

The substantia nigra is a curved plate of grey matter lying between the crus cerebri and the tegmentum. It contains large nerve cells with a considerable amount of melanin in their cytoplasm. These cells have connections with the tegmentum of the midbrain and with the corpus striatum (part of the deep nuclei in the cerebrum) in the ipsilateral hemisphere. They play an important part in the control of muscle tone and activity, and produce dopamine which is passed along their axons to the corpus striatum. The substantia nigra extends from the superior border of the pons into the inferolateral part of the subthalamus, superior to the midbrain [Figs. 28.17, 28.18].

## Tegmentum

The tegmentum of the midbrain consists of a thick column of grey and white matter. It is continuous inferiorly with the dorsal part of the pons, and superiorly with the hypothalamus and subthalamus. Posteriorly, it is continuous with the tectum around the cerebral aqueduct. The cerebral aqueduct is surrounded by a thick layer of grey matter (the **central grey substance**), in which lie the nuclei of the oculomotor and trochlear nerves and the mesencephalic nucleus of the trigeminal nerve [Figs. 28.16, 28.17, 28.18].

In addition, the tegmentum contains a number of important nuclei and tracts which are best seen in microscopic section and are described below.

## Tectum

The two superior and two inferior colliculi are rounded elevations of the grey matter on the posterior surface of the tectum [Fig. 28.3]. They overlie the nucleus of the superior and inferior colliculi described below.

## White matter of the midbrain

Many of the tracts seen in the spinal cord, medulla, and pons continue into the midbrain and are seen here.

### Corticospinal, corticopontine, and corticonuclear fibres

The majority of fibres in the crus cerebri end in the pontine nuclei in the ventral part of the pons. They constitute the **corticopontine fibres**. A smaller number of fibres—the **corticospinal fibres**—run longitudinally through the pons and form the pyramid on the medulla oblongata. A still smaller number end in the motor cranial nerve nuclei in the brainstem—the **corticonuclear fibres**. The majority of corticospinal and corticonuclear fibres cross to the opposite side before they end [Fig. 28.19].

### Medial lemniscus and spinothalamic tracts

The **medial lemniscus** and **spinothalamic tracts** [Figs. 28.16, 28.17, 28.18] ascend through the tegmentum from the dorsal part of the pons. They

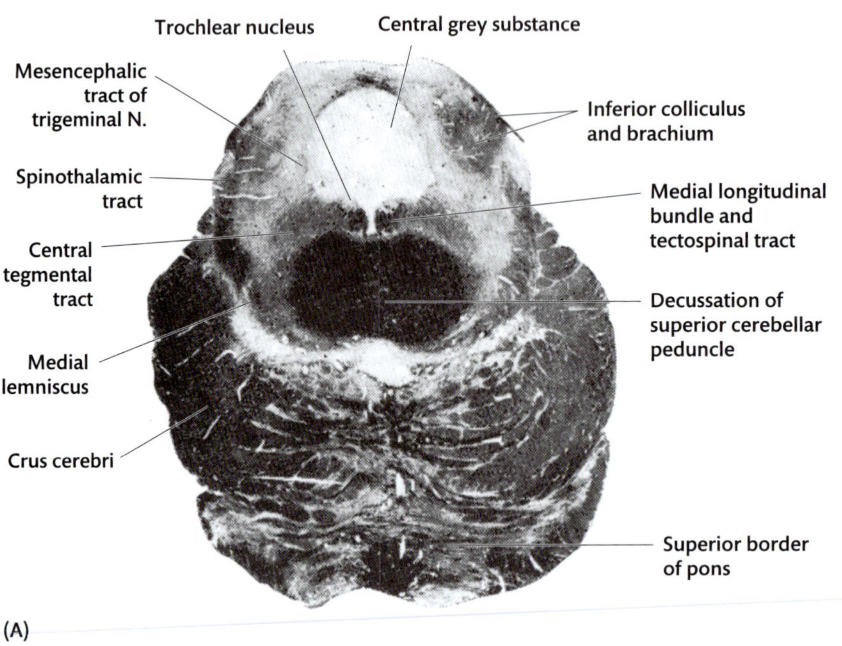


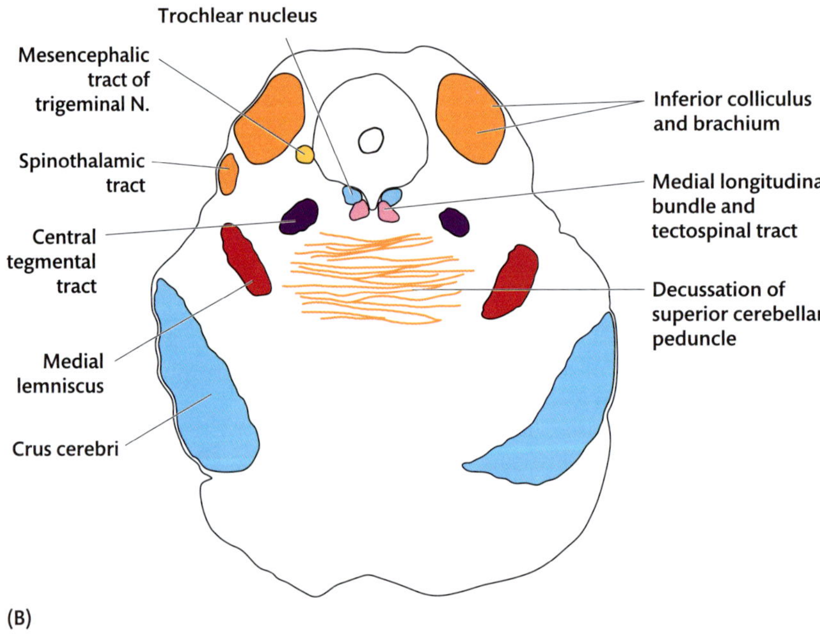


**Fig. 28.16** Transverse section through the lowest part of the midbrain. (A) Histology section. Grey matter = white; white matter = grey to black. (B) Structures of interest in (A) are highlighted.

pass further laterally, as they ascend (the spinothalamic tract intermingling with the medial lemniscus) and lie deep to the brachium of the inferior colliculus in the upper midbrain. At this level, the spinothalamic tract gives off fibres to the superior colliculus—the **spinotectal tract**. In addition to the fibres which these tracts contain in the medulla oblongata, fibres from the sensory nucleus of the trigeminal nerve—the **trigeminothalamic tract**—come to lie medial to them at the midbrain level [Fig. 28.5].

## Superior cerebellar peduncle

The superior cerebellar peduncle connects the cerebellum to the midbrain. The fibres cross the midline at the level of the inferior colliculus in the **decussation of the superior cerebellar peduncle** [Fig. 28.16]. Most of the fibres in this peduncle originate in the dentate nucleus of the cerebellum. A large number of these dentato-rubral fibres end in the red nucleus of the midbrain. Some fibres pass directly on to the thalamus (dentato-thalamic tract).

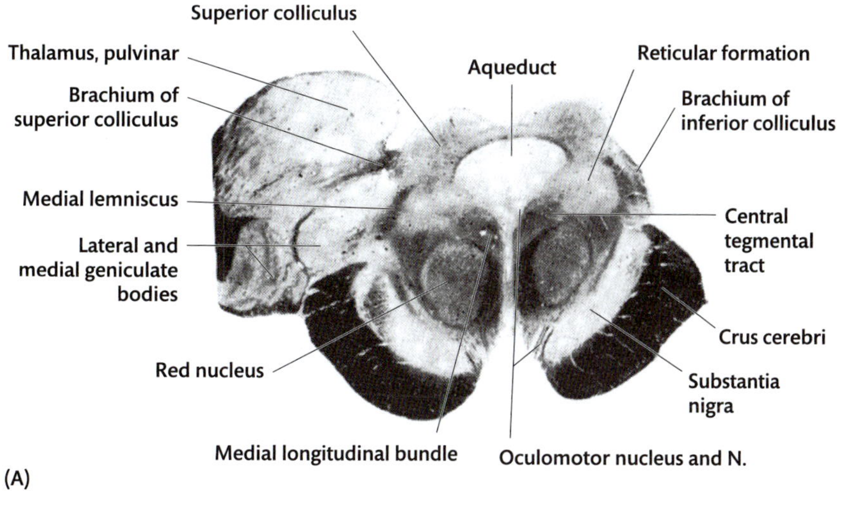


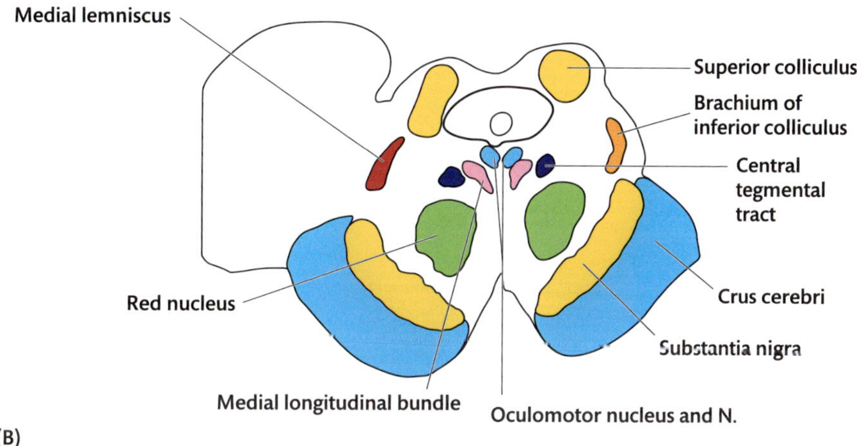


**Fig. 28.17** Transverse section through the upper part of the midbrain. (A) Histology section. Grey matter = white; white matter = grey to black. (B) Structures of interest in (A) are highlighted.

## Rubrospinal tract

The **rubroreticular and rubrospinal tracts** arise in the red nucleus. The rubrospinal tracts decussate in the ventral part of the tegmentum (**ventral tegmental decussation**) at the level of the superior colliculus and descend through the dorsal part of the pons to the lateral part of the medulla oblongata and upper spinal cord.

## Medial longitudinal fasciculus

The **medial longitudinal fasciculus** is a small, compact bundle which extends from the upper part of the midbrain to the spinal cord. It lies adjacent to the midline and the nuclei of the oculomotor and trochlear nerves, and maintains this position throughout the brainstem. It is an intersegmental bundle which connects various levels of the brainstem and receives its major single contribution from the vestibular nuclei. In the spinal cord, it is continuous with the anterior intersegmental tract or medial vestibulospinal tract [Figs. 28.6, 28.7, 28.8, 28.9, 28.13, 28.12, 28.14, 28.16, 28.17, 28.18].

## Dorsal longitudinal fasciculus

The **dorsal longitudinal fasciculus** lies posterior to the nuclei of the third and fourth cranial nerves in the central grey matter. It connects the hypothalamus with the reticular formations of the midbrain and pons.

## Tectospinal tract

The **tectospinal tract** consists of fibres which arise in the deeper layer of the superior colliculus. They curve around the margin of the central grey substance, decussate anterior to the medial longitudinal fasciculus in the **dorsal tegmental decussation**, and descend through the dorsal part of the pons, medulla oblongata, and spinal cord. Fibres of the tectospinal tract end in the reticular formation of the brainstem and spinal cord, and produce reflex movements in response to visual stimuli reaching

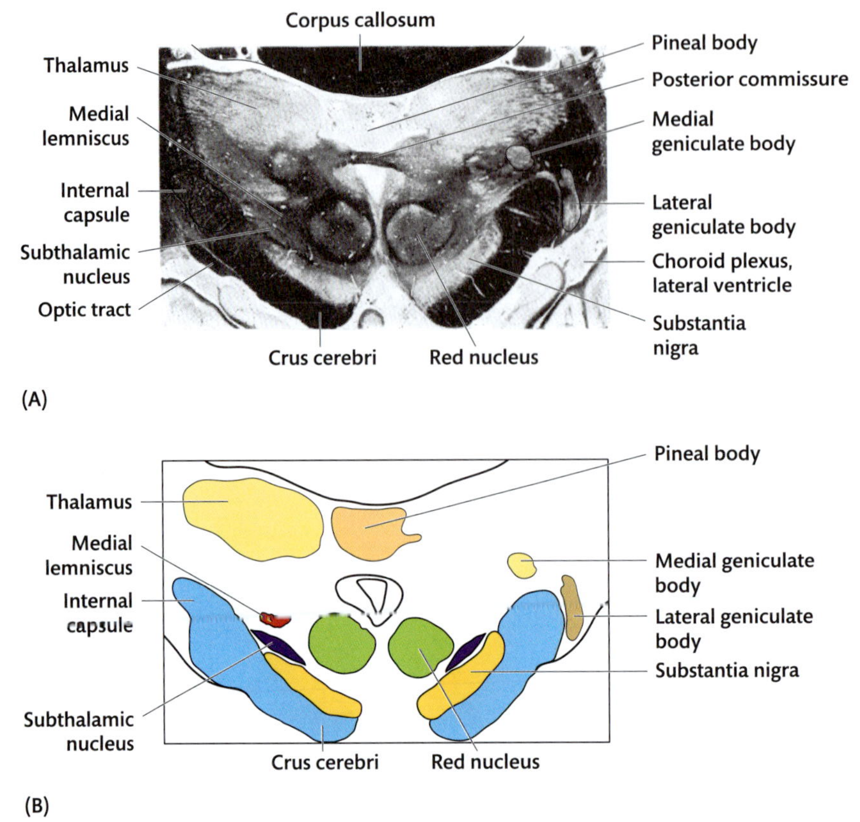


**Fig. 28.18** Transverse section through the junction between the midbrain and diencephalon. (A) Histology section. Grey matter = white; white matter = grey to black. (B) Structures of interest in (A) are highlighted.

the superior colliculus (e.g. turning of the head and eyes towards a sudden flash of light) [see Fig. 31.35].

## Central tegmental tract

The **central tegmental tract** is a large, diffuse bundle of fibres, dorsolateral to the red nucleus. It can be traced from the upper midbrain, through the dorsal part of the pons to end in the capsule of the olivary nucleus [Figs. 28.9, 28.12, 28.13, 28.14, 28.16, 28.17, 28.18; see also Fig. 29.8]. It probably transmits a number of different fibres in both directions and forms a pathway uniting the parts of the reticular formation with each other and with the thalamus, subthalamus, and olivary nucleus. It is one of the pathways for the brainstem ascending activating system to reach the intralaminar thalamic nuclei. It also carries cerebello-olivary fibres and may form a link between the corpus striatum and the cerebellum via the reticular formation and olivary nucleus.

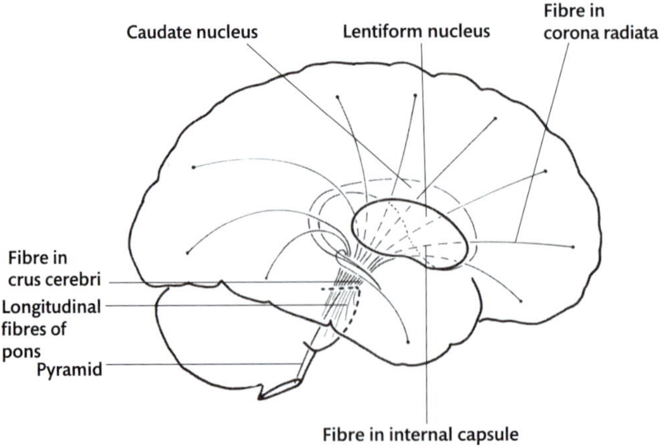


**Fig. 28.19** Diagram to show the arrangement of fibres in the corona radiata, internal capsule, crus cerebri, pons, and pyramid.

## Lateral lemniscus

The lateral lemniscus is formed in the pons by fibres which arise in the cochlear nucleus [Fig. 28.14]. It contains fibres from the ipsilateral cochlear nucleus (uncrossed fibres) and from the contralateral cochlear nucleus (fibres which have crossed in the trapezoid body [Fig. 28.12]). It ends by synapsing in cells of the inferior colliculus.

# Grey matter of the midbrain

The nuclear masses in the midbrain include the nuclei of cranial nerves III and IV, the red nucleus, and the nucleus of the superior and inferior colliculi.

## Cranial nerve nuclei in the midbrain

The cranial nerve nuclei in the midbrain are: (1) the motor nucleus of the trochlear nerve (CN IV); (2) the motor nucleus of the oculomotor nerve (CN III); (3) the Edinger–Westphal nucleus of the oculomotor nerve (CN III); and (4) the mesencephalic nucleus of the trigeminal nerve (CN V).

## Trochlear nucleus

The **trochlear nucleus** is the motor nucleus of the trochlear nerve. It lies on the ventral aspect of the peri-aqueductal grey matter at the level of the inferior colliculus, close to the midline [Fig. 28.16]. The nerve emerges from the dorsal surface of the brainstem, immediately inferior to the inferior colliculi. It supplies the superior oblique muscle.

## Oculomotor nucleus

The **oculomotor nucleus** lies at the level of the superior colliculus, on the ventral aspect of the central grey matter [Fig. 28.17]. It gives motor fibres to the extraocular muscles of the eyeball and preganglionic parasympathetic fibres to the ciliary ganglion.

## Mesencephalic nucleus of the trigeminal

The **mesencephalic tract of the trigeminal nerve** [see Fig. 31.27] ascends from the pons. It contains the proprioceptive sensory fibres from the muscles of mastication. It differs from all other peripheral sensory neurons in that its cells of origin are situated along the tract within the brainstem and are not situated in the trigeminal ganglion.

## Summary of cranial nerves CN III and CN IV

Cranial nerve nuclei in the midbrain with their functional group:

The **oculomotor nerve** (CN III):

1. Supplies the levator palpebrae superioris, inferior oblique, and superior, medial, and inferior rectus muscles in the orbit (GSE) through fibres which arise in the oculomotor nucleus.
2. Supplies preganglionic parasympathetic fibres to the sphincter pupillae and ciliaris muscle through fibres which arise in the Edinger–Westphal component of the oculomotor nucleus (GVE).

The **trochlear nerve** (CN IV):

1. Supplies the superior oblique (GSE) through fibres which arise in the trochlear nucleus.

## Other nuclei in the midbrain

### Nucleus of the superior colliculus

In the **superior colliculus**, the grey matter is on the surface and consists of many layers. It receives a bundle of visual fibres from the optic tract through the **brachium of the superior colliculus** which also sends fibres to the pretectal region, immediately in front of the superior colliculus [see Fig. 30.5]. The nucleus of the superior colliculus and the pretectal region are concerned with visual reflexes. The nucleus of the superior colliculus is connected to the cranial nerve nuclei and to the motor cells of the spinal cord through the **tectospinal tract** [see Fig. 27.3, 31.35; Figs. 28.8, 28.16], and is responsible for the reflex turning of the head and eyes towards a source of light.

### Nucleus of the inferior colliculus

The **nucleus of the inferior colliculus** is oval. It receives the lateral lemniscus which transmits impulses from the cochlear nuclei. On the side of the midbrain, a ridge—the **brachium of the inferior colliculus** [Figs. 28.2, 28.17]—passes anterosuperiorly from the inferior colliculus to the **medial geniculate body** of the thalamus [Fig. 28.2]. It transmits auditory impulses to the medial geniculate body for relay to the cerebral cortex.

### Red nucleus

The **red nucleus** is a cylindrical, rod-shaped collection of reddish grey matter in the medial part of the tegmentum at the superior colliculus level. It extends cranially into the subthalamus [Fig. 28.18].

The fibres of the oculomotor nerve run through it, to emerge between the crus cerebri [Figs. 28.17, 28.18]. The majority of the cells of the red nucleus send their axons to the thalamus. Other small neurons in the caudal part of the red nucleus give origin to the **rubroreticular** and **rubrospinal tracts**.

## Neurological lesions in midbrain

### Benedikt's syndrome

➲ **Benedikt's syndrome** is a neurological condition typically caused by a stroke in the posterior cerebral artery or its branches. A patient with left-sided infarction would present with the following signs and symptoms:

1. Inability to move the left eye inwards or upwards, and ptosis and mydriasis on the left due to damage to the oculomotor nerve.
2. Weakness or paralysis of the arm and leg of the right side (extrapyramidal symptoms) due to damage to the red nucleus.
3. Involuntary, writhing movements of the limbs due to disruption of the dentato-rubral fibres.
4. Loss of pain and temperature on the right side may be seen if the medial lemniscus is affected.

Note the proximity of the damaged structures in the midbrain [Fig. 28.20].

### Weber's syndrome

➲ Like Benedikt's syndrome, **Weber's syndrome** is a neurological disease caused by interruption to blood flow to parts of the cerebral peduncle of the midbrain. A patient with a left-sided lesion would present with the following signs and symptoms:

1. Inability to move the left eye inwards or upwards, and ptosis and mydriasis on the left due to damage to the oculomotor nerve.
2. Weakness or paralysis of the face and arms on the right side due to damage to the corticonuclear and corticospinal fibres in the crus cerebri.

Note the proximity of the damaged structures in the midbrain [Fig. 28.20].

Note that the sensory deficit and involvement of the red nucleus seen in Benedikt's syndrome are not seen in Weber's syndrome.

## Reticular formation in brainstem

The **reticular formation** consists of numerous neurons arranged in ill-defined groups, mingled with fine bundles of nerve fibres which run mainly in the longitudinal direction. Fibres arising in the reticular formation of the pons and medulla oblongata descend in the spinal cord as the **reticulospinal tract**. Other fibres ascend into the diencephalon—the thalamus and hypothalamus.

The reticular formation receives collaterals of ascending pathways (e.g. spinothalamic tracts) and sensory information from some cranial nerves. It has extensive reciprocal connections with the cerebellum and other parts of the central nervous system. The reticular formation of the midbrain occupies the lateral parts of the tegmentum between the central grey substance and the medial lemniscus and spinothalamic tract. It is continuous with the reticular formation of the dorsal part of the pons and with the lateral part of the hypothalamus.

See Clinical Application 28.1 for the practical implications of the anatomy discussed in this chapter.

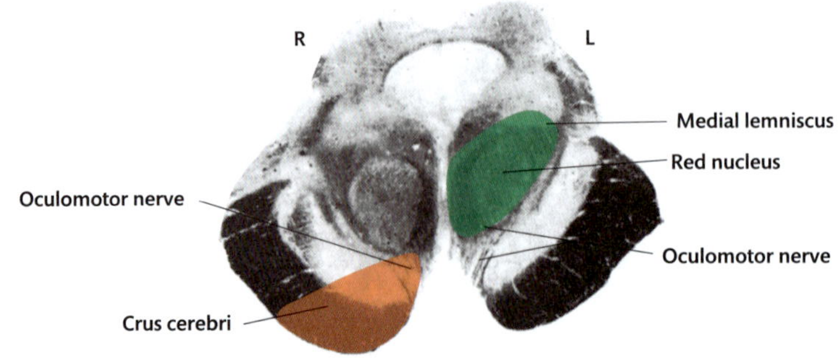


**Fig. 28.20** Diagram to show the structures affected in Benedikt's syndrome (left) and Weber's syndrome (right)

**CLINICAL APPLICATION 28.1 Herpes zoster ophthalmicus**

A 58-year-old male on immunosuppressive therapy developed painful vesicular eruptions on the right side of the face, involving the tip and side of the nose, the forehead, and the upper eyelid. This was preceded with fever and malaise for a few days. The vesicles initially contained clear fluid, and later became cloudy and ruptured to form dry plaques. The pain over the above region persisted for several weeks.

Study question 1: what is the likely diagnosis? (Answer: the clinical presentation is typical of herpes zoster ophthalmicus. The varicella-zoster virus causes overt or subclinical chickenpox infection in childhood and remains latent in some of the trigeminal ganglion cells. The latent virus can be reactivated in elderly, poorly nourished, or immunosuppressed individuals. The virus damages the nerves by causing severe perineural and intraneural inflammation.)

Study question 2: what is the nerve supply to the affected region? (Answer: the nose, upper eyelid, and forehead are supplied by the ophthalmic division of the trigeminal nerve. Herpes zoster characteristically affects the skin supplied by the ophthalmic division of the trigeminal nerve.)

Other complications of this condition include conjunctivitis, keratitis, and uveitis.

Herpes zoster can affect the maxillary and mandibular dermatomes of the trigeminal nerve, and dermatomes of the trunk and other cranial nerves. It is treated with antiviral drugs and topical steroids.

Ramsay Hunt syndrome is herpes zoster infection involving the facial nerve, causing vesicular eruptions of the skin of the external ear, ipsilateral anterior two-thirds of the tongue, severe ear pain, and facial nerve neuropathy. The prognosis is worse than that of Bell's palsy.

# CHAPTER 29
# The cerebellum



## External features of the cerebellum

The cerebellum consists of the two **cerebellar hemispheres** and a median part—the **vermis** [see Figs. 24.1, 24.2; Fig. 29.1]. It surrounds the posterior surface of the brainstem [Fig. 29.2]. The two cerebellar hemispheres lie inferior to the posterior part of the cerebrum and are separated from it by the tentorium cerebelli. The cerebellum has a superior [Fig. 29.2] and an anteroinferior surface [Fig. 29.3]. The superior aspect of the vermis is the median ridge on the superior surface [Fig. 29.2]. The vermis is more clearly separated from the cerebellar hemispheres on the anteroinferior surface, as it lies in a deep median hollow between the two cerebellar hemispheres (the **vallecula of the cerebellum**) [Fig. 29.3]. Each part of the vermis is continuous with a part of the hemispheres—a feature which is more obvious on the superior surface.

The **superior and inferior medullary vela** are thin layers of tissue on the anterior aspect of the cerebellum which sweep superiorly and inferiorly from the apex of the cerebellar recess [Figs. 29.1, 29.4A]. They form the roof of the fourth ventricle.

### Lobes and lobules of the cerebellum

The cerebellum becomes greatly folded during development, so that the surface is irregular with transversely running **fissures** and **folia** (the cortex between the fissures) [Fig. 29.2]. Of the great number of fissures formed in the cerebellum, three are of particular importance: (1) the **primary fissure**

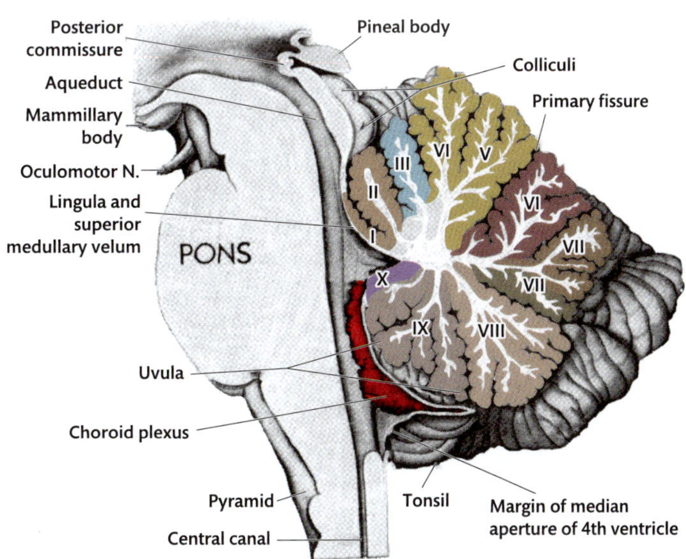


**Fig. 29.1** Median section through the brainstem and cerebellum. The lobules of the vermis are numbered using Roman numerals.

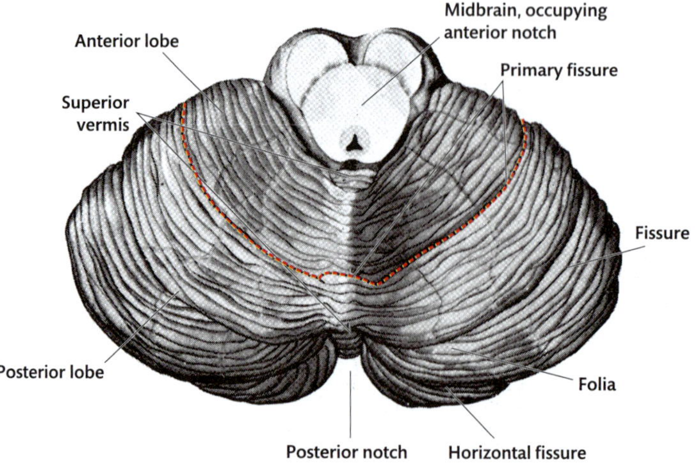


**Fig. 29.2** Superior surface of the cerebellum.





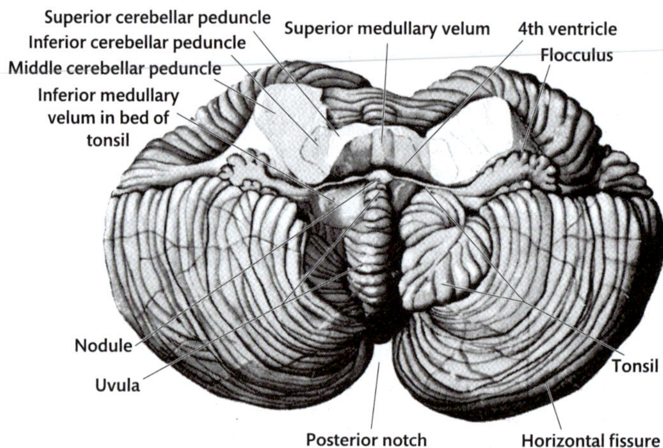


**Fig. 29.3** Anteroinferior surface of the cerebellum. The right tonsil has been removed to show more of the inferior medullary velum.

[Figs. 29.1, 29.2]—this deep fissure cuts across the superior surface of the cerebellum and separates the anterior and posterior lobes; (2) the **horizontal** (or intercrural) **fissure** which extends from one middle cerebellar peduncle to the other and lies close to the junction of the superior and anteroinferior surfaces of the cerebellum [Fig. 29.3]; and (3) the **posterolateral fissure** on the anteroinferior surface of the cerebellum [Fig. 29.3]. The vermis and cerebellar hemispheres are subdivided into three lobes by the three fissures. The **anterior lobe** lies in front of the primary fissure. The **posterior lobe** lies between the primary and posterolateral fissures [Fig. 29.2]. The **flocculonodular lobe** lies beyond the posterolateral fissure. It is made up of the nodule of the vermis and the flocculus of the cerebellar hemisphere [Fig. 29.3]. The lobes are further subdivided into ten **lobules** which are continuous across the vermis from one hemisphere to the other. Lobules I–V lie in the anterior lobe; lobules VI–VIII lie in the posterior lobe, and lobule X lies in the flocculonodular lobe [Fig. 29.1]. A detailed description of the lobules is beyond the scope of this book. However, you should note the position of the: (1) lingula, a part of the vermis which lies on the superior medullary velum [Fig. 29.1]; (2) uvula, a part of the inferior vermis that lies between the tonsils; and (3) tonsils, a part of the cerebellar hemispheres that lie in continuity with the uvula on the anteroinferior aspect [Fig. 29.3]. ➲ The tonsils lie close to the foramen magnum and are forced down into the vertebral canal when there is a sudden increase in intracranial pressure—a condition known as **tonsillar herniation**.

Using the instructions given in Dissection 29.1, identify the main parts of the cerebellum.

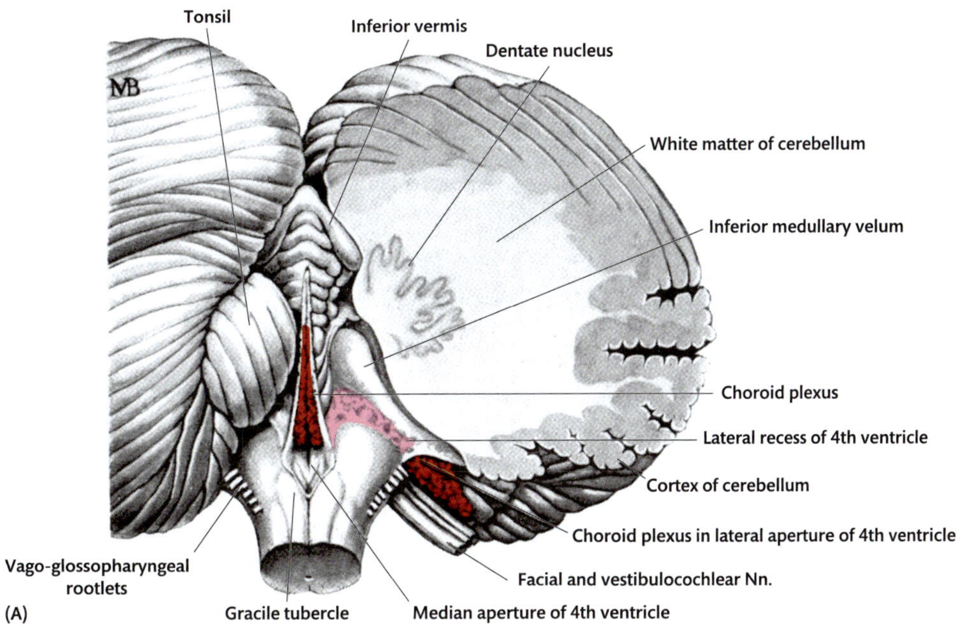


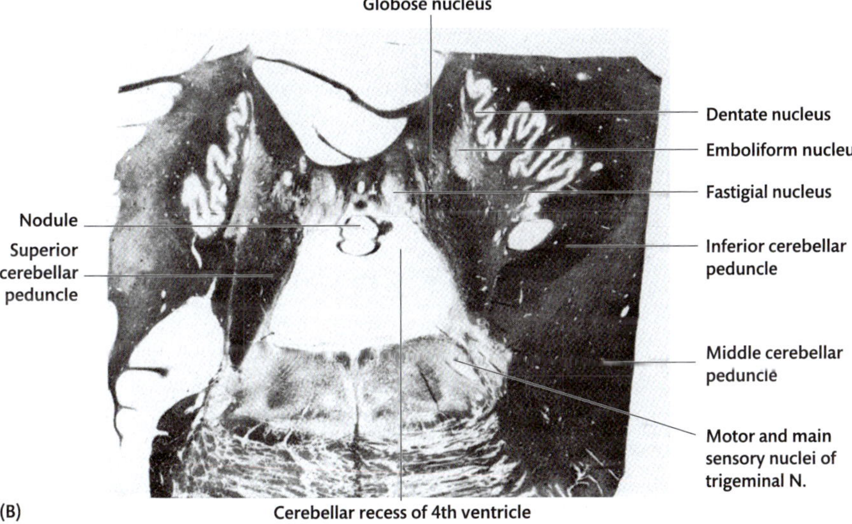


**Fig. 29.4** (A) Dissection of the left inferior surface of the cerebellum to show the median and lateral apertures of the fourth ventricle. The medulla oblongata has been displaced anteriorly so as to open up the median aperture. Note the choroid plexus which is visible at both apertures and can also be seen through the thin roof of the fourth ventricle. (B) Oblique transverse section, parallel to the cerebellar recess of the fourth ventricle, to show the cerebellar nuclei. [Compare with Fig. 12.11.]

### DISSECTION 29.1 Parts of the cerebellum

**Objective**

**I.** To identify the main parts of the cerebellum.

**Instructions**

1. Remove the meninges from the superior and posterior surfaces of the cerebellum, but avoid depressing the cerebellum too strongly to expose all of its superior surface.
2. With the assistance of Figs. 29.2 and 29.3, identify its main parts, including the primary fissure, horizontal fissure, superior and inferior vermis, hemispheres, tonsils, and flocculonodular lobe.

## Cerebellar peduncles

The cerebellum receives and sends information to other parts of the brain and spinal cord through nerve fibres which enter and leave through cerebellar peduncles. There are three pairs of peduncles—the **inferior**, **middle**, and **superior cerebellar peduncles**. Note the relative positions of these, as they enter the cerebellum, in Fig. 28.3.

### Inferior cerebellar peduncle

The inferior cerebellar peduncle connects the medulla to the cerebellum. It forms on the posterolateral surface of the medulla oblongata [see Fig. 28.2] and passes posteromedially into the vermis of the cerebellum. (Some of its fibres enter the cerebellar hemispheres.) **Afferent fibres**: the inferior cerebellar peduncle contains mainly afferent fibres to the cerebellum—the **posterior spinocerebellar tract** (from the spinal cord), **cuneocerebellar fibres** from the accessory cuneate nucleus, **olivocerebellar fibres** from the inferior olivary nucleus, **vestibulocerebellar fibres** from the vestibular nuclei and nerve, and fibres from the **reticular system**. **Efferent fibres**: it also transmits efferent cerebellar fibres to the **vestibular nuclei** and the **reticular formation** of the medulla oblongata [see Fig. 28.3].

### Middle cerebellar peduncle

This is the largest and most lateral of the three peduncles and connects the cerebellum to the pons. **Afferent fibres**: it contains **pontocerebellar fibres** which arise in the opposite half of the pons from the pontine nuclei and pass to the cerebellum. They transmit impulses which reach the pons from the cerebral cortex through the corticopontine fibres. The peduncle enters the cerebellum through the anterior end of the horizontal fissure [see Figs. 28.1, 28.2, 28.3]. Note: there are no efferent fibres in the middle cerebellar peduncle.

### Superior cerebellar peduncle

The superior cerebellar peduncle connects the cerebellum to the midbrain. Each of these peduncles begins in the roof of the fourth ventricle and passes anteriorly as it ascends, forming the lateral wall of the superior part of the fourth ventricle. It is the principal efferent pathway from the cerebellum. **Efferent fibres**: it contains the dentato-thalamic and dentato-rubro-thalamic tracts. Its fibres arise mainly from the dentate nucleus. The fibres of the superior cerebellar peduncle decussate in the tegmentum of the midbrain at the level of the inferior colliculus, and pass to the thalamus and to the red nucleus of the opposite side. Some fibres descend into the pons in the central tegmental fasciculus [see Figs. 28.9A, 28.9B; see also Fig. 29.5]. **Afferent fibres**: the anterior spinocerebellar tract enters the cerebellum in the superior cerebellar peduncle.

## Interior of the cerebellum

The surface of the cerebellum is covered by a thin layer of grey matter—the **cerebellar cortex**—which overlies the deeper **white matter**. The **deep nuclei of the cerebellum** are situated deep in the white matter of the cerebellum. They are the **dentate**, **globose**, **fastigial**, and **emboliform** nuclei [Figs. 29.4A, 29.4B].

Using the instructions given in Dissection 29.2, cut the cerebellum to expose the white matter and deep nuclei.

### Deep nuclei of the cerebellum

There are four nuclei of the cerebellum which lie deep in the white matter. The **dentate nucleus** is the largest and most lateral of the group. It lies close to the cerebellar recess of the fourth ventricle. It has the shape of a thin, crinkled lamina of grey matter, very similar in appearance to the inferior olivary nucleus in the medulla. Like the inferior olivary nucleus, it has a wide mouth, or hilus, which faces anterosuperiorly. Fibres from the dentate nucleus cross the midline and project to the red nucleus of the opposite side in the superior cerebellar peduncle [Fig. 29.5]. The other three deep nuclei—the **emboliform**, **globose**, and **fastigial**—lie between the dentate nucleus and the midline [Fig. 29.4B].

### Cerebellar cortex

The cerebellar cortex has a uniform structure throughout and consists of three layers—(1) the granular layer; (2) the Purkinje cell layer; and (3) the molecular layer. The deepest layer is the **granular**

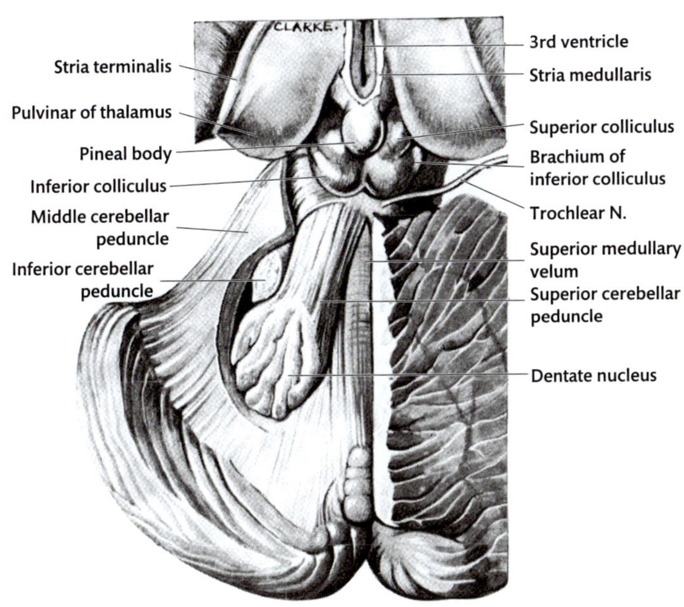


**Fig. 29.5** Dissection to show the dentate nucleus, cerebellar peduncles, tectum of the midbrain, and superior surface of the diencephalon.





**layer** which contains small granule cells. The axons of the granule cells go superficially to the molecular layer. The middle layer—the **Purkinje cell layer**—has a single row of large cell bodies of the **Purkinje cells**; they send their axons into the white matter, and their branching dendrites superficially into the molecular layer where they spread out in a plane at right angles to the folia. The surface layer is the **molecular layer** which has stellate and basket cells. This layer also contains the dendrites of the Purkinje cells, and the axons of the granule cells pass running parallel to the folia [Fig. 29.6].

## DISSECTION 29.2 Vermis and dentate nucleus

### Objectives

**I.** To remove the right half of the cerebellum and examine the cut surface of the vermis. **II.** To make a horizontal section through the cerebellar hemisphere and identify the dentate nucleus.

### Instructions

1. Split the cerebellum into two equal parts by a midline sagittal section through the vermis. Make this incision carefully, separating the two parts as the incision is deepened.
2. Note that approximately halfway between the superior and inferior margins of the cerebellum, a narrow slit is opened into. This is the **cerebellar recess of the fourth ventricle**.
3. Identify the cerebellar peduncles of the right side, and make a vertical incision through them, just posterior to the brainstem.
4. Remove the right half of the cerebellum from the remainder of the brain.
5. Examine the mid-sagittal section of the vermis, and note the folded grey matter of the cortex and the white matter deep to it. The white matter fits the complex folds of the cortex and has the appearance of a branching tree—the **arbor vitae cerebelli** [Fig. 29.1].
6. Make a transverse incision midway through the right half of the cerebellum.
7. Identify the **dentate nucleus**, a crinkled bag of grey matter within the central mass of white matter. It lies relatively close to the midline. It is the largest of the deep nuclei of the cerebellum [Fig. 29.4].
8. Remove the remains of the membranes from the surface of the midbrain, avoiding, if possible, damage to the trochlear nerves.
9. Identify the pineal body between the superior colliculi [see Fig. 28.3], and note that it is attached to the dorsal surface of the brain at the junction of the midbrain and diencephalon, inferior to the splenium of the corpus callosum.

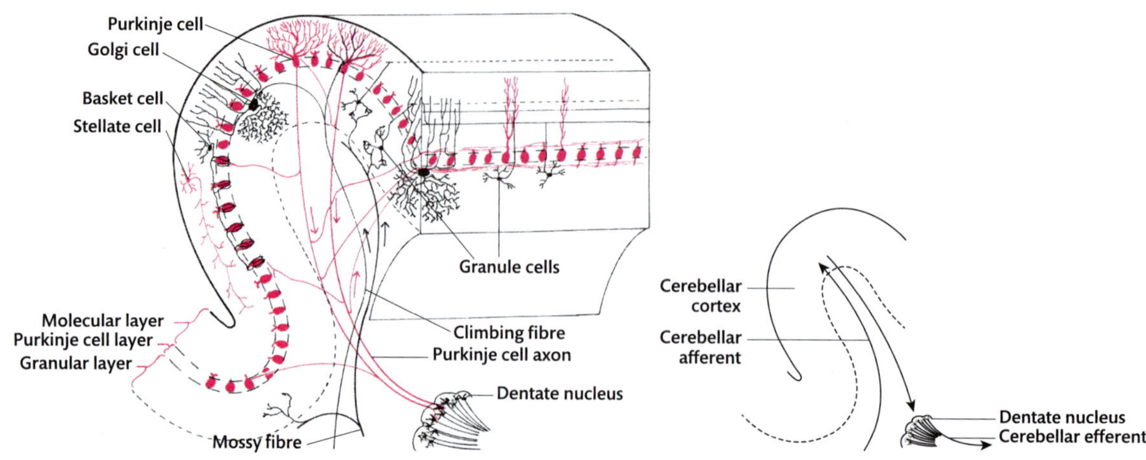


**Fig. 29.6** A diagram of the main nerve cells and their processes in the cerebellar cortex. A single folium is shown cut longitudinally (right) and transversely (left). Both mossy and climbing fibres send collaterals to the cerebellar nuclei. Inset: cerebellar circuitry in brief.





## Cerebellar circuitry

All fibres entering the cerebellum project to the cerebellar cortex. The cerebellar cortex projects to the deep nuclei. All fibres leaving the cerebellum arise in the deep nuclei [Fig. 29.5].

### Cerebellar afferents

The cerebellum receives sensory impulses from the spinal cord and vestibular nuclei, and motor information from the cerebral cortex and basal ganglia [Chapter 31]. All afferent fibres end by synapsing with cells in the cerebellar cortex. There are two types of afferent fibres—the mossy fibres and climbing fibres. Fibres from the inferior olivary nucleus (the olivocerebellar fibres) are the **climbing fibres**. They ascend through the deeper layers and end by synapsing in the molecular layer with the dendrites of the Purkinje cells. All other fibres (spinocerebellar, pontocerebellar, and others) are **mossy fibres**. They end in the granular layer by synapsing with the granule cells. The axons of the granule cells synapse with the dendrites of the Purkinje cells in the molecular layer. All the afferents to the cerebellum send their impulses directly or indirectly to the Purkinje cell dendrites in the molecular layer. The axons of the Purkinje cells project to the deep nuclei of the cerebellum.

### Efferents of cerebellum

The deep nuclei of the cerebellum give rise to all the efferent fibres of the cerebellum [Fig. 29.6]. The following flow chart illustrates the path of the impulses entering the cerebellum as mossy and climbing fibres:

Afferent, mossy fibres →granule cell →Purkinje cell dendrites →Purkinje cell axon →Deep nuclei →Efferent

## Functional subdivisions of the cerebellum

Based on the functions and connections, the cerebellum is divided into three parallel sagittal regions—the **spinocerebellum**, **cerebrocerebellum**, and **vestibulocerebellum** [Fig. 29.7]. Each of these regions includes an area of the cortex and an underlying deep nucleus. The spinocerebellum includes the vermis and paravermal cortex, and globose and emboliform nuclei. The remaining lateral area of the cortex and the dentate nucleus form the neocerebellum or pontocerebellum. The flocculonodular lobe with the fastigial nucleus forms the vestibulocerebellum.

### Connections of the vestibulocerebellum

The cortex of the flocculonodular lobe (vestibulocerebellum) receives fibres from the vestibular nuclei and projects to the fastigial nucleus. Efferents of the fastigial nuclei hook over the superior cerebellar peduncle and descend in the inferior cerebellar peduncle to the vestibular nuclei and the reticular formation of the medulla oblongata.

### Connections of the spinocerebellum

The cortex of the vermis and paravermal regions (spinocerebellum) receive the spinocerebellar and

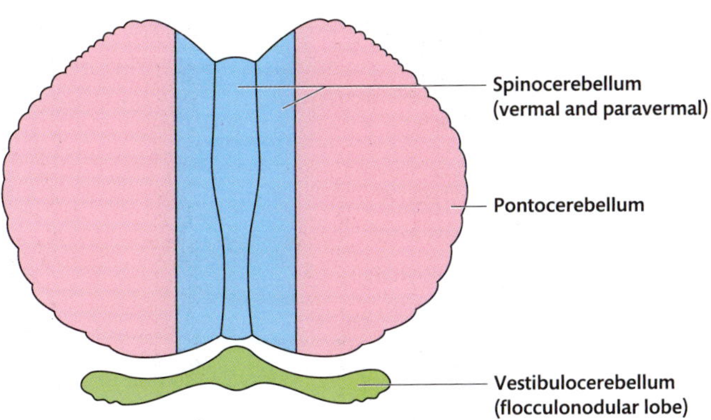


**Fig. 29.7** Schematic representation of the function areas of the cerebellum. The cerebellum is shown 'opened out'. The superior surface on the upper half, and the anteroinferior surface on the lower half of the image.

cuneocerebellar fibres, and project to the globose and emboliform nuclei. These nuclei project to the reticular formation and vestibular nuclei.

## Connections of the neocerebellum

The cerebellar cortex of the lateral sides of the hemisphere (neocerebellum) receives the pontocerebellar fibres and projects to the dentate nucleus. The axons of the dentate nucleus emerge from its medial side to form the superior cerebellar peduncle [Fig. 29.5]. The fibres of the superior cerebellar peduncle go to the red nucleus and thalamus. The major output from the cerebellum is from the neocerebellum.

The main afferent and efferent pathways of the cerebellum are shown in Fig. 29.8.

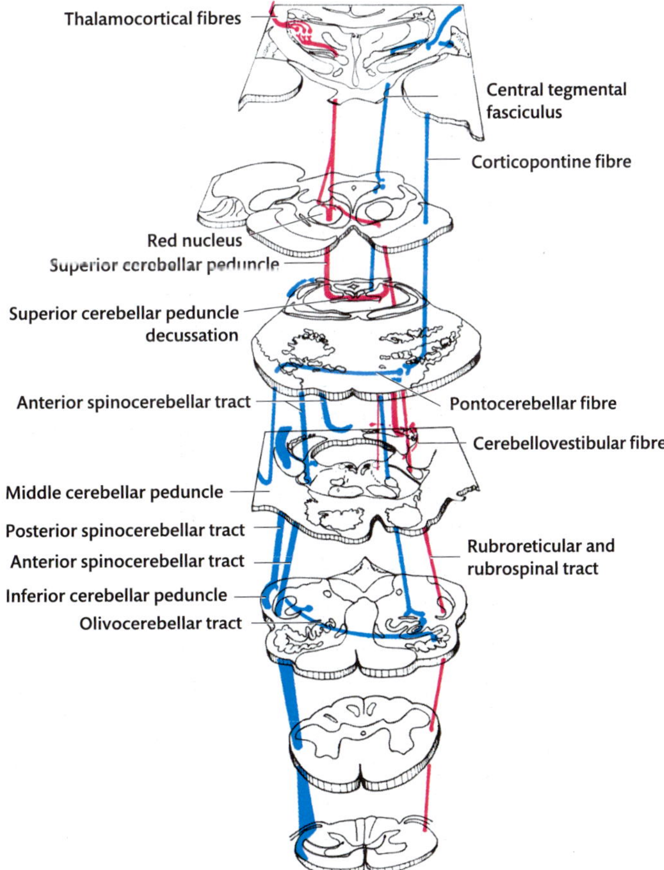


**Fig. 29.8** A diagram to show the main afferent (pontocerebellar, olivocerebellar, and anterior and posterior spinocerebellar pathways = blue) and efferent (to the red nucleus and thalamus = red) connections of the cerebellum. Serial sections are shown through the spinal cord, lower medulla, upper medulla, medulla-pons junction, pons, midbrain, and thalamus.

## Overview of the spinocerebellar fibres

The spinal input to the cerebellum consists mostly of subconscious proprioception from the limbs and trunk. The fibre tracts conveying these impulses are the: (1) posterior spinocerebellar tract; (2) cuneocerebellar tract; and (3) anterior spinocerebellar tract. (The less important rostral spinocerebellar tract carries fibres from the upper trunk and limbs to the ipsilateral cerebral hemisphere.)

### Posterior spinocerebellar tract

The **posterior spinocerebellar tract** transmits proprioceptive information from the inferior half of the same side of the body to the cerebellum. The tract arises from the cells of the thoracic nucleus (lamina VII) and ascends in the posterolateral part of the lateral column of the same side [see Figs. 27.4, 27.6]. In the medulla oblongata, the posterior spinocerebellar tract lies anterior to the spinal tract of the trigeminal nerve. It then passes posteriorly over the lateral surface of the spinal tract of the trigeminal and enters the inferior cerebellar peduncle [Fig. 29.8].

### Cuneocerebellar tract

The **cuneocerebellar tract** arises from the cells of the accessory cuneate nucleus [see Fig. 28.7] and enters the ipsilateral cerebellum through the inferior cerebellar peduncle. It transmits proprioceptive information from the upper limb, which reach the accessory cuneate nucleus through the fasciculus cuneatus.

### Anterior spinocerebellar tracts

Fibres of the **anterior spinocerebellar tract** arise from laminae V to VII of the lumbosacral spinal cord and carry information from the lower limb. The fibres cross the midline in the spinal cord, ascend in the lateral column anterior to the posterior spinocerebellar tract [see Figs. 27.4, 27.6], pass through the medulla oblongata and pons anterior to the spinal tract of the trigeminal nerve, and turn posteriorly into the cerebellum over the superior cerebellar peduncle [see Fig. 28.2]. They cross the midline a second time to enter the cerebellar hemisphere on the same side as the origin of the fibres [Fig. 29.8].

## Cerebellar lesions

### Lesions in the vestibulocerebellum

➲The vestibulocerebellum consists of the flocculonodular lobe and has two-way connections with the vestibular nuclei. Lesions in this part of the cerebellum would result in **loss of balance**, **dizziness**, and **nystagmus** (a condition where the eyes make involuntary repetitive movements from side to side).

### Lesions in the spinocerebellum

➲The spinocerebellum consists of the vermis and paravermal region. Lesions in the vermis result in **truncal ataxia**—an inability to stand without support.

### Lesions in the neocerebellum

➲Diseases of the neocerebellum or pontocerebellum result in problems with motor planning and ipsilateral coordination. When fine, purposeful movements are attempted, the hand trembles as it reaches the target. This is known as **intention tremor** and is due to lack of coordination between the agonists and antagonists acting on the elbow and wrist. For the same reason, the hand may go past the target object—**overshoot**. Another sign of inability to plan movements accurately and incoordination is **dysdiadochokinesis**—an inability to perform alternating movements, such as pronation and supination, smoothly.

Coordination is tested using the 'finger to nose' test where the patient is asked to alternately touch their nose and the physician's outstretched finger; and the 'heel to knee' test where the patient is asked to lie supine, place the heel of one foot on the opposite knee, and move it down the shin. An inability to execute these movements smoothly is a sign of cerebellar disease.

CHAPTER 30

# The diencephalon

## Diencephalon

The diencephalon develops from the primitive forebrain vesicle and encloses the third ventricle [see Table 24.1]. It is made up of the thalamus (or dorsal thalamus), epithalamus, hypothalamus, metathalamus, and subthalamus.

### Epithalamus

The epithalamus consists of the **pineal gland** and **habenular nuclei** [Fig. 30.1]. The **pineal gland** is a small structure attached to the habenular and posterior commissures by its stalk. It secretes melatonin, a hormone implicated in the sleep–wake cycle. The **habenular nuclei** lie in the habenular triangle, a small area between the medial aspect of the thalamus, the pineal stalk, and the superior colliculus [Fig. 30.2]. **Afferents**: the nuclei receive fibres from the septal nuclei (in the frontal lobe, anterior to the lamina terminalis) through the **stria medullaris thalami** [Fig. 30.2].

**Efferents**: they give rise to a small bundle of fibres—the fasciculus retroflexus—which runs through the upper part of the tegmentum of the midbrain and ends in the interpeduncular nucleus, a small collection of cells in the posterior perforated substance [see Fig. 30.7].

### Thalamus

The **thalamus** is a large mass of grey matter on the dorsal part of the diencephalon. It is concerned with processing of sensory information. Many of its cells transmit impulses to the sensory areas of the cortex, but it also has reciprocal connections with most parts of the cerebral cortex and with a number of subcortical masses of grey matter [see Fig. 30.6A].

#### Surfaces of the thalamus

The thalamus has four surfaces—medial, lateral, superior, and inferior; and two ends—anterior and posterior [Fig. 30.3].

The **anterior end** is narrow and rounded. It lies just posterior to the interventricular foramen and the column of the fornix. The **posterior end** of the thalamus is wide and overhangs the superior part of the midbrain. It is known as the **pulvinar** [Fig. 30.2].

The anterior two-thirds of the **medial surface** of the two thalami are covered with the ependyma. They form the lateral walls of the third ventricle, superior to the hypothalamic sulcus [Fig. 30.1]. The two thalami are frequently fused across the cavity of the third ventricle by the **interthalamic adhesion**. The posterior thirds are widely separated from each other and abut medially on the superior part of the midbrain [see Fig. 28.3].

The **superior surface** is limited laterally by the stria terminalis and the thalamostriate vein, and medially by the stria medullaris thalami [Fig. 30.2]. It tapers anteriorly to end in the rounded **anterior tubercle** of the thalamus. The groove for the fornix courses obliquely across the superior surface. The area lateral to the groove is covered with the ependyma of the floor of the lateral ventricle. The groove and the area medial to it are covered by the tela choroidea of the lateral ventricle. Where the superior and medial surfaces

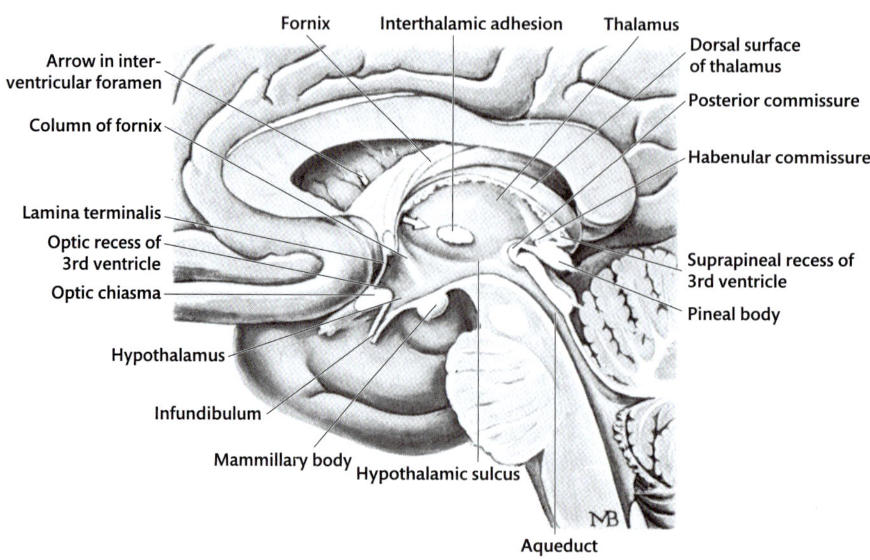


**Fig. 30.1** Median section through the brain to show parts of the diencephalon.

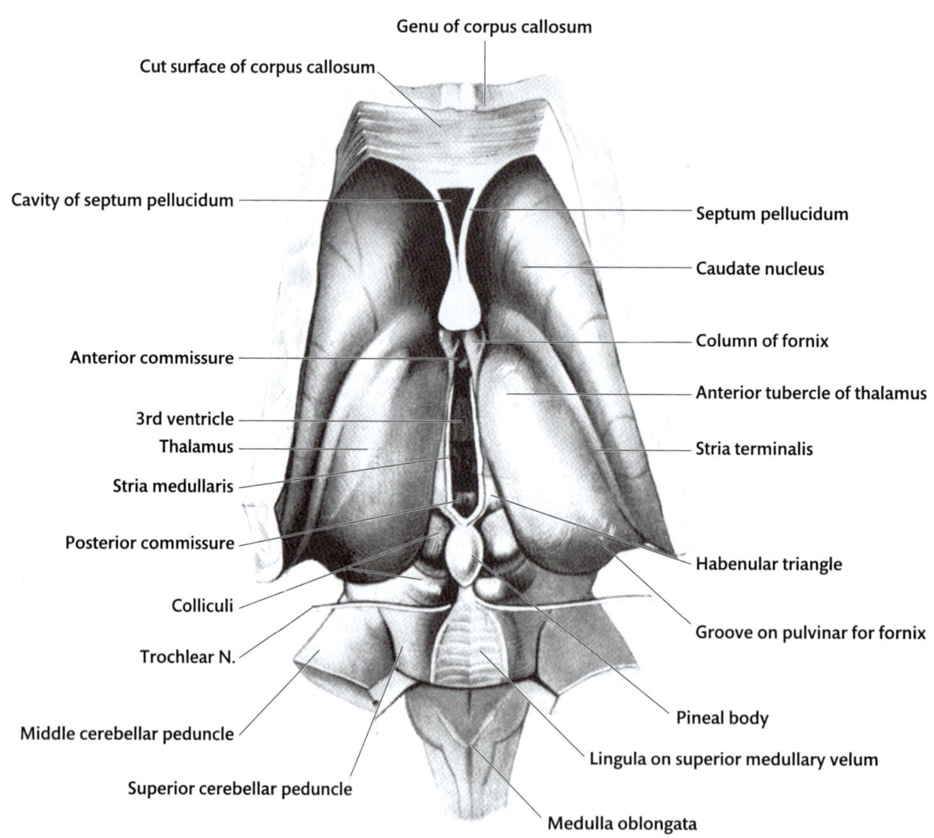


**Fig. 30.2** The thalami and third ventricle seen from above after removal of the overlying tela choroidea. [Compare with Fig. 32.7.]

meet, a delicate ridge of white matter—the **stria medullaris thalami**—run anteroposteriorly on the thalamus [Fig. 30.2]. The stria has the ependymal roof of the third ventricle attached to its medial margin, posterior to the interventricular foramen [Fig. 30.2].

The **lateral surface** of the thalamus is in contact with the internal capsule [Fig. 30.4].

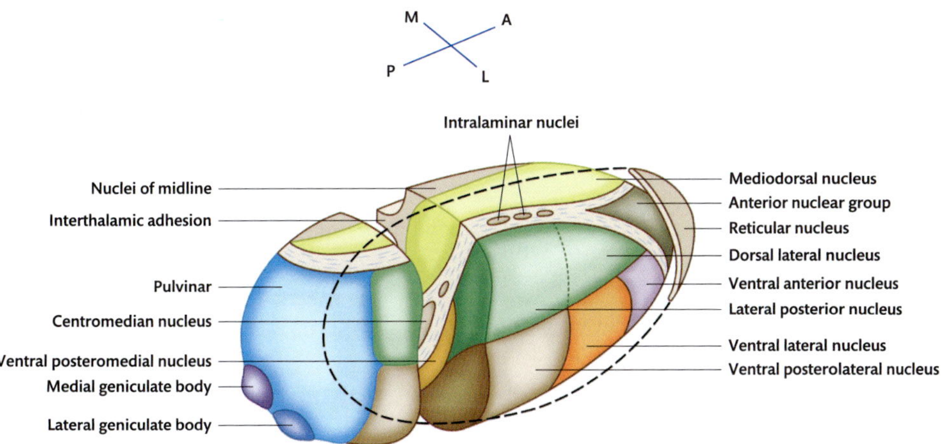


**Fig. 30.3** Main nuclear masses of the thalamus, viewed from the lateral side. (Only the anterior extent of the reticular nucleus is shown; its full extent is depicted by the interrupted black line.)





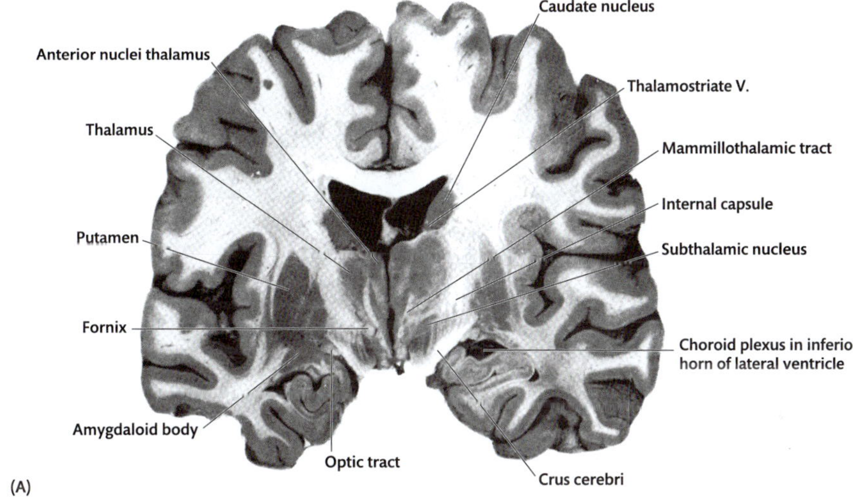


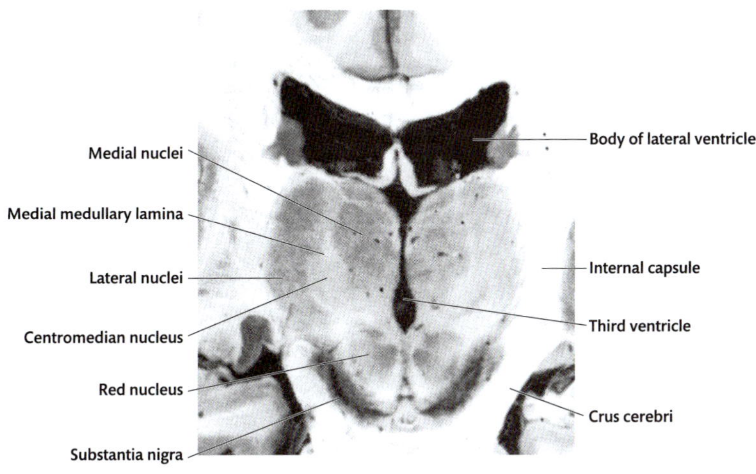


**Fig. 30.4** (A) Coronal section through the brain at the level of the mammillary bodies. (B) Coronal section through the brain, passing through the basilar part of the pons. Note the division of the thalamus into the medial and lateral nuclei.

Most of the **inferior surface** rests on the hypothalamus. The posterior part—the pulvinar—is free and exhibits two rounded swellings—the medial and lateral geniculate bodies [see Fig. 28.2].

### Laminae and nuclei of the thalamus

The thalamus is subdivided into a number of separate cell groups or nuclei by two layers of white matter—the medial and lateral medullary laminae—which run approximately in the sagittal plane.

The **medial medullary lamina** lies midway between the third ventricle and the internal capsule. It divides the thalamus into **medial** and **lateral nuclei** [Fig. 30.3]. Inferiorly, the medial medullary lamina curves medially under the medial nuclei. Anteriorly, the medial medullary lamina splits into two to enclose the **anterior nucleus** [Fig. 30.4]. Posteriorly, the medial medullary lamina encloses the **centromedian nucleus** [Fig. 30.3] and a number of other small **intralaminar nuclei**.

The **lateral medullary lamina** lies close to the internal capsule. A thin, broken lamina of grey matter—the **reticular nucleus** of the thalamus—lies between the lateral medullary lamina and the internal capsule [Fig. 30.4].

The **medial nuclei** (**mediodorsal nuclei**) lie between the third ventricle and the medial medullary lamina. The lateral nuclear mass is further subdivided into lateral and ventral nuclear masses. The **lateral nuclei** consist of the **lateral posterior** and **dorsal lateral nuclei**. The **ventral nuclei** consist of the **ventral anterior**, **ventral lateral**, **ventroposterior lateral**, and **ventroposterior medial** nuclei [Fig. 30.4]. There is no clear line of demarcation between the lateral and ventral nuclei.

The **pulvinar** lies behind the ventral nucleus, lateral to the medial medullary lamina. It is best seen on the inferior and lateral aspects of the thalamus [Fig. 30.2]. The **medial geniculate** and **lateral geniculate bodies** lie on the inferior surface of the pulvinar.

## Metathalamus

The medial and lateral geniculate bodies constitute the **metathalamus**. They are located on the inferior aspect of the pulvinar.

The **medial geniculate body** is a well-defined oval mass [Fig. 30.3]. The **lateral geniculate body** lies anterolateral to the medial geniculate body [Figs. 30.4B, 30.3, 30.5] and is directly continuous anteriorly with the **optic tract**.

## Connections of the thalamus and metathalamus

### Overview of thalamic and metathalamic connections

**Afferents**: the thalamus and metathalamus together receive sensory input from: (1) the **body** through the spinothalamic tract, medial lemniscus, and fibres from the trigeminal nuclei; (2) the **eyes** through the

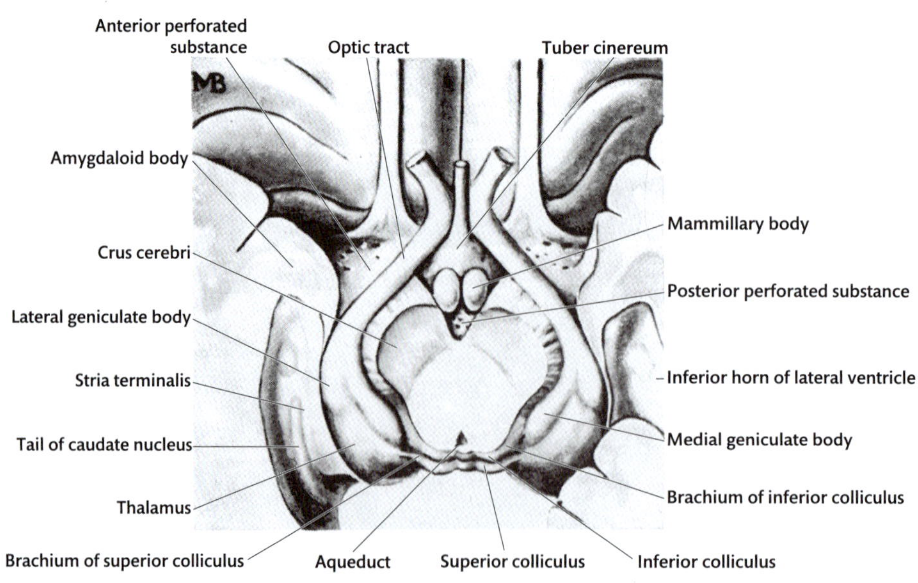


**Fig. 30.5** Base of the brain seen from below to show the optic tracts.

optic tract; (3) the **inner ear** through the brachium of the inferior colliculus; (4) the **hypothalamus** through the mammillothalamic tract; (5) the **cerebellum** either directly from the dentate nucleus or through the red nucleus; and (6) the **globus pallidus** of the corpus striatum. In addition to these, most of the thalamic nuclei receive: (7) reciprocal fibres from the area of the **cerebral cortex** to which they project; and (8) other **thalamic nuclei** through intrathalamic connections.

**Efferents**: the thalamus sends efferent fibres to almost all parts of the **cerebral cortex** [Fig. 30.6]. In addition, it sends fibres to the **hypothalamus**, **corpus striatum**, and **reticular formation** of the brainstem. The **thalamocortical fibres** form the **sensory radiations** which transmit sensory information to the cerebral cortex through the internal capsule and corona radiata [Fig. 30.6].

## Specific thalamic and metathalamic connections

### Anterior nucleus

**Afferents**: the **anterior nucleus** of the thalamus receives the **mammillothalamic tract** from the mammillary nuclei in the hypothalamus [see Fig. 32.5]. **Efferents**: it sends efferent fibres to the cingulate gyrus. The anterior nucleus is part of the limbic system which connects the hippocampus, hypothalamus, thalamus, and other parts of the limbic lobe [Chapter 32].

### Ventral posterior nucleus

**Afferents**: the **ventral posterior nucleus** of the thalamus receives fibres from the spinothalamic tract, medial lemniscus, and trigeminothalamic tract (from the sensory nuclei of the trigeminal nerve). The spinothalamic tract and medial lemniscus convey sensory impulses from the opposite side of the body and end in the **ventroposterior lateral** nucleus of the thalamus. The trigeminothalamic tract conveys sensory impulses from the opposite half of the face and ends in the **ventroposterior medial** nucleus of the thalamus [see Fig. 31.29]. **Efferents**: fibres from these two nuclei project to the sensory cortex of the cerebrum through the thalamocortical radiations.

## Medial geniculate body

The medial geniculate body is part of the auditory pathway. **Afferents**: it receives the brachium





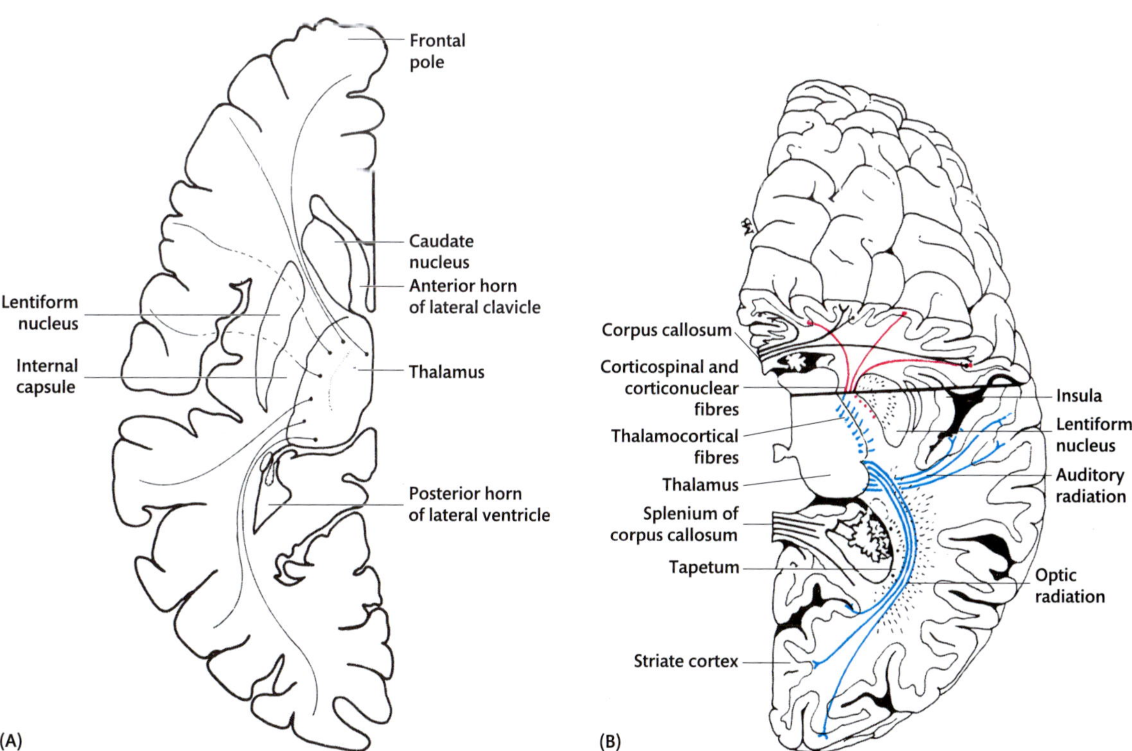


**Fig. 30.6** (A) Thalamocortical radiations to the cerebral cortex. The broken lines indicate fibres arching superiorly out of the section over the lentiform nucleus. (B) Diagrammatic representation of projection fibres. Pink = descending 'motor' fibres; blue = ascending sensory fibres; black = commissural fibres of the corpus callosum.

of the inferior colliculus, which carries auditory impulses from the inferior colliculus [see Fig. 29.2]. **Efferents**: it sends efferent fibres to the transverse temporal gyrus through the auditory radiation [see Fig. 24.5; Figs. 30.5, 30.6].

### Lateral geniculate body

The lateral geniculate body is part of the visual pathway. **Afferents**: each lateral geniculate body receives fibres from the contralateral visual field through the optic tract. **Efferents**: it gives rise to fibres of the **optic radiation** which convey visual impulses to the occipital lobe of the cerebral cortex [Fig. 30.6; see Fig. 31.37].

### Role of geniculate bodies

➲ The geniculate bodies are metathalamic nuclei concerned with the auditory and visual pathways. They differ from each other in that the lateral geniculate body is the only route through which impulses generated in the opposite half of the field of vision can reach the cerebral cortex, whereas each medial geniculate body carries auditory impulses originating in both cochleae. Thus, destruction of one lateral geniculate body produces blindness in the opposite half of the field of vision, but destruction of one medial geniculate body has little effect on hearing.

# Hypothalamus

The hypothalamus forms the lateral wall of the third ventricle, inferior to the hypothalamic sulcus [Fig. 30.1]. Parts of the hypothalamus—the mammillary bodies and infundibulum—appear on the inferior surface of the brain in the interpeduncular fossa [Fig. 30.5]. Laterally, the hypothalamus extends to the lower part of the internal capsule. Inferiorly, it is continuous with the tegmentum of the midbrain, without any line of demarcation.

## Nuclei of the hypothalamus

The nuclei of the hypothalamus are arbitrarily divided into three groups, from anterior to posterior: (1) the **chiasmatic** or **supraoptic group of nuclei**, in the region above the optic chiasma. They include the **supraoptic**, **anterior**, and **paraventricular nuclei**; (2) the **tuberal group of nuclei** above the infundibulum. They include the **arcuate**, **ventromedial**, and **dorsomedial nuclei**; and (3) the **posterior** or **mammillary group of nuclei** above the mammillary bodies. They include the **mammillary body nucleus** and the **posterior nucleus**. The **preoptic nucleus** lies anterior to the supraoptic group of nuclei. These groups are also classified according to their distance from the midline into the most medial or **periventricular group**, the middle or **medial group**, and the **lateral group**.

## Connections of the hypothalamus

The connections of the hypothalamus are complex, and only a few important ones are mentioned here. **Afferents**: the hypothalamus receives input from the hippocampus, thalamus, and brainstem. **Efferents**: it gives efferent fibres to other parts of the brain and to the pituitary.

### Connections of the mammillary body

The mammillary body is part of the limbic system. **Afferents**: it receives input from the hippocampal formation through the fornix. **Efferents**: it gives fibres to the anterior nucleus of the thalamus through the mammillothalamic tract [Fig. 30.7] and to the tegmentum of the midbrain through the mammillotegmental tract [Fig. 30.7].

### Connections of the supraoptic and paraventricular nuclei

Cells in the supraoptic and paraventricular nucleus have axons extending into the posterior pituitary to end in relation to vascular sinusoids there. They carry neurosecretions produced in these nuclei to the blood vessels of the posterior pituitary. They form the hypothalamohypophyseal tract.

### Vascular connections

The hypothalamus and hypophysis are also connected by the hypothalamohypophyseal portal system. Through this vascular system, secretions of the arcuate, preoptic, and other nuclei of the hypothalamus reach the anterior pituitary and influence secretion of hormones produced in it.

## Functions of the hypothalamus

The hypothalamus is concerned with a number of visceral functions. It controls the autonomic nervous system, regulates temperature, and regulates eating, drinking, sleeping and waking, sexual arousal, fear, and rage.

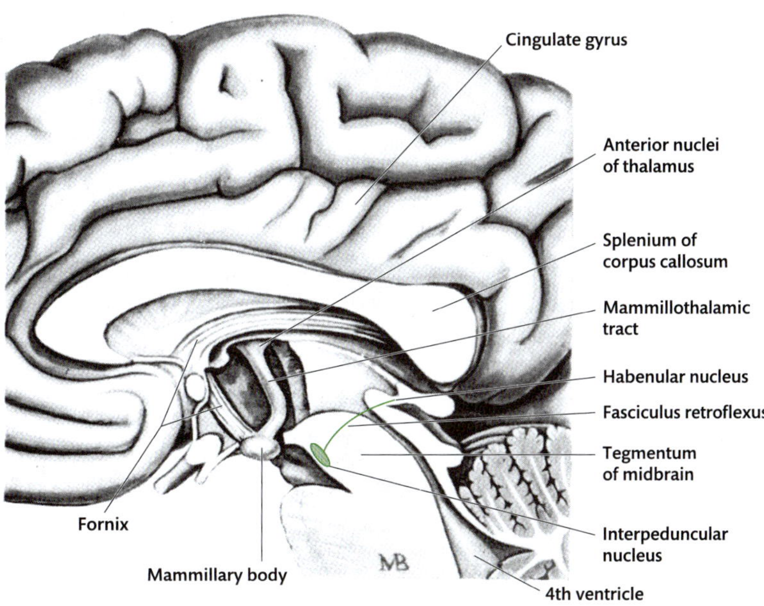


**Fig. 30.7** Dissection to show the fornix and mammillothalamic tract.



## Subthalamus

The subthalamus lies just rostral to the tegmentum of the midbrain, lateral to the hypothalamus [Fig. 30.4B]. **Afferents**: it receives fibres from the globus pallidus through the subthalamic fasciculus. **Efferents**: most of its efferent fibres pass back to the globus pallidus, but some probably descend into the midbrain. ➲ Lesions of the subthalamic nucleus give rise to hemiballism, a condition marked by abrupt onset of wild, flailing movement of the opposite upper limb.

See Clinical Application 30.1 for the practical implication of the anatomy discussed in this chapter.

### CLINICAL APPLICATION 30.1 Thalamic infarct

A 72-year-old woman presented in the Neurology clinic with a two-day history of numbness on the right side of her face, decreased sensation in her right arm, and loss of sensation in her right foot. A computerized tomography (CT) scan revealed a small lacunar infarct in the left thalamus.

Study question 1: which nucleus in the thalamus receives sensory input from the right side of the face? (Answer: the left ventroposterior medial (VPM) nucleus.)

Study question 2: trace the pathway from the right side of the face to the left VPM nucleus. (Answer: right side of face > trigeminal nerve > main sensory and spinal nuclei of trigeminal > trigeminothalamic tract on left side > ascends in pons and midbrain > ends in VPM nucleus of thalamus [see Fig. 28.5B].)

Study question 3: which nucleus in the thalamus receives sensory input from the right leg? (Answer: the left ventroposterior lateral (VPL) nucleus.)

Study question 4: trace the pathway from the right leg to the left VPL nucleus. (Answer: (1) pathway for crude touch, vibration, and position sense: sensory nerves of leg > dorsal root ganglion > fasciculus gracilis > nucleus gracilis > internal arcuate fibres > medial lemniscus on left side > VPL nucleus of thalamus; (2) pathway for pain and temperature: sensory nerves of leg > dorsal root ganglion > cells in posterior grey horn > spinothalamic tract of left side > VPL nucleus of thalamus.)

CHAPTER 31

# The cerebrum

## External features of the cerebral hemisphere

Begin your study of this region by reviewing the relationship between the skull and the brain, with the help of a dry skull. Note the relationship of the parts of the brain to the folds of the dura mater (the falx cerebri and the tentorium cerebelli) in a cadaver where the brain has been removed. Also review the external features of the cerebrum described in Chapter 24.

The **longitudinal fissure** is the narrow cleft between the two cerebral hemispheres. It is occupied by: (1) the falx cerebri; (2) the fold of the arachnoid which follows the surface of the falx; (3) the pia mater covering the medial surfaces of the hemispheres; and (4) the arteries and veins which lie in the subarachnoid space. (The falx was removed when the brain was taken from the skull, but the other structures are still *in situ*.)

### Surfaces and borders of the cerebral hemisphere



**Surfaces**: each cerebral hemisphere has three surfaces: (1) the convex **superolateral surface** [Fig. 31.1]; (2) the **medial** surface; and (3) the **inferior surface** [Fig. 31.2]. The inferior surface has an anterior **orbital part** which rests on the floor of the anterior cranial fossa, and a posterior **tentorial part** which rests on the floor of the middle cranial fossa and the tentorium cerebelli. The medial

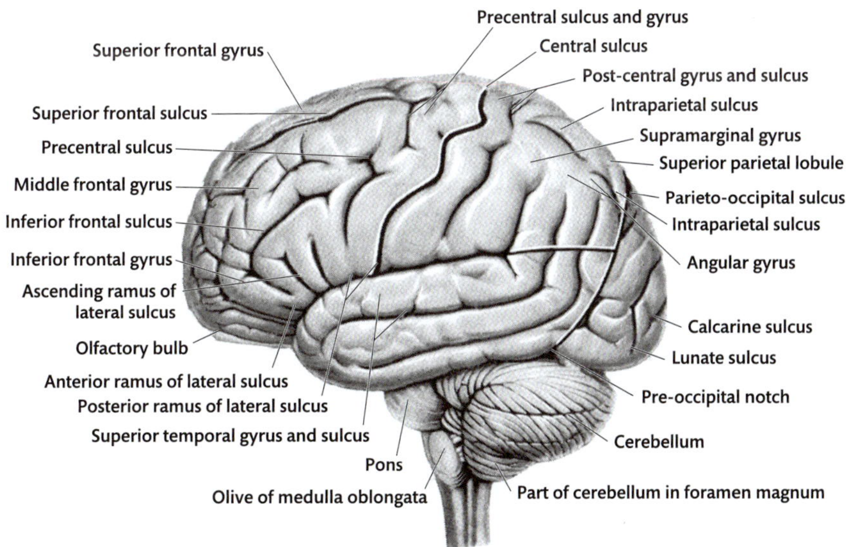


**Fig. 31.1** Lateral surface of the brain to show the sulci and gyri. The division of the superolateral surface into lobes by the central sulcus and two arbitrary lines is shown.

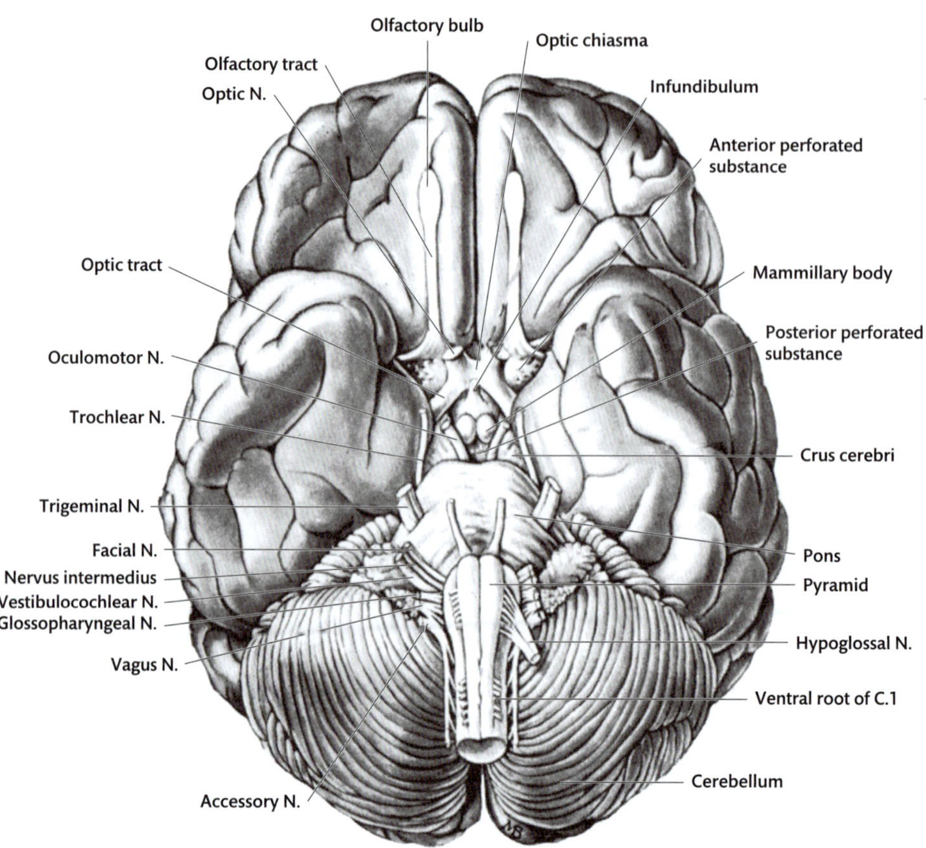


**Fig. 31.2** The base of the brain and the cranial nerves.

surface is flat and vertical, and lies against the falx cerebri [Fig. 31.3].

**Borders**: the three borders of the cerebral hemisphere are the: (1) **superomedial** border; (2) **inferolateral** border; and (3) **medial** border. The superomedial border lies along the longitudinal fissure. The anterior part of the inferolateral border is the **superciliary border** which lies at the junction of the superolateral and orbital surfaces. About 3 cm from the occipital pole, the inferolateral border exhibits a notch—the **preoccipital notch** [Fig. 31.1]—where the inferior anastomotic vein enters the transverse sinus. The border at the junction of the medial and orbital surfaces is the **medial orbital border**, and that at the junction of the medial and tentorial surfaces is the **medial occipital border**. Together the medial orbital and medial occipital borders form the medial border.

Using the instructions given in Dissection 31.1, section the cerebrum in the midline [Fig. 31.3].

## Cerebral cortex

Start your study of the cerebral cortex by removing the arachnoid mater from the surface of the cerebrum and identifying the lobes, poles, and main sulci and gyri of the cerebral cortex.

Remove the arachnoid mater of the brain, following the instructions provided in Dissection 31.2.

### Lobes of cerebrum

The cerebrum is divided into four lobes—the **frontal lobe** anteriorly, the **parietal lobe** laterally, the **occipital lobe** posteriorly, and the **temporal lobe** inferiorly. Using Fig. 31.4, identify the sulci and imaginary lines which separate one lobe from the other on the superolateral and medial surfaces. (Detailed descriptions of the sulci are given later.) (1) The central sulcus and an imaginary line extending down from it to the posterior ramus of the lateral sulcus separate the

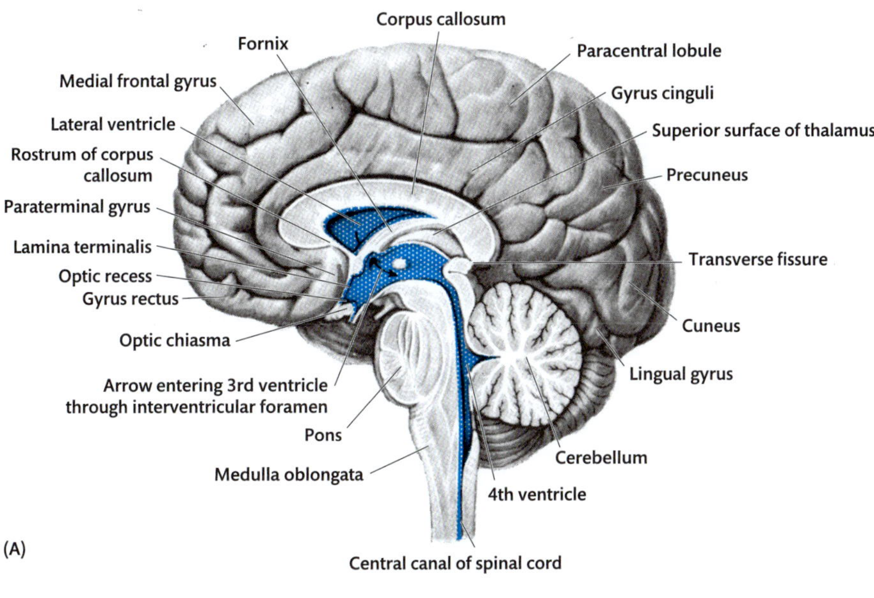


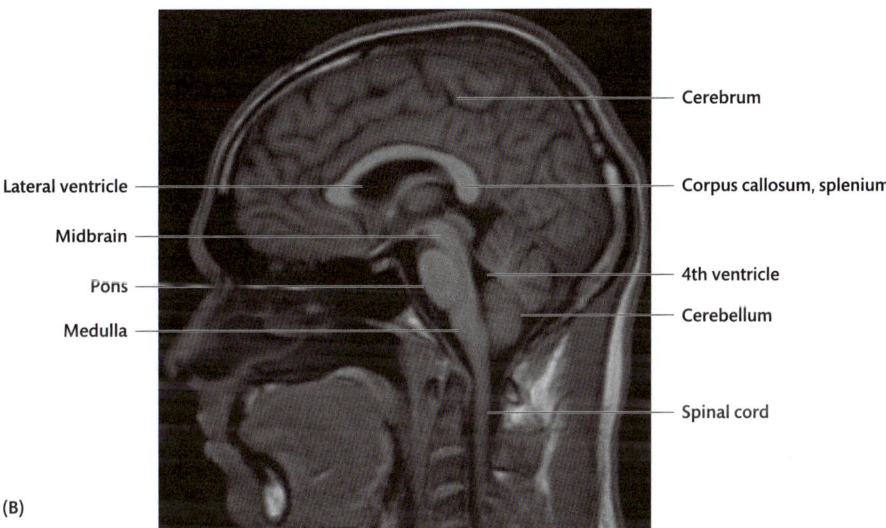


**Fig. 31.3** (A) Medial surface of the right hemisphere. The septum pellucidum has been removed to expose the lateral ventricle. The arrow passes through the interventricular foramen from the lateral to the third ventricle. Ependymal lining of ventricles = blue. (B) T1-weighted sagittal magnetic resonance imaging (MRI) of the brain.

frontal lobe in front from the parietal lobe behind. (2) The posterior ramus of the lateral sulcus and a line extending posteriorly from it separates the parietal lobe from the temporal lobe. (3) An imaginary line joining the parieto-occipital sulcus and the pre-occipital notch separates the temporal and parietal lobes in front from the occipital lobe behind [Fig. 31.4].

## Poles of cerebrum

The most anterior extent of the frontal lobe forms the **frontal pole**. The most posterior extent of the occipital lobe forms the **occipital pole**, and the most anterior extent of the temporal lobe forms the **temporal pole** [Fig. 31.4].

## General features of cerebral sulci and gyri

The cerebral cortex extends as an uninterrupted sheet over the whole surface of the hemisphere and consists of nerve cells which are arranged in layers parallel to the surface [Fig. 31.5]. These layers are differentiated from each other in a microscopic section by their different cell

## DISSECTION 31.1 Hemisection of the cerebrum

### Objectives

**I.** To remove the right half of the cerebral hemisphere. **II.** To identify the features seen on the medial side of the cerebral hemisphere.

### Instructions

1. Separate the two cerebral hemispheres at the longitudinal fissure, and expose the mass of white matter which joins them deep in the fissure. This is the **corpus callosum**, the posterior part of which (**splenium**) has already been seen as a thick, rounded mass superior to the pineal body.
2. At the splenium of the corpus callosum, identify the **great cerebral vein** emerging between the pineal body and the splenium of the corpus callosum.
3. Divide the corpus callosum in the midline, starting at the splenium. Proceed carefully, noting that the corpus callosum is much thinner immediately anterior to the splenium and that a thin layer of pia mater lies inferior to the corpus callosum in this part.
4. Divide the right posterior cerebral artery close to its origin from the basilar artery.
5. Turn to the right side of the brain, and make a transverse cut through the upper part of the right half of the midbrain so as to join the two ends of the median cut. Now lift away the right hemisphere.
6. Examine the medial aspect of the hemisphere.
7. Pass a fine probe through the cerebral aqueduct from the posterosuperior part of the third ventricle to the fourth ventricle.
8. Identify the features on the medial surface of the cerebrum, using Fig. 31.3. The cut surface of the corpus callosum is seen near the middle. Identify its parts: the rostrum, genu, body, and splenium.
9. The third ventricle lies inferior to the body of the corpus callosum.
10. The fornix—an arch of white matter—lies in close apposition to the corpus callosum posteriorly. Anteriorly, it curves downwards as the column of the fornix.
11. The septum pellucidum is a thin vertical sheet of white matter which stretches from the corpus callosum to the fornix. The septum is made up of two laminae (the **laminae of the septum pellucidum**) which enclose a narrow space—the **cavum septi pellucidi**—between them [see Fig. 30.2].
12. Follow the rostrum of the corpus callosum downwards. At its lower extremity, a round bundle of fibres will be seen in the midline, immediately anterior to the columns of the fornix. This is the **anterior commissure** [see Fig. 31.8].
13. Identify the thin lamina terminalis which extends inferiorly from the anterior commissure and forms the anterior wall of the third ventricle.
14. Trace the lamina terminalis down to the cut end of the optic chiasma.
15. Turn to the inferior surface of the brain, and identify the optic chiasma and the cut end of the anterior communicating artery which unites the two anterior cerebral arteries above the chiasma.
16. Identify the interventricular foramen, as it lies inferior to the fornix, and pass a probe through it into the lateral ventricle.
17. Identify the choroid plexus in the roof of the third ventricle.
18. Identify the thalamus on the lateral wall of the third ventricle and the bridge of tissue crossing the third ventricle—the interthalamic adhesion.
19. Identify the infundibulum and mammillary bodies on the inferior aspect of the third ventricle.

## DISSECTION 31.2 Removal of the arachnoid mater

### Objectives

**I.** To remove the arachnoid from the surface of the cerebrum. **II.** To identify and trace the middle cerebral artery and its branches.

### Instructions

1. Review the vessels on the surfaces of the cerebral hemisphere, and then proceed to strip the arachnoid from its surface.
2. On the superolateral surface of the brain, strip the arachnoid towards the lateral sulcus [Fig. 31.1], pulling it off along the line of the other sulci.
3. Note the large branches of the middle cerebral artery which arise from the lateral sulcus.
4. Remove the arachnoid mater from the medial and inferolateral surfaces.

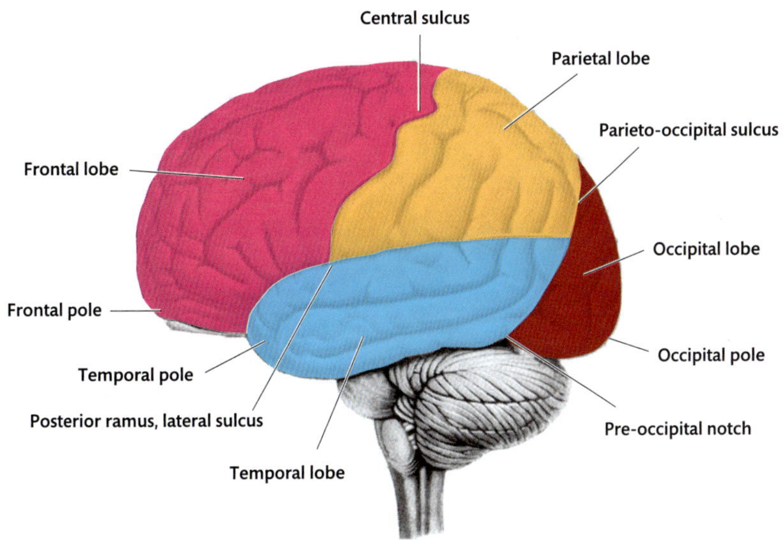


**Fig. 31.4** Lateral surface of the brain to show the main sulci and gyri. The division of the superolateral surface into lobes by the central sulcus and two arbitrary lines is shown.

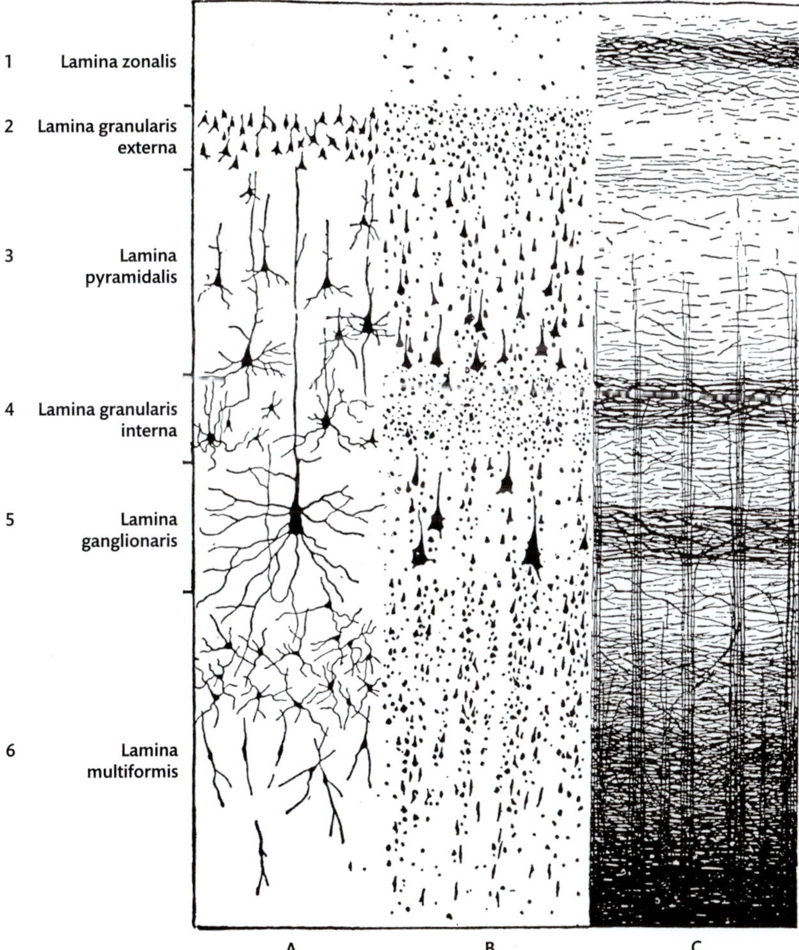


**Fig. 31.5** Arrangement of cells and myelinated nerve fibres in the cerebral cortex. (A) Cells shown by the Golgi method; (B) cells shown by the Nissl method; (C) nerve fibres shown by the Weigert method.

Reprinted from *An Introduction to Neurology*, 5th edition, Herrick, CJ. W.B. Saunders (Elsevier) 1938.

contents. The cortex is thicker on the summits of the gyri than in the depths of the sulci. There are great individual variations in the details of the sulci and gyri, so attention should be given mainly to the major sulci and gyri. These can be identified with the help of Figs. 31.6, 31.7, 31.8, 31.9 and 31.10.

The **sulci** vary in depth, from slight grooves to deep fissures. Some sulci, like the calcarine and collateral sulci, are sufficiently deep to indent the wall of the lateral ventricle. The **gyri** consist of a central core of white matter (nerve fibres running to and from the overlying cortex), covered by a layer of grey matter—the **cerebral cortex** [see Fig. 31.13].

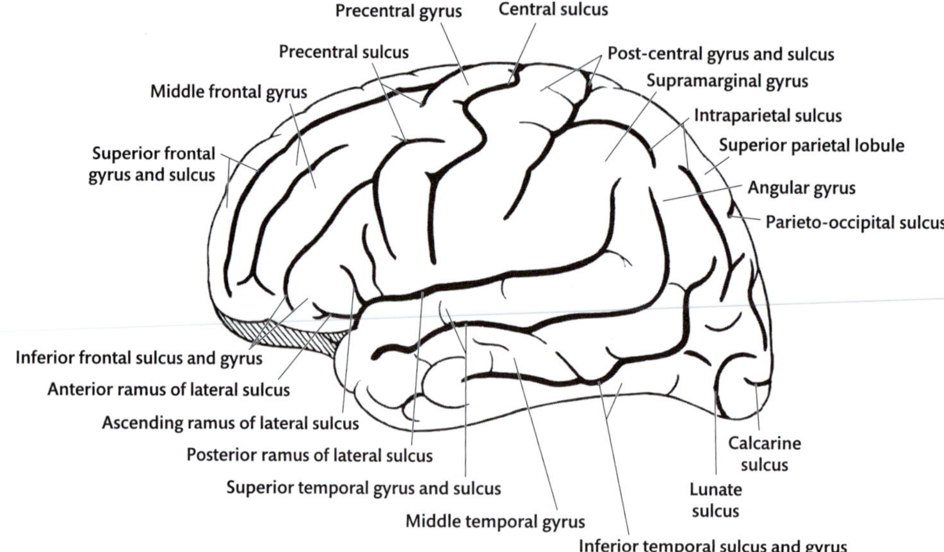


**Fig. 31.6** Sulci and gyri of the superolateral surface of the left hemisphere.

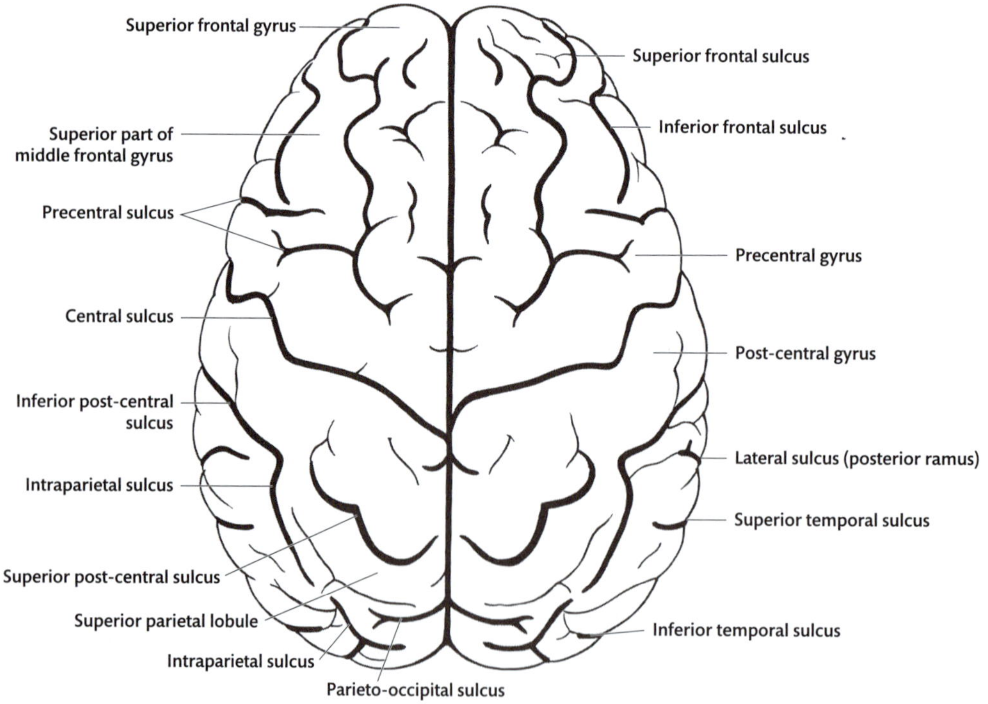


**Fig. 31.7** Sulci and gyri of the cerebral hemispheres viewed from above.

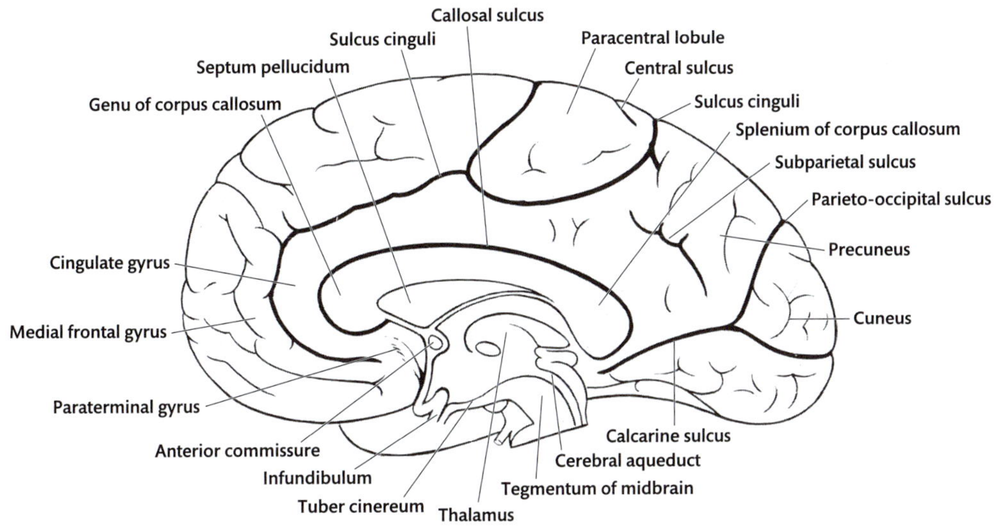


**Fig. 31.8** Sulci and gyri of the medial surface of the right cerebral hemisphere.

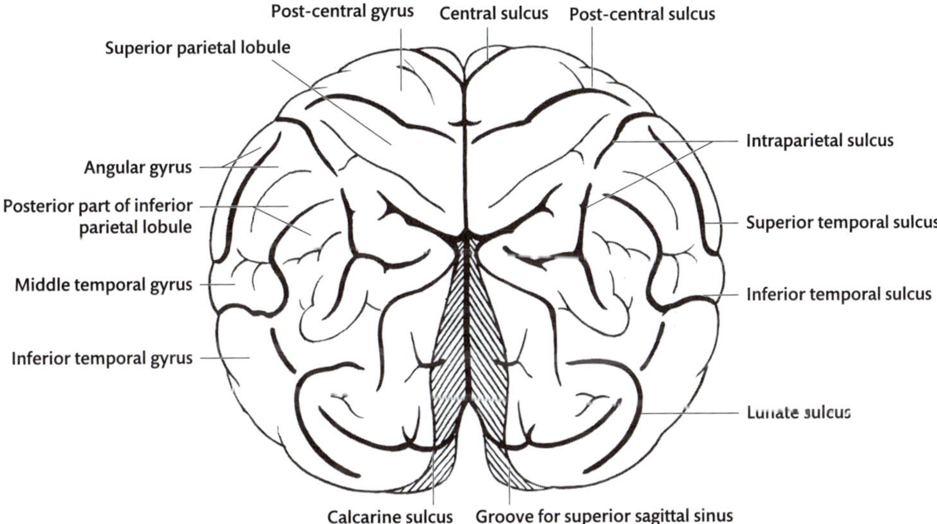


**Fig. 31.9** Sulci and gyri of the posterior view of the cerebral hemispheres.



## Sulci and gyri on the superolateral surface

### Central sulcus

The important **central sulcus** begins superiorly on the medial surface of the hemisphere, approximately midway between the frontal and occipital poles [Fig. 31.6]. It crosses the superomedial border and extends anteroinferiorly on the superolateral surface to end just above the posterior ramus of the lateral sulcus, 2–3 cm behind its origin. The central sulcus separates the frontal and parietal lobes of the hemisphere [Figs. 31.6, 31.7]. It is of special importance because it separates the main '**motor**' and '**sensory**' **areas** of the cerebral cortex.

### Lateral sulcus

For the most part, the stem of the lateral sulcus lies on the inferior surface of the brain. It ends on the superolateral surface by dividing into **anterior**, **ascending**, and **posterior rami** [Fig. 31.6]. The anterior and ascending rami extend into the inferior frontal gyrus. The posterior ramus runs backwards and separates the frontal and parietal lobes of the brain from the temporal lobe inferiorly. The terminal part of the posterior ramus curves upwards

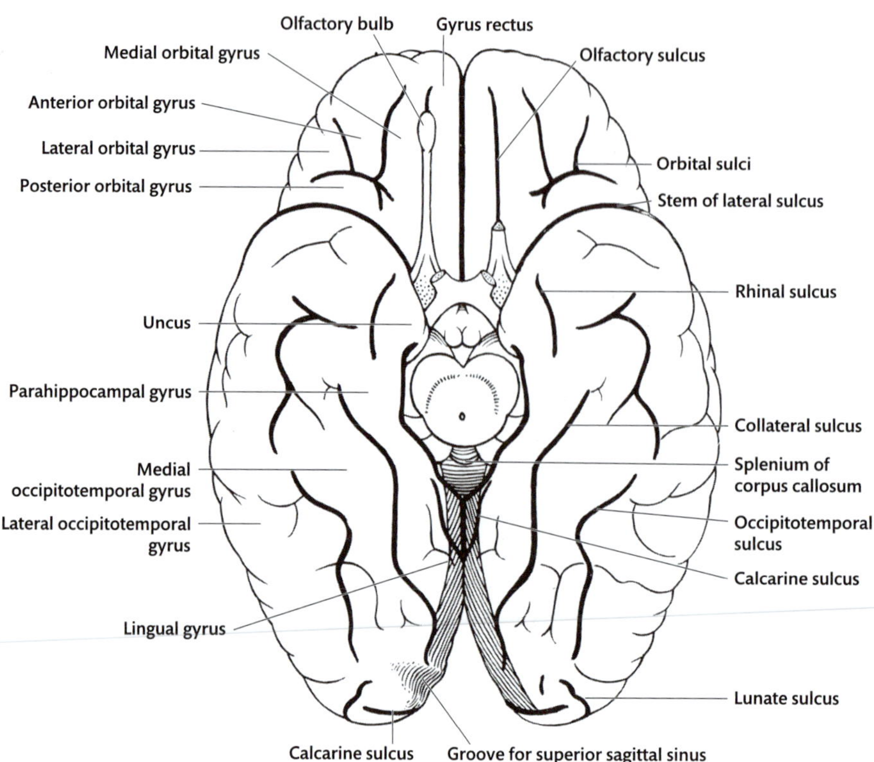


**Fig. 31.10** Sulci and gyri of the inferior surface of the cerebral hemispheres.

into the parietal lobe. When the lips of the lateral sulcus are pulled apart, the **insular cortex** is exposed. The main branches of the middle cerebral artery can be seen running over it before emerging from the sulcus onto the superolateral surface of the hemisphere.

### Sulci and gyri on the frontal lobe

In front of, and parallel to, the central sulcus is the **precentral sulcus**, with the **precentral gyrus** between the two [Figs. 31.6, 31.7].

The anterior part of the frontal lobe, the part in front of the precentral gyrus, has the **superior** and **inferior frontal sulci**, which divide the cortex of this area into **superior**, **middle**, and **inferior frontal gyri** [Figs. 31.6, 31.7].

### Sulci and gyri on the parietal lobe

The **post-central gyrus** and **post-central sulcus** lie immediately behind the central sulcus in the parietal lobe [Figs. 31.6, 31.7]. Behind the post-central sulcus, the **intraparietal sulcus** divides this part of the parietal lobe into **superior** and **inferior parietal lobules** [Fig. 31.6]. The posterior ramus of the lateral sulcus and the superior and inferior temporal sulci sweep superiorly into the inferior parietal lobule and divide it into three parts arranged around the ends of these three sulci. The two anterior parts are the **supramarginal** and **angular gyri** [Fig. 31.6].

### Sulci and gyri on the temporal lobe

The superolateral surface of the temporal lobe is divided into the **superior**, **middle**, and **inferior temporal gyri** by the **superior** and **inferior temporal sulci** [Figs. 31.1, 31.7].

### Sulci and gyri on the occipital lobe

The terminal part of the **calcarine sulcus** curves around the superomedial border of the cerebrum and appears on the superolateral surface of the occipital lobe. The short **lunate sulcus** surrounds the end of the calcarine sulcus [Fig. 31.6].

## Sulci and gyri on the medial surface

### Parieto-occipital and calcarine sulci

These two deep sulci form a Y-shaped depression on the medial aspect of the posterior part of the hemisphere [Fig. 31.8].

The **calcarine sulcus** begins just below the splenium of the corpus callosum and extends backwards and slightly upwards. The posterior end of the calcarine may extend round the occipital pole on the superolateral surface. When the **calcarine sulcus** extends to the superolateral surface, the end is surrounded by the **lunate sulcus** [Figs. 31.6, 31.9].

The **parieto-occipital sulcus** begins at the middle of the calcarine sulcus and extends upwards and backwards to the superomedial border. The superior end of the parieto-occipital sulcus reaches the superolateral surface. An imaginary line joining the superior end of the parieto-occipital sulcus to the pre-occipital notch separates the occipital lobe from the parietal and temporal lobes.

### Sulci and gyri on the frontal lobe

The **callosal sulcus** lies immediately adjacent to the corpus callosum. The **cingulate sulcus** (**sulci cinguli**) lies parallel to the callosal sulcus. It begins inferior to the genu of the corpus callosum and curves forwards, upwards, and backwards to run posteriorly in the frontal lobe. At its posterior end, the cingulate sulcus curves upwards towards the superomedial border [Fig. 31.8]. The **cingulate gyrus** lies between the callosal and cingulate sulci. The **medial frontal gyrus** lies in front of, and superior to, the cingulate sulcus as it curves [Figs. 31.3, 31.8]. The cortex immediately anterior to the lamina terminalis is the **paraterminal gyrus**. The cortex on either side of the central sulcus on the medial surface of the brain is the **paracentral lobule** and contains the parts of the frontal and parietal lobes.

### Sulci and gyri on the parietal lobe

The cerebral cortex in front of the parieto-occipital sulcus is the **precuneus**, and the area between the parieto-occipital sulcus and calcarine sulcus is the **cuneus**.

### Sulci and gyri on the occipital lobe

The **lingual gyrus** lies inferior to the calcarine sulcus and extends onto the inferior surface of the cerebrum [Fig. 31.8].

## Sulci and gyri on the inferior surface

### Lateral sulcus

The **stem of the lateral sulcus** lies in the depression which runs laterally between the temporal pole and the posterior part of the orbital surface of the hemisphere [Fig. 31.10]. It contains the middle cerebral artery and veins. The stem ends on the superolateral surface of the cerebrum.

### Sulci and gyri on the frontal lobe

The H-shaped **orbital sulcus** on the orbital surface of the frontal lobe divides the major part of this surface into the **anterior**, **medial**, **posterior**, and **lateral orbital gyri** [Fig. 31.10]. The **olfactory sulcus** lies on the medial side of the medial orbital gyrus and separates it from the **gyrus rectus**. The **olfactory bulb** and **tract** lie in the **olfactory sulcus**.

### Sulci and gyri on the temporal lobe

The **uncus** is a raised area on the inferior surface of the temporal lobe. It is separated from the remainder of the temporal lobe by the **rhinal sulcus** [Fig. 31.10]. The uncus is continuous posteriorly with the **parahippocampal gyrus**, which is separated from the remainder of the temporal lobe by the **collateral sulcus**. The collateral sulcus is often continuous with the rhinal sulcus. The uncus and parahippocampal gyrus form the **inferomedial border** of the hemisphere and lie close to the free margin of the tentorium. The remainder of the inferior surface of the temporal lobe is divided into the **medial** and **lateral occipitotemporal gyrus** by the **occipitotemporal sulcus**.

# Functional areas of cerebral cortex

Areas of the cortex subserve specific functions. Based on the functions, the cerebral cortex can be divided into **motor areas**, **sensory areas**, and **association areas**. Motor areas control voluntary movements; sensory areas process sensory information, and association areas integrate information for higher cognitive functions.

## Motor cortex

### Primary motor area

The '**primary motor**' area, the area responsible for movement of skeletal muscles of the opposite side of the body, lies in the anterior wall of the central sulcus and the adjacent part of the precentral gyrus. Most of the corticospinal and corticonuclear fibres arise from the motor cortex. Within the motor cortex, there is a further functional subdivision—movements of the opposite side of the head and neck are brought about by neurons lying in the inferior precentral region, and neurons controlling movements of the upper limb, trunk, lower limb, and perineum follow in sequence superiorly. The area for the lower limbs and genitalia lies in the part of the post-central gyrus on the medial surface of the cerebrum, in the paracentral lobule [Fig. 31.8].

➲ The frontal branch of the **middle meningeal artery** runs on the dura mater, parallel to, and a short distance anterior to, the central sulcus [see Fig. 7.17]. Haemorrhage from this artery is likely to press on this region of the brain and interfere with the voluntary movements in the opposite half of the body.

### Premotor area

The premotor cortex is situated in front of the motor cortex and helps to plan and coordinate movements.

### Motor speech area (Broca's area)

The '**motor speech area**' lies in the inferior frontal gyrus [Figs. 31.6, 31.11]. This region is intimately connected with the control of movements of the larynx and tongue through connections with the motor area immediately posterior to it. The complex mechanism which subserves speech involves many other regions of the brain, most commonly in the left hemisphere.

## Sensory cortex

### Primary somatosensory cortex

The '**sensory**' area lies in the posterior wall of the central sulcus and the adjacent part of the post-central gyrus. It receives sensory stimuli from the opposite side of the body through the thalamic radiations. Similar to the arrangement of motor neurons in the motor cortex, sensory fibres from the opposite side of the head end in the inferior post-central region and the other regions of the body are represented in sequence superiorly [Figs. 31.6, 31.8, 31.11].

The cortex on either side of the central sulcus on the medial surface of the brain is the **paracentral lobule**, and contains the parts of the frontal and parietal lobes. It contains the sensory and motor cortices of the lower limbs.

### Primary auditory cortex

The **auditory area** is the cortical area to which auditory impulses are primarily relayed. It lies on the middle of the superior surface of the superior temporal gyrus—the **transverse temporal gyrus**—and extends onto the lateral surface, inferior to the post-central gyrus [Fig. 31.11]. If the superior temporal gyrus is pulled inferiorly, the transverse temporal gyrus will be seen running across its superior surface.

### Primary visual cortex

The visual cortex lies on the upper and lower banks of the calcarine sulcus, in the cuneus and lingual gyrus [Fig. 31.12]. This cortex has a very well-defined white stria running through it and is called the **striate cortex**. The cerebral cortex enclosed by the lunate sulcus is part of the visual cortex [Figs. 31.6, 31.11].

## Association cortex

Association areas integrate sensory information and memory, facilitating higher-order cognitive

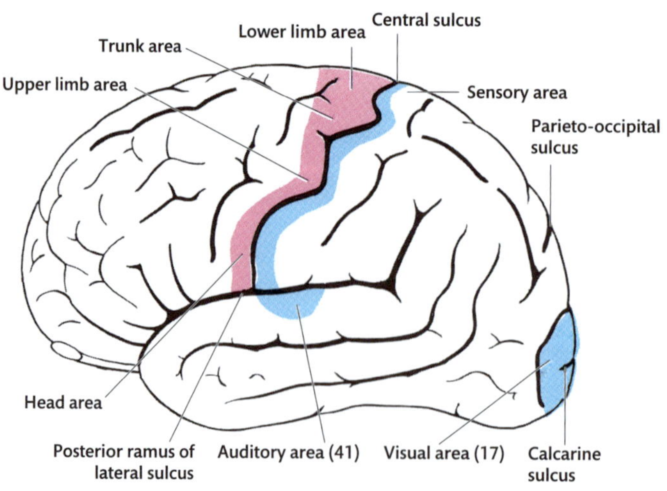


Fig. 31.11 Diagram of the superolateral surface of the left hemisphere. 'Motor' area = red; 'sensory' area = blue.

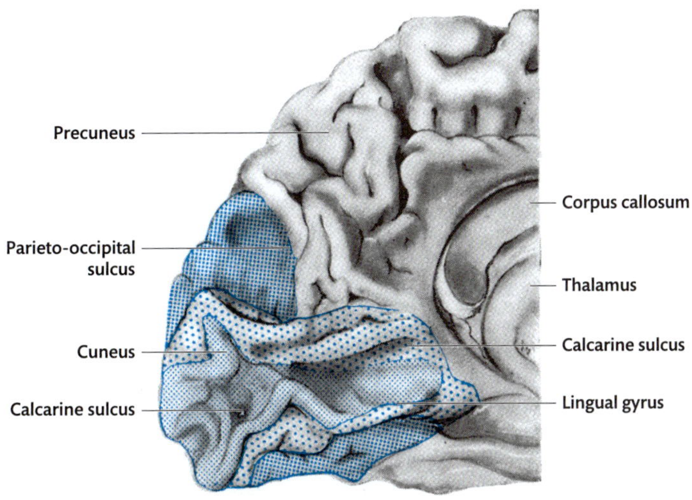


**Fig. 31.12** Posterior part of the medial surface of the left hemisphere. The calcarine sulcus has been forced open to expose the cortex lying in its depths. Fine blue dots = visual receptive area; coarse blue dots = visual association area; upper and lower dark blue areas have long association connections with other parts of the cortex.



**DISSECTION 31.3 Examination of the visual cortex**

**Objective**

I. To examine the visual cortex.

**Instructions**

1. Cut a slice through the calcarine sulcus, posterior to its junction with the parieto-occipital sulcus, and examine the cortex for the presence of the stria.

functions. The **supramarginal** and **angular gyri** are important in the recognition of structures and symbols, and body image. The cortex bordering the visual cortex on the occipital lobe contains the visual association area [Fig. 31.12].

Using the instructions given in Dissection 31.3, incise the visual cortex and inspect it.

## Insular cortex

The insula is that part of the cerebral cortex which is submerged in the lateral sulcus. It is roughly triangular in shape, and its margin is formed by the **circular sulcus**. The insula is hidden from view by parts of the frontal, parietal, and temporal lobes which are known as the **frontal**, **frontoparietal**, and **temporal opercula**. The cortex of the insula is continuous with the cortex on the deep surfaces of the **opercula**. The apex of the insula is known as the **limen insulae** [Fig. 31.13]. The surface of the insula is marked by a number of sulci and gyri radiating superiorly from the stem of the lateral sulcus, which lies at the apex. The middle cerebral artery lies on the limen insulae, as it passes laterally onto the surface of the insula. Medial to the limen insulae is the **anterior perforated substance**, through which the central branches of the middle and anterior cerebral arteries pass into the substance of the brain [Fig. 31.10].

Dissection 31.4 provides instructions on dissection of the insula.

## Olfactory pathway

The olfactory bulb and tract lie in the olfactory sulcus on the inferior aspect of the frontal lobe [Fig. 31.14]. The **olfactory bulb** is a narrow, oval body which lies on the dura mater, immediately above the cribriform plate of the ethmoid. It receives the 12–20 olfactory nerves from the olfactory mucosa in the nasal cavity. ➲ Fractures of the anterior cranial fossa are likely to damage the olfactory bulb and lead to anosmia.

The **olfactory tract** extends posteriorly in the olfactory sulcus [Fig. 31.14]. Posteriorly, it splits into the **medial** and **lateral olfactory striae**

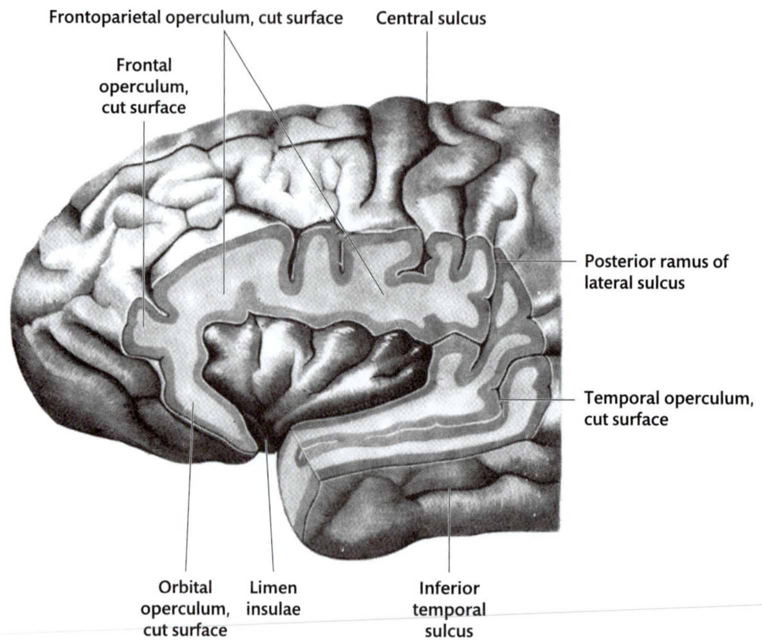


**Fig. 31.13** Dissection of the superolateral surface of the left hemisphere to show the insula.

> **DISSECTION 31.4 The insula**
>
> **Objective**
>
> I. To remove the opercula and expose the insula.
>
> **Instructions**
>
> 1. Expose the insula on the right cerebral hemisphere by removing the frontal, frontoparietal, and temporal opercula.
> 2. The greater part of the insula and the posterior part of the **superior longitudinal bundle** are now seen in the root of the operculum [see Fig. 31.23A].

at the anterior margin of the anterior perforated substance. Between the two striae, there is a small grey elevation—the **olfactory trigone**. The medial olfactory stria curves round the posterior end of the gyrus rectus to the medial side of the hemisphere and ends in the region of the **paraterminal gyrus** [Figs. 31.3, 31.15]. The lateral olfactory stria runs posterolaterally on the margin of the anterior perforated substance, curves round the stem of the lateral sulcus, and enters the uncus and anterior part of the parahippocampal gyrus. The uncus and anterior part of the parahippocampal gyrus constitute the piriform lobe.

## Limbic lobe

The **limbic lobe** is formed by a rim of the cerebral cortex adjacent to the corpus callosum and diencephalon. The limbic lobe is made up of the cingulate gyrus, parahippocampal gyrus, hippocampus, dentate gyrus, paraterminal gyrus, and uncus, and the bundles of white matter associated with them. The term **limbic system** includes the limbic cortex, as well as related subcortical nuclei, including the **amygdala**.

### Hippocampus

The **hippocampus** lies deep within the parahippocampal gyrus in the floor of the inferior horn of the lateral ventricle [Fig. 31.15]. Anteriorly, it turns medially near the tip of the inferior horn and becomes continuous with the uncus. This part of the hippocampus is ridged and known as the pes hippocampi [Fig. 31.16]. The hippocampus tapers posteriorly and is continuous with a small ridge—the **gyrus fasciolaris**—which curves round the inferior surface of the splenium [Fig. 31.15].

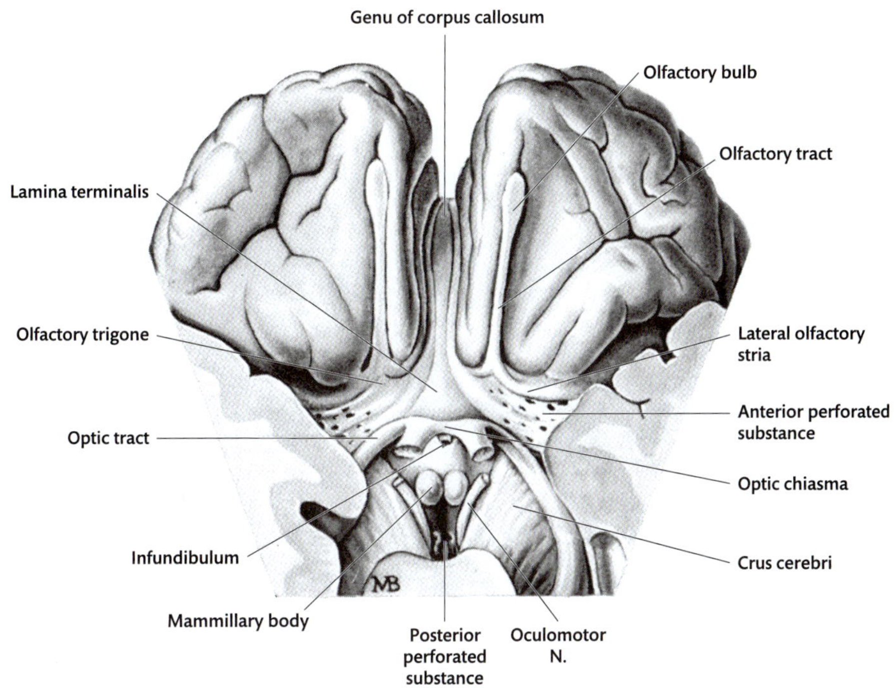


**Fig. 31.14** Orbital surfaces of the hemispheres and the interpeduncular fossa. The frontal lobes have been separated slightly to show the genu of the corpus callosum, and the optic chiasma has been pulled inferiorly to uncover the lamina terminalis.

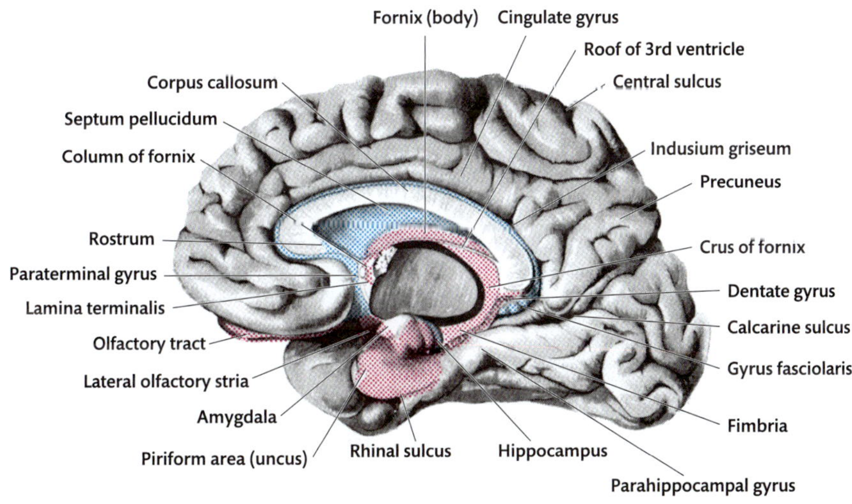


**Fig. 31.15** Medial aspect of the right cerebral hemisphere, with the limbic parts coloured. The olfactory bulb, tract, and lateral stria, the uncus, and the dentate gyrus are shown in red. The hippocampus, indusium griseum, paraterminal gyrus, septum pellucidum, and medial olfactory stria are shown in blue.

## Connection of the hippocampus

**Afferents**: the hippocampus receives afferents from the parahippocampal gyrus and the amygdala. **Efferents**: the hippocampus projects to the mammillary body, anterior nucleus of the thalamus, and septal region. Efferent fibres from the hippocampus run across the floor of the inferior horn of the lateral ventricle as the **alveus**. They then form the **fimbria** of the hippocampus on the medial margin of the hippocampus and continue posteriorly as the **crus of the fornix** [Fig. 31.17]. The alveus, fimbria, and fornix together form the efferent pathway for the hippocampus.

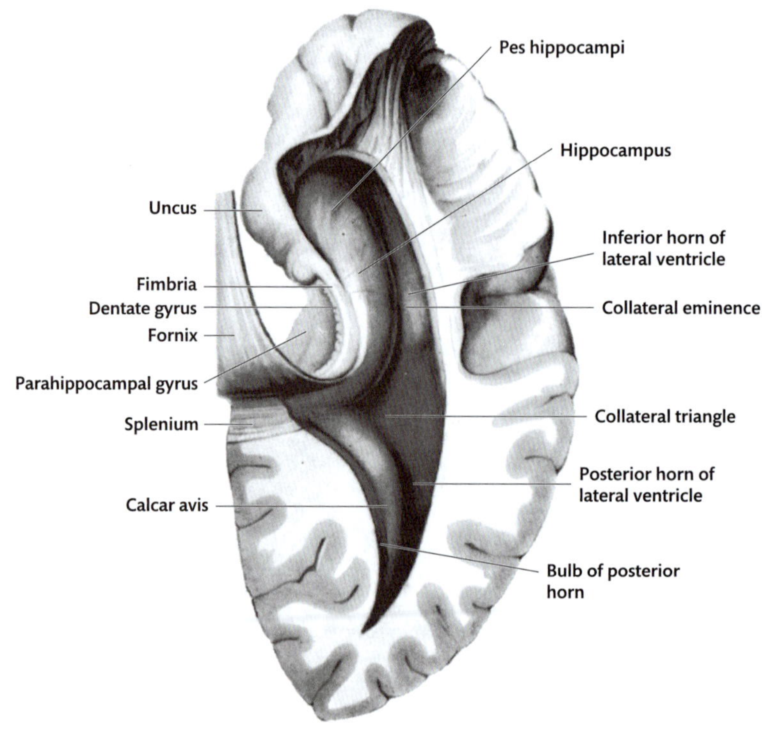


**Fig. 31.16** Posterior and inferior horns of the right lateral ventricle, viewed from above.

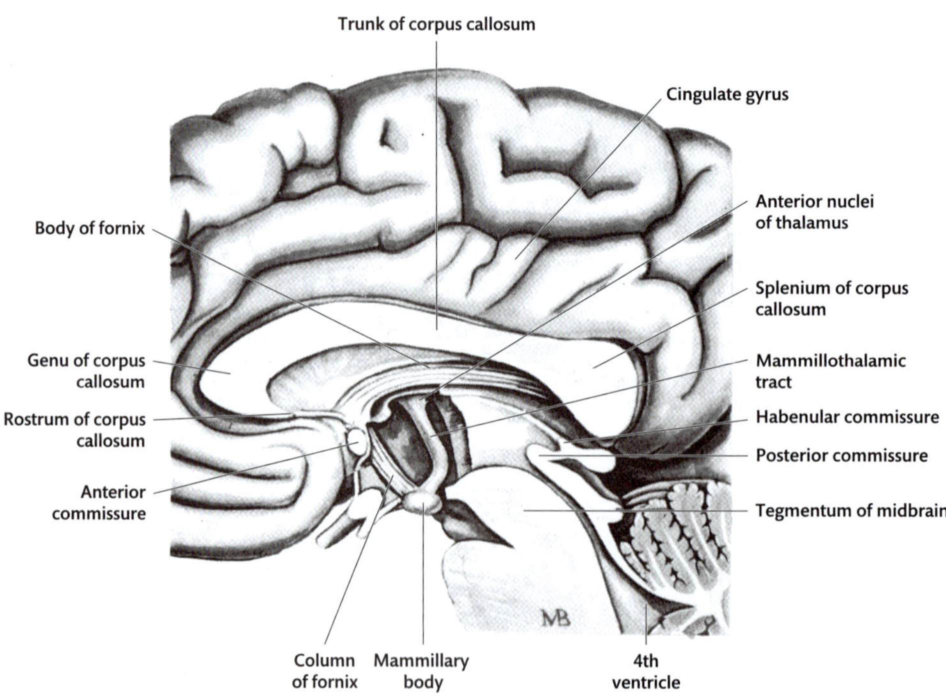


**Fig. 31.17** Medial surface of the cerebrum showing the commissures, fornix, and mammillothalamic tract.

## Fornix

The main efferent pathway from the hippocampus is the **fornix**, a C-shaped white fibre bundle which, together with the fimbria, forms almost one complete turn of a spiral. There is one fornix in each hemisphere, but the two are so closely fused beneath the middle of the trunk of the corpus callosum that they are usually described as a single structure [Figs. 31.16, 31.17].

**Parts of the fornix**: the fornix is made up of the two **crura**, **body**, and **column** of the fornix. The crus of the fornix is a flattened strip which arches upwards, medially, and forwards under the splenium of the corpus callosum to become continuous with that of the other side to form the **body of the fornix**. Anteriorly, the body becomes more cylindrical and separates to form the **columns of the fornix**. The columns run inferiorly between the anterior commissure and the interventricular foramen, curve posteriorly through the anterior hypothalamus, and end in the mammillary body [Figs. 31.16, 31.17].

The fibres in the fornix pass to: (1) the opposite hippocampus through the **commissure of the fornix**, which is situated where the two crura meet, inferior to the corpus callosum [see Fig. 32.5]; (2) the septal and anterior hypothalamic regions; and (3) the mammillary body. In addition, (4) a few of its fibres may pass directly to the anterior nuclei of the thalamus. The fornix also contains fibres which pass from the cells in the region of the anterior commissure—the septal nuclei—to the hippocampus.

Impulses from the hippocampus reach the mammillary body, anterior nucleus of the thalamus, and cingulate gyrus in series. Some fibres which arise in the cingulate gyrus pass through the cingulum to the parahippocampal gyrus and the hippocampus, thus producing feedback to the hippocampus. This entire circuit on the margin of the hemisphere (including parts of the hypothalamus) has been called the **limbic lobe**.

**Relations of the fornix**: the fornix forms the margin of the **choroid fissure** between the beginning of the fimbria and the interventricular foramen. It has the ependyma of the choroid plexus attached to its sharp lateral margin throughout this length [see Fig. 32.9].

The crura and body of the fornix groove the posterior and superior surfaces of the thalamus, respectively, and lie in the medial part of the floor of the lateral ventricle [see Fig. 30.2]. The columns of the fornix form slight ridges on the lateral wall of the third ventricle, inferior to the interventricular foramen [see Fig. 30.1].

## Dentate gyrus

The **dentate gyrus** lies in the depths of the hippocampal sulcus—the sulcus lying medial to the parahippocampal gyrus [Fig. 31.15]. It is a small gyrus, transversely ridged to give the appearance of 'teeth'. It continues anteriorly with the uncus. Posteriorly, the dentate gyrus is continuous with the gyrus fasciolaris and, through it, with the thin layer of grey matter on the superior surface of the corpus callosum—the **indusium griseum**. The indusium griseum follows the curve of the corpus callosum to the paraterminal gyrus, inferior to the rostrum of the corpus callosum [Fig. 31.15].

In addition to the specific connections mentioned earlier, all parts of the cerebral cortex are connected to the thalamus, striatum, brainstem reticular formation, and claustrum.

# Arterial supply to the cerebral cortex

Review the details of the arterial supply to the cerebral cortex described in Chapter 26. The cortex is supplied by the anterior, middle, and posterior cerebral arteries [see Figs. 26.3, 26.4, 26.5]. All three arteries supply parts of the three surfaces. The superolateral surface is mainly supplied by the middle cerebral artery [see Fig. 26.5], the medial surface by the anterior cerebral artery [see Fig. 26.4], and the inferior surface by the posterior cerebral artery [see Fig. 26.3].

# White matter of the cerebrum

The white matter of the cerebrum consists of the nerve fibres which lie deep to the cerebral cortex. They connect the various parts of the cortex with each other and with the other parts of the central nervous system. The white matter is classified as: (1) **association fibres**, which connect parts of the cerebral cortex within one hemisphere; (2) **commissural fibres**, which cross the midline and connect corresponding parts of the two cerebral cortices; and (3) **projection fibres**, which connect the cerebral cortex with other regions of the central nervous system. All three types of fibre bundles contain fibres passing in both directions.

## Association fibres

Association fibres are of two types—short and long association fibres. **Short association fibres** pass from one part of a gyrus to another part of the same gyrus, or loop around one sulcus to an adjacent gyrus [Fig. 31.18]. **Long association fibres** connect distant parts of the cortex. The long association fibre bundles are: (1) the **cingulum** on the medial aspect of the brain [Fig. 31.19]; (2) the **superior longitudinal bundle**, or **fasciculus**, on the superolateral aspect [Fig. 31.18]; (3) the **fasciculus uncinatus** on the superolateral and orbital aspects [Fig. 31.18]; and (4) the **inferior longitudinal bundle** on the tentorial aspect. (5) The external capsule is a thin layer of white matter on the lateral surface of the lentiform nucleus (a deep nucleus of the cerebrum). It contains corticocortical association fibres.

### Cingulum

Dissection 31.5 provides instructions on dissection of the cingulum and superior longitudinal bundle.

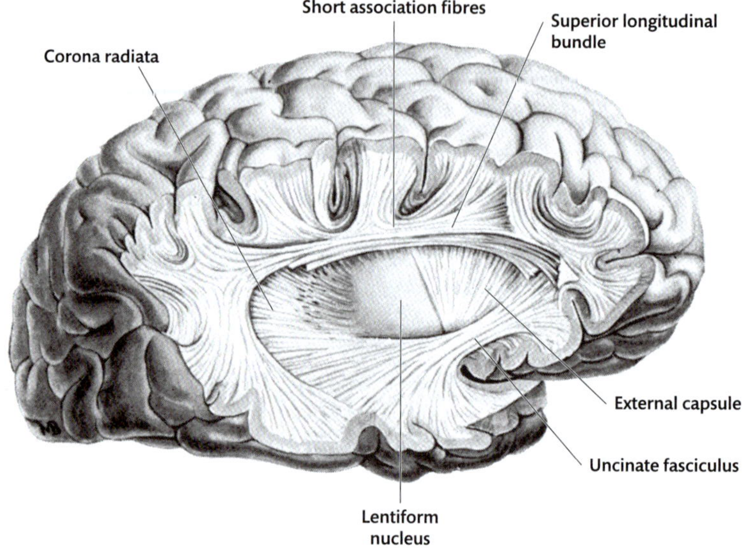


**Fig. 31.18** Dissection of the superolateral surface of the right hemisphere to show the white fibre bundles deep to the cortex.

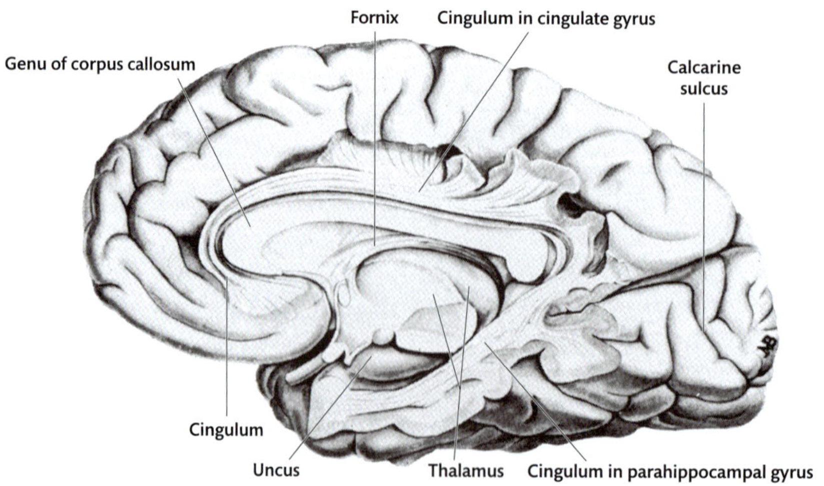


**Fig. 31.19** Dissection of the medial aspect of the right hemisphere to show the cingulum.

## DISSECTION 31.5 The cingulum and superior longitudinal bundle

**Objectives**

**I.** To expose the cingulum. **II.** To expose the superior longitudinal bundle.

**Instructions**

1. On the right hemisphere, scrape away the grey matter of the cingulate gyrus, and expose a rounded bundle of white matter lying longitudinally within it. It is simplest to determine the edge of the cingulum by removing the cortex between it and the superior surface of the corpus callosum, and then extending the removal superiorly.
2. Tear away the parts of the frontal lobe which still cover the anterior parts of the insula, and uncover the anterior part of the superior longitudinal bundle. This part is less clearly seen than the posterior part because it is traversed by many fibres of the corona radiata passing laterally through it.

The cingulum is a thick bundle of long association fibres which connects all parts of the cerebral cortex on the medial aspect of the hemisphere. It extends from the region of the paraterminal gyrus to the uncus and forms an almost complete circle (cingulum means a girdle) [Fig. 31.19].

### Fasciculus uncinatus

The fasciculus uncinatus is a thick bundle of association fibres which passes between the frontal and temporal lobes of the brain [Fig. 31.18]. Its inferior fibres hook round the stem of the lateral sulcus into the anterior part of the temporal lobe. The superior fibres pass directly backwards and downwards towards the posterior part of the temporal lobe. It is narrow in the middle, but at both ends, the fibres spread out, giving it the shape of a bent bundle [Fig. 31.18].

### Superior longitudinal bundle

The superior longitudinal bundle is a thick bundle of longitudinal association fibres. It lies immediately external to the circular sulcus of the insula [Fig. 31.18]. It extends around the insula from the frontal pole to the tip of the temporal pole and is thickest superior to the posterior half of the insula. Fibres enter and leave its external surface throughout its length, and it occupies approximately the same position on the lateral surface of the brain as the cingulum does on the medial surface. It connects the various parts of the cerebral cortex on the superolateral surface of the cerebral hemisphere.

### Inferior longitudinal bundle

The inferior longitudinal bundle is a bundle of association fibres which runs horizontally through the temporal and occipital lobes, near their inferior surfaces. It connects the various parts of the cerebral cortex on the tentorial surface of the hemisphere.

## Commissural fibres

The commissural fibres connect corresponding parts of the brain across the midline. The largest commissure is the **corpus callosum**. Other commissures of the forebrain are the: (1) **anterior commissure**; (2) **posterior commissure**; (3) **habenular commissure**; and (4) **commissure of the fornix**.

### Corpus callosum

#### Relations and parts of the corpus callosum

The corpus callosum unites the medial surfaces of the two cerebral hemispheres. Its upper surface forms the floor of part of the longitudinal fissure [Fig. 31.20]. The anterior cerebral vessels lie on the pia mater covering it, and the falx cerebri touches it posteriorly. It is covered on each side by the cingulate gyrus. Attached to the inferior surface of the corpus callosum in each hemisphere is the septum pellucidum, with the fornix attached to its inferior margin. The **septum pellucidum** is made up of neural tissue. It consists of two thin parallel laminae, each of which connects the fornix to the corpus callosum and fills the interval in the concavity of its genu. Its two laminae may be separated by the **cavity of the septum pellucidum**.

In the midline, the corpus callosum overlies a thin sheet of pia mater—the **tela choroidea of the third** and **lateral ventricles** above the roof of the median, slit-like third ventricle [see Fig. 32.7].

The parts of the corpus callosum are the: (1) rostrum; (2) genu; (3) body or trunk; and (4) splenium. The main part, or **trunk**, of the corpus callosum is thinner than the extremities [Fig. 31.17]. The

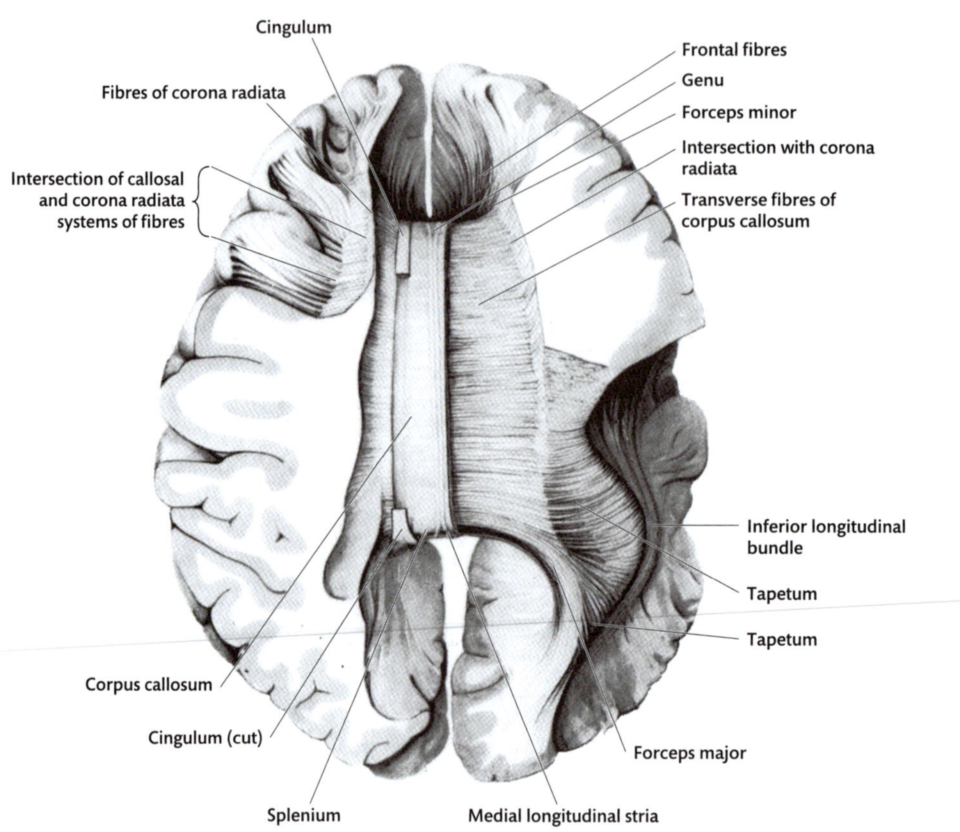


**Fig. 31.20** The corpus callosum exposed from above. The course of its fibres is seen in the right half.

posterior end, or **splenium**, is thick and rounded because of the large number of fibres which it transmits from the parietal, occipital, and temporal lobes. It overlies the upper part of the midbrain and extends posteriorly to the highest part of the cerebellum [Fig. 31.17]. Anteriorly, the corpus callosum is folded back on itself to form the **genu**, the lower, recurved portion of which—the **rostrum**—thins rapidly as it passes posteriorly. The tip of the rostrum is usually connected by neuroglia to the superior end of the lamina terminalis, anterior to the anterior commissure [Fig. 31.8].

The corpus callosum is formed by cortical fibres which converge in the midline and then fan out into the opposite hemisphere [Fig. 31.20]. Fibres of the corpus callosum radiate into the part of the hemisphere which lies adjacent to it. Fibres in the rostrum extend inferiorly to the orbital surface of the frontal lobe. Fibres from the genu pass to the anterior part of the frontal lobe, forming the **forceps minor**. Fibres from the trunk go to the remainder of the frontal lobe and to the parietal lobe, and fibres from the splenium radiate to the posterior parts of the parietal lobe and to the occipital and temporal lobes. Fibres connecting the medial surface of the two occipital lobes form the **forceps major**. Fibres connecting the inferior parts of the temporal and occipital lobes form a sheet of white matter on the roof and lateral wall of the posterior horn of the lateral ventricle—the **tapetum** [Figs. 31.20, 31.21]. The individual fibres retain the same relationship to each other throughout their course and connect similar parts of the two hemispheres.

## Anterior commissure

The anterior commissure is a bundle of fibres which crosses the midline in the superior part of the lamina terminalis, immediately anterior to the column of the fornix and the interventricular foramen [Figs. 31.17, 31.21]. The fibres in this commissure arise mainly in the temporal lobe and olfactory bulbs.

## Posterior commissure

The slender posterior commissure crosses the midline, immediately dorsal to the upper part of the

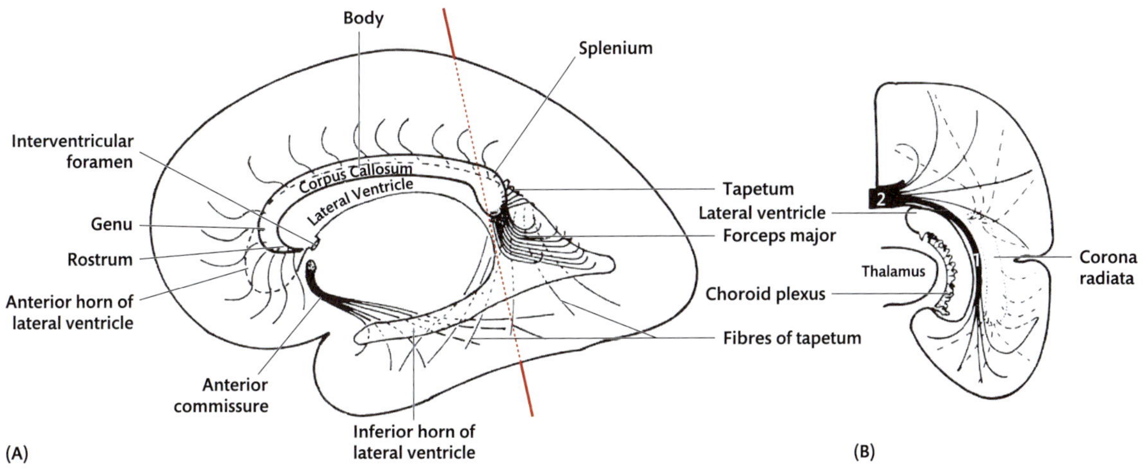


**Fig. 31.21** Diagram to illustrate the course and position of the major commissural fibres of the hemisphere. Figure (B) is a coronal section along the red line in figure (A). 1 = the tapetum; 2 = the splenium of the corpus callosum.

aqueduct and inferior to the root of the pineal body. It is composed mainly of fibres from the superior colliculi, the medial longitudinal bundle, and a number of nuclei associated with the superior part of that bundle [Fig. 31.17].

### Habenular commissure

The habenular commissure lies at the root of the pineal body and is separated from the posterior commissure by the small pineal recess of the third ventricle. The commissure unites the two habenular nuclei [see Fig. 30.2; Fig. 31.17].

## Projection fibres

Projection fibres connect the cerebral cortex with other regions of the central nervous system like the deep nuclei, brainstem, cerebellum, and spinal cord. The important bundles of projection fibres are the: (1) corona radiata; (2) internal capsule; and (3) optic and (4) auditory radiations. These fibres lie among, and in close relation to, the deep nuclei of the cerebrum—the caudate nucleus, globus pallidus, and putamen. The globus pallidus and putamen together make up the lentiform nucleus. The relationship between the deep nuclei and the projection fibres is best studied by examining a horizontal section through them [Fig. 31.22]. A horizontal section of the brain is made by following the instructions given in Dissection 31.6.

### Corona radiata

The corona radiata is a collection of projection fibres passing from the cerebral cortex to other parts of the central nervous system [Figs. 31.18, 31.21, 31.23, 31.24]. It consists of fibres passing inferiorly from the cortex and fibres passing superiorly to the cortex. Fibres of the corona radiata are continuous with the internal capsule around the periphery of the putamen, and spread out in a fan-like fashion into the cerebral cortex [Figs. 31.23, 31.24].

### Internal capsule

Certain gross features of the internal capsule are clear from the study of Figs. 31.22, 31.23, 31.24, and 31.25. (1) It has an **anterior limb**, a **posterior limb**, and the **genu**, which lie medial to the globus pallidus and putamen. These parts are best seen in Fig. 31.22. The anterior limb lies between the head of the caudate nucleus and lentiform nucleus, and the posterior limb between the lentiform nucleus and thalamus. The genu is the part where the anterior and posterior limbs meet. (2) The internal capsule is continuous superiorly with the corona radiata, and inferiorly with the crus cerebri [Figs. 31.23D, 31.24, 31.25]. (3) Its fibres radiate in a fan-shaped manner, so that fibres from the frontal lobe enter its anterior limb, run a long course in it, and enter the medial part of the crus cerebri. The temporal fibres enter it posteriorly, just superior to the optic tract, run a very short distance in it, and enter the posterolateral part of the crus with the occipital fibres. It follows from this that the position of the various groups of fibres in the internal capsule and crus is determined by their point of origin in the hemisphere. Motor fibres which arise in the precentral gyrus

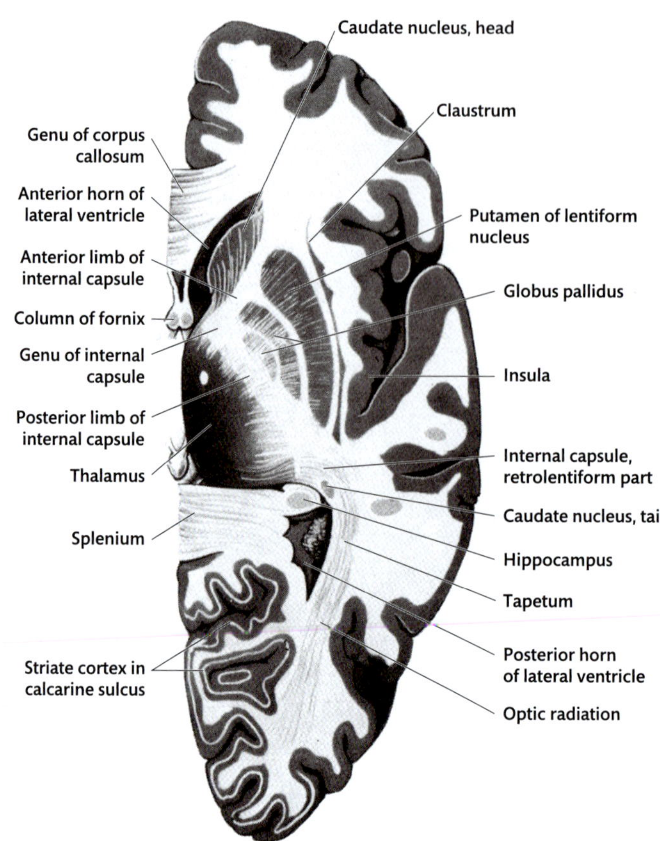


**Fig. 31.22** Horizontal section through the cerebral hemisphere at the level of the interventricular foramen.

## DISSECTION 31.6 Horizontal section of the brain

### Objective

**I.** To cut the brain horizontally, and identify the deep nuclei and white matter on the section.

### Instructions

Sections of the hemisphere can be carried out on the left side which is nearly intact. It is desirable to have both horizontal and coronal sections for study. For this purpose, groups of students should combine their specimens.

1. Make a horizontal cut through the left hemisphere, passing through the interventricular foramen and the inferior half of the splenium of the corpus callosum. This is best carried out with a long knife pulled through the brain in a single sweep.
2. Examine the cut surface of the cerebrum, and identify the structures shown in Fig. 31.22. Start by identifying the grey matter: (1) the cortex; (2) the **putamen** and **globus pallidus**; (3) the **head** and **tail** of the **caudate nucleus**; and (5) the **thalamus**.
3. Identify the parts of the **lateral ventricle** which have been opened—the **anterior horn** and **posterior horn**.
4. Identify the V-shaped **internal capsule** lying medial to the lentiform nucleus. It is divisible into **anterior** and **posterior limbs** which meet at the **genu**.
5. Identify the **external capsule** (white matter) between the putamen and the claustrum.
6. Medial to the **anterior limb of the internal capsule**, identify the **head of the caudate nucleus** in relation to the anterior horn of the lateral ventricle. Medial to the **posterior limb of the internal capsule**, identify the thalamus, and further posteriorly the tail of the caudate nucleus. Note that, in the posterior limb, the fibres are cut transversely and appear darker in colour than the fibres of the anterior limb which are cut longitudinally.
7. Identify the **optic radiation** passing towards the occipital lobe. It is lighter in colour than the tapetum which separates it from the posterior horn of the lateral ventricle [see Fig. 31.32].
8. Identify the **genu** and **splenium** of the **corpus callosum**.
9. Note the position and extent of the **striate cortex**.

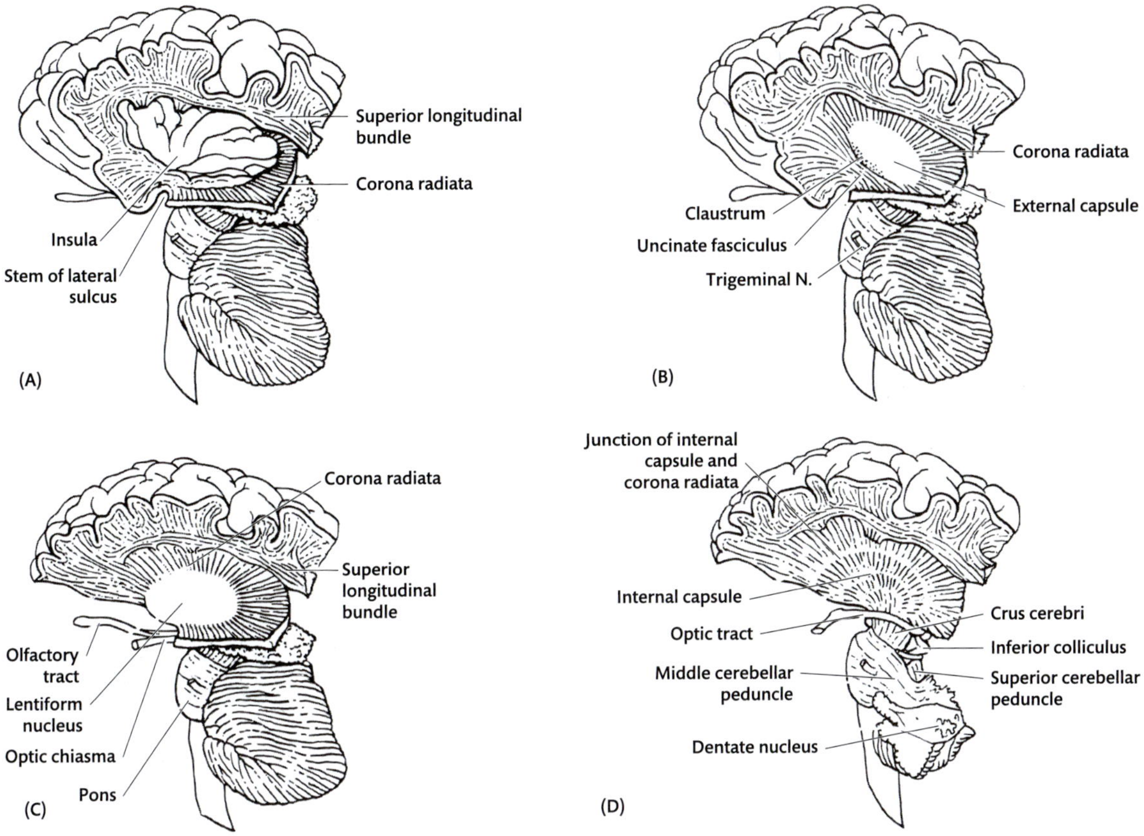

(A)
Superior longitudinal bundle
Corona radiata
Insula
Stem of lateral sulcus

(B)
Corona radiata
External capsule
Claustrum
Uncinate fasciculus
Trigeminal N.

(C)
Corona radiata
Superior longitudinal bundle
Olfactory tract
Lentiform nucleus
Optic chiasma
Pons

(D)
Junction of internal capsule and corona radiata
Internal capsule
Optic tract
Middle cerebellar peduncle
Dentate nucleus
Crus cerebri
Inferior colliculus
Superior cerebellar peduncle

**Fig. 31.23** Diagrammatic representations of the deep dissection of the cerebrum from the lateral side. (A) The frontal and parietal parts of the operculum have been removed to expose the insula and superior longitudinal bundle. (B) The insula has been removed, and the external capsule, claustrum, and fasciculus uncinatus are shown. (C) The structures exposed in (B) are removed to expose the lentiform nucleus. The fibres of the corona radiata (around the lentiform nucleus) are seen. (D) The lentiform nucleus has been removed to expose the internal capsule. The continuity of the internal capsule with the crus cerebri and corona radiata is seen.

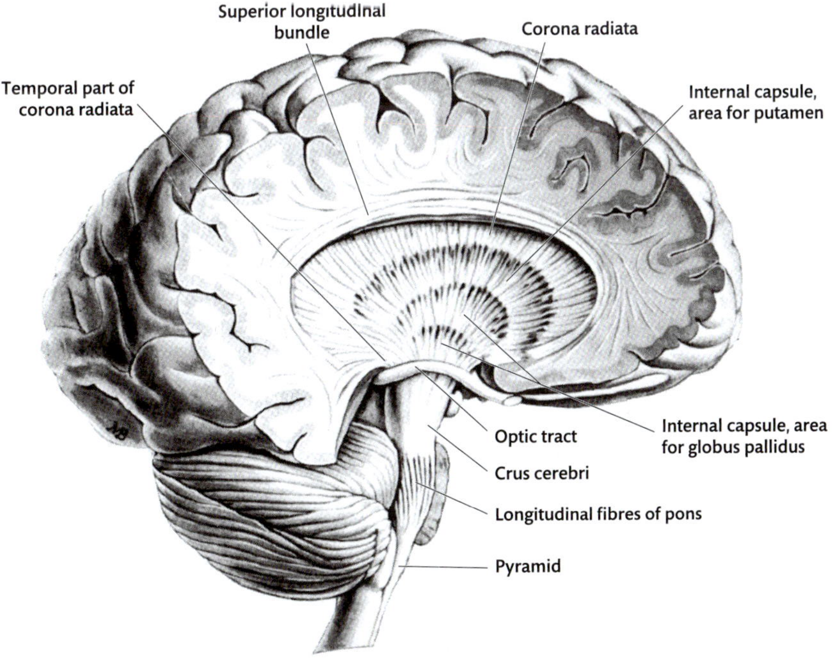


**Fig. 31.24** Dissection to show the continuity of the corona radiata, internal capsule, crus celebri, longitudinal fibres of the pons, and the pyramid.

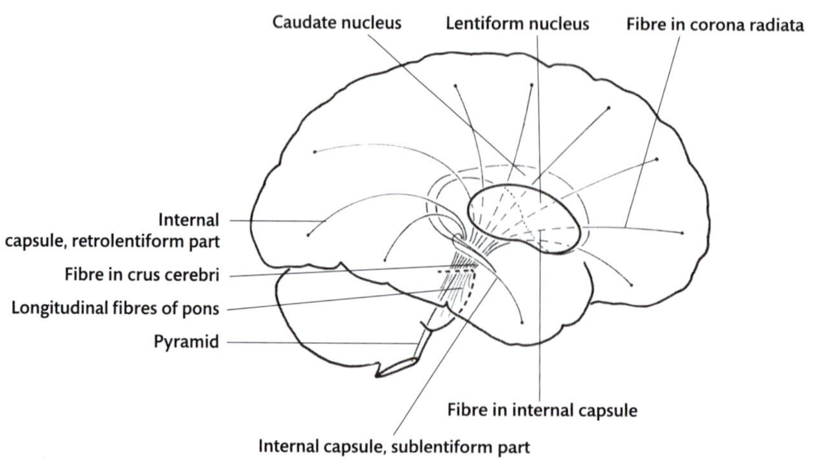


**Fig. 31.25** Diagram to show the arrangement of fibres in the corona radiata, internal capsule, crus cerebri, pons, and pyramid.





(**corticonuclear** and **corticospinal fibres**), near the midpoint between the frontal and occipital poles, will enter the middle of the internal capsule and crus [Fig. 31.22].

Fibres of the internal capsule which emerge posterior to the lentiform nucleus (**retrolentiform part**) pass to and from the occipital lobe [Figs. 31.22, 31.25]. Fibres which emerge beneath the posterior end of the lentiform nucleus (**sublentiform part**) pass to and from the temporal lobe [Fig. 31.25].

## Optic radiation

The optic radiation is made up of fibres which arise from the **lateral geniculate body** [Fig. 31.22]. They sweep forwards into the retrolentiform part of the internal capsule, spread out into a broad sheet which turns around the lateral surface of the lateral ventricle, and pass towards the occipital lobe, lateral to the tapetum and the posterior horn of the lateral ventricle. The inferior fibres sweep far forwards on the superior surface of the inferior horn of the lateral ventricle (close to the optic tract) before turning backwards [Figs. 31.22, 31.26].

## Auditory radiation

Fibres of the auditory radiation arise in the medial geniculate body. They pass anterolaterally into the sublentiform part of the internal capsule, between the roof of the inferior horn of the lateral ventricle and the lentiform nucleus. They end on the transverse temporal gyrus and, to a small extent, on its lateral surface [see Figs. 30.6B; Figs. 31.11, 31.25].

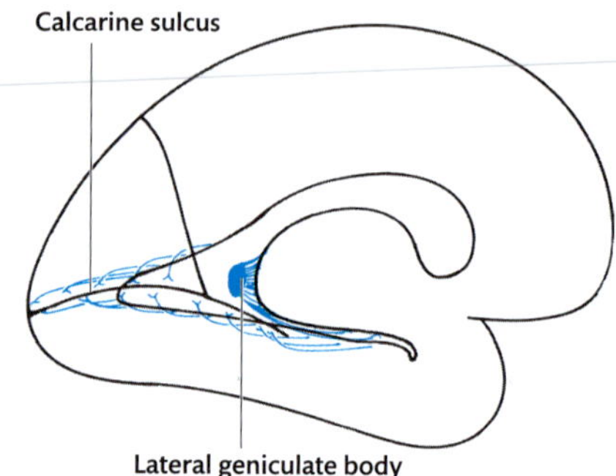


**Fig. 31.26** Medial view of the left cerebral hemisphere showing the relation of the optic radiation to the lateral ventricle and calcarine sulcus.

# Deep nuclei of the cerebrum

A number of nuclear masses are seen deep in the cerebrum. They include the: (1) caudate nucleus; (2) putamen; (3) globus pallidus; (4) claustrum [Fig. 31.22]; and (5) amygdala. These nuclei are grouped together under certain names. The term **basal ganglia** include the caudate nucleus, putamen, globus pallidus, and amygdala. The term **corpus striatum** refers to the caudate nucleus, putamen, and globus pallidus. The putamen and lentiform nucleus together make up the **lentiform nucleus**. The corpus striatum, along with other nuclei in the diencephalon and midbrain, is involved in control of movement. The amygdala is part of the limbic lobe.

Before studying the deep nuclei, complete Dissection 31.7 on coronal sections through the brain (Figs. 31.27, 31.28, 31.29, 31.30, 31.31, and 31.32)

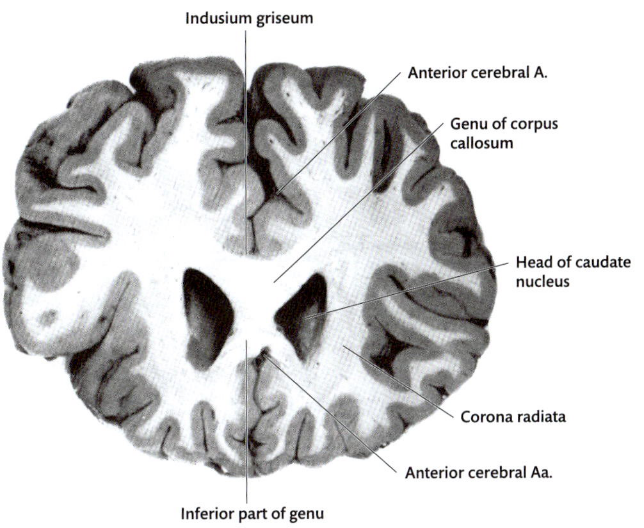


**Fig. 31.27** Coronal section through the genu of the corpus callosum and the anterior horns of the lateral ventricles, anterior view.

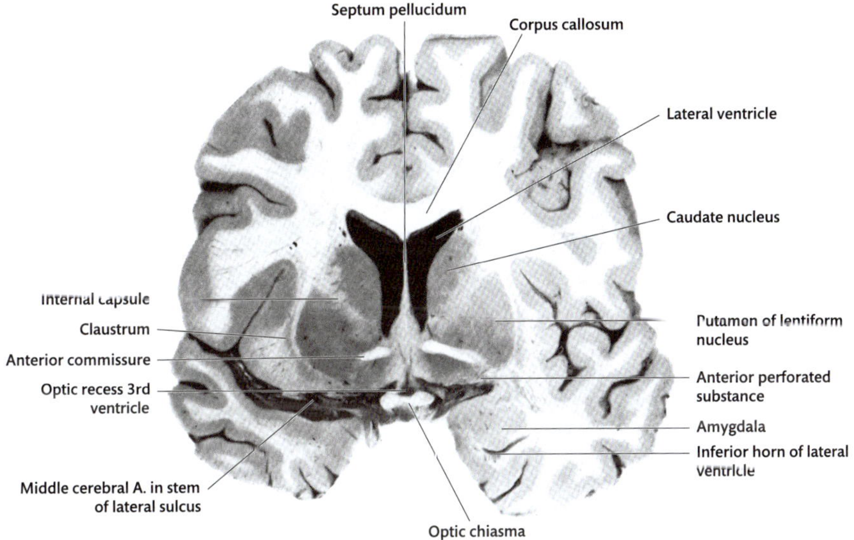


**Fig. 31.28** Coronal section through the brain at the level of the optic chiasma. On the right, the section is slightly posterior to that on the left half.

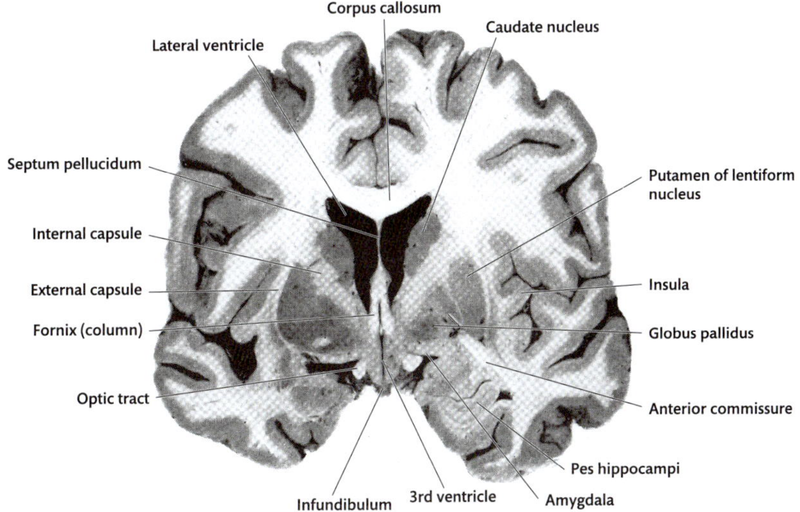


**Fig. 31.29** Coronal section through the brain at the level of the infundibulum.

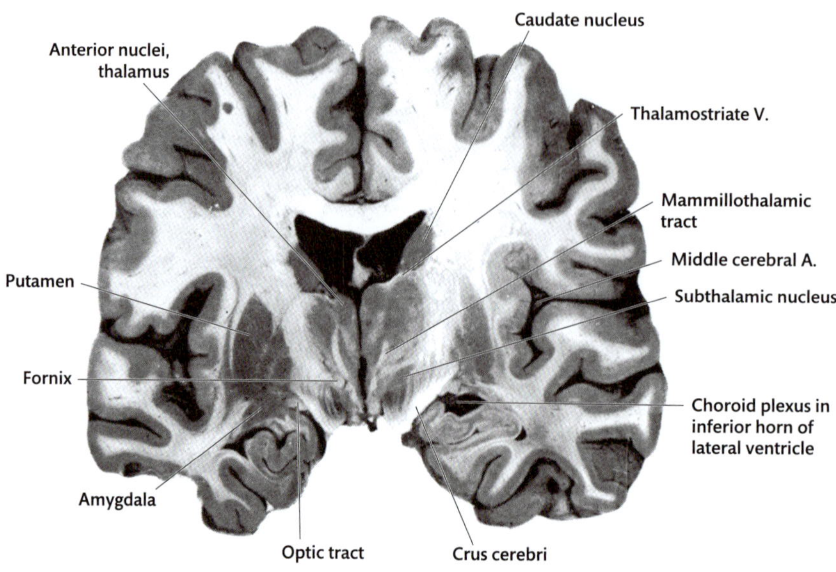


**Fig. 31.30** Coronal section through the brain at the level of the mammillary bodies.

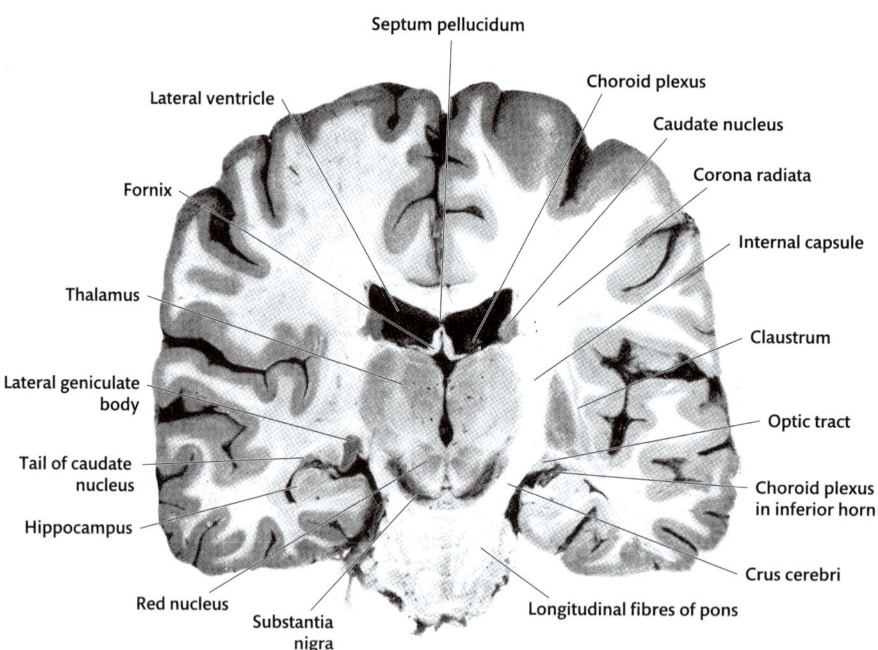


**Fig. 31.31** Coronal section through the brain passing through the basilar part of the pons. Note the division of the thalamus into anterior, medial, lateral, and centromedian nuclei on the left.

## Corpus striatum

The **corpus striatum** consists of the **caudate nucleus**, **putamen**, and **globus pallidus**. The putamen and globus pallidus together form the **lentiform nucleus**. The caudate nucleus and putamen together are known as the **striatum**. The striatum can be considered as one mass, partially separated by the fibres of the internal capsule. The head of the caudate nucleus is fused to the putamen, below the anterior limb of the internal capsule. The body and tail of the caudate nucleus are connected to the putamen by strands of grey matter between the bundles of the internal capsule [see Fig. 34.4A]. The caudate nucleus and putamen

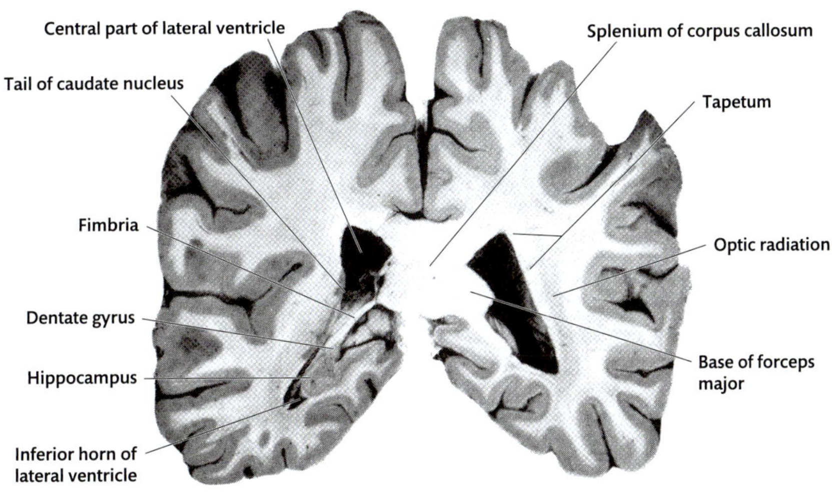


**Fig. 31.32** Coronal section through the splenium of the corpus callosum to show the continuity of the central part and inferior horn of the lateral ventricle. Note how the fibres of the splenium and its tapetum virtually surround the posterior part of the lateral ventricle, as the fibres of the genu surround the anterior horn. Compare with Fig. 31.27.





**DISSECTION 31.7 Coronal sections of the brain**

**Objective**

**I.** To cut the brain in coronal slices to see the arrangement of the deep nuclei and white matter around the ventricles.

**Instructions**

1. Make a series of coronal sections as follows: (1) through the posterior part of the genu of the corpus callosum [Fig. 31.27]; (2) through the anterior perforated substance [Fig. 31.28]; (3) immediately anterior to the infundibulum [Fig. 31.29]; (4) immediately anterior to the mammillary bodies [Fig. 31.30]; (5) obliquely downwards through the crus cerebri and pons (if present) [Fig. 31.31]; and (6) through the splenium of the corpus callosum [Fig. 31.32].
2. With the assistance of Figs. 31.27, 31.28, 31.29, 31.30, 31.31 and 31.32, identify the structures seen in the coronal sections. These are the head and body of the caudate nucleus, putamen, globus pallidus, thalamus, parts of the corpus callosum, parts of the internal capsule, internal and external medullary laminae of the lentiform nucleus, and anterior horn, body, and posterior horn of the lateral ventricle. Relate the position of these structures to those seen in the horizontal section. In this manner, try to build a mental three-dimensional picture of the internal structures of the cerebral hemisphere. (Place the sections together to reconstruct the hemisphere, and take them apart several times to familiarize yourself with the internal arrangement.)

are identical in histological structure and have similar connections, in contrast to the globus pallidus which is very different.

## Caudate nucleus

The caudate nucleus is comma-shaped [Fig. 31.25]. It has a wide, thick **head** anteriorly, followed by a short **body** and a long, thin **tail**. The head lies in the lateral wall of the anterior horn of the lateral ventricle [Figs. 31.25, 31.27, 31.28]. It is fused with the anterior end of the lentiform nucleus, inferior to the anterior limb of the internal capsule. This part of the head is also fused with the anterior perforated substance, and the striate branches of the middle and anterior cerebral arteries enter it [Fig. 31.28]. The head tapers rapidly to the narrow **body**, which runs posteriorly in the lateral part of the floor of the central portion of the lateral ventricle [Figs. 31.25, 31.29, 31.30]. The **tail of the caudate nucleus** is narrow and flat, and continues posteriorly from the body. It turns inferiorly and runs anteriorly in the roof of the inferior horn of the lateral ventricle to end in relation to the amygdala [Figs. 31.25, 31.31, 31.32].

The ventricular surface of the caudate nucleus is covered with ependyma. The deep surface of the head is fused anteriorly with the putamen. Posteriorly, it is applied to the anterior limb of the internal capsule. The deep surfaces of the body and tail lie on the internal capsule.

## Lentiform nucleus

The lentiform nucleus is a large, lens-shaped mass of grey matter which lies lateral to the internal capsule. It is divided into three parts by two vertical sheets of white matter—the **lateral** and **medial medullary laminae**. The lateral, darker part of the lentiform nucleus is the **putamen**; the two paler medial parts are the segments of the **globus pallidus**. The lentiform nucleus has three surfaces—lateral, medial, and inferior surfaces.

The **lateral surface** is smooth and convex, and is grooved by the lateral striate vessels. It is separated from the claustrum by the external capsule [Fig. 31.22].

The **medial surface** projects medially and comes to a point opposite the interventricular foramen [Fig. 31.22]. This point lies on the genu of the internal capsule, between the head of the caudate nucleus anteriorly and the thalamus posteriorly. The striate arteries traverse and supply the lentiform nucleus and continue through the internal capsule, to supply the caudate nucleus and the lateral part of the thalamus.

The **inferior surface** is fused anteriorly with the anterior perforated substance and, through it, is continuous with the amygdala [Fig. 31.29]. In this part, the lentiform nucleus is pierced by the anterior commissure [Fig. 31.28]). Posteriorly, the lentiform nucleus lies on the white matter which passes laterally into the temporal lobe. This white matter contains the **sublentiform part of the internal capsule** (auditory radiation) and separates the lentiform nucleus from the tail of the caudate nucleus, the optic [see Fig. 31.31] tract, and the inferior horn of the lateral ventricle [see Fig. 31.31].

## Connections of the corpus striatum (basal ganglion)

The main connections of the corpus striatum are shown in Fig. 31.33.

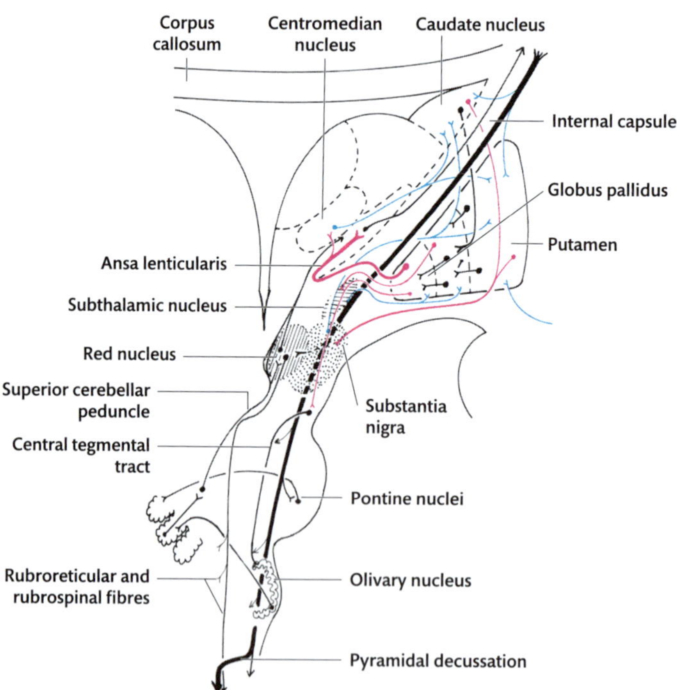


Fig. 31.33 Diagram to show some of the principal connections of the basal ganglia. Afferent fibres to the striatum from the thalamus and cortex = blue; efferent fibres from the globus pallidus to the thalamus, substantia nigra, and reticular formation = red; internal capsule and connections between the putamen and globus pallidus = black.

### Connections of the caudate nucleus and putamen

**Afferents**: the caudate nucleus and putamen receive a considerable number of fibres from the cerebral cortex, thalamus, and substantia nigra.

**Efferents**: efferent fibres from the caudate nucleus and putamen pass to the globus pallidus and substantia nigra.

### Connections of the globus pallidus

**Afferents**: the globus pallidus gets fibres from the caudate nucleus and putamen.

**Efferents**: the main efferent fibre from the globus pallidus—the **ansa lenticularis**—passes medially through and around the inferior part of the internal capsule to the thalamus. Other fibres pass to the subthalamus and the tegmentum of the midbrain [Fig. 31.33].

From the thalamus, impulses are conveyed to the posterior part of the frontal lobe (motor area).

### Functions of the corpus striatum

The corpus striatum is concerned with the regulation of muscle tone and control of associated movements, and has a part in the control of voluntary movements. ➲ Damage to the corpus striatum leads to a state of increased muscle tone, the disappearance of associated movements like swinging of the arms in walking, and tremor at rest.

## Claustrum

The **claustrum** is a thin sheet of grey matter which lies between the external capsule and the white matter of the insula. It belongs to the deep nuclei of the forebrain [Figs. 31.22, 31.28, 31.29, 31.30, 31.31].

## Amygdala

The **amygdala** is made up of a group of nuclei which lies at the tip of the inferior horn of the lateral ventricle. It is continuous with the tail of the caudate nucleus posteriorly, and with the cortex of the uncus medially. **Afferents**: it receives afferent fibres from the thalamus, the hypothalamus, and various parts of the cerebral cortex. **Efferents**: its main efferent is the stria terminalis. The **stria terminalis** is a delicate bundle of fibres which arises in the amygdala, follows the curve of the caudate nucleus with the thalamostriate vein, and ends in the anterior hypothalamus and septal nuclei [Fig. 31.30; see also Fig. 32.6].

## Blood supply of deep structures

The **lateral striate arteries** (also known as lenticulostriate arteries) are branches of the middle cerebral artery. They enter the brain through the anterior perforated substance. The **medial striate arteries** arise from the anterior cerebral artery, usually near the anterior communicating artery, and run a recurrent course to the anterior perforated substance [see Fig. 26.2]. Both sets of arteries ascend through the anterior perforated substance to enter and supply the caudate nucleus, lentiform nucleus, and internal capsule which runs between them [Fig. 31.29]. They also pierce the internal capsule and supply the lateral surface of the thalamus. The **recurrent artery** also arises from the anterior cerebral artery and supplies parts of the head of the caudate nucleus, putamen, globus pallidus, and internal capsule. Small central branches of the posterior cerebral artery (**thalamoperforate arteries**) supply the thalamus and some parts of the posterior limb of the internal capsule.

## Overview of motor and sensory pathways

Having now completed the study of the major parts of the central nervous system, the tracts extending from the cerebral cortex to the spinal cord, or vice versa, can be reviewed in entirety.

### Corticospinal tracts

The corticospinal tract is the motor pathway through which the cerebral cortex acts on the spinal cord. The majority of fibres in the corticospinal tract arise in the motor cortex and descend in the corona radiata and internal capsule [Fig. 31.34]. They are located in the crus cerebri in the midbrain, ventral part of the pons, and pyramids in the medulla. In the ventral part of the upper

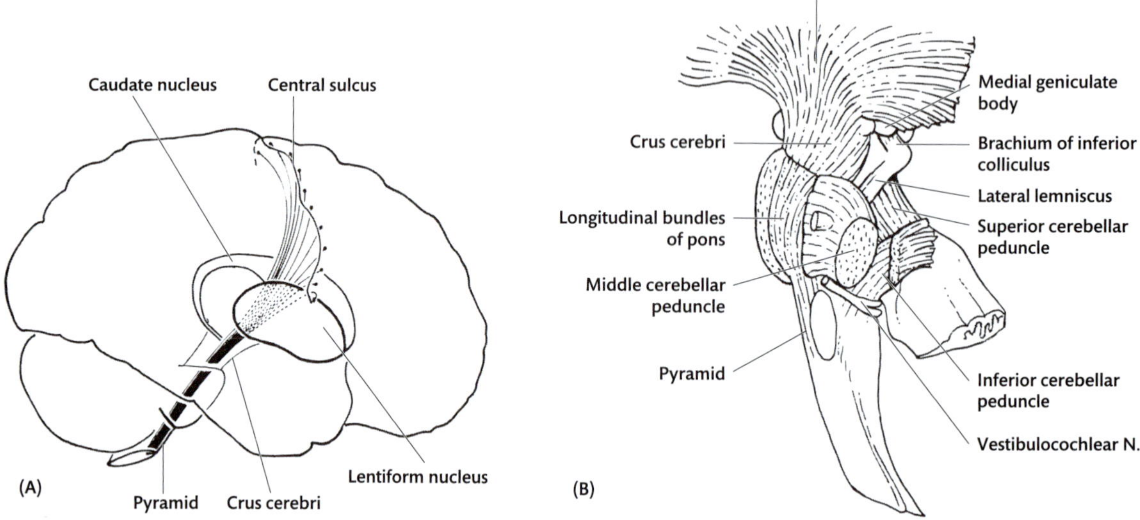


**Fig. 31.34** (A) Diagram to show the course of fibres arising in the precentral gyrus (motor cortex) and passing through the corona radiata, internal capsule, crus cerebri, pons, and pyramid. (B) Deep dissection of the brainstem. The left half of the pons has been removed to show the longitudinal fibres passing through it to become continuous with the pyramid in the medulla oblongata.





medulla, they form the pyramids. The majority of fibres decussate in the pyramidal decussation to form the lateral corticospinal tract in the lateral column of the spinal cord. The fibres of the lateral corticospinal tract end in the grey matter of the spinal cord on the anterior horn cells. They control the movement of skeletal muscles of the trunk and limbs [Fig. 31.35]. ➲ Damage to the corticospinal tract anywhere along its course will cause an upper motor neuron type of paralysis of the muscles supplied by it.

## Dorsal column–medial lemniscus pathway

The dorsal column–medial lemniscus pathway is concerned with appreciation of crude touch, two-point discrimination, and proprioception. The first-order neurons are located in the dorsal root ganglion, from which the fibres enter the spinal cord at the dorsal root entry zone and ascend in the posterior column [see Fig. 27.3]. These fibres end in the nuclei gracilis and cuneatus in the lower part of the medulla [see Figs. 28.3, 28.7; Fig. 31.36]. Second-order neurons arise from the nuclei gracilis and cuneatus, cross the midline as internal arcuate fibres, and ascend in the medial lemniscus through the upper medulla, pons, and midbrain. They end in the ventroposterior lateral (VPL) nucleus of the thalamus. Third-order neurons from the VPL nucleus ascend to the sensory cortex in the thalamocortical or sensory radiations [see Fig. 30.6B; Fig. 31.11].

## Spinothalamic tract

The spinothalamic tract carries sensation of fine touch and pain from the body to the thalamus. The first-order neurons are located in the dorsal root ganglion. Their fibres end in the posterior grey horn of the spinal cord. The second-order neurons arise from the posterior horn cells, cross the midline in the white commissure, and ascend in the anterolateral column of the spinal cord [see Fig. 27.6] and through the brainstem [Fig. 31.36]. They end in the VPL nucleus of the thalamus. The third-order neurons from the thalamus ascend to the sensory cortex through the sensory radiation. (Note: the thalamic nuclei of termination and the final pathway for the dorsal column–medial lemniscus pathway and spinothalamic tract are the same.)

## Visual pathway

The visual pathway from the retina to the visual cortex in the occipital lobe consists of the optic nerve, optic chiasma, optic tract, lateral geniculate body, optic radiation, and visual cortex [Fig. 31.37]. Visual impulses received in the retina of both eyes are transmitted to the brain through the **optic nerve** [Chapter 11]. The optic nerve leaves the orbit in the optic canal and enters the middle

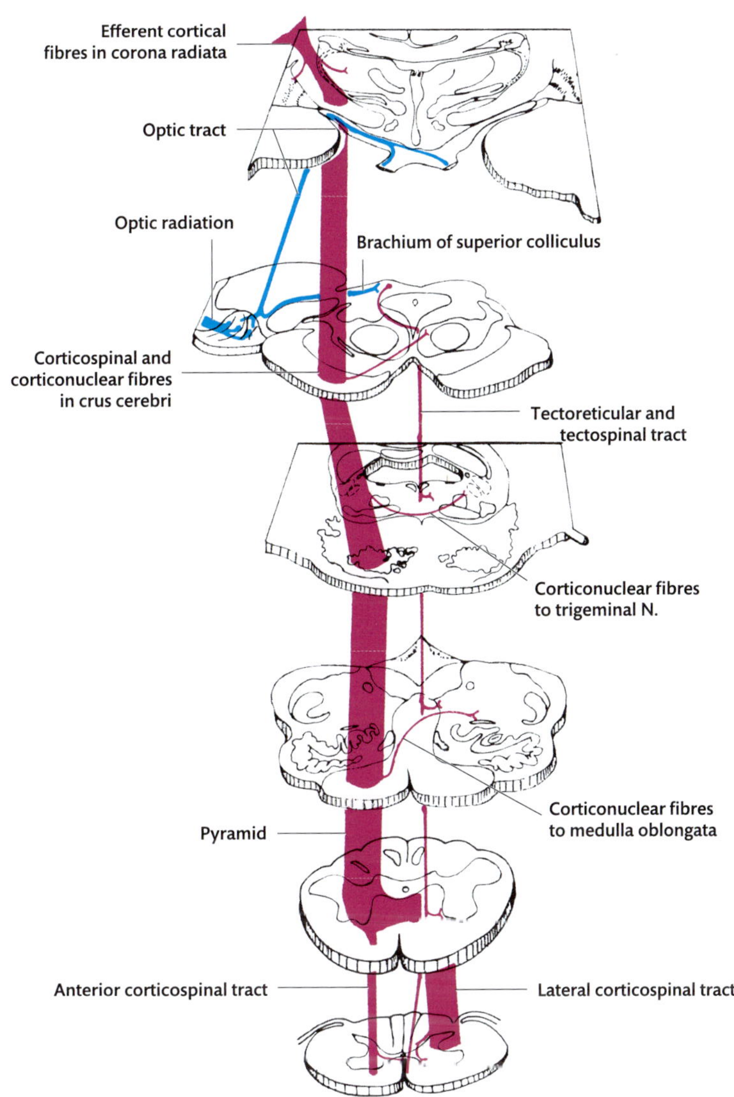


**Fig. 31.35** A diagram to show the course of the corticonuclear and corticospinal fibres (red) through the brainstem. Serial sections are shown through the spinal cord, lower medulla, upper medulla, pons, midbrain, and thalamus.

cranial fossa. At the **optic chiasma**, optic nerve fibres from the nasal half of each retina cross the midline and join the **optic tract** of the opposite side. Fibres from the temporal half of the retina continue in the optic tract of the same side. Thus, each optic tract contains fibres from the temporal half of the ipsilateral retina and from the nasal half of the contralateral retina—the opposite visual field. Most of the fibres of the optic tract end in the lateral geniculate body. From the lateral geniculate body, fibres project to the visual cortex through the optic radiation. In the optic radiation, fibres from the superior quadrants of the retina sweep superiorly to reach the visual cortex above the calcarine sulcus, and fibres from the inferior quadrants of the retina reach the visual cortex below the calcarine sulcus. Fibres from the inferior quadrant take an indirect course. They run anteriorly in the temporal lobe, curve around the inferior horn of the lateral ventricle, and then reach the cerebral cortex [Fig. 31.26].

Some fibres in the optic tract bypass the lateral geniculate body and enter the superior colliculus. These fibres form the **brachium of the superior colliculus** and are concerned with the production of visual reflexes such as turning of the head and eyes towards a sudden flash of light, and constriction of the pupil when light is shone into the eye [see Fig. 30.5; Fig. 31.37]. See Clinical Application 31.3 for signs of visual field defects.

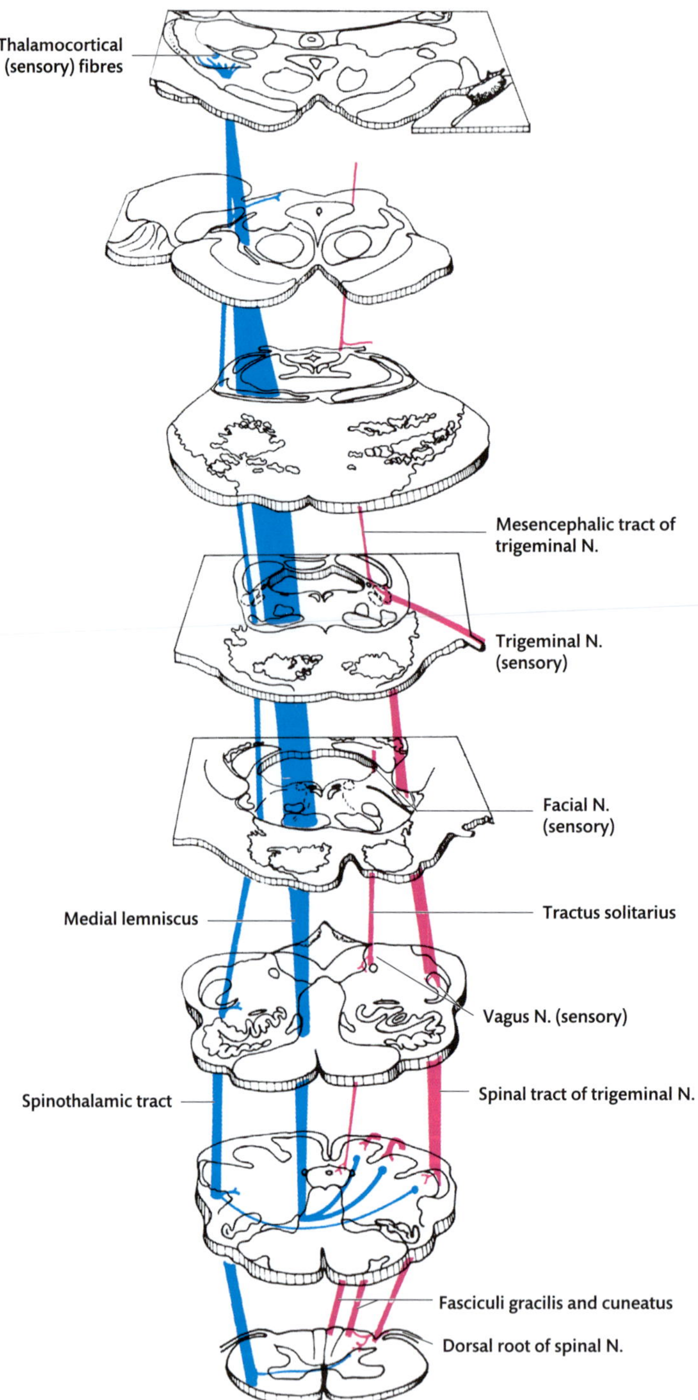


**Fig. 31.36** An outline diagram to show the spinothalamic and dorsal column–medial lemniscus pathway. Serial sections are shown through the spinal cord, mid-medulla, upper medulla, lower and upper pons, lower and upper midbrain, and thalamus.

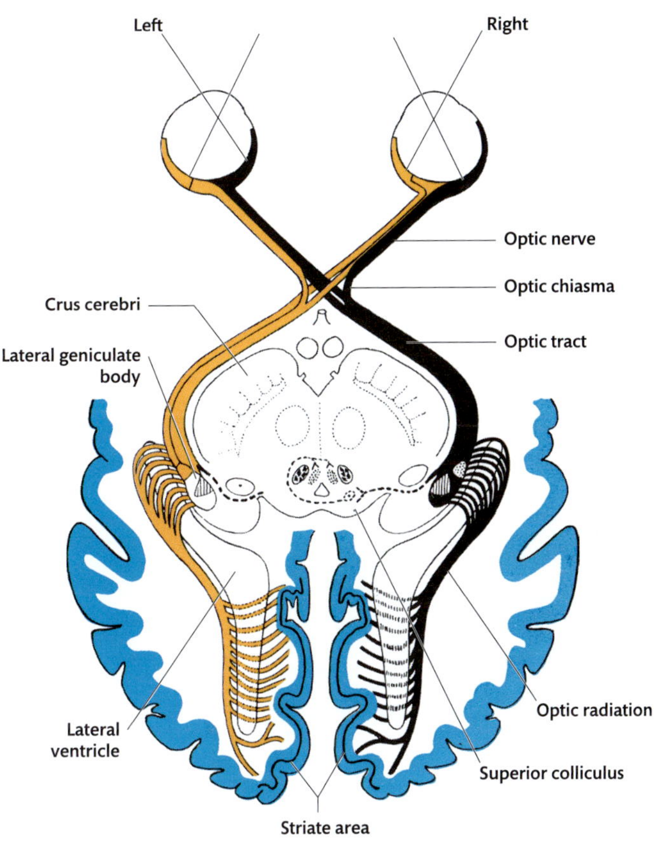


**Fig. 31.37** Composite diagram to show the projection of the visual field upon the retinae, and the visual pathway.

## Auditory pathway

The auditory impulses from the internal ear reach the cochlear nucleus which lies on either side of the inferior cerebellar peduncle at the junction of the medulla and pons [see Fig. 28.9]. Some fibres from the cochlear nucleus cross the midline in the trapezoid body. They form the lateral lemniscus at the lateral end of the trapezoid body and are joined by uncrossed fibres from the cochlear nucleus of that side. The lateral lemniscus ascends with the medial lemniscus and spinothalamic tract. (The lateral lemniscus contains crossed and uncrossed fibres and receives input from both ears.) It ends in the inferior colliculus. The inferior colliculus sends impulses through the **brachium of the inferior colliculus** to the medial geniculate body. From the medial geniculate body, the auditory impulses reach the transverse temporal gyrus through the auditory radiation [Fig. 31.38].

➲ From the above description, it is clear that each lateral lemniscus and parts of the auditory pathway superior to it carry impulses from both ears. This arrangement enables the appreciation of time difference in the arrival of sounds at the two ears and sound localization. It also explains why damage to this pathway on one side does not cause hearing loss on that side. By contrast, injury to the vestibulocochlear nerve would result in hearing loss on that side.

See Clinical Applications 31.1, 31.2, 31.3, 31.4, and 31.5 for the practical implications of the anatomy discussed in this chapter.

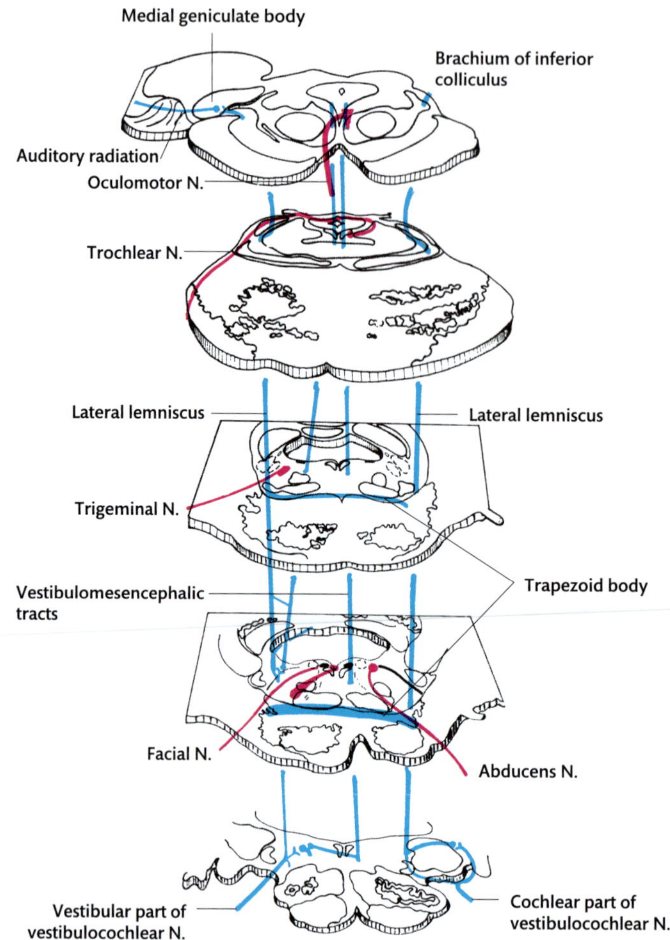


**Fig. 31.38** An outline diagram to show the ascending connections of the cochlear part of the vestibulocochlear nerve (blue). Serial sections are shown through the upper medulla, lower and upper pons, lower midbrain, and junction of the midbrain and thalamus.

## CLINICAL APPLICATION 31.1 Middle cerebral artery stroke

A 60-year-old woman on irregular treatment for diabetes mellitus, hypertension, and hypercholesterolaemia was taking her regular evening walk when she suddenly developed right-sided hemiparesis, hemianaesthesia, loss of consciousness, and seizures. On awakening, she had severe weakness of the right arm and right leg, and an inability to express herself verbally (motor aphasia). Imaging studies showed features of a stroke caused by a middle cerebral artery (MCA) territory infarct [Fig. 31.39].

Study question 1: what is an infarct? (Answer: an infarct is an acute shortage of blood supply to tissue or an organ, resulting in focal death of tissue—in this case, to the region of the brain supplied by the MCA.)

Study question 2: what is the cause for a cerebral stroke? (Answer: there are two main causes for strokes, and strokes are classified accordingly as: (1) ischaemic strokes; and (2) haemorrhagic strokes. Ischaemic strokes are more common and caused by obstruction of blood vessels, either by a thrombus within a cerebral blood vessel or an embolus (dislodged thrombus) from another vessel outside the cranial cavity. Haemorrhagic strokes are caused by rupture of cerebral blood vessels.)

Study question 3: on which side is the lesion? (Answer: sensory and motor fibres cross in the spinal cord or medulla oblongata. To cause signs on the right side of the body, as seen in this case, the MCA infarct would have to be on the left. Also, the motor speech centre situated in the left cerebral hemisphere (dominant hemisphere) is affected in this patient.) Motor aphasia suggests that the anterior branch of the MCA is probably affected in this patient. Posterior branch lesions would cause sensory aphasia with deficits in reception of verbal commands. Main trunk lesions would cause extensive sensorimotor deficit and global aphasia.

Study question 4: what symptoms would be seen in a stroke affecting the right MCA territory? (Answer: a right MCA stroke would cause left-sided hemiparesis, hemianaesthesia, and other specific deficits such as inattention to a sensory stimulus on the left side, dressing apraxia (an inability to use familiar items of clothing to dress oneself), constructional apraxia (an inability to draw or construct simple configurations), and topographic memory deficit where an individual gets lost in familiar surroundings. These are all functions of the right (non-dominant) hemisphere.)

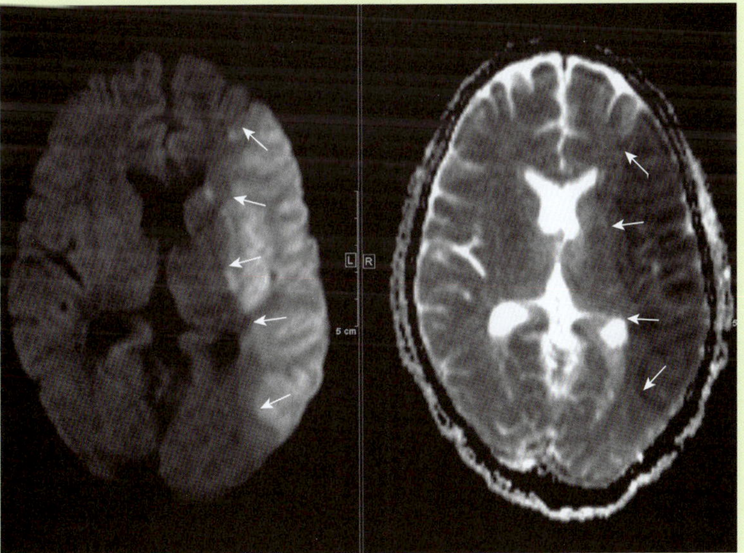


**Fig. 31.39** Diffusion-weighted magnetic resonance image showing an infarct in the middle cerebral artery. Arrows indicate the boundary of the infarcted area.

**CLINICAL APPLICATION 31.2 Brain tumour**

A 48-year-old man presented with complaints of persistent headache, vomiting, and loss of appetite. Magnetic resonance imaging revealed an astrocytoma in the medial part of the parietal lobe [Fig. 31.40].

Study question 1: given the location of the tumour, which part of the body is likely to exhibit a sensory loss? (Answer: the right lower limbs and perineum.)

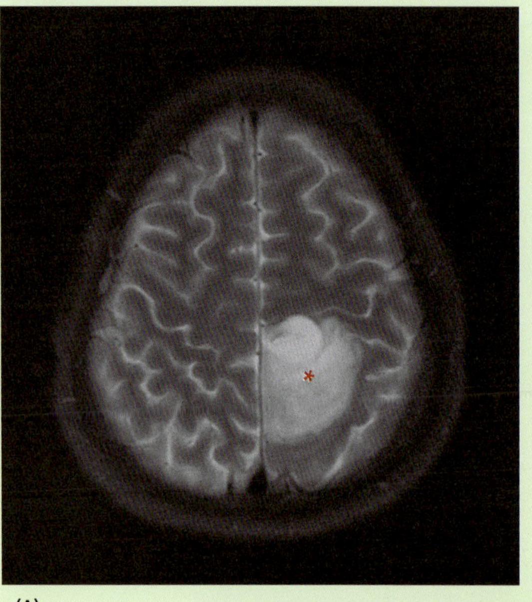

(A)

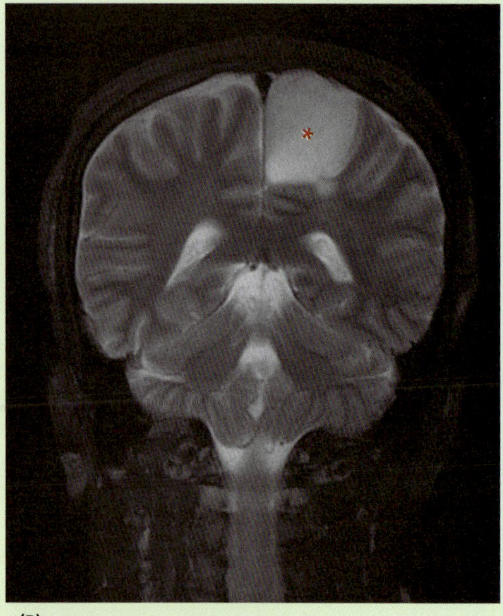

(B)

(C)

**Fig. 31.40** A brain tumour—astrocytoma—in the parietal lobe (asterisk). (A) T2-weighted axial magnetic resonance imaging (MRI). (B) T2-weighted coronal MRI. (C) T1-weighted sagittal post-contrast MRI.

## CLINICAL APPLICATION 31.3 Visual field defects

The visual field is divided into four quadrants—right upper, right lower, left upper, and left lower quadrants. Impulses from the visual field pass through the eye and fall on a segment of the retina. (1) Visual impulses from the left half of the field of vision fall on the right half of the retinae (the temporal half of the right retina and the nasal half of the left retina). (2) Visual impulses from the right half of the field of vision fall on the left half of the retinae (the temporal half of the left retina and the nasal half of the right retina). (3) Visual impulses from the upper half of the field of vision fall on the lower half of the retinae. (4) Visual impulses from the lower half of the field of vision fall on the upper half of the retinae.

Damage to any part of the visual pathway will lead to a defect in the field of vision. The type of visual field defect will depend on the site and size of the lesion. Fig. 31.41A shows the location of six lesions in the visual pathway, indicated by letters A–F. Fig. 31.41B shows the visual field defect in each of these lesions.

Lesion A: damage to a small part of the right retina on the temporal side. Visual field defect: monocular scotoma (focal loss of vision) in the right eye, affecting part of the left field of vision.

Lesion B: damage to the right optic nerve. Visual field defect: blindness in the right eye.

Lesion C: damage to the optic chiasma. Visual field defect: bitemporal hemianopia. Severing of fibres from the nasal halves of both retinae will lead to loss of the temporal half of the field of vision in both eyes. Further fibres from parts of the retinae cross in the upper part of the chiasma. Therefore, damage to the upper part of the chiasma will result in a lower bitemporal visual field defect, and damage to the lower part of the chiasma will result in an upper bitemporal visual field defect.

Lesion D: damage to the optic tract. Visual field defect: contralateral homonymous hemianopia. Each optic tract contains fibres from the temporal half of the ipsilateral retina and the nasal half of the contralateral retina—parts of the retinae receiving impulses from the opposite half of the visual field. As such, destruction of one optic tract will result in loss of the opposite half of the field of vision—contralateral homonymous hemianopia.

Lesion F: damage to the entire optic radiation. Visual field defect: contralateral homonymous hemianopia—same as the result of damage to the optic tract.

Lesion E: damage confined to the optic radiation fibres which curve around the inferior horn of the lateral ventricle. Visual field defect: contralateral homonymous superior quadrantanopia—due to damage to fibres carrying impulses from the superior quadrants of the opposite visual fields.

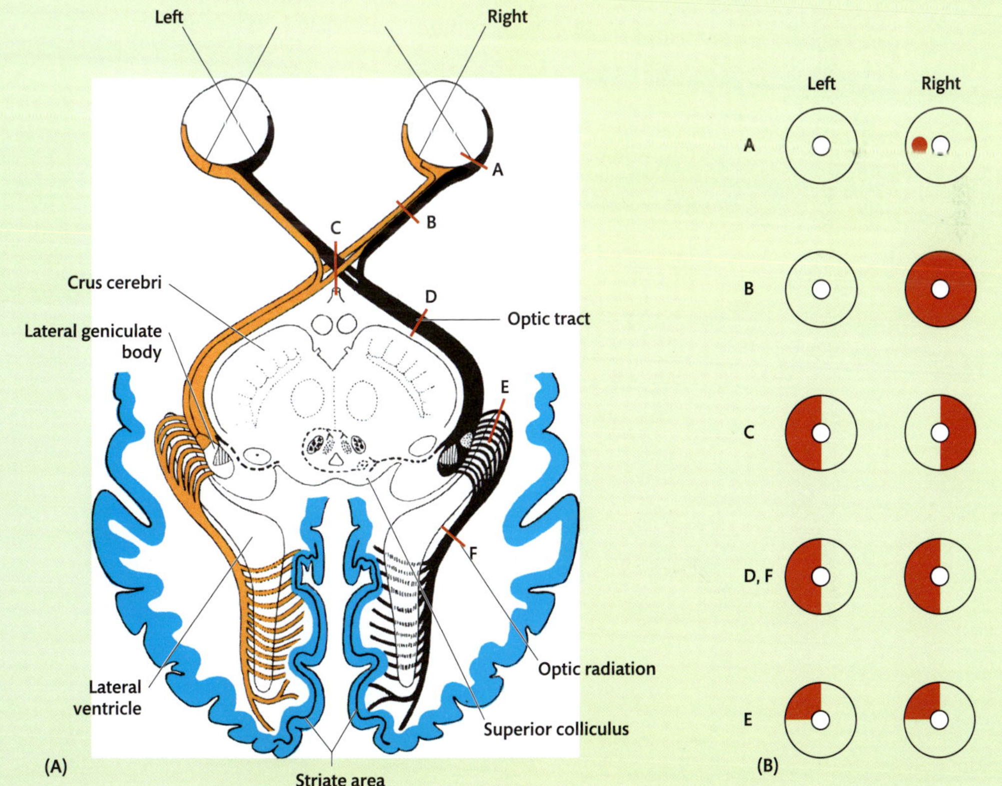


Fig. 31.41 (A) Visual pathway with lesions at different sites. (B) Visual field defects arising from visual pathway lesions.

**CLINICAL APPLICATION 31.4 Scotomata**

Fibres carrying impulses from corresponding points of the two retinae lie together in the optic radiation. Hence a small injury in the radiation produces a blind spot (*scotoma*) in the contralateral half of the field of vision in the corresponding area of both eyes. It is more obvious to the patient than a scotoma produced by a small retinal lesion in one eye, as the latter is covered by the image on the intact retina of the other eye.

Scotomata produced by injuries to the upper part of the radiation or striate cortex are seen in the lower half of the field of vision, and vice versa, but both are in the contralateral field.

**CLINICAL APPLICATION 31.5 Basal ganglia infarct**

The head of the caudate nucleus, putamen, and globus pallidus are supplied mainly by the deep branches of the middle cerebral artery. Fig. 31.42 is a diffusion-weighted magnetic resonance (MR) image of an acute infarct of the left basal ganglia. Such cases may be asymptomatic. Signs of contralateral upper motor neuron type of hemiparesis due to involvement of the corticospinal and corticonuclear tracts, and sensory loss due to involvement of thalamocortical fibres may be present.

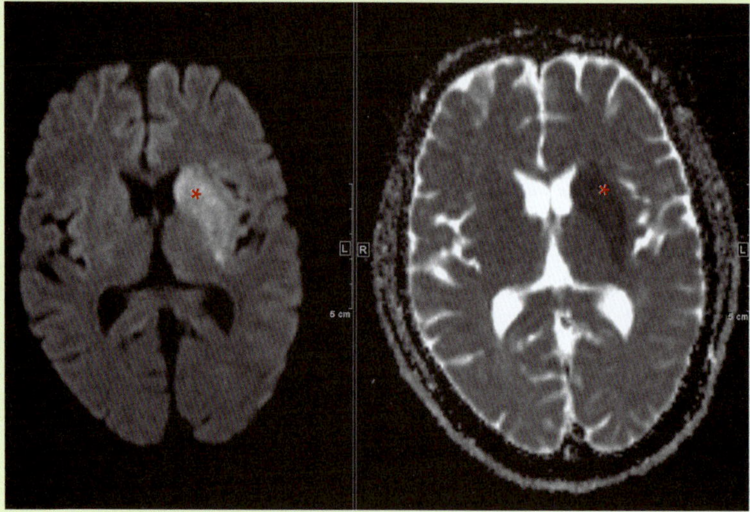


**Fig. 31.42** Diffusion-weighted magnetic resonance imaging (MRI) showing an acute infarct in the left basal ganglia (asterisk).

CHAPTER 32

# The ventricular system

## Introduction

The ventricular system is a hollow, fluid-filled space derived from the cavities of the primitive brain vesicles. It is lined by ependyma. It consists of four ventricles: two **lateral ventricles**—one in each cerebral hemisphere—the **third ventricle** in the diencephalon, and the **fourth ventricle** between the pons, medulla, and cerebellum. The ventricles contain cerebrospinal fluid (CSF) and the choroid plexus which produces it. The four ventricles are interconnected by the **interventricular foramen**, or **foramen of Monro**, between the two lateral ventricles and the third ventricle, and the **cerebral aqueduct** between the third and fourth ventricles. Inferiorly, the cavity of the fourth ventricle is continuous with the central canal in the inferior part of the medulla and, through that, with the central canal of the spinal cord. The roof of the fourth ventricle has **one median** and **two lateral apertures** which open into the subarachnoid cistern [Figs. 32.1, 32.2].

## Circulation of cerebrospinal fluid



The CSF is a clear fluid produced in the choroid plexus of the lateral, third, and fourth ventricles by the choroid plexus. It circulates through the ventricles and enters the subarachnoid space through the median and lateral apertures on the roof of the fourth ventricle. In the subarachnoid space, the CSF cushions the brain against the skull and provides buoyancy. It also plays a role in maintaining the homeostasis of the brain's interstitial fluid and in waste removal. The CSF from the subarachnoid space drains into the superior sagittal sinus through the arachnoid villi and arachnoid granulations [Fig. 32.2].

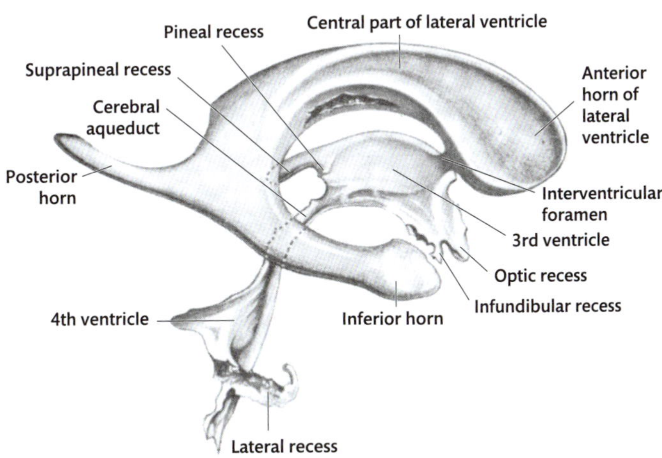


Fig. 32.1 Cast of the ventricles of the brain.

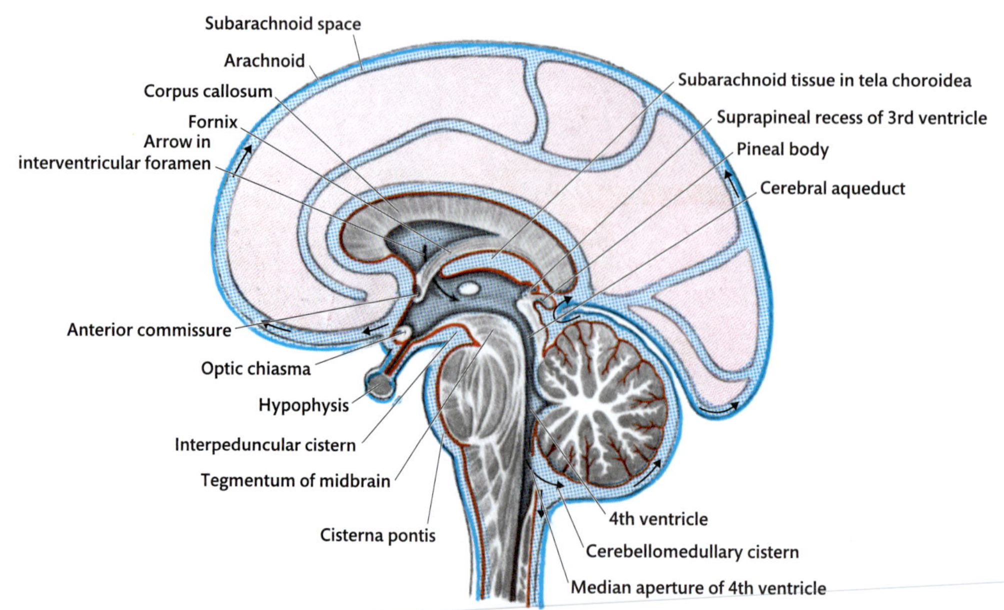


**Fig. 32.2** Median section of the brain to show membranes and cisterns. Red = pia mater; blue stipple = subarachnoid space and ventricles; blue = arachnoid; pink = surface view of the shallow subarachnoid space. The lines of blue stipple running over the pink area indicate the places where the subarachnoid space is deeper around the branches of the anterior and posterior cerebral arteries. The arrows in the subarachnoid space show and direction of flow of CSF.

## Formation of the choroid plexus

The choroid plexus lies within the ventricles and produces CSF. In specific locations of the developing brain, the pia mater covering the surface of the brain is invaginated into the ventricles and carries with it a covering of the ependymal lining of the ventricles. The invaginating pia mater is vascularized by a tuft of choroidal vessels and is known as the **tela choroidea**. The choroid plexus is formed by: (1) the invaginating vascularized pia mater; and (2) the ependymal covering [Fig. 32.3].

## Lateral ventricle

The lateral ventricle is a C-shaped cavity which lies in the cerebrum [Figs. 32.1, 32.4A]. It has an **anterior horn**, a **central part** or **body**, an **inferior horn**, and a **posterior horn**. The anterior end of the C—the anterior horn—extends into the frontal lobe and is continuous behind with the central part. The lower limb of the C runs forwards as the inferior horn in the temporal lobe. The posterior horn projects backwards from the convexity of the

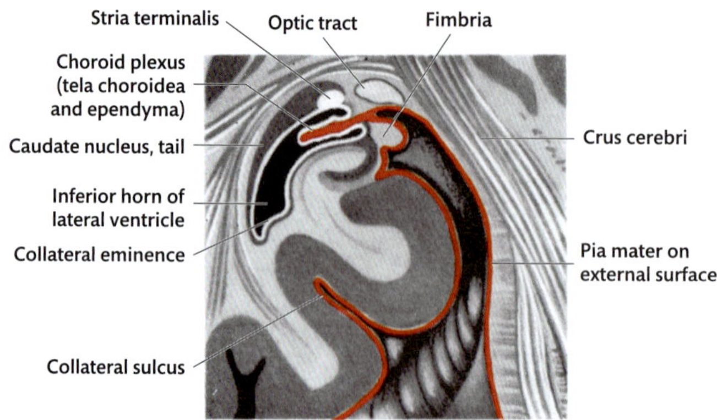


**Fig. 32.3** Coronal section through the inferior horn of the lateral ventricle.

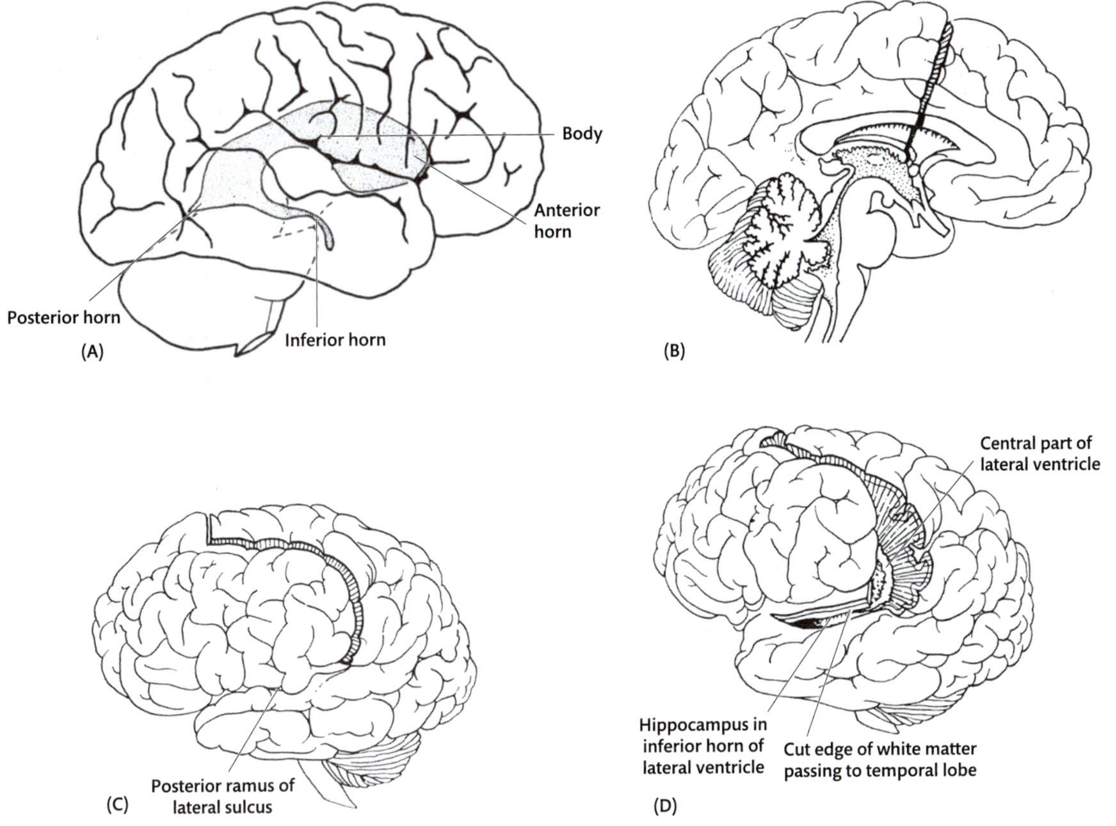


Fig. 32.4 (A) Drawing to show the parts and position of the lateral ventricle (shaded) in the cerebral hemisphere. (B), (C), and (D) Drawings to show the first, second, and third incisions to be made in Dissection 32.1.

C into the occipital lobe [Fig. 32.1]. The size and shape of the lateral ventricle are very variable. The two lateral ventricles communicate with each other and with the third ventricle through the **interventricular foramen**, or foramen of Monro. ➲ In young children, a prolonged increase in pressure in the ventricles causes the brain and skull to expand, as the sutures are not closed (hydrocephalus). In older children and adults, no such expansion is possible and distension of the ventricle results in the loss of nervous tissue.

Using the instructions given in Dissection 32.1, divide the hemisphere to open the lateral ventricle [Fig. 32.5].

## Transverse fissure, choroid fissure, and choroid plexus

The transverse fissure lies between the splenium of the corpus callosum and the dorsal surface of the thalamus [Fig. 32.2]. The tela choroidea common to the central part of the lateral ventricle and the third ventricle extends anteriorly through the transverse fissure below the fornix and superior to the roof of the third ventricle [Fig. 32.2]. It contains the internal cerebral veins and posterior choroidal branches of the posterior cerebral arteries [Fig. 32.6]. The tela choroidea narrows anteriorly, as the two lateral ventricles and their choroid plexuses approach one another, and ends in an apex at the interventricular foramen. The choroid plexus of the lateral ventricle becomes continuous with the corresponding choroid plexus of the third ventricle through the interventricular foramen [Figs. 32.6, 32.7]. These two strips of the choroid plexus in the third ventricle lie side by side on the inferior surface of the tela choroidea, close to the midline [Fig. 32.7].

The choroid fissure is the space along which the vascular pia mater enters into the lateral ventricle to form the choroid plexus of the lateral ventricle. No nervous tissue is developed in this narrow strip of the ventricular wall, so that the vascular pia mater is applied directly to the ependymal lining. The choroid fissure of the lateral ventricle follows the line of the C and lies in the concavity of the

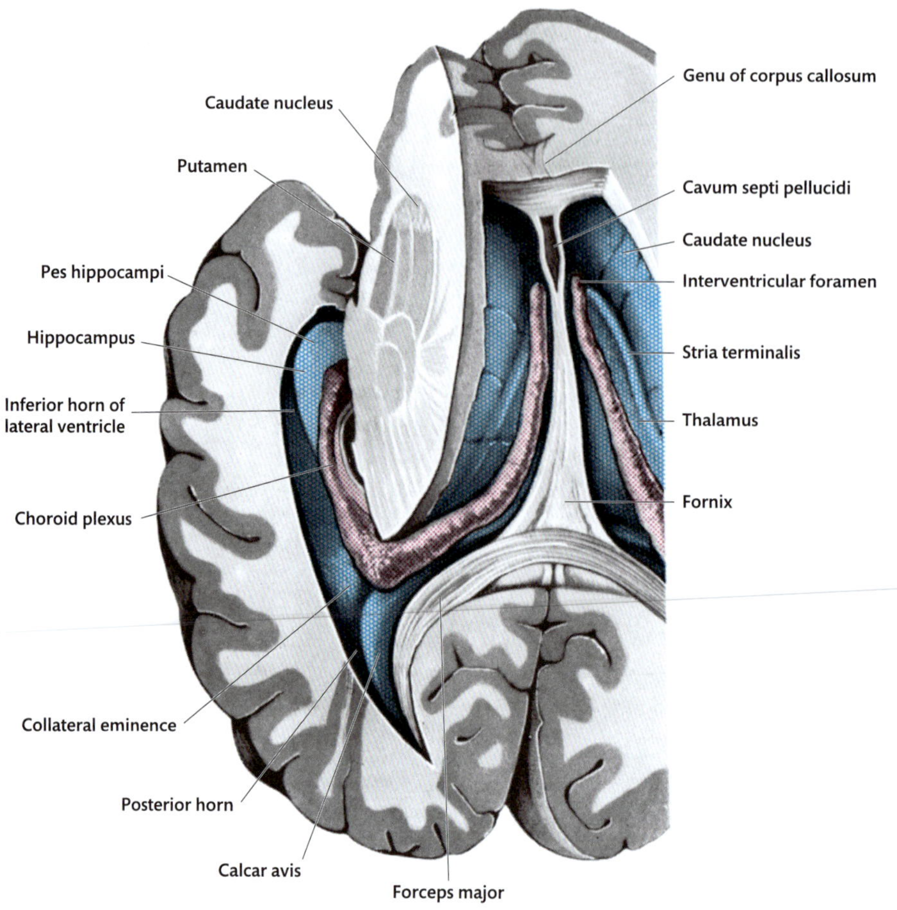


**Fig. 32.5** Dissection from above to show the lateral ventricles. Ependyma = blue; choroid plexus = red. (The ependyma covering the choroid plexus is not shown.)

## DISSECTION 32.1 Opening of the lateral ventricle

### Objective

I. To open into the lateral ventricle.

### Instructions

Dissection 32.1 is illustrated in Fig. 32.4. It exposes the entire lateral ventricle by dividing the brain into two parts which may be readily fitted together again, so that the form and position of the ventricle and the choroid fissure may be appreciated.

1. Study Fig. 32.4A to gauge the approximate position of the lateral ventricle.
2. Place the point of a knife in the interventricular foramen, and make a vertical cut through the fornix, septum pellucidum, and medial aspect of the hemisphere, as shown in Fig. 32.4B.
3. Open the cut as it is made, and carry the point of the knife as far as the lateral edge of the lateral ventricle, but avoid cutting into its floor.
4. Now turn the knife, so that its edge faces posteriorly, and cut backwards and then downwards, following the curve of the lateral ventricle with the point of the knife. Extend the incision as far as the posterior ramus of the lateral sulcus [Fig. 32.4C], and open the cut as you proceed.
5. Note the ridge of the choroid plexus protruding into the ventricle from its floor [Fig. 32.5].
6. Depress the temporal lobe strongly, exposing the inferior part of the insula.
7. Keeping the knife in the ventricle and holding it as nearly vertical as possible, cut forwards through the medial part of the transverse temporal gyri on the

superior surface of the temporal lobe, and enter the sulcus (circular sulcus) which separates the insula from the temporal lobe. This cut divides the white matter passing horizontally into the temporal lobe and opens into the roof of the inferior horn of the lateral ventricle.

8. Carry the cut anteriorly along the circular sulcus to the stem of the lateral sulcus [Fig. 32.4D], opening the cut and confirming that it enters the inferior horn of the lateral ventricle as you proceed.
9. The hemisphere is now separated into two parts which are held together by the ependyma which passes over the choroid plexus between them. The two parts are: (1) an anterior part, with the brainstem attached to it; and (2) a posterior part which includes parts of the frontal and parietal lobes, the arch of the fornix, the fimbria, the hippocampus, and the trunk and splenium of the corpus callosum.
10. Turn to the medial side, and lift the fornix away from the superior surface of the thalamus. Separate the choroid plexus from the fornix, and leave it attached to the thalamus.
11. Note the position of the choroid plexus of the lateral ventricle, and follow it from the interventricular foramen into the inferior horn of the ventricle.
12. Slowly separate the two parts of the cerebrum along the line of the choroid fissure, between the fornix and the thalamus, and note the posterior choroidal branches of the posterior cerebral artery passing to the choroid plexus. Divide these vessels to prevent them from pulling the choroid plexus from the surface of the thalamus.
13. When the two parts have been separated, they may be replaced as often as necessary to relate the internal appearances to the surface structures.





curve of the **fimbria** and **fornix**, between the fornix and the thalamus in the central part of the ventricle [Fig. 32.8] and below the fimbria in the inferior horn. (The choroid fissure should be distinguished from the transverse fissure [see Fig. 24.7], through which the tela choroidea of the third and central parts of the lateral ventricles is continuous with the pia mater on the surface of the midbrain.)

In the central part of each lateral ventricle, the choroid plexus of the lateral ventricle lies at the lateral extremity of a continuous sheet of the pia mater—**tela choroidea of the third and**

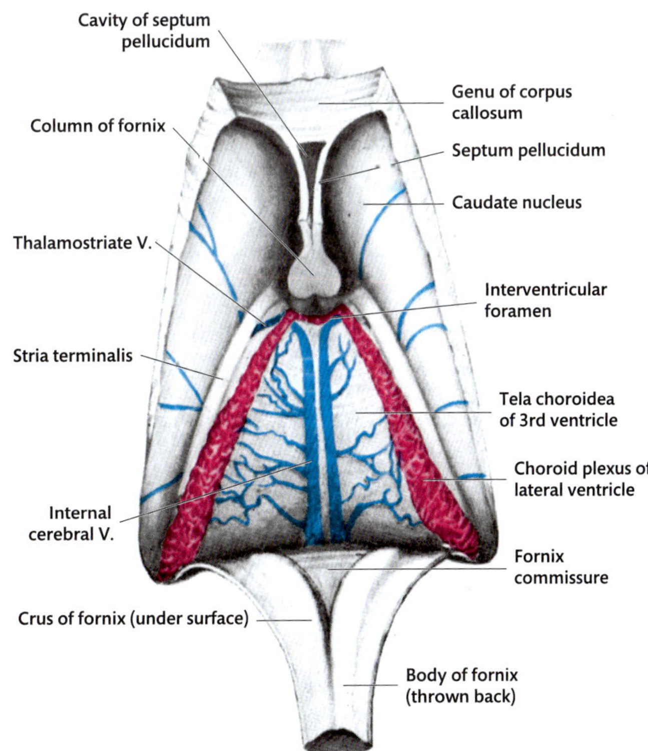


**Fig. 32.6** Tela choroidea of the third and lateral ventricles exposed from above, by dividing the columns of the fornix and turning them backwards.

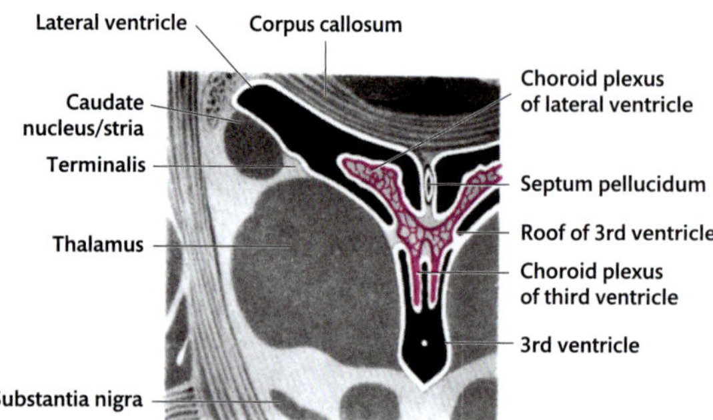


**Fig. 32.7** Coronal section through the thalamus and associated structures, just posterior to the interventricular foramen. Note the choroid plexuses of the third and lateral ventricles.





**lateral ventricles**. This sheet covers the dorsal surface of the thalamus and the roof of the third ventricle [Figs. 32.6, 32.7]. As the ventricles turn downwards, this pia mater is continuous with the pia mater on either side of the upper midbrain. In the inferior horn, each choroid fissure passes forwards to the posterior margin of the uncus, parallel to the optic tract and between it and the margin of the hemisphere [Figs. 32.3, 32.9].

## Parts of the lateral ventricle

The lateral ventricle has an **anterior horn**, a **central part** or **body**, an **inferior horn**, and a **posterior horn**. The anterior horn of the lateral ventricle curves inferiorly into the frontal lobe from the interventricular foramen. It is triangular-shaped in coronal section. The narrow floor is formed by the genu and rostrum, the roof by the trunk, and the anterior wall by the genu of the corpus callosum. The vertical medial wall is formed by the septum pellucidum and the column of the fornix, and the lateral wall by the bulging head of the caudate nucleus [see Figs. 31.22, 31.27, 31.28; Fig. 32.10].

The **central part** of the lateral ventricle is roofed by the trunk of the corpus callosum. The medial wall is formed by the fornix and septum pellucidum anteriorly, and the fornix posteriorly [see Figs. 31.30, 31.31]. The floor is made up of the following structures from lateral to medial: (1) the **caudate nucleus**, which lies in the angle between the floor and the roof and narrows rapidly as it is traced posteriorly [see Figs. 30.2, 31.29, 31.30, 31.31; Figs. 32.5, 32.6]; (2) the **thalamostriate vein**, which runs anteriorly in the groove between the thalamus and the caudate nucleus and passes medially beneath the ependyma to join the internal cerebral vein at the interventricular foramen. A number of tributaries enter it from the centre of the hemisphere by running across the caudate nucleus, deep to the ependyma [Fig. 32.6]; (3) the **stria terminalis**, which runs with the thalamostriate vein; it is a slender bundle of fibres running from the amygdala to the grey matter around

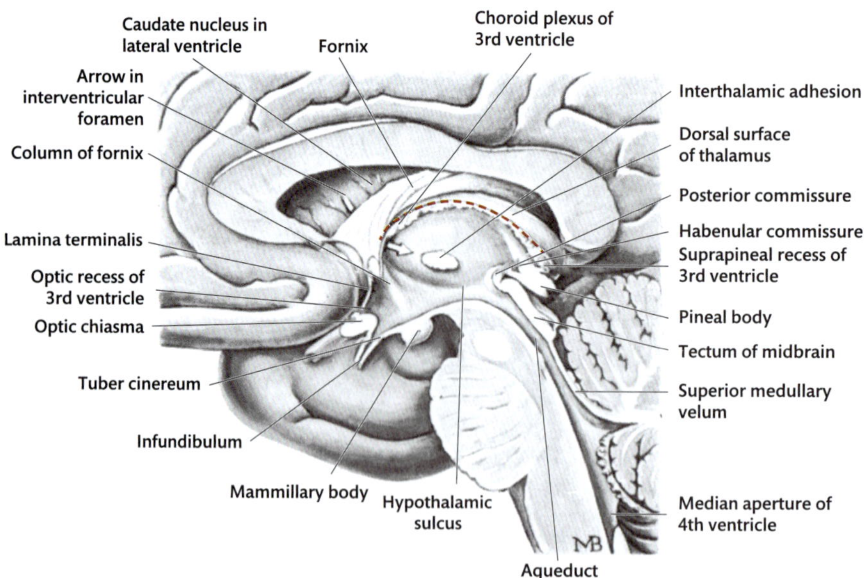


**Fig. 32.8** Median section through the third and fourth ventricles of the brain. The septum pellucidum has been removed to expose the lateral ventricle. Red line = choroid fissure in the central part of the lateral ventricle.

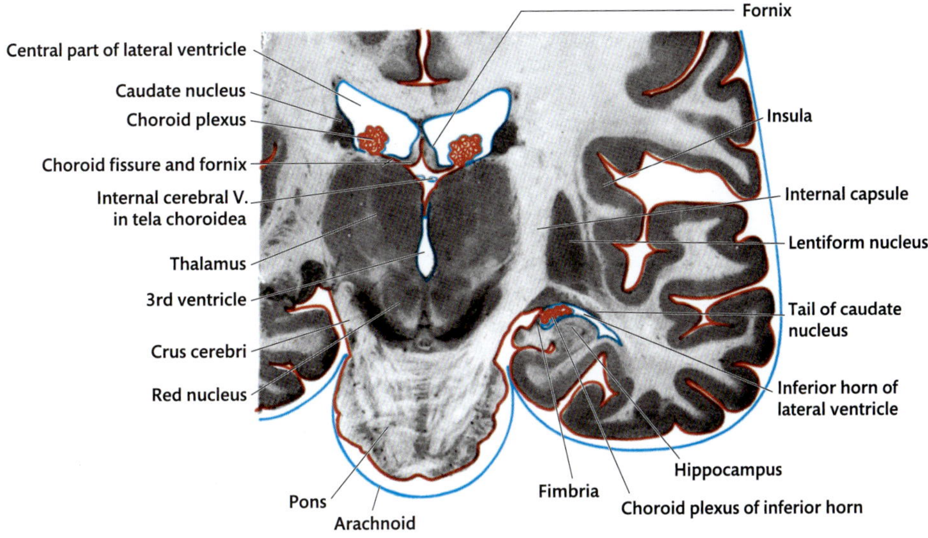


**Fig. 32.9** Coronal section through the cerebrum, midbrain, and pons to show the arrangement of the pia mater and the choroid plexuses of the lateral ventricle. Pia mater = red; arachnoid mater, ependyma, and internal cerebral veins = blue.

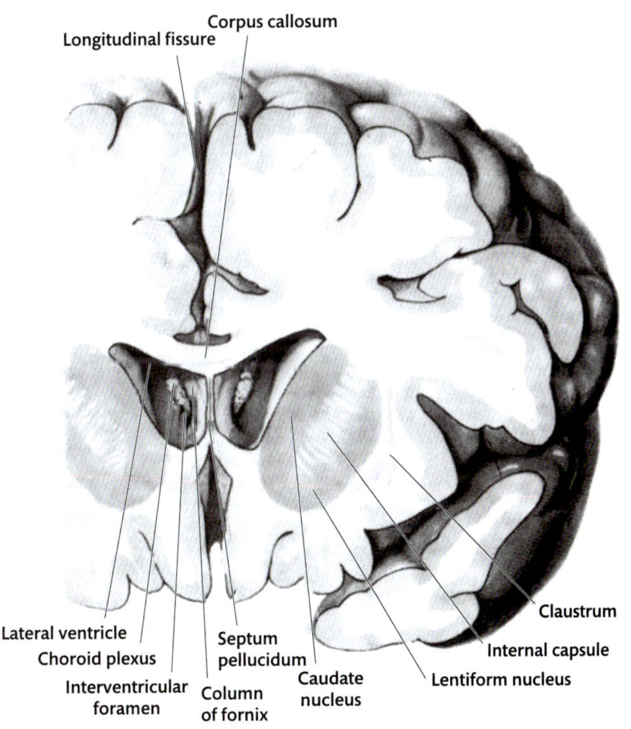


**Fig. 32.10** Coronal section through the hemispheres behind the genu of the corpus callosum, seen from in front.

the anterior commissure [see Fig. 30.2]; (4) a narrow strip of the dorsal surface of the thalamus; (5) the choroid plexus [Fig. 32.7]; and (6) the **fornix** [Fig. 32.5].

The **posterior horn** begins inferior to the splenium of the corpus callosum and extends posteriorly into the occipital lobe. The roof, lateral wall, and floor are formed by a sheet of fibres from the splenium of the corpus callosum—the tapetum—which arches over it and passes inferiorly to the lower parts of the occipital lobe [see Fig. 31.21; Fig. 32.11]. The medial wall is invaginated by two ridges; the upper

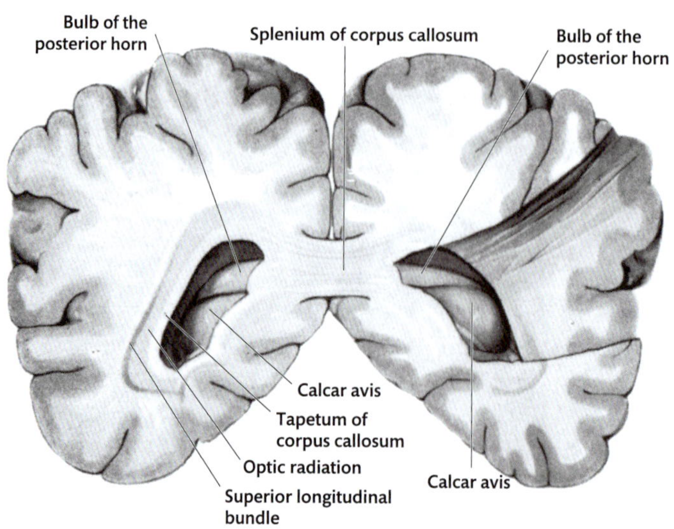


**Fig. 32.11** Coronal section through the posterior horns of the lateral ventricles.





of these—the **bulb of the posterior horn**—is formed by the fibres of the forceps major. The lower ridge—the **calcar avis**—is produced by the calcarine sulcus which extends into it from the medial surface of the occipital lobe [Figs. 32.11, 32.12].

The **inferior horn** is the continuation of the ventricular cavity into the temporal lobe [Fig. 32.1; Figs. 31.30, 31.31, 31.32]. It runs inferiorly, posterior to the thalamus, and then passes anteriorly, curving medially to end at the uncus. The lateral wall is formed by the tapetum of the corpus callosum. The roof consists of the white matter which passes laterally into the temporal lobe (including the sublentiform part of the internal capsule), the

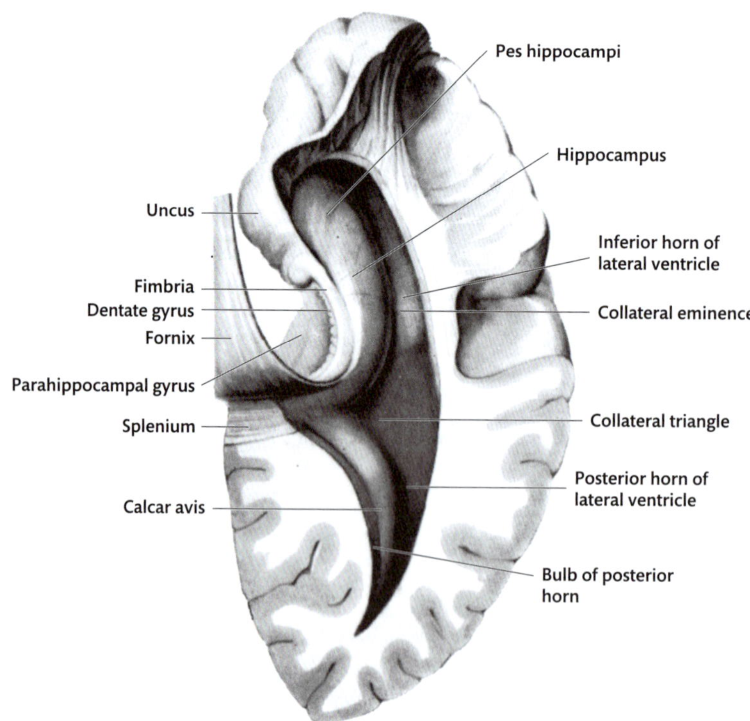


**Fig. 32.12** Posterior and inferior horns of the right lateral ventricle, viewed from above.

stria terminalis, and the tail of the caudate nucleus [Fig. 32.9]. The stria terminalis and the caudate nucleus can be followed from the floor of the central part of the ventricle to the amygdala at the tip of the inferior horn. The floor is broad posteriorly where the inferior and posterior horns meet, and is often raised—the **collateral triangle**—by the collateral sulcus [Fig. 32.12]. Anteriorly, the medial part is formed by the **hippocampus** covered by the **alveus**. The **amygdala** overlies the tip of the inferior horn of the lateral ventricle.

## The third ventricle

The narrow, slit-like third ventricle lies in the midline within the diencephalon. It extends from the lamina terminalis anteriorly to the superior end of the aqueduct and root of the pineal posteriorly [Fig. 32.13].

The **roof** of the third ventricle consists of a layer of ependyma, which is invaginated on each side by the overlying vascular pia mater to form the linear choroid plexus on either side [Fig. 32.8]. The roof is attached on both sides to the stria medullaris thalami. It extends from the interventricular foramen to the habenular commissure and curves over the superior surface of the pineal body to form the suprapineal recess of the ventricle [Figs. 32.2, 32.8].

The **floor** of the third ventricle extends posteriorly from the **optic recess** on the superior surface of the optic chiasma into the **infundibular recess**, and then passes above the mammillary bodies and the tegmentum of the midbrain to the aqueduct [Fig. 32.8].

The **anterior wall** is formed by the lamina terminalis. The anterior commissure lies at the superior end of this wall.

The **lateral wall** of the third ventricle is marked by a shallow groove—the **hypothalamic sulcus**—which extends from the interventricular foramen to the cerebral aqueduct. This sulcus separates the thalamus above from the hypothalamus below. Immediately above the sulcus, the two thalami bulge towards each other and may fuse, forming the **interthalamic adhesion**. This adhesion has no functional significance, is variable in size, and is not a commissure. Immediately posterior to the anterior commissure, the column of the fornix forms a low ridge on the lateral wall. Posterior to the column of the fornix, and almost hidden by it, is a small, obliquely placed **interventricular foramen** which opens into the lateral ventricle. On each side, the narrow strip of choroid plexus in the roof of the third ventricle becomes continuous with the choroid plexus of the corresponding lateral ventricle through the interventricular foramen. The foramen is often so narrow that it is nearly filled by the choroid plexus. ➲ Any hypertrophy of the plexus in this situation blocks the





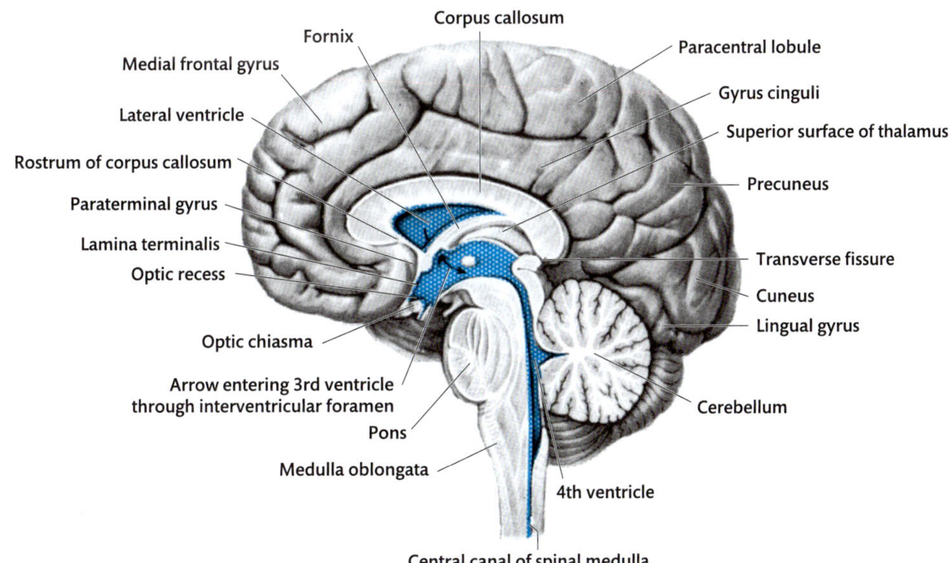


**Fig. 32.13** Medial surface of the right half of a bisected brain. The septum pellucidum has been removed to expose the lateral ventricle. The arrow passes through the interventricular foramen from the lateral to the third ventricle. Ependymal lining of ventricles = blue.

communication between the two ventricles, causing an increase in pressure in the lateral ventricle. If this is unilateral, it may be sufficient to cause compression of the opposite hemisphere and a shift of the midline structures towards that side.

The tela choroidea and choroid plexus of the third ventricle have been described earlier.

## The fourth ventricle

The fourth ventricle is the cavity of the hindbrain. It extends from the superior border of the pons to the middle of the medulla oblongata. It lies behind the pons and the upper part of the medulla, and in front of the cerebellum and the medullary vela. It narrows above to the superior angle where it becomes continuous with the cerebral aqueduct. Inferiorly, it continues with the small central canal of the inferior half of the medulla oblongata and spinal cord [Fig. 32.2].

The fourth ventricle is widest at the level of the junction of the pons and the medulla oblongata [Fig. 32.14]. At this point, it extends laterally on each side to form a tubular **lateral recess**. The lateral recess curves over the posterior aspect of the inferior cerebellar peduncle, extends as far laterally as the tip of the flocculus, and opens into the subarachnoid space through the **lateral aperture** of the fourth ventricle. The lateral aperture lies posterior to the ninth and tenth cranial nerves [see Fig. 29.4A]. The deepest part of the ventricle is opposite the inferior part of the pons where the tent-like cerebellar recess extends posteriorly almost to the level of the dentate nuclei. Immediately inferior to this, the inferior medullary velum passes anteriorly, and the ventricle becomes a shallow slit. Its depth again increases towards the inferior angle, as the median part of the thin roof curves posteriorly on the anterior surface of the cerebellum to the margin of the **median aperture** of the fourth ventricle [see Fig. 29.4A; Fig. 32.13].

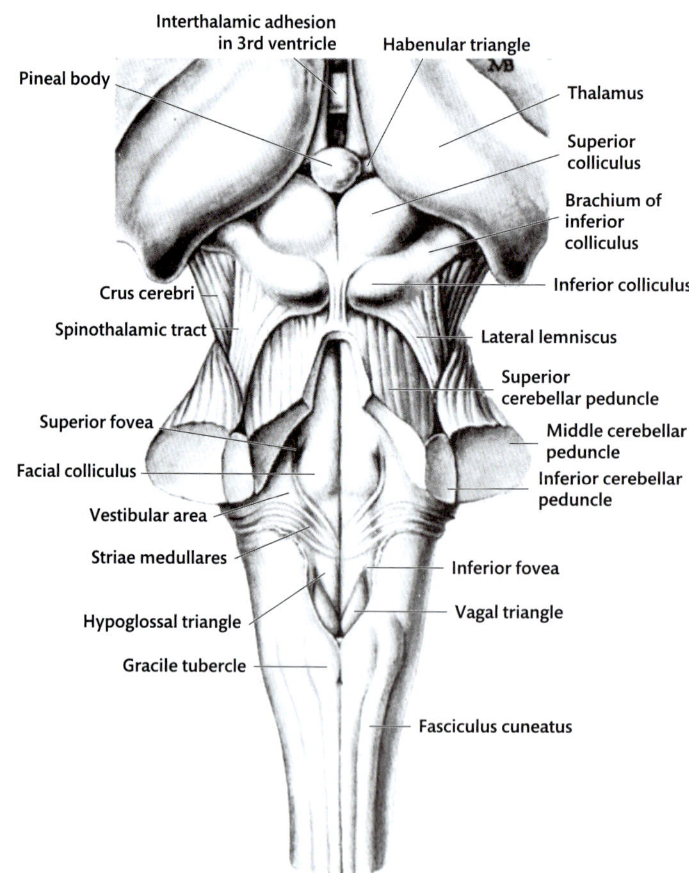


**Fig. 32.14** Posterior view of the brainstem, showing the floor of the fourth ventricle.

➲ Blockage of the median and lateral apertures by scar tissue following an injury or infection prevents the flow of CSF into the subarachnoid space and causes it to accumulate in the cavities of the brain. This results in raised intracranial pressure. Similar scar tissue in the subarachnoid space can impede the flow of CSF through it.

## Roof of the fourth ventricle

Superior to the cerebellar recess, the superior medullary velum forms the greater part of the roof. This velum extends transversely between the two superior cerebellar peduncles and gradually narrows as it approaches the tectum of the midbrain. Inferior to the cerebellar recess, the thin roof of the fourth ventricle extends in the midline from its cerebellar attachment to the margin of the median aperture [see Fig. 29.1] on the anteroinferior surface of the cerebellum. Laterally, the roof forms the bed of the cerebellar tonsil and is attached to the posterior surface of the medulla oblongata. The lateral attachments converge towards the median aperture inferiorly, but superiorly they pass laterally over the posterior surface of the inferior cerebellar peduncle to form the inferior limit of the lateral recess [see Fig. 29.4A].

## Tela choroidea and choroid plexuses of the fourth ventricle

The pia mater on the surface of the brain passes between the thin roof of the fourth ventricle and the cerebellum. It contains the posterior inferior cerebellar artery and forms the tela choroidea of the choroid plexus of the fourth ventricle. Each half of the choroid plexus is shaped like an inverted L. The two vertical limbs of the L lie on the roof of the fourth ventricle, on each side of the midline, from the margin of the median aperture to the level of the lateral recess. From this point, the horizontal limbs of the L extend laterally into the roof of the corresponding lateral recess as far as the lateral aperture. At the lateral aperture, the extremities of the choroid plexus protrude as miniature cauliflower-like tufts, immediately inferior to the flocculus of the cerebellum. The extremities of both limbs of the L can be seen in the intact brain at the median and lateral apertures of the fourth ventricle [see Fig. 29.4].

## Floor of the fourth ventricle

The floor of the fourth ventricle is diamond-shaped and covered by ependyma. It extends from the aqueduct superiorly to the central canal inferiorly. It is formed by the posterior surfaces of the pons and the superior half of the medulla oblongata. Its lateral boundaries are formed by the superior cerebellar peduncles, the inferior cerebellar peduncles, and the cuneate and gracile tubercles [Fig. 32.14]. For details on the other features of the floor of the fourth ventricle, see p. 315 and p. 316.

# Hydrocephalus

➲ Hydrocephalus literally means 'water in the head' and is due to excess fluid in the intracranial cavity. In infants with hydrocephalus, the fontanelles are bulged and the cranial cavity may expand to accommodate the excess fluid. The reasons for hydrocephalus are varied: (1) due to excess production of CSF, as in the case of a choroid plexus papilloma—a rare tumour; (2) obstruction of CSF due to a mass or some congenital malformation. Obstruction could be at the interventricular foramen, cerebral aqueduct, or fourth ventricle, or in the subarachnoid space; and (3) decreased CSF absorption, due to damage or block of arachnoid granulations.

Clinically, hydrocephalus is classified as: (1) **communicating hydrocephalus**—when it is due to impaired CSF absorption or obstruction to flow in the subarachnoid space; and (2) **non-communicating hydrocephalus** when it is due to obstruction to flow in the ventricular system.

## Congenital hydrocephalus

➲ Congenital hydrocephalus is present at birth and is due to brain malformation or block in the flow of CSF. The primary cause could be due to genetic abnormalities or maternal infections. If left untreated, congenital hydrocephalus can cause brain damage or developmental delays.

See Clinical Application 32.1 for the practical implications of the anatomy discussed in this chapter.




**CLINICAL APPLICATION 32.1 CSF rhinorrhoea**

Fractures of the anterior cranial fossa could result in blood and CSF leaking into the nose and/or the orbit. In addition, infection from the nose could spread to the meninges, and also into the frontal air sinus if the sinus invades the orbital part of the frontal bone.

CHAPTER 33

# MCQs on brain and spinal cord

Each of the following questions have four options. Please choose the most correct answer.

**1. The lower extent of the spinal dura mater is at the level of the**

A. L. 1 vertebra
B. L. 3 vertebra
C. S. 2 vertebra
D. Coccyx



**2. Which of the following statements is NOT true about the thoracic nucleus of the spinal cord?**

A. It extends through the thoracic and upper lumbar segments
B. It is present in the ventral grey column
C. It receives afferents from the fasciculus gracilis
D. It sends axons to the cerebellum through the posterior spinocerebellar tract

**3. The nervus intermedius carries**

A. Motor fibres
B. Sensory fibres
C. Parasympathetic fibres
D. Both sensory and parasympathetic fibres

**4. Which one of the following is a branch of the vertebral artery?**

A. Posterior inferior cerebellar artery
B. Posterior cerebral artery
C. Anterior inferior cerebellar artery
D. Anterior cerebral artery

**5. The posterior external arcuate fibres arise from the**

A. Arcuate nucleus
B. Gracile nucleus
C. Cuneate nucleus
D. Accessory cuneate nucleus

**6. Fibres arising from pontine nuclei traverse the**

A. Cerebral peduncle
B. Superior cerebellar peduncle
C. Middle cerebellar peduncle
D. Inferior cerebellar peduncle

**7. The cranial nerve nucleus underlying the facial colliculus is the**

A. Motor nucleus of the trigeminal nerve
B. Chief sensory nucleus of the trigeminal nerve
C. Abducens nucleus
D. Motor nucleus of the facial nerve

**8. The climbing fibres are the**

A. Olivocerebellar fibres
B. Cerebello-olivary fibres
C. Pontocerebellar fibres
D. Cerebellorubral fibres

**9. Which one of the following is a component of the tegmentum of the midbrain?**

A. Red nucleus
B. Substantia nigra
C. Corticopontine fibres
D. Corticonuclear fibres

**10. The artery that lies on the stem of the lateral sulcus is the**

A. Anterior cerebral artery
B. Middle cerebral artery
C. Posterior cerebral artery
D. Posterior communicating artery

**11. The name 'striate cortex' is given to the**

A. Visual area
B. Auditory area
C. Motor area
D. Broca's area

**12. The fibre bundle on the floor of the lateral ventricle between the thalamus and the caudate nucleus is the**

A. Stria medullaris thalami
B. Stria medullaris
C. Stria terminalis
D. Linea terminalis

**13. Which one of the following is NOT true regarding the geniculate bodies?**

A. The medial geniculate body receives the brachium of the inferior colliculus
B. The lateral geniculate body is continuous anteriorly with the optic tract
C. Destruction of the lateral geniculate body of one side will result in loss of vision in the same half of the field of vision
D. Destruction of the medial geniculate body of one side has little effect on hearing

**14. Which one of the following is true regarding the uncinate fasciculus?**

A. It is a commissure
B. The fibre bundle passes between the temporal lobe and the frontal lobe
C. The fibre bundle passes between the temporal lobe and the occipital lobe
D. The fibre bundle passes between the frontal lobe and the occipital lobe

**15. The afferent to the anterior nucleus of the thalamus is the**

A. Mammillothalamic tract
B. Medial lemniscus
C. Spinal lemniscus
D. Trigeminal lemniscus





Please see Chapter 35 for the answers.

Find additional MCQs online by searching for *Cunningham's Manual of Practical Anatomy Volume 3 Head, Neck and Brain, 17th edition* at https://academic.oup.com/ and go to the endmatter to find the free online appendix at the end of the book.

PART 3

# Cross-sectional anatomy

CHAPTER 34

# Cross-sectional anatomy of the head and neck

## Cross-sectional anatomy of the head and neck

In this chapter, serial sections through the head and neck are presented alongside computerized tomography (CT) and magnetic resonance imaging (MRI) scans at approximately the same level. The relationship of the brain to the surrounding skull and soft tissue is shown. Fig. 34.1 is a sagittal section through the head on which the planes of Figs. 34.2, 34.3, 34.4, 34.5, 34.6, 34.7, 34.8, 34.9, 34.10, 34.11, and 34.12 are shown. Figs. 34.13, 34.14, and 34.15 are sections through the neck at sequentially lower levels. The CT and MRI scans are matched to the closest image available in the Visible Human Project.

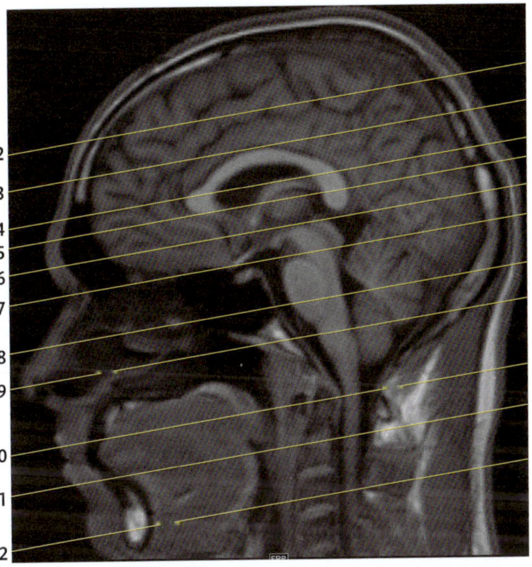


**Fig. 34.1** Oblique lines on the sagittal section of the head to show the approximate plane of section for Figs. 34.2, 34.3, 34.4, 34.5, 34.6, 34.7, 34.8, 34.9, 34.10, 34.11, and 34.12.

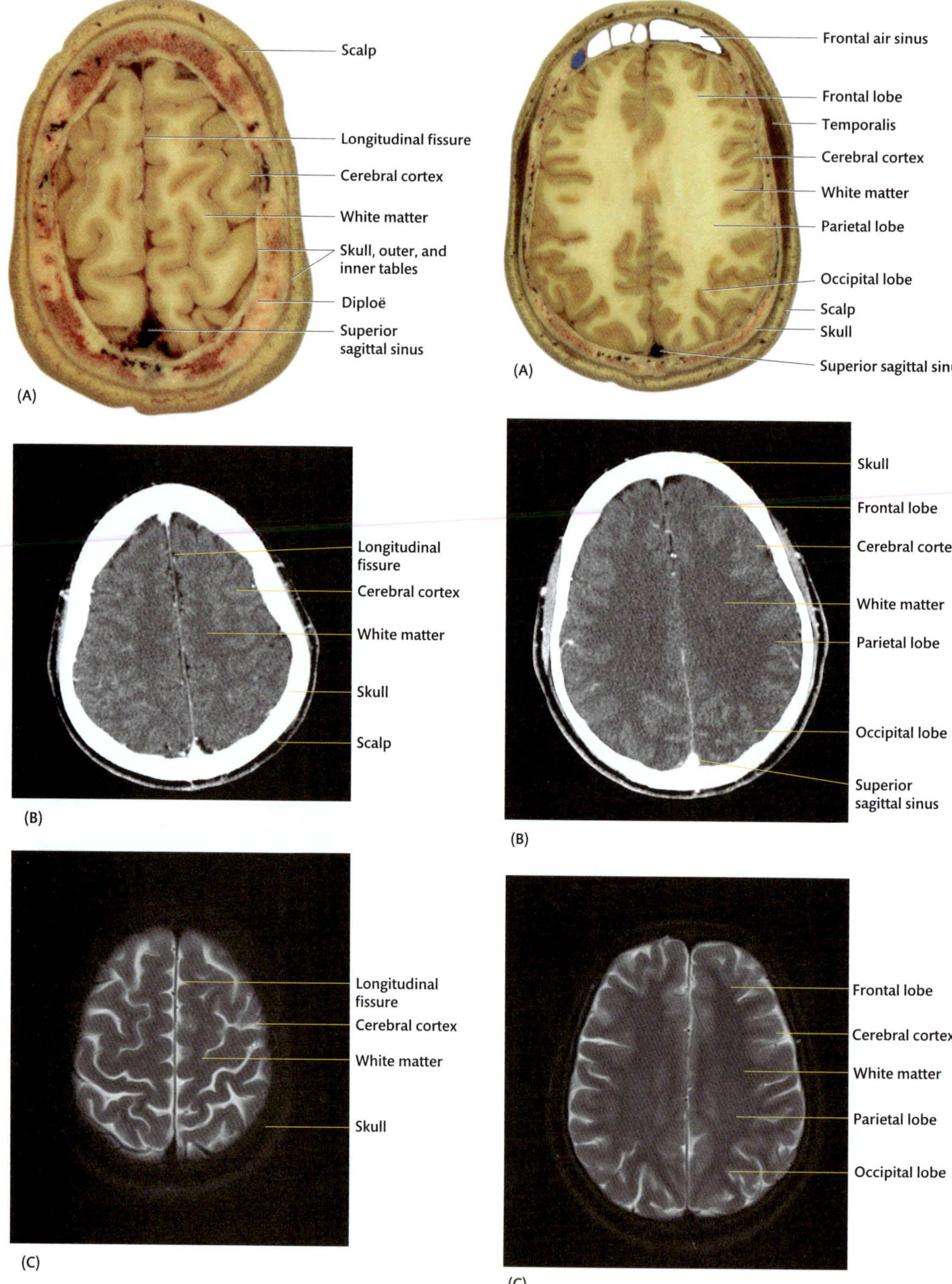


**Fig. 34.2** (A) Cross-section through the upper part of the head, showing the scalp, skull, and cerebral hemisphere. (B) Post-contrast axial CT of the brain. (C) T2-weighted axial MRI.

(A) Image courtesy of the Visible Human Project of the US National Library of Medicine.

**Fig. 34.3** (A) Cross-section through the upper part of the head at a slightly lower level than Fig. 34.2. The scalp, skull, and cerebral hemisphere are shown. (B) Post-contrast axial CT of the brain. (C) T2-weighted axial MRI.

(A) Image courtesy of the Visible Human Project of the US National Library of Medicine.

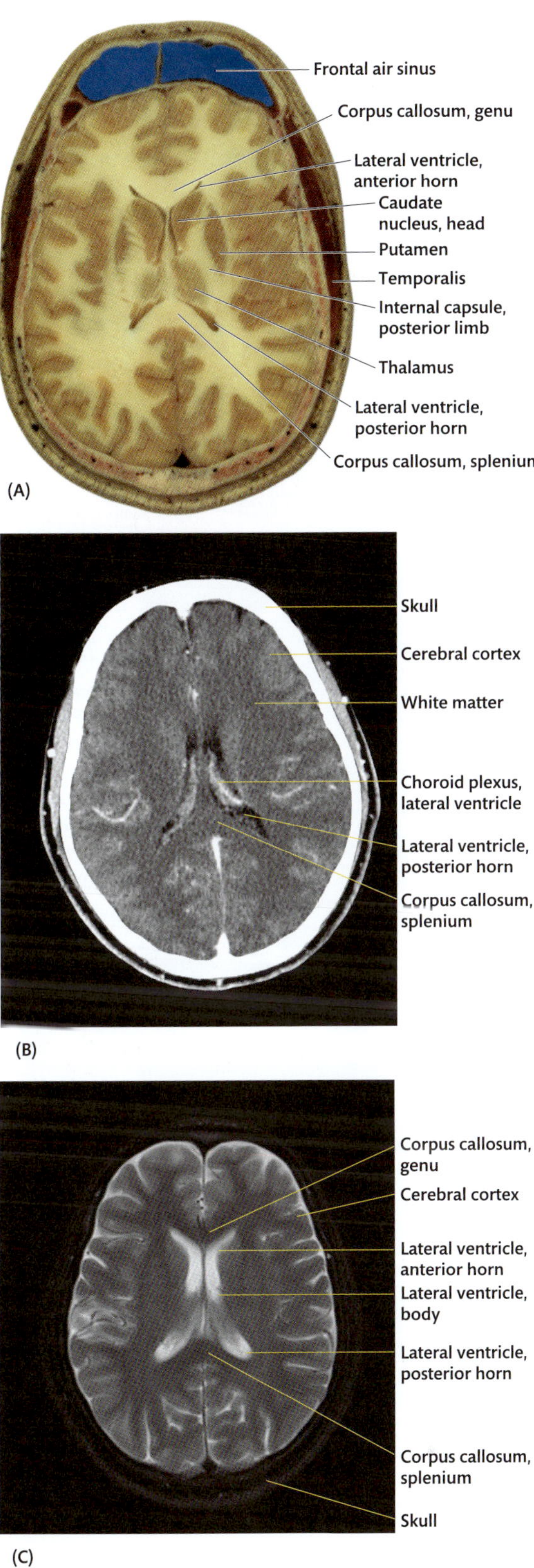


**Fig. 34.4** (A) Cross-section through the head at a slightly lower level than Fig. 34.3. The cerebral hemispheres, lateral ventricles, and a small part of the thalamus are seen. (B) Post-contrast axial CT of the brain, showing parts of the lateral ventricle and the choroid plexus. (C) T2-weighted axial MRI. The lateral ventricle is seen clearly.

(A) Image courtesy of the Visible Human Project of the US National Library of Medicine.

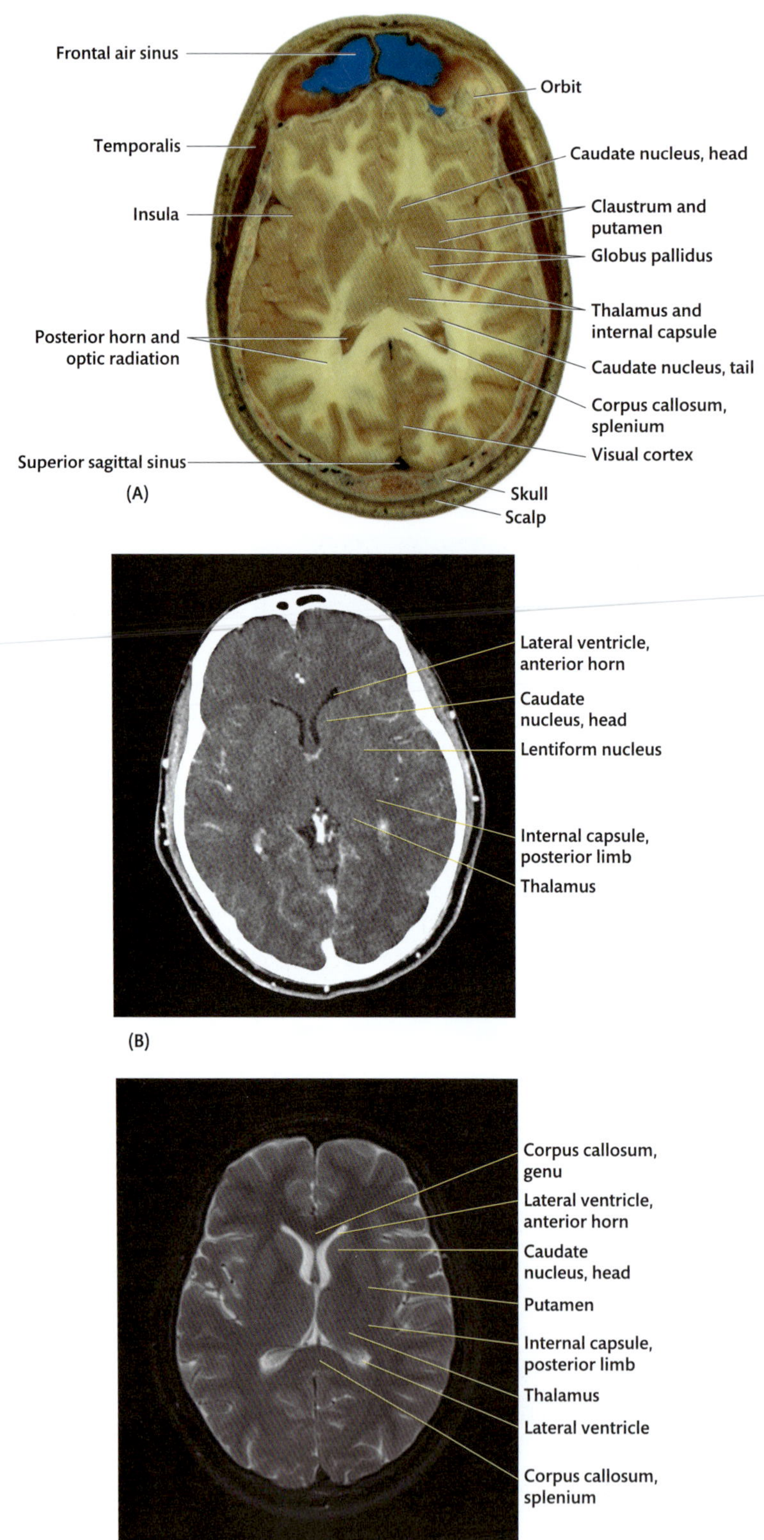


**Fig. 34.5** (A) Cross-section through the head at a slightly lower level than Fig. 34.4. The frontal air sinus, cerebrum, and thalamus are seen. (B) Post-contrast axial CT. (C) T2-weighted axial MRI.

(A) Image courtesy of the Visible Human Project of the US National Library of Medicine.

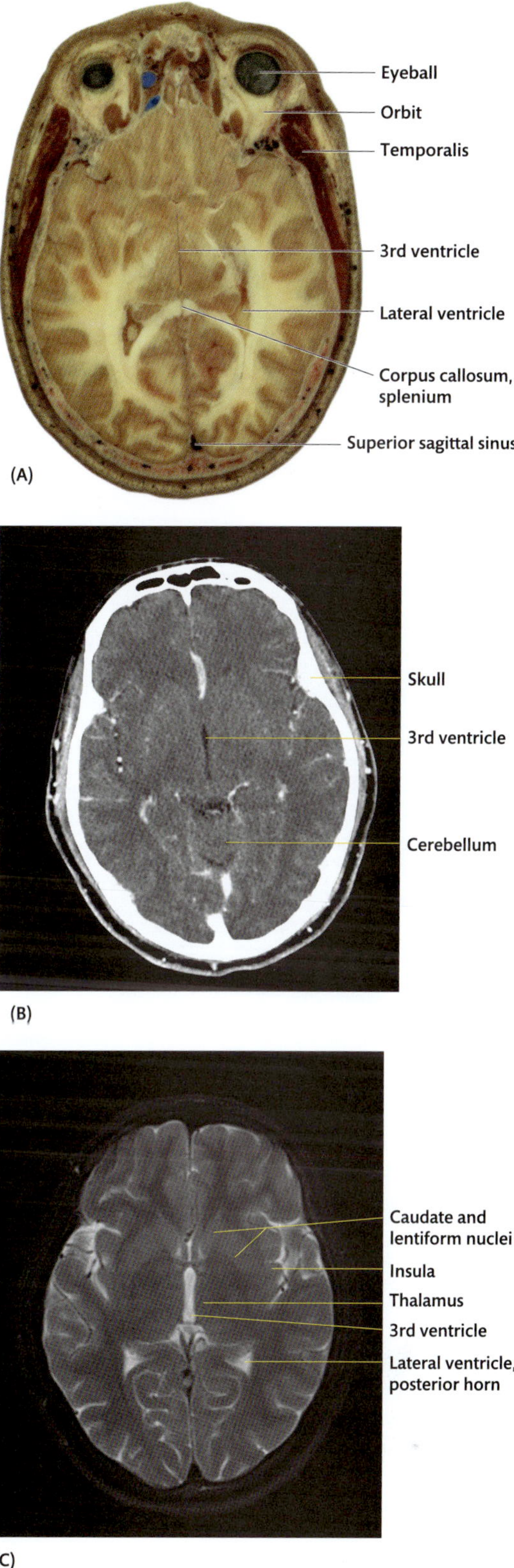


**Fig. 34.6** (A) Cross-section through the head at a slightly lower level than Fig. 34.5. The orbit, nasal cavity, and cerebral hemispheres are seen. (B) Post-contrast axial CT. (C) T2-weighted axial MRI. The CT and MRI images are taken above the orbit.

(A) Image courtesy of the Visible Human Project of the US National Library of Medicine.

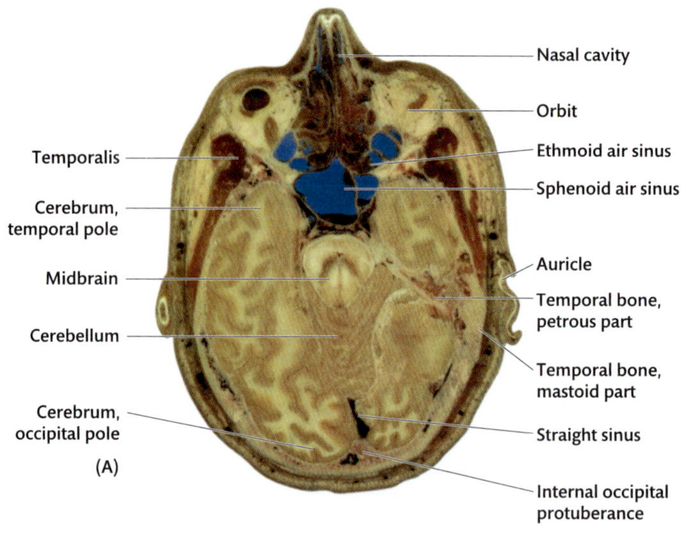


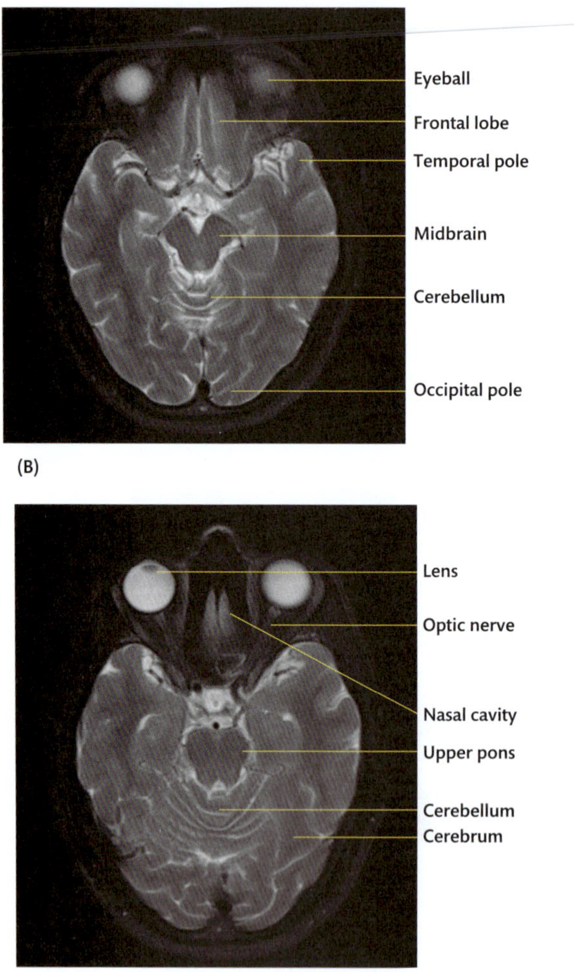


**Fig. 34.7** (A) Cross-section through the head at a slightly lower level than Fig. 34.6. The nasal cavity, orbit, auricle, cerebrum, midbrain, and part of the cerebellum are seen. (B) T2-weighted axial MRI. (C) T2-weighted axial MRI at a slightly lower level than Fig. 34.7B. The upper pons and cerebellum are seen.

(A) Image courtesy of the Visible Human Project of the US National Library of Medicine.

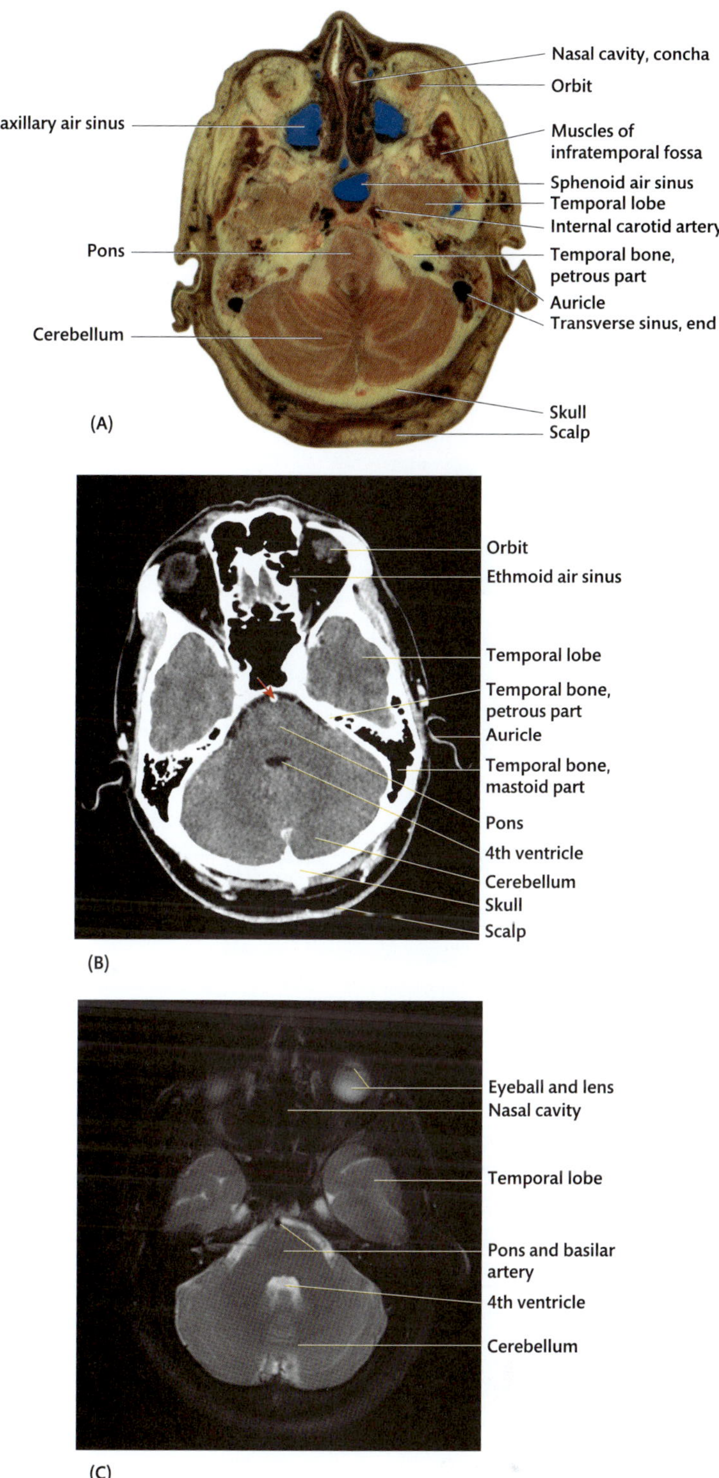


**Fig. 34.8** (A) Cross-section through the head at a slightly lower level than Fig. 34.7. The lower part of the orbit, nasal cavity, upper part of the sphenoid and maxillary air sinuses, infratemporal fossa, pons, and cerebellum are seen. (B) Post-contrast axial CT. Red arrow = basilar artery. (C) T2-weighted axial MRI.

(A) Image courtesy of the Visible Human Project of the US National Library of Medicine.

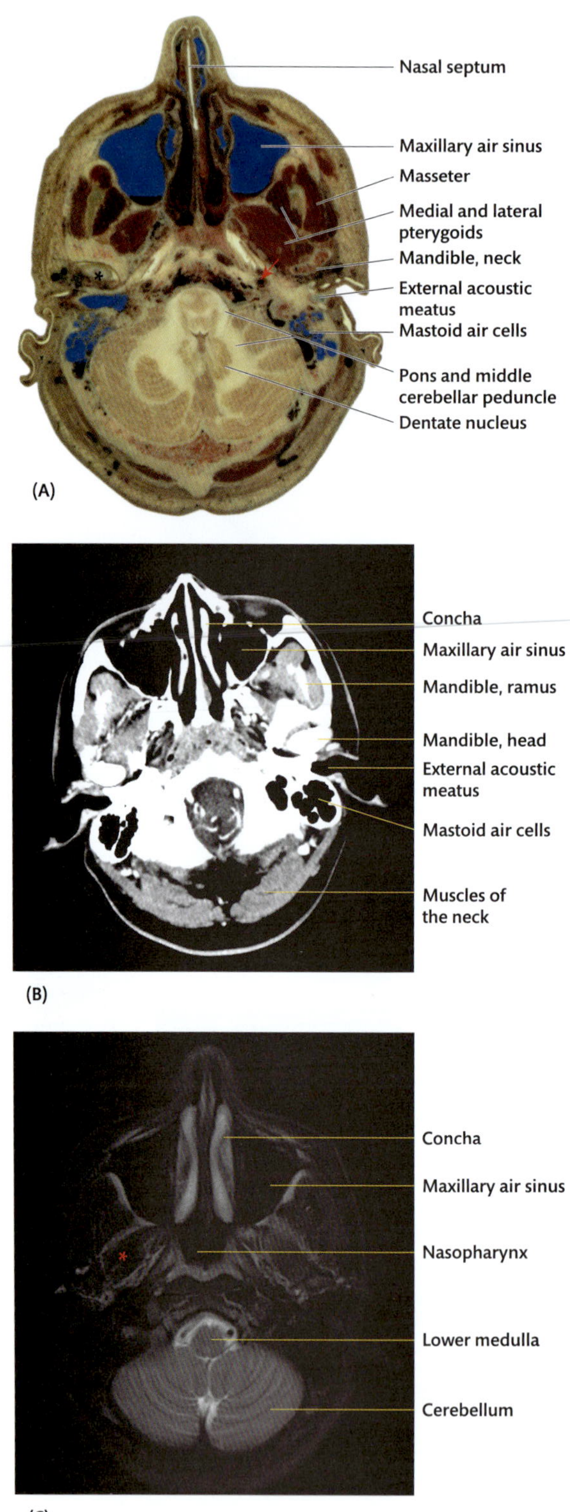


**Fig. 34.9** (A) Cross-section through the head at a slightly lower level than Fig. 34.8. The nasal cavity, maxillary air sinus, right temporomandibular joint (= asterisk), muscles of mastication, external ear, mastoid air cells, pons, cerebellum, and middle cerebellar peduncle are seen. Red arrow = right internal carotid artery. (B) Post-contrast axial CT. (C) T2-weighted axial MRI. Asterisk = right lateral pterygoid.

(A) Image courtesy of the Visible Human Project of the US National Library of Medicine.

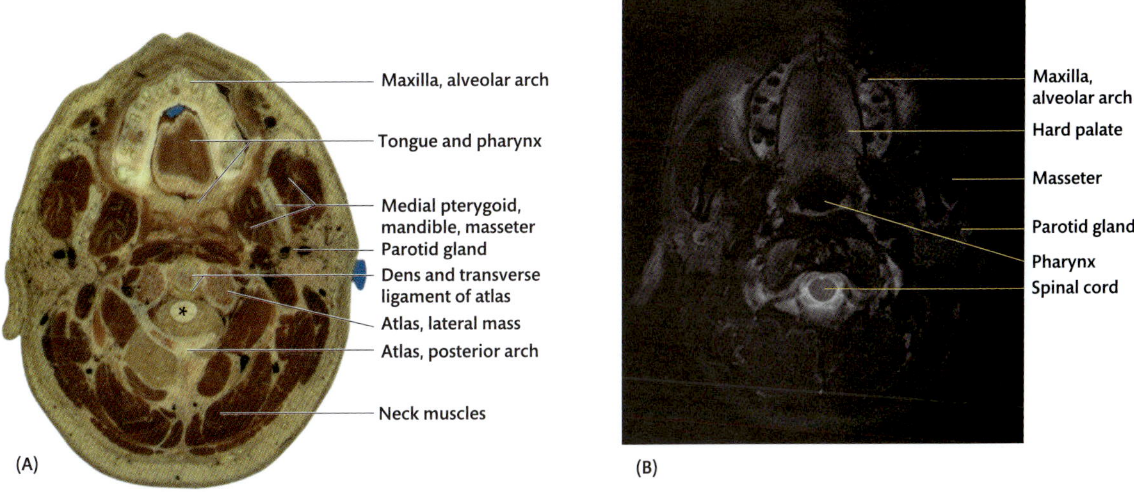


**Fig. 34.10** (A) Cross-section through the head at a slightly lower level than Fig. 34.9. The alveolar arch of the maxilla, oral cavity, parotid gland, atlanto-axial joint, and neck muscles are seen. Asterisk = spinal cord. (B) T2-weighted axial MRI.

(A) Image courtesy of the Visible Human Project of the US National Library of Medicine.

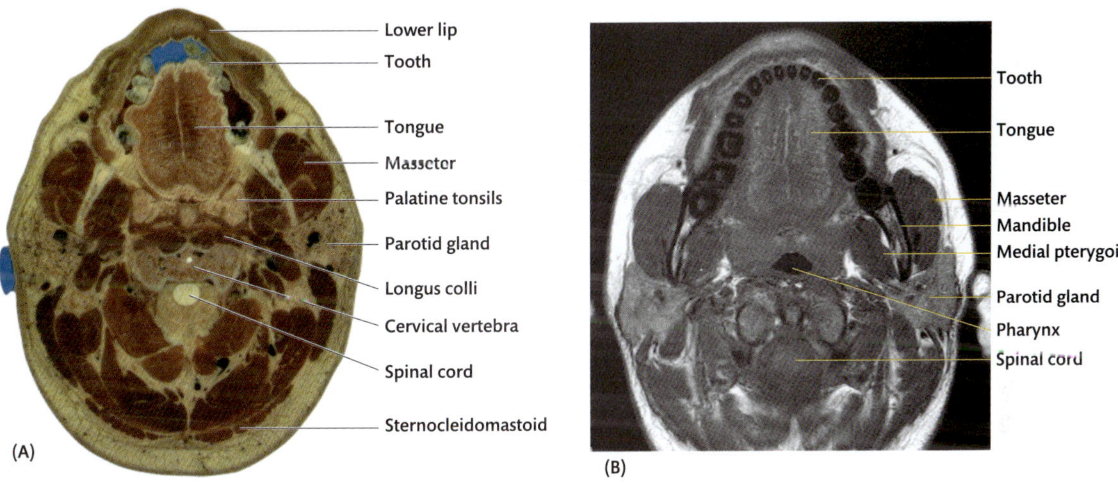


**Fig. 34.11** (A) Cross-section through the head at a slightly lower level than Fig. 34.10. The alveolar arch of the mandible, oral cavity, and parotid gland are seen. (B) Axial MRI.

(A) Image courtesy of the Visible Human Project of the US National Library of Medicine.

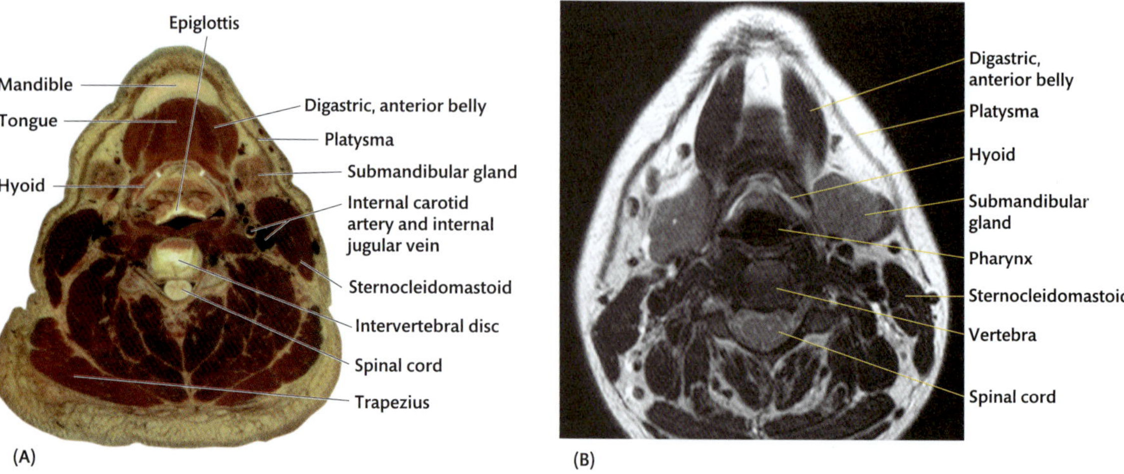


**Fig. 34.12** (A) Cross-section through the head at the lower level of the chin, submandibular gland, and hyoid bone. (B) Axial MRI.

(A) Image courtesy of the Visible Human Project of the US National Library of Medicine.

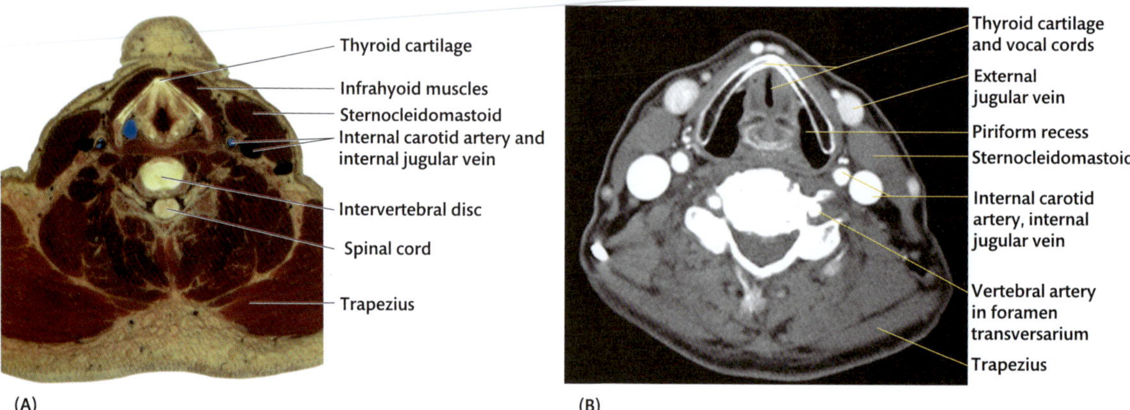


**Fig. 34.13** (A) Cross-section through the neck at the level of the thyroid cartilage. (B) Axial CT.

(A) Image courtesy of the Visible Human Project of the US National Library of Medicine.

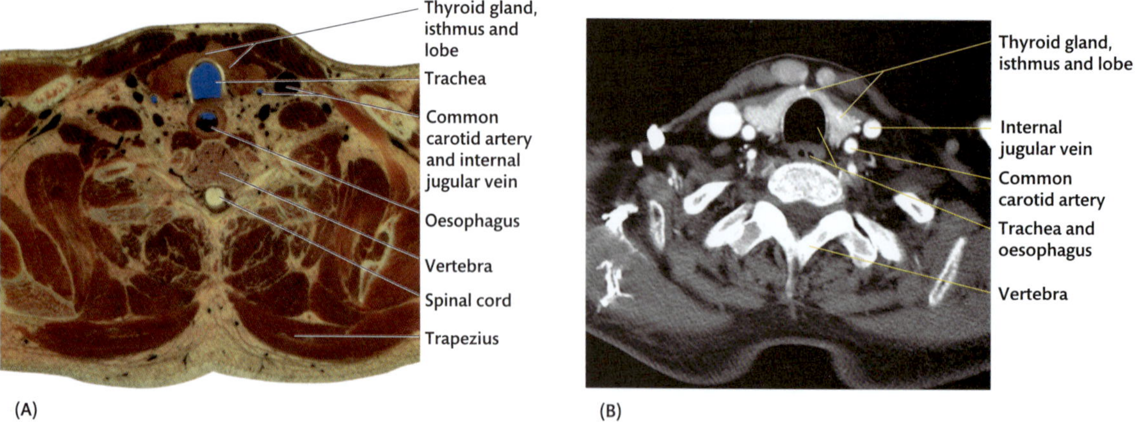


**Fig. 34.14** (A) Cross-section through the neck at the level of the isthmus of the thyroid gland. (B) Axial CT.

(A) Image courtesy of the Visible Human Project of the US National Library of Medicine.

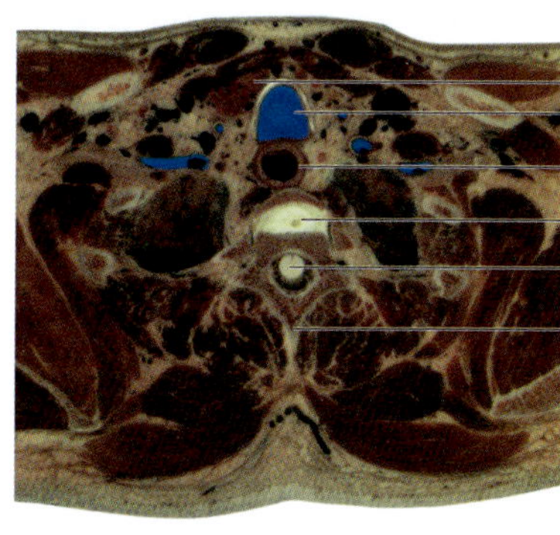


(A)

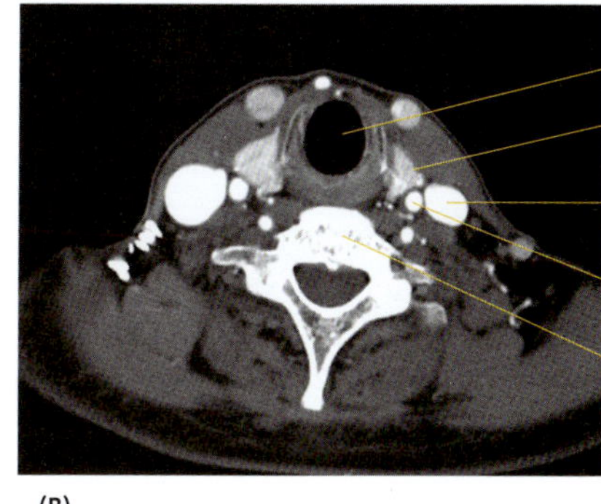


(B)

**Fig. 34.15** (A) Cross-section through the neck at a level slightly lower than Fig. 34.14. (B) Axial CT.

(A) Image courtesy of the Visible Human Project of the US National Library of Medicine.

CHAPTER 35

# Answers to MCQs

Answers to Chapter 23—MCQs on head and neck

1. C
2. A
3. B
4. A
5. D
6. C
7. D
8. D
9. C
10. B
11. D
12. C
13. C
14. A
15. A

Answers to Chapter 33—MCQs on brain and spinal cord

1. C
2. B
3. D
4. A
5. A
6. C
7. C
8. A
9. A
10. B
11. A
12. C
13. C
14. B
15. A

# Index

*For the benefit of digital users, indexed terms that span two pages (e.g., 52–53) may, on occasion, appear on only one of those pages*

Tables are indicated by an italic *t* following the page number.

## O



## P